Clinical Psychopharmacology in the Medically Ill

Third Edition

Clinical Manual of Psychopharmacology in the Medically Ill

Third Edition

Edited by

James L. Levenson, M.D.

Stephen J. Ferrando, M.D.

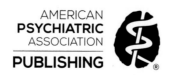

AMERICAN
PSYCHIATRIC
ASSOCIATION
PUBLISHING

Manufactured in the United States of America on acid-free paper

27   26   25   24   23   5   4   3   2   1

American Psychiatric Association Publishing
800 Maine Avenue SW, Suite 900
Washington, DC 20024-2812
www.appi.org

Library of Congress Cataloging-in-Publication Data
Names: Levenson, James L., editor. | Ferrando, Stephen J., editor. |
   American Psychiatric Association, issuing body.
Title: Clinical manual of psychopharmacology in the medically ill / edited
   by James L. Levenson, Stephen J. Ferrando.
Description: Third edition. | Washington, DC : American Psychiatric
   Association Publishing, [2024] | Includes bibliographical references and index.
Identifiers: LCCN 2023003642 (print) | LCCN 2023003643 (ebook) | ISBN
   9781615375134 (paperback : alk. paper) | ISBN 9781615375141 (ebook)
Subjects: MESH: Psychotropic Drugs—pharmacokinetics | Psychotropic
   Drugs—adverse effects | Drug Interactions | Comorbidity
Classification: LCC RM315 (print) | LCC RM315 (ebook) | NLM QV 77.2 |
   DDC 615.7/88--dc23/eng/20230802
LC record available at https://lccn.loc.gov/2023003642
LC ebook record available at https://lccn.loc.gov/2023003643

British Library Cataloguing in Publication Data
A CIP record is available from the British Library.

Contents

James L. Levenson, M.D.
Stephen J. Ferrando, M.D.

Part 1
General Principles

Ericka L. Crouse, Pharm.D.
Jonathan G. Leung, Pharm.D.

Contributors

Katie S. Adams, Pharm.D.
Clinical Pharmacy Specialist—Psychiatry; and Clinical Assistant Professor, Departments of Pharmacy and Psychiatry, Virginia Commonwealth University Health System, Richmond, Virginia

Syed Rashdi Ahmed, M.D.
Attending Consultation-Liaison Psychiatrist, West Los Angeles VA, Greater Los Angeles Health System, Los Angeles, CA

Margaret Altemus, M.D.
Associate Professor, Department of Psychiatry, Yale University School of Medicine, and VA Connecticut Health Care System, West Haven, Connecticut

Rosalind M. Berkowitz, M.D.
Private Practice, Hematology and Oncology, Moorestown, New Jersey

Philip A. Bialer, M.D.
Attending Psychiatrist, Memorial Sloan Kettering Cancer Center; and Associate Professor of Clinical Psychiatry, Weill Cornell Medical College, New York, New York

Jozef Bledowski, M.D.
Consultation-Liaison Psychiatrist, Arlington, Virginia

Melissa P. Bui, M.D.
Assistant Professor of Psychiatry, Department of Psychiatry, Virginia Commonwealth University School of Medicine, Richmond, Virginia

xiv   Clinical Manual of Psychopharmacology in the Medically Ill

E. Cabrina Campbell, M.D.
Robert L. Sadoff Professor and Vice Chair of Education; and Director, Psychiatry Residency Program, Department of Psychiatry, University of Pennsylvania Perelman School of Medicine, Corporal Michael J. Crescenz VA Medical Center, Philadelphia, Pennsylvania

Jason P. Caplan, M.D.
Chair of Psychiatry, St. Joseph's Hospital and Medical Center, Phoenix, Arizona; and Professor of Psychiatry, Creighton University School of Medicine, Phoenix, Arizona

Stanley N. Caroff, M.D.
Emeritus Professor, Department of Psychiatry, University of Pennsylvania Perelman School of Medicine, Corporal Michael J. Crescenz VA Medical Center, Philadelphia, Pennsylvania

Catherine C. Crone, M.D.
Associate Professor, Department of Psychiatry and Behavioral Sciences, George Washington University, Washington, D.C.

Ericka L. Crouse, Pharm.D.
Associate Professor, Department of Pharmacotherapy and Outcomes Science, Virginia Commonwealth University School of Pharmacy; and Clinical Associate Professor, Department of Psychiatry, Virginia Commonwealth University Health System, Richmond, Virginia

Catherine Daniels-Brady, M.D.
Assistant Clinical Professor, Department of Psychiatry and Behavioral Science, New York Medical College at Westchester Medical Center, Valhalla, New York

Elisabeth A. Dietrich, M.D.
Chief Psychiatry Resident, Department of Psychiatry, Virginia Commonwealth University School of Medicine, Richmond, Virginia

Andrea F. DiMartini, M.D.
Professor of Psychiatry and Professor of Surgery, Western Psychiatric Institute; and Consultation Liaison to the Liver Transplant Program, Starzl Transplant Institute, University of Pittsburgh Medical Center, Pittsburgh, Pennsylvania

Andrew Drysdale, M.D., Ph.D.
Postdoctoral Fellow; and Assistant in Clinical Psychiatry, Department of Psychiatry, Columbia University, New York, New York

Stephen J. Ferrando, M.D.
Director, Department of Psychiatry, Westchester Medical Center Health System; and Edith Har Esh, M.D., Professor and Chairman, Department of Psychiatry and Behavioral Sciences, New York Medical College, Valhalla, New York

Marian Fireman, M.D.
Professor of Psychiatry, Oregon Health & Science University, Portland, Oregon

Madhulika A. Gupta, M.D., M.Sc., FRCPC
Professor, Department of Psychiatry, Schulich School of Medicine and Dentistry, University of Western Ontario, London, Ontario, Canada

Jennifer Kraker, M.D., M.S.
Private Practice in Psychiatry, New York, New York

Alba Lara, M.D.
Associate Medical Director for Behavioral Health, Babylon Health; and Volunteer Faculty, Department of Psychiatry and Behavioral Sciences, The University of Texas at Austin Dell Medical School, Austin, Texas

Jonathan G. Leung, Pharm.D.
Clinical Pharmacy Specialist—Psychiatry, Department of Pharmacy; and Clinical Associate Professor of Psychiatry, Associate Professor of Pharmacy, Mayo Clinic College of Medicine & Science, Mayo Clinic, Rochester, Minnesota

James L. Levenson, M.D.
Rhona Arenstein Professor of Psychiatry, Professor of Medicine and Surgery, Chair of the Division of Consultation-Liaison Psychiatry, and Vice-Chair, Department of Psychiatry, Virginia Commonwealth University School of Medicine, Richmond, Virginia

Stephan C. Mann, M.D.
Private Practice, Psychiatry, Harleysville, Pennsylvania

Michael Marcangelo, M.D.
Professor, Department of Psychiatry and Behavioral Sciences, Northwestern University Feinberg School of Medicine, Chicago, Illinois

Curtis A. McKnight, M.D.
Psychiatrist, St. Joseph's Hospital and Medical Center, Phoenix, Arizona; and Associate Professor, Creighton University Arizona Health Education Alliance, Phoenix, Arizona

Sahil Munjal, M.D.
Assistant Professor, Psychiatry and Behavioral Medicine, Wake Forest School of Medicine, Winston-Salem, North Carolina

Mallay Occhiogrosso, M.D.
Clinical Assistant Professor, Department of Psychiatry, Weill Cornell Medical College, New York, New York

Kimberly N. Olson, CRNP
Private Practice, Main Line Healthcare Endocrinology, Wynnewood, Pennsylvania

Jacqueline Posada, M.D.
Assistant Professor, Department of Psychiatry and Behavioral Sciences, Dell Medical School, The University of Texas at Austin, Austin, Texas

Peter A. Shapiro, M.D.
Professor of Psychiatry, Columbia University Medical Center, Columbia University; and Director, Consultation-Liaison Psychiatry Service, New York Presbyterian Hospital–Columbia University Irving Medical Center, New York, New York

Yvette L. Smolin, M.D.
Director, Consultation-Liaison Psychiatry Service, and Fellowship, Department of Psychiatry and Behavioral Science, New York Medical College at Westchester Medical Center, Valhalla, New York

Cullen Truett, D.O.
Instructor, Department of Psychiatry and Behavioral Sciences, George Washington University, Washington, D.C.

Christina M. van der Feltz-Cornelis, M.D., Ph.D.
Professor, Department of Health Sciences, University of York, Heslington, York, United Kingdom

Robert M. Weinrieb, M.D., FACLP
Professor and Chief Psychiatric Consultant, Penn Transplant Institute; and Program Director, Penn/VA Consultation-Liaison Psychiatry Fellowship, Department of Psychiatry, University of Pennsylvania Perelman School of Medicine, Philadelphia, Pennsylvania

Shirley Qiong Yan, Pharm.D., BCOP
Pediatric Hematology/Oncology Clinical Pharmacy Specialist, Department of Pharmacy, Memorial Sloan Kettering Cancer Center, New York, New York

Disclosure of Interests

The following contributors to this book have indicated a financial interest in or other affiliation with a commercial supporter, manufacturer of a commercial product, and/or provider of a commercial service as listed below:

Stanley N. Caroff, M.D.
Research grants: Neurocrine Biosciences, Eagle Pharmaceuticals; *Consultant:* Neurocrine Biosciences, Teva Pharmaceuticals, Adamas Pharmaceuticals.

Ericka L. Crouse, Pharm.D.
Compensation: Editorial Board, *The Medical Letter; Consultant:* Wolters Kluwer/Lexi-Drugs.

Jonathan G. Leung, Pharm.D.
Consultant: Saladax Biomedical.

Peter A. Shapiro, M.D.
Stock: Pfizer, 2020 to present.

Christina M. van der Feltz-Cornelis, M.D., Ph.D.
Research funding: In 2007, my then employer (National Institute of Mental Health and Addiction/Trimbos Instituut, Utrecht, the Netherlands) received €180,000 funding from Eli Lilly for an Investigator Initiated Trial for which I was the main applicant, titled: "Cost Effectiveness of Transmural Collaborative Care Versus Duloxetine in Major Depressive Disorder With Concomitant Chronic Pain." Eli Lilly had no influence on the design, conduct, analysis, or reporting of the results of this trial.

The following contributors have indicated that they have no financial interests or other affiliations that represent or could appear to represent a competing interest with their contributions to this book:

Katie S. Adams, Pharm.D.; Syed Rashdi Ahmed, M.D.; Margaret Altemus, M.D.; Rosalind M. Berkowitz, M.D.; Jozef Bledowski, M.D.; Melissa P. Bui, M.D.; E. Cabrina Campbell, M.D.; Catherine Daniels-Brady, M.D.; Elisabeth A. Dietrich, M.D.; Andrea F. DiMartini, M.D.; Andrew Drysdale, M.D., Ph.D.; Stephen J. Ferrando, M.D.; Marian Fireman, M.D.; Madhulika A. Gupta, M.D., M.Sc., FRCPC; Jennifer Kraker, M.D., M.S.; Alba Lara, M.D.; James L. Levenson, M.D.; Stephan C. Mann, M.D.; Michael Marcangelo, M.D.; Curtis A. McKnight, M.D.; Sahil Munjal, M.D.; Mallay Occhiogrosso, M.D.; Jacqueline Posada, M.D.; Cullen Truett, D.O.; Robert M. Weinrieb, M.D., FACLP; Shirley Qiong Yan, Pharm.D., BCOP.

Acknowledgments

The editors would collectively like to acknowledge multiple individuals for their support, encouragement, and thoughtful input during the preparation of this book. We thank our original contributors, who have undertaken to update their original contributions, and welcome our newest authors for their high-quality contributions. We continue to appreciate the wisdom and dedication of Dr. Laura Roberts, Editor-in-Chief of American Psychiatric Association (APA) Publishing, as well as the editorial staff of APA Publishing for their enthusiastic encouragement to produce a third edition.

Dr. Levenson would like to thank his wife, Janet, his family, and his colleagues for their support.

Dr. Ferrando would like to thank his wife, Maria, and his children, Luke, Nicole, Marco, and David, for all their support.

Introduction

James L. Levenson, M.D.
Stephen J. Ferrando, M.D.

We are very happy with the publication of this third edition of the *Clinical Manual of Psychopharmacology in the Medically Ill*, the collective effort of many expert clinicians, including 11 new authors. The mission of this third edition is the same as that of the first two: to serve as a clinical manual and educational tool for specialist and nonspecialist clinicians for the psychopharmacological treatment of patients with medical illness. Every chapter has been thoroughly updated, with thousands of new references. Nineteen new psychiatric drugs have been approved by the U.S. FDA since the publication of the second edition, and we and the other contributors have incorporated them in the manual whenever relevant. There have also been 19 new forms or routes of administration introduced for previously approved psychiatric drugs (e.g., transdermal, intranasal, long-acting injection), which can be particularly important for patients who cannot take a pill or capsule, a common occurrence in the medically ill (see Chapter 3, "Alternative Routes of Drug Administration"). We are also pleased that many fellowship programs approved by the Accreditation Council for Graduate Medical Education have adopted this book as a core reference and text for teaching the principles and practice of prescribing psychotropic medication to psychiatrically and medically ill patients. Furthermore, physicians in other specialties of medicine, including primary care specialties, have found the manual to be useful.

Since the publication of the first two editions, the importance of the co-occurrence of psychiatric and medical illness has become even more evident (van Niekerk et al. 2022). There is increasing recognition that patients with medical and psychiatric comorbidity have more functional impairment, disability days, emergency department use, rehospitalization, and other medical care costs than do those without such comorbidity. Many studies have found that collaborative and integrated models of care that address patients' medical and psychiatric needs together improve outcomes (Bartels et al. 2018). Health care systems are developing new and innovative models of population-based care that integrate medical and psychiatric care in an effort to increase quality and prevention while decreasing use of expensive services such as emergency department visits and hospitalizations. In this context, a broader array of physician and nonphysician practitioners will be called on to prescribe psychiatric medications to individuals with medical illness, taking into account neuropsychiatric, metabolic, and other side effects as well as drug-drug and drug-disease interactions. Of further importance is the fact that outpatient practitioners will be called on to take care of sicker patients more than ever before, making issues of safe prescribing even more critical. It is our hope that this manual will continue to fill a key need for up-to-date and practical information.

How to Use This Manual

The organization of the third edition is the same as that of the first two. We aim to provide clinically relevant information regarding psychopharmacology in patients who are medically ill, including pharmacokinetic and pharmacodynamic principles, drug-drug interactions, and organ system disease–specific issues. Chapters are authored and updated by experts in the field, with editorial input to maintain consistency of format and style.

The manual has two parts. Part 1, "General Principles," provides fundamental background information for prescribing psychotropic drugs across medical disease states and is suggested reading prior to advancing to the disease-specific information in the second part. Part 1 includes discussion of pharmacodynamics and pharmacokinetics, principles of drug-drug interactions, major systemic adverse effects of psychotropic drugs, and alternative routes of psychotropic drug administration.

Part 2, "Psychopharmacology in Organ System Disorders and Specialty Areas," includes chapters on psychopharmacological treatment in specific organ system diseases, such as renal and cardiovascular disease, as well as other relevant subspecialty areas, such as critical care, organ transplantation, pain, and substance use disorders. With some variation, chapters are structured to include the following elements: key differential diagnostic considerations, including adverse neuropsychiatric side effects of disease-specific medications; disease-specific pharmacokinetic principles in drug prescribing; review of evidence for psychotropic drug treatment of psychiatric disorders in the specific disease state or specialty area; disease-specific adverse psychotropic drug side effects; and interactions between psychotropic drugs and disease-specific drugs. Each chapter has tables that summarize information on adverse neuropsychiatric side effects of disease-specific medications, adverse disease-specific side effects of psychotropic drugs, and drug-drug interactions. Chapters are heavily referenced with source information should readers wish to expand their knowledge in a specific area. Finally, each chapter ends with a list of key points pertaining to psychotropic prescribing in the specific medical disease(s) or specialty area covered in the chapter.

With this structure, we hope that we have contributed a comprehensive yet practical guide for psychotropic prescribing for patients who are medically ill. We will consider this manual a success if it proves useful for a broad range of specialists, such as the consultation-liaison psychiatrist caring for a delirious patient with cancer, the general psychiatrist in the community mental health clinic whose patient with schizophrenia develops liver disease in the setting of alcohol use disorder and hepatitis C infection, and the general medical practitioner prescribing an antidepressant to a diabetic patient who recently had a myocardial infarction. We hope that this manual, beyond serving as a clinical guide, will also become a mainstay of curricula in general psychiatric residency programs, in consultation-liaison psychiatry fellowships, and in nonpsychiatric residency training programs that seek to provide training in psychopharmacology for medically ill patients.

References

Bartels SJ, DiMilia PR, Fortuna KL, Naslund JA: Integrated care for older adults with serious mental illness and medical comorbidity: evidence-based models and future research directions. Psychiatr Clin North Am 41(1):153–164, 2018 29412843

van Niekerk M, Walker J, Hobbs H, et al: The prevalence of psychiatric disorders in general hospital inpatients: a systematic umbrella review. J Acad Consult Liaison Psychiatry 63(6):567–578, 2022 35491011

PART 1

General Principles

1

Pharmacokinetics, Pharmacodynamics, and Principles of Drug-Drug Interactions

Ericka L. Crouse, Pharm.D.

Jonathan G. Leung, Pharm.D.

Psychotropic drugs are commonly used in the management of patients who are medically ill. Depending on the setting, 30%–100% of psychiatric consultations to hospitals, primary care, and nursing homes include recommendations for psychiatric medication (Lowenstein et al. 2017; Pezzia et al. 2018).

The authors acknowledge James A. Owen, Ph.D., for his original authorship of this chapter.

The appropriate use of psychopharmacology in medically ill patients requires careful consideration of the underlying medical illness, potential alterations to pharmacokinetics, drug-drug interactions, drug-disease interactions, drug-gene interactions, and contraindications. In this chapter, we review drug action, drug pharmacokinetics, and drug interactions to provide a basis for drug-drug and drug-disease interactions presented in later disease-specific chapters.

The effects of a drug—that is, the magnitude and duration of its therapeutic and adverse effects—are determined by the drug's pharmacodynamic and pharmacokinetic properties. *Pharmacodynamics* describes the effects of a drug on the body. Pharmacodynamic processes determine the relationship between drug concentration and response for both therapeutic and adverse effects. *Pharmacokinetics* describes what the body does to the drug. It characterizes the rate and extent of drug absorption, distribution, metabolism, and excretion. These pharmacokinetic processes determine the rate of drug delivery to and the drug's concentration at the sites of action. The relationship between pharmacokinetics and pharmacodynamics is diagrammed in Figure 1–1.

Pharmacodynamics

For most drugs, the pharmacological effect is the result of a complex chain of events, beginning with the interaction of drug with receptor. Pharmacodynamic response is further modified—enhanced or diminished—by disease states, aging, and other drugs. For example, the presence of Parkinson's disease increases the incidence of movement disorders induced by selective serotonin reuptake inhibitors (SSRIs). Pharmacodynamic drug-disease interactions are reviewed in the relevant chapters; pharmacodynamic drug-drug interactions are discussed later in this chapter in the subsection "Pharmacodynamic Drug Interactions."

A drug's spectrum of therapeutic and adverse effects is due to its interaction with multiple receptor sites and other downstream effects. The effects produced depend on which receptor populations are occupied by the drug; some receptor populations are readily occupied at low drug concentrations, whereas other receptor sites require high drug levels for interaction. In this way, different responses are recruited in a stepwise manner with increasing drug concentration. As drug levels increase, each effect will reach a maximum as all active receptors responsible for that effect are occupied by the drug. Fur-

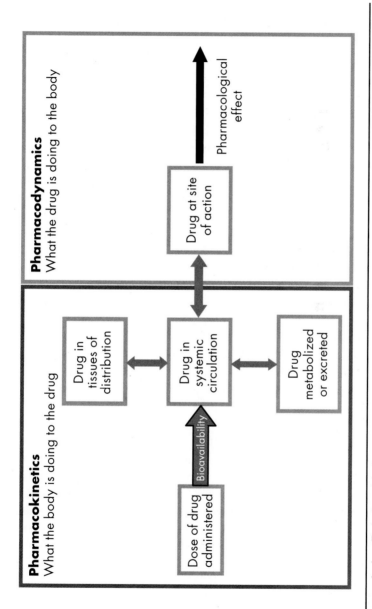

Figure 1–1.   Relationship between pharmacokinetics and pharmacodynamics.

ther increases in drug concentration will not increase the intended therapeutic response but may elicit other effects, usually adverse ones. Figure 1–2 illustrates three pharmacological effects produced by a drug in a concentration-dependent manner. In this example, *Effect B* is the primary therapeutic effect, *Effect A* is a minor adverse effect, and *Effect C* is a significant toxic effect. Low drug concentrations recruit only Effect A; the patient experiences a nuisance side effect without any therapeutic gain. As drug concentration increases, Effect B is engaged and Effect A is maximized. Clearly, for this drug, except in the rare situation when Effect B antagonizes Effect A (e.g., when the initial sedating effect of a drug is counteracted by stimulating effects recruited at a higher concentration), Effect A will always accompany a therapeutically effective dose because it is recruited at a lower concentration than that required for the therapeutic effect. Further increases in drug concentration improve the therapeutic effect until the therapeutic effect reaches its maximum, but these increases also introduce toxic Effect C.

Optimum therapy requires that drug concentrations be confined to a therapeutic range to maximize the therapeutic effect and minimize any adverse and/or toxic effects. Many psychotropic agents have well-established therapeutic drug levels (Hiemke et al. 2018); however, routine therapeutic drug monitoring is primarily reserved for those drugs with narrow therapeutic indexes. Developing a dosage regimen to maintain drug levels within this therapeutic range requires consideration of pharmacokinetic processes, drug-drug interactions, and patient-specific parameters.

Drug-receptor interactions produce effects on several timescales. Immediate effects are the result of a direct receptor interaction. Several psychoactive drugs, including benzodiazepines, have immediate therapeutic effects and therefore are useful on an acute or as-needed basis. However, many psychoactive drugs, such as antidepressant and antipsychotic agents, require chronic dosing over several weeks for a significant therapeutic response. These drugs appear to alter neuronal responsiveness by modifying slowly adapting cellular processes. Unfortunately, many adverse effects appear immediately—the result of a direct receptor interaction. Medication adherence may be significantly affected when a patient experiences adverse effects before the benefits of the medication's therapeutic effects. Table 1–1 lists strategies to maximize medication adherence.

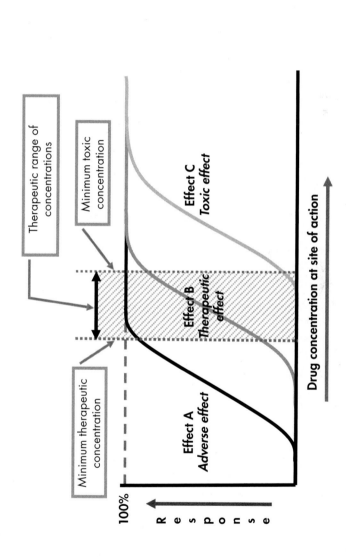

Figure 1–2. Concentration-response relationship (see text for details). Optimum therapy dose occurs during Effect B, when therapeutic effect is achieved, adverse effects are minimized, and toxicity has not occurred.

Table 1–1.   Strategies to maximize medication adherence

Provide patient education

Inform the patient about potential adverse effects, their speed of onset, and whether tolerance will develop over time.

Indicate the time for onset of the therapeutic effect. Many psychotropic drugs have a considerable delay (weeks) before the appearance of significant therapeutic effects yet give rise to adverse effects immediately. Patients not aware of this temporal disconnect between adverse and therapeutic effects may consider the medication a failure and discontinue the drug if only adverse effects and no therapeutic effects are initially experienced.

Select drugs with a convenient dosing schedule

Select drugs with once-daily dosing (i.e., those with a suitably long half-life or available in an extended-release formulation) to maximize adherence.

Consider the use of long-acting injectable formulations for antipsychotic agents. Depending on the agent, they may be dosed every 2 or 4 weeks. Extended interval formulations of aripiprazole lauroxil (every 6 weeks or 2 months) and paliperidone palmitate (every 3 months or 6 months) are also available. Adherence can be confirmed from administration records. However, the patient must have undergone a successful trial of the equivalent oral formulation to verify therapeutic response and tolerance to adverse effects and to establish the appropriate dose. Confirm date of previous injection before administering a maintenance dose.

Minimize adverse effects

Select drugs with minimal pharmacokinetic interaction whenever possible (e.g., avoid potent cytochrome P450 inhibitors or inducers).

Gradually increase drug dosage to therapeutic levels over several days or weeks ("start low, go slow") so that patients experience minimal adverse effects while gradually developing tolerance. For example, antidepressants do not have a substantially faster onset of action with a rapid titration. Adverse effects such as orthostasis are minimized with slower titrations.

Use the minimum effective dose.

Select a drug with an adverse-effect profile the patient can best tolerate. Drugs within a class may be similar therapeutically but differ in their adverse-effect profile. Patients may vary in their tolerance of a particular effect.

Table 1–1.   Strategies to maximize medication
adherence *(continued)*

Reduce peak drug levels following absorption of oral medications. Many adverse effects are concentration dependent and are exacerbated as drug levels peak following oral dosing. Consider administering the drug with food or using divided doses or extended-release formulations to reduce and delay peak drug levels and diminish adverse effects.

Schedule the dose so the side effect is less bothersome. If possible, prescribe activating drugs in the morning and sedating drugs or those that cause gastrointestinal distress in the evening.

Use therapeutic drug monitoring

Keep in mind that therapeutic drug monitoring is available for many psychotropic drugs. This is valuable for monitoring adherence and ensuring that drug levels are within the therapeutic range.

Check for patient adherence

Schedule office or telephone visits to discuss adherence and adverse effects for newly prescribed drugs. Explore strategies such as alarms or pillboxes.

Pharmacokinetics

Drug response, including the magnitude and duration of the drug's therapeutic and adverse effects, is significantly influenced by the drug's pharmacokinetics (absorption from administration sites, distribution throughout the body, and metabolism and excretion). Individual differences in constitutional factors, compromised organ function, and disease states and the effects of other drugs and food all contribute to the high variability in drug response observed across patients. Understanding the effect of these factors on a drug's pharmacokinetics will aid in drug selection and dosage adjustment in a therapeutic environment complicated by polypharmacy and medical illness.

Absorption and Bioavailability

The speed of onset and, to a certain extent, the duration of the pharmacological effects of a drug are determined by the route of administration. *Bioavailability of a drug formulation* describes the rate and extent of drug delivery to the systemic circulation from the formulation. Intravenous or intra-arterial administration delivers 100% of the drug dose to the systemic circulation (100% bioavailability) at a rate that can be controlled if necessary. For drugs delivered by other routes, bioavailability is typically less than 100%, and often much less.

Drug absorption is influenced by the characteristics of the absorption site and the physiochemical properties of a drug. Specific site properties affecting absorption include surface area, ambient pH, mucosal integrity and function, and local blood flow, all of which may be altered by, for example, peptic ulcer disease or inflammatory bowel disease and the drugs used to treat the disease.

Orally administered drugs face several pharmacokinetic barriers that limit drug delivery to the systemic circulation. Drugs must dissolve in gastric fluids to be absorbed, and drug dissolution in the stomach and gut may be incomplete (e.g., after gastric bypass surgery). Drugs may be acid labile and degrade in the acidic stomach environment, or they may be partially metabolized by gut flora. Use of acid suppression agents (e.g., proton pump inhibitors) and aluminum- or magnesium-containing antacids may affect absorption of lipophilic basic medications (Yoshida et al. 2019). Specifically, magnesium oxide decreases the solubility and intestinal absorption of risperidone, zotepine, biperiden, and gabapentin (Yagi et al. 2012; Yoshida et al. 2019). Use of antacids does not appear to alter lithium concentrations (Goode et al. 1984) or duloxetine absorption (Knadler et al. 2011). Conversely, absorption of some medications (e.g., ibuprofen) could potentially be enhanced with magnesium-containing, but not aluminum-containing, antacids (Neuvonen and Kivistö 1994). Little is known about the extent to which antacids may reduce or enhance absorption of psychotropics, but on theoretical grounds such effects may be significant and vary depending on the specific antacid (Neuvonen and Kivistö 1994). Even as benign a substance as the fiber supplement psyllium has been reported to reduce absorption of olanzapine (Merrick et al. 2021) and lithium (Toutoungi et al. 1990). Some medications require food to enhance absorption. For example, the bioavailability of ziprasidone is enhanced almost twofold with food, and lurasidone exposure (area under the curve [AUC]) is doubled in the presence of food. Conversely, some medications (e.g., levothyroxine, alendronate) require an empty stomach to enhance absorption. Drugs absorbed through the gastrointestinal tract may be extensively altered by first-pass metabolism before entering the systemic circulation (Figure 1–3). *First-pass metabolism* refers to the transport and metabolism of drugs from the gut lumen to the systemic circulation via the portal vein and

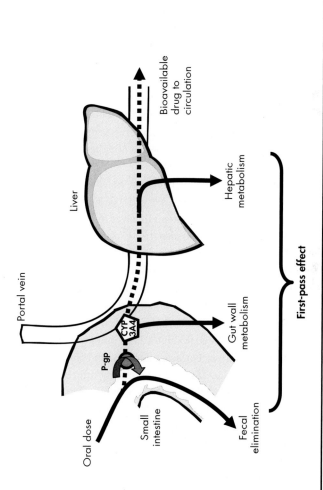

Figure 1–3. First-pass metabolism of orally administered drugs.

Many drugs undergo a first-pass effect as they are absorbed from the intestinal lumen before they are delivered to the systemic circulation. The first-pass effect limits oral bioavailability through countertransport by P-glycoprotein (P-gp) back into the intestinal lumen and by gut wall (mainly cytochrome P450 3A4 [CYP3A4]) and hepatic metabolism.

liver. Drug passage from the gut lumen to the portal circulation may be limited by two processes: 1) a P-glycoprotein (P-gp) efflux transport pump, which serves to reduce the absorption of many compounds (some P-gp substrates are listed in Appendixes A and B to this chapter) by countertransporting them back into the intestinal lumen, and 2) metabolism within the gut wall by cytochrome P450 (CYP) 3A4 enzymes. Because P-gp is co-localized with and shares similar substrate affinity with CYP3A4, drug substrates of CYP3A4 typically have poor bioavailability. Bioavailability may be further decreased by hepatic extraction of drugs as they pass through the liver before gaining access to the systemic circulation. Sublingual and topical drug administration minimizes this first-pass effect. Rectal delivery, although often resulting in erratic absorption, may reduce first-pass effect by 50%.

Bioavailability can be markedly altered by disease states and drugs that alter gut and hepatic function. As with the CYP and uridine 5′-diphosphate glucuronosyltransferase (UGT) enzyme systems involved in drug metabolism, drugs can also inhibit or induce the P-gp transporter. Common P-gp inhibitors include paroxetine, sertraline, trifluoperazine, verapamil, and proton pump inhibitors. Because intestinal P-gps serve to block absorption in the gut, inhibition of these transporters can dramatically increase the bioavailability of poorly bioavailable drugs. For example, oral fentanyl absorption in humans is increased 2.7-fold when the drug is administered with quinidine, a known intestinal P-gp inhibitor (Kharasch et al. 2004). P-gp inhibitors are listed in Appendixes A and B to this chapter. For drugs administered chronically, the *extent* of drug absorption is the key factor in maintaining drug levels within the therapeutic range. In situations when bioavailability may be significantly altered, parenteral administration of drugs may be preferable.

Drug formulation, drug interactions, gastric motility, and the characteristics of the absorptive surface all influence the *rate* of absorption, a key factor when rapid onset is desired. Oral medications are absorbed primarily in the small intestine because of its large surface area. Delayed gastric emptying or drug dissolution will slow absorption and therefore blunt the rise in drug levels following an oral dose. In this way, the occurrence of transient concentration-related adverse effects following an oral dose may be reduced by administering a medication with food, whereas the common practice of dissolving medications in juice may produce higher peak levels and exacerbate these transient adverse reactions.

Distribution

Following absorption into the systemic circulation, the drug is distributed throughout the body in accordance with its physiochemical properties and the extent of protein binding. *Volume of distribution* describes the relationship between the bioavailable dose and the plasma concentration. Lipophilic drugs, including most psychotropic medications, are sequestered into lipid compartments of the body. Because of their low plasma concentrations relative to dose, these drugs appear to have a large volume of distribution. In contrast, hydrophilic drugs (e.g., lithium, oxazepam, valproate), being confined mainly to the intravascular volume and other aqueous compartments, have a high plasma concentration relative to dose, suggesting a small volume of distribution. Volume of distribution is often unpredictably altered by disease-related changes in organ and tissue perfusion or body composition. Edema (e.g., in congestive heart failure, cirrhosis, or nephrotic syndrome) causes expansion of the extracellular fluid volume and may significantly increase the volume of distribution for hydrophilic drugs. Lipophilic drugs experience an increase in volume of distribution with obesity, which is sometimes iatrogenic (e.g., with corticosteroids or antipsychotics), and age-related increases in body fat. P-gp, a major component of the blood-brain barrier, may limit entry of drugs into the CNS. Many antiretroviral agents have limited CNS penetration because they are P-gp substrates (see Appendix B to this chapter). Besides the P-gp efflux transport pump, the blood-brain barrier itself presents a physical barrier through tight junctions that limit the movement of agents into the CNS.

Most drugs bind, to varying degrees, to the plasma proteins albumin or α_1-acid glycoprotein. Acidic drugs (e.g., valproic acid, barbiturates) bind mostly to albumin, and more basic drugs (e.g., phenothiazines, tricyclic antidepressants, amphetamines, most benzodiazepines) bind to globulins.

Drug in plasma circulates in both bound and free (unbound to plasma proteins) forms. Generally, only free drug is pharmacologically active. The amount of drug bound to plasma proteins is dependent on the presence of other compounds that displace the drug from its protein-binding sites (a protein-binding drug interaction) and the plasma concentration of albumin and α_1-acid glycoprotein. Medical conditions may alter plasma concentrations of albumin or α_1-acid glycoprotein (Table 1–2) or increase the levels of endogenous displacing compounds. For example, uremia, chronic liver disease, and hypoalbuminemia may significantly increase the proportion of free drug rel-

Table 1–2.   Conditions that alter plasma levels of albumin and α_1-acid glycoprotein

Decrease albumin

Surgery

Burns

Trauma

Pregnancy

Alcohol use disorder

Sepsis, systemic inflammatory response syndrome

Bacterial pneumonia

Acute pancreatitis

Uncontrolled diabetes

Hepatic cirrhosis

Nephritis, nephrotic syndrome, and renal failure

Older age

Malnutrition

Pulmonary edema

Malignancy

Increase albumin

Hypothyroidism

Decrease α_1-acid glycoprotein

Pancreatic cancer

Pregnancy

Uremia

Hepatitis, cirrhosis

Cachexia, malnutrition

Hyperthyroidism

Nephrotic syndrome

Table 1–2. Conditions that alter plasma levels of albumin and α_1-acid glycoprotein *(continued)*

Increase α_1-acid glycoprotein

Stress response to disease states

Inflammatory bowel disease

Acute myocardial infarction

Trauma, injury

Epilepsy

Stroke

Surgery

Burns

Cancer (except pancreatic)

Acute glomerulonephritis

Rheumatoid arthritis and systemic lupus erythematosus

Organ transplantation

Obesity

Source. Compiled in part from Dasgupta 2007; di Masi et al. 2016; Israili and Dayton 2001; Ulldemolins et al. 2011.

ative to total drug in circulation (Dasgupta 2007). The free drug also is correlated with toxic adverse effects (Charlier et al. 2021).

Changes in drug protein binding, either disease induced or the result of a protein-binding drug interaction, were once considered a common cause of drug toxicity because therapeutic and toxic effects increase with increasing concentrations of free drug. These interactions are now seen as clinically significant in only very limited cases (e.g., malnourished patients) involving rapidly acting, highly protein bound (>80%), narrow therapeutic index drugs with high hepatic extraction (e.g., propafenone, verapamil, intravenous lidocaine) (Benet and Hoener 2002; Rolan 1994). For drugs with low hepatic extraction, such as warfarin (Greenblatt and von Moltke 2005) and phenytoin (Tsanaclis et al. 1984) (see Table 1–3 later in this chapter), metabolism is not limited by hepatic blood flow, and a reduction in protein binding serves to increase the amount of free drug available for metabolism and excretion. Consequently, hypoalbuminemia or the presence of a displacing drug enhances drug elimination, which generally limits changes in circulating unbound drug levels to only a transient, and clinically insignificant, increase. (Many warfarin drug interactions previously thought to be protein-binding interactions are now recognized as pharmacodynamic and CYP2C9 and CYP1A2 metabolic interactions.) Therapeutic drug monitoring procedures that measure total drug levels could mislead the clinician by suggesting lower, possibly subtherapeutic, levels and might prompt a dosage increase with possible toxic effects. For this reason, in patients with uremia, chronic hepatic disease, hypoalbuminemia, or a protein-binding drug interaction, the use of therapeutic drug monitoring for dose adjustment requires caution; clinical response to the drug (e.g., international normalized ratio for warfarin), rather than laboratory-determined drug levels, should guide dosage (Nadkarni et al. 2011). When therapeutic drug monitoring is used, methods selective for unbound (free) drug should be used, if available, for phenytoin, valproate, tacrolimus, cyclosporine, amitriptyline, haloperidol, and possibly carbamazepine (Charlier et al. 2021; Dasgupta 2007; Madan et al. 2021; Patsalos et al. 2018). Clinically free phenytoin levels are the most widely used, especially in the older adult, malnourished, and critically ill populations. Free valproate levels (which is ≥90% protein bound) have been increasingly used in clinical practice, especially in intensive care patients when protein binding may be highly variable. As free fraction increases, metabolism increases, potentially leading to lower-than-expected total valproate concentrations. Continuing to increase the dose of valproate has been shown to lead to higher free fraction concentrations, despite what appears to be low total concentrations (Charlier et al. 2021).

Disease-related changes to a drug's protein binding have little effect on steady-state plasma concentrations of free drug as long as the disease does not affect metabolic and excretory processes (Benet and Hoener 2002). However, most diseases that affect protein binding also affect metabolism and excretion, with clinically significant consequences, especially for drugs with a low therapeutic index.

Drug Elimination: Metabolism and Excretion

The kidney is the primary organ of drug excretion, with fecal and pulmonary excretion being of less importance. Hydrophilic compounds are removed from the body through excretion into the aqueous environment of urine and feces. In contrast, lipophilic drugs, including most psychoactive medications, are readily reabsorbed through the intestinal mucosa (enterohepatic recirculation) and renal tubules, which limits their excretion. Because all drugs undergo glomerular filtration, lipophilic drugs would experience significant renal elimination were it not for renal resorption. Renal resorption, and thus the elimination, of several drugs, including amphetamines, meperidine, and methadone, can be significantly changed by altering urine pH (discussed later in the subsection "Pharmacokinetic Drug Interactions").

The general function of metabolism is to convert lipophilic molecules into more polar water-soluble compounds that can be readily excreted. Although biotransformation often results in less active or inactive metabolites, this is not always true. For some drugs, metabolites have pharmacological activities similar to, or even greater than, those of the parent compound, and thus contribute to the therapeutic effect. Indeed, some metabolites are separately marketed, including paliperidone (principal active metabolite of risperidone), desvenlafaxine (metabolite of venlafaxine), and temazepam and oxazepam (both metabolites of diazepam). Some drugs are administered as prodrugs—inactive compounds requiring metabolic activation—including lisdexamfetamine (metabolized to dextroamphetamine), serdexmethylphenidate (metabolized to dexmethylphenidate), tramadol, codeine (metabolized to morphine), clopidogrel, fosphenytoin, primidone (metabolized to phenobarbital), and tamoxifen (metabolized to endoxifen). Other drug metabolites may have pharmacological effects considerably different from those of the parent drug and may cause unique toxicities (e.g., the meperidine metabolite normeperidine has proconvulsant activity, and carbamazepine-10,11-epoxide is a toxic metabolite of carbamazepine).

Metabolism

Biotransformation occurs throughout the body, with the greatest activity in the liver and gut wall. Most psychotropic drugs are eliminated by hepatic metabolism followed by renal excretion. Hepatic biotransformation processes are of two types, identified as Phase I and Phase II reactions. Phase I reactions typically convert the parent drug into a more polar metabolite by introducing or unmasking a polar functional group in preparation for excretion or further metabolism by Phase II pathways. Phase II metabolism conjugates the drug or

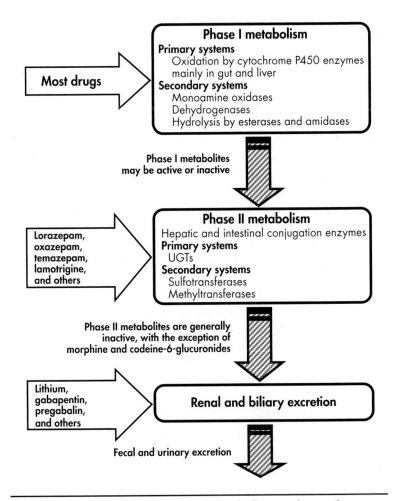

Figure 1–4. General pathways of metabolism and excretion.

UGTs=uridine 5'-diphosphate glucuronosyltransferases.

Phase I metabolite with an endogenous acid such as glucuronate, acetate, or sulfate. The resulting highly polar conjugates are usually inactive and are rapidly excreted in urine and feces (see Figure 1–4).

Phase I metabolism.   Phase I reactions include oxidation, reduction, and hydrolysis. Most Phase I oxidation reactions are carried out by the hepatic

CYP system, with a lesser contribution from the monoamine oxidases (MAOs). CYP enzymes exist in a variety of body tissues, including the gastrointestinal tract, liver, lung, and brain. Approximately 12 enzymes within three main families, CYP1, CYP2, and CYP3, are responsible for the majority of drug metabolism (Zanger and Schwab 2013). These families are divided into subfamilies identified by a capital letter (e.g., CYP3A). Subfamilies are further subdivided into isozymes on the basis of the homology between subfamily proteins. Isozymes are denoted by a number following the subfamily letter (e.g., CYP3A4, CYP2J2).

In humans, CYP1A2, CYP2C9, CYP2C19, CYP2D6, and CYP3A4 are the most important enzymes for drug metabolism. These enzymes exhibit substrate specificity. Functional deficiencies in one CYP enzyme will affect the metabolism of only those compounds that are substrates for that enzyme. Because some of these enzymes exist in a polymorphic form, a small percentage of the population, varying with ethnicity, has one or more CYP enzymes with significantly altered activity. For example, polymorphisms of the 2D6 gene give rise to populations with the capacity to metabolize CYP2D6 substrates extensively (normal condition), poorly (5%–14% of whites, ~1% of Asians), or ultraextensively (1%–3% of the population) (Zanger and Schwab 2013; Zanger et al. 2004). Certain Asian populations are more likely to be 2C19 poor metabolizers (18%–23%) as compared with populations characterized as white or Black (1%–5%) (Belle and Singh 2008). The FDA has suggested that as many as 30% of certain Asians may actually be lacking the 2C19 enzyme (U.S. Food and Drug Administration 2016). CYP enzyme activity can also be altered (inhibited or enhanced through induction) by environmental compounds or drugs, giving rise to many drug-drug interactions (discussed in the section "Drug-Drug Interactions" later in this chapter).

Several genetic tests assessing variations in CYP enzymes and other genetic factors are available or marketed to physicians and to consumers to guide prescribing of antidepressants and psychotropic medication. Several guidelines exist to help implement pharmacogenomic information into clinical practice, but evidence is insufficient for this testing to predict positive response or adverse effects for most psychotropics (Hicks et al. 2015, 2017; Solomon et al. 2019; Zeier et al. 2018). Although the FDA approved the tests, it has stated that "the relationship between genetic (DNA) variations and the medication's effects has not been established" (U.S. Food and Drug Administration 2019).

However, it should be noted that there are already drug-gene interactions noted in FDA prescribing information of many medications. Specific examples include dosing recommendations or warnings when there are known genetic alterations for aripiprazole (i.e., CYP2D6), brivaracetam (i.e., CYP2C19), citalopram (i.e., CYP2C19), codeine (i.e., CYP2D6), deutetrabenazine (i.e., CYP2D6), and valbenazine (i.e., CYP2D6). Additionally, testing for HLA-B*1502 is recommended prior to starting carbamazepine in patients of Asian descent to minimize the risk of Stevens-Johnson syndrome. The combination of drug-gene interactions plus other drug-drug or drug–disease state interactions may also increase the risk of adverse events or poor outcomes, but confirmatory studies are lacking.

Phase II metabolism.   Phase II conjugation reactions mainly involve enzymes belonging to the superfamily of UGTs. UGT enzymes are located hepatically (primarily centrizonal) (Debinski et al. 1995) and in the kidney and small intestine (Fisher et al. 2001). The UGT enzyme superfamily is classified in a manner similar to the CYP system. There are four UGT subfamilies (1, 2, 3, and 8). Two clinically significant UGT subfamilies—1A and 2B—are best characterized in terms of medication effects. As with the CYP system, there can be substrates, inhibitors, and inducers of UGT enzymes. For example, those benzodiazepines that are primarily metabolized by conjugation (oxazepam, lorazepam, and temazepam) are glucuronidated by UGT2B7. Lamotrigine is metabolized by UGT1A4 and UGT2B7. Valproic acid, tacrolimus, cyclosporine, and several nonsteroidal anti-inflammatory drugs (NSAIDs), including diclofenac, flurbiprofen, and naproxen, are competitive inhibitors of UGT2B7. Carbamazepine, phenytoin, rifampin (rifampicin), phenobarbital, and oral contraceptives are general inducers of UGTs (Kiang et al. 2005; Meech et al. 2019).

Drug interactions involving Phase II UGT-mediated conjugation reactions are increasingly becoming recognized. These interactions between critical substrates, inducers, and inhibitors follow the same rationale as for CYP interactions (discussed later in the section "Drug-Drug Interactions").

Effect of disease on metabolism.   Hepatic clearance of a drug may be limited by either the rate of delivery of the drug to the hepatic metabolizing enzymes (i.e., hepatic blood flow) or the intrinsic capacity of these enzymes to metabolize the substrate. Reduced hepatic blood flow impairs the clearance of drugs with high hepatic extraction (>6 mL/min/kg; flow-limited drugs) but has little effect on drugs with low hepatic extraction (<3 mL/min/kg; capacity-limited drugs), whose clearance depends primarily on hepatic function. Table 1–3 lists psychotropic drugs according to their degree of hepatic extraction.

Clinically significant decreases in hepatic blood flow, which occur in severe cardiovascular disease, chronic pulmonary disease, and severe cirrhosis, impair the clearance of flow-limited drugs. A reduction in the metabolic capacity of hepatic enzymes, as often accompanies congestive heart failure, renal disease, or hepatic disease, mainly impairs the clearance of capacity-limited drugs. Renal disease can significantly reduce hepatic Phase I and Phase II metabolism and increase intestinal bioavailability by reducing metabolic enzyme and P-gp gene expression (Pichette and Leblond 2003). Hepatic disease may preferentially affect anatomical regions of the liver, thereby altering specific metabolic processes. For example, oxidative metabolic reactions are more concentrated in the pericentral regions affected by acute viral hepatitis or alcohol-related liver disease. Disease affecting the periportal regions, such as chronic hepatitis (in the absence of cirrhosis), may spare some hepatic oxidative function. Acute and chronic liver diseases generally do not impair glucuronide conjugation reactions.

Severity of hepatic disease may be calculated with the Child-Pugh score. Five markers are used to calculate the score: serum bilirubin, serum albumin, prothrombin time, presence of encephalopathy, and the presence of ascites; scores of 5–6 are considered mild and 10–15 are considered severe hepatic dysfunction. Psychotropic medications with dosage adjustment recommendations based on Child-Pugh score include eszopiclone, venlafaxine, galantamine, and atomoxetine (Spray et al. 2007).

Excretion

The kidney's primary pharmacokinetic role is drug excretion. However, renal disease may also affect drug absorption, distribution, and metabolism. Reduced renal function, due to age or disease, results in the accumulation of drugs and active metabolites predominantly cleared by renal elimination. Dosage reduction may be required for narrow therapeutic index drugs that undergo significant renal excretion.

For renally eliminated drugs, a 24-hour urine creatinine clearance determination is a more useful indicator of renal function than is serum creatinine,

Table 1–3.   Systemic clearance of hepatically metabolized psychotropic drugs

High extraction ratio (clearance >6 mL/min/kg)

Amitriptyline	Flumazenil	Olanzapine
Asenapine	Fluoxetine	Paroxetine
Bupropion	Fluvoxamine	Quetiapine
Buspirone	Haloperidol	Rizatriptan
Chlorpromazine	Hydrocodone	Ropinirole
Clozapine	Hydromorphone	Sertraline
Codeine	Imipramine	Sumatriptan
Desipramine	Meperidine	Venlafaxine
Diphenhydramine	Midazolam	Zaleplon
Doxepin	Morphine	Zolmitriptan
Fentanyl	Nortriptyline	

Intermediate extraction ratio (clearance 3–6 mL/min/kg)

Bromocriptine	Flunitrazepam	Risperidone
Citalopram	Flurazepam	Triazolam
Clonidine	Protriptyline	Zolpidem

Low extraction ratio (clearance <3 mL/min/kg)

Alprazolam	Lamotrigine	Paliperidone
Carbamazepine	Levetiracetam	Phenytoin
Chlordiazepoxide	Lorazepam	Temazepam
Clonazepam	Methadone	Tiagabine
Clorazepate	Modafinil	Topiramate
Diazepam	Nitrazepam	Trazodone
Donepezil	Oxazepam	Valproate
Ethosuximide	Oxcarbazepine	Vilazodone

Source.   Compiled from Thummel et al. 2018.

but this is often not practical. In older adult patients, reduced creatinine production because of decreased muscle mass and possibly reduced exercise and dietary meat intake causes the calculation of creatinine clearance from serum creatinine levels by the Cockcroft-Gault formula to overestimate glomerular filtration rate (GFR; Sokoll et al. 1994). Many medication recommendations for renal dosage adjustments were based on Cockcroft-Gault estimation of creatinine clearance. Calculations of creatinine-based estimated GFR (eGFR) are increasingly reported within the electronic health record. The Modification of Diet in Renal Disease four-variable equation to estimate GFR was studied primarily in a white chronic kidney disease population (Levey et al. 2006; National Institute of Diabetes and Digestive and Kidney Diseases 2021). The more recent Chronic Kidney Disease Epidemiology Collaboration equations are suggested to estimate GFR even more accurately and have been evaluated in large, diverse populations (Levey et al. 2014; National Institute of Diabetes and Digestive and Kidney Diseases 2021).

A limitation of any serum creatinine–based eGFR is that it may be less accurate in persons of extreme body size or muscle mass (National Institute of Diabetes and Digestive and Kidney Diseases 2021). In patients with severe liver disease, estimates of GFR must be interpreted with caution. The reduced muscle mass and impaired metabolism of creatine associated with severe liver disease often results in inaccurate estimates of GFR when estimates are based on either serum creatinine levels (Cockcroft-Gault method) or creatinine clearance (Papadakis and Arieff 1987). Other populations with low muscle mass include frail older adults, critically ill patients, malnourished individuals, and oncology patients (National Institute of Diabetes and Digestive and Kidney Diseases 2021).

Drug-Drug Interactions

Polypharmacy is common in medically ill patients and frequently leads to clinically significant pharmacokinetic or pharmacodynamic drug-drug interactions. Pharmacokinetic interactions alter drug absorption, distribution, metabolism, or excretion and change the drug concentration in tissues. These interactions are most likely to be clinically meaningful when the drug involved has a low therapeutic index. Pharmacodynamic interactions alter the pharmacological response to a drug. These interactions may be additive, synergistic, or antagonistic. Pharmacodynamic interactions may occur directly by altering drug binding to the receptor site or indirectly through other mechanisms.

Use of resources to help determine clinical significance of drug-drug interactions is recommended when prescribing in a polypharmacy environment. Many hospital electronic health records include built-in drug-drug or drug-disease interaction checking software; however, limitations of these alerts include that some may have been turned off, downgraded, or not activated; they may not be characterized by severity; or they may be overlooked given the number of alerts a provider has to navigate or the fact that some may warn against use of combinations routinely used in clinical practice (e.g., SSRI plus trazodone, SSRI plus quetiapine, SSRI plus bupropion). When medications with known drug-drug interactions are being prescribed, databases such as Wolters Kluwer/Lexi-Drugs (within www.uptodate.com), Micromedex, or Epocrates, or even the prescribing information of individual agents, may provide clinical significance and severity of drug-drug interactions. Additional websites are listed in Appendix C to this chapter. It is important to review and determine whether the interaction is contraindicated or whether increased monitoring of adverse effects or reduction or increase in dosage is needed.

Pharmacokinetic Drug Interactions

Most drugs are substrates for metabolism by one or more CYP enzymes. The most common pharmacokinetic drug-drug interaction involves changes in the CYP-mediated metabolism of the substrate drug by an interacting drug. The interacting drug may be either an inducer or an inhibitor of the specific CYP enzymes involved in the substrate drug's metabolism. In the presence of an *inducer*, CYP enzyme activity and the rate of metabolism of the substrate are increased. Enzyme induction is not an immediate process but occurs over several days to weeks. Induction will decrease the amount of circulating parent drug and may cause a decline in or loss of therapeutic efficacy. Consider a patient, stabilized on olanzapine (a CYP1A2 substrate), who begins to smoke (a CYP1A2 inducer). Smoking will increase olanzapine metabolism, and unless drug dosage is suitably adjusted, olanzapine levels will decrease and psychotic symptoms may worsen. If the interacting drug is a metabolic *inhibitor* (e.g., fluvoxamine or ciprofloxacin, both potent CYP1A2 inhibitors), drug metabolism mediated through the inhibited CYP isozyme will be impaired. The resulting rise in substrate drug levels may increase drug toxicity and prolong the pharmacological effect. Ciprofloxacin added to clozapine (a CYP1A2 substrate) has resulted in significant increases in clozapine levels, resulting in syncope and even death

(Meyer et al. 2016). Although enzyme inhibition is a rapid process, substrate drug levels respond more slowly, taking five half-lives to restabilize.

Not all combinations of substrate drug and interacting drug will result in clinically significant drug-drug interactions. For a drug eliminated by several mechanisms, including multiple CYP enzymes or non-CYP routes (e.g., UGTs, renal elimination), the inhibition of a single CYP isozyme serves only to divert elimination to other pathways, with little change in overall elimination rate. For these interactions to be clinically relevant, a critical substrate drug must have a narrow therapeutic index and one primary CYP isozyme mediating its metabolism. For example, aripiprazole is metabolized primarily by the CYP3A4 and CYP2D6 isozymes. The addition of a potent CYP3A4 inhibitor, such as voriconazole or ritonavir, will inhibit aripiprazole's metabolism. Without a compensatory reduction in aripiprazole dose, aripiprazole levels will rise and toxicity may result. Aripiprazole, brexpiprazole, and iloperidone require dosage adjustment with concurrent CYP2D6 or CYP3A4 inhibitors. When prescribing in a polypharmacy environment, the clinician should minimize use of medications that significantly inhibit or induce CYP enzymes and should prefer those that are eliminated by multiple pathways and have a wide safety margin. Attention to drug interactions should occur in the polypharmacy environment of HIV because many protease inhibitors (e.g., ritonavir, darunavir) are potent CYP3A4 inducers. Drugs that are significant CYP isozyme inhibitors, inducers, and critical substrates are listed in Appendixes A and B to this chapter.

The abundance of clinically significant pharmacokinetic interactions involving monoamine oxidase inhibitors (MAOIs), especially inhibitors of MAO-A, has limited their therapeutic use. Many of these interactions involve foods containing high levels of tyramine (e.g., pickled herring, aged cheeses), a pressor amine metabolized by gut MAO-A. Several drugs, including some sympathomimetics and triptan antimigraine medications (e.g., sumatriptan, rizatriptan), are also metabolized by MAO (Eadie 2001). The average population can tolerate 800–2,000 mg of tyramine per meal; for those taking an MAOI such as tranylcypromine, 35 mg of tyramine has been shown to increase systolic blood pressure by 30 mm Hg. Therefore, from a safety standpoint, 6 mg of tyramine is considered the threshold for mild symptoms, and 25 mg of tyramine per meal is the threshold for severe reactions (Shulman and Walker 1999; Ulrich et al. 2017). Newer low-tyramine diets are thought to be less restrictive than previously recommended (Gardner et al. 1996). Drugs and foods associated with MAO-related interactions are listed in Appendixes A and B to this chapter. Normal servings of bottled beer and chocolate are thought to be less likely to have a high tyramine content (Gardner et al. 1996; Ricken et al. 2017). Cheeses differ in their tyramine content, and part-skim mozzarella cheese has significantly less tyramine (0.5 mg/serving) than cheddar cheese stored in the refrigerator for 7 days (~<10 mg/serving) (Shulman and Walker 1999). Linezolid and tedizolid are antibiotics with reversible, non-selective MAOI properties and carry a potential risk for serotonin syndrome if combined with serotonergic antidepressants or methadone (Douros et al. 2015; Flanagan et al. 2013; Gatti et al. 2021; Woytowish and Maynor 2013). The antineoplastic agent procarbazine is also an MAOI. Concomitant use of VMAT-2 (vesicular monoamine transporter 2) inhibitors (e.g., valbenazine, deutetrabenazine) with MAOIs should be avoided.

Although the role of Phase II UGT-mediated conjugation is being increasingly recognized in clinical pharmacology, surprisingly few clinically significant drug interactions are known to involve UGTs. The clinically significant interaction between valproate and lamotrigine is considered a consequence of valproate inhibition of lamotrigine glucuronidation. In patients taking lamotrigine, the addition of valproate resulted in a dose-dependent increase in systemic exposure (AUC) to lamotrigine ranging from 84% at a valproate dosage of 200 mg/day to 160% at 1,000 mg/day. Correspondingly, lamotrigine half-life increased from prevalproate values 2.5-fold in the presence of 1,000 mg/day of valproate (Morris et al. 2000). In human participants, the addition of the UGT inducer rifampicin (600 mg/day) produced the opposite effect on lamotrigine levels. In comparison to the pre-rifampicin condition, lamotrigine half-life declined by more than 40%, accompanied by a similar decrease in AUC (Ebert et al. 2000). Another potentially UGT-mediated interaction is between carbapenem antibiotics and valproate, but this interaction is complex and not fully understood. Seizures have occurred when a carbapenem antibiotic was added in stable patients taking valproate because of reduced plasma valproate levels to subtherapeutic concentrations. Increasing valproate does not compensate for this interaction; thus, this combination should be avoided (Al-Quteimat and Laila 2020).

Only those drugs dependent on UGT biotransformation for their elimination and having no other significant metabolic or excretory routes are candidates for clinically important UGT-based drug interactions. Most drugs undergoing conjugation by UGTs are also substrates for Phase I metabolism and other metabolic and excretory processes and therefore are little affected by the addition of UGT inhibitors or inducers. Some UGT substrates, inducers, and inhibitors are listed in Appendixes A and B to this chapter.

Metabolic drug interactions are most likely to occur in three situations: when an interacting drug (inhibitor or inducer) is added to an existing critical substrate drug, when an interacting drug is withdrawn from a dosing regimen containing a substrate drug, and when a substrate drug is added to an existing regimen containing an interacting drug. The addition of an interacting drug to a medication regimen containing a substrate drug at steady-state levels will dramatically alter substrate drug levels, possibly resulting in toxicity (addition of an inhibitor) or loss of therapeutic effect (addition of an inducer).

A much-overlooked interaction involves the withdrawal of an interacting medication from a regimen that includes a critical substrate drug. Previously, the substrate drug dosage will have been titrated, in the presence of the interacting drug, to optimize therapeutic effect and minimize adverse effects. Withdrawal of an enzyme inhibitor will allow metabolism to return (increase) to normal levels. This increased metabolism of the substrate drug will lower its levels and decrease therapeutic effect. In contrast, removal of an enzyme inducer will result in an increase in substrate drug levels and drug toxicity as metabolism of the drug decreases to the normal rate over a period of several days to weeks. For example, discontinuation of carbamazepine can result in increased sedation with diazepam if the diazepam dose is not subsequently reduced. Stopping a medication that is an inducer does not quickly result in a return to baseline CYP function. This outcome is dependent on several factors such as half-life and clearance of the medication itself and natural degradation of the enzymes. As an example, 2 weeks after the discontinuation of rifampin (a CYP inducer), midazolam levels were at only 80% of baseline, and they continued to increase over a total of 4 weeks. The half-life of rifampin is approximately 3 hours and thus would be expected to be completely cleared in less than 1 day after discontinuing the medication (Reitman et al. 2011). Deinduction after carbamazepine discontinuation may take up to 2 weeks, despite a half-life of close to 15 hours with repeated doses (Punyawudho et al. 2009). Lastly, the CYP1A2 inducing effects of cigarettes may persist for days into inpatient admission following smoking cessation (Faber and Fuhr 2004; Hiemke et al. 2018).

The addition of a critical substrate drug to an established drug regimen containing an interacting drug can result in a clinically significant interaction if the substrate is dosed according to established guidelines. Dosing guidelines do not account for the presence of a metabolic inhibitor or inducer and thus may lead to substrate concentrations that are toxic or subtherapeutic, respectively.

Metabolic drug interactions can be minimized by avoiding drugs that are known critical substrates or potent inhibitors or inducers. Although avoiding these drugs is not always possible, adverse effects of these metabolic interactions can be reduced by identifying potentially problematic medications, making appropriate dosage adjustments, and monitoring drug levels (when possible).

An appreciation of drug interactions with the P-gp efflux transporter system is now emerging. P-gps influence the distribution and elimination of many clinically important hydrophobic compounds by transporting them out of the brain (P-gps are a major component of the blood-brain barrier), gonads, and other organs and into urine, bile, and the gut. Inhibition of P-gps can lead to drug toxicity as a result of dramatic increases in the oral bioavailability of poorly bioavailable drugs and to increased drug access to the CNS. Itraconazole, a CYP3A4 and P-gp inhibitor, has been shown to increase the bioavailability of paroxetine, a P-gp substrate, in human participants. The addition of itraconazole to an existing paroxetine regimen increased paroxetine AUC 1.5-fold and peak blood levels 1.3-fold in spite of only a 10% increase in half-life (Yasui-Furukori et al. 2007). Other psychotropic drugs transported by P-gp include opioids, risperidone, paliperidone, olanzapine, nortriptyline, imipramine, citalopram, escitalopram, and fluvoxamine (Moons et al. 2011). Some drug interactions with P-gp are listed in Appendixes A and B to this chapter. Rodent models are exploring the role of verapamil (a P-gp inhibitor) in increasing antidepressant (imipramine and escitalopram) levels in the brain to enhance antidepressant effects (Clarke et al. 2009; O'Brien et al. 2013).

Drug interactions that affect renal drug elimination are clinically significant only if the parent drug or its active metabolite undergoes appreciable renal excretion. By reducing renal blood flow, some drugs, including many NSAIDs, decrease GFR and impair renal elimination. This interaction is often responsible for lithium toxicity. Other drug interactions that increase lithium levels include thiazide diuretics, angiotensin converting enzyme inhibitors, and angiotensin receptor blockers (Finley 2016).

Changes in urine pH can modify the elimination of those compounds whose ratio of ionized to un-ionized forms is dramatically altered across the physiological range of urine pH (4.6–8.2) (i.e., the compound has a pK_a

within this pH range). Common drugs that alkalinize urine include antacids and carbonic anhydrase inhibitor diuretics. Un-ionized forms of drugs undergo greater glomerular resorption, whereas ionized drug forms have less resorption and greater urinary excretion. For a basic drug, such as amphetamine, alkalinization of urine increases the un-ionized fraction, enhancing resorption and prolonging activity. Other basic drugs, such as amitriptyline, imipramine, meperidine, methadone (Nilsson et al. 1982), and memantine (Freudenthaler et al. 1998), may be similarly affected.

Pharmacodynamic Drug Interactions

Pharmacodynamic interactions occur when drugs with similar or opposing effects are combined. The nature of the interaction relates to the addition or antagonism of the pharmacological and toxic effects of each drug. Generally, pharmacodynamic interactions are most apparent in individuals who have compromised physiological function, such as cardiovascular disease, or in older adults.

For example, drugs with anticholinergic activity cause a degree of cognitive impairment or delirium, an effect that is exacerbated when several anticholinergic agents are combined, referred to as *anticholinergic drug burden* (Egberts et al. 2021; Salahudeen et al. 2015). Several scales are available to help quantify this anticholinergic burden and associated risk (Egberts et al. 2021; Lavrador et al. 2021; Salahudeen et al. 2015). Unfortunately, anticholinergic activity is an underrecognized property of many common drugs, such as diphenhydramine, hydroxyzine, loperamide, olanzapine, and paroxetine (for a listing, see American Geriatrics Society 2019 Beers Criteria® Update Expert Panel 2019; Durán et al. 2013). This additive interaction is most disruptive in older adults or patients with cognitive impairment, such as those with Alzheimer's disease, and forms the basis for many cases of delirium.

Often, additive pharmacodynamic interactions are used therapeutically to enhance a drug response—this is the use of adjunctive medications. Antagonistic pharmacodynamic interactions are sometimes used deliberately to diminish a particular adverse effect. Unintentional antagonistic interactions may be countertherapeutic, as with the reduction of asthma control in a patient who has successfully used a β-agonist inhaler and is recently prescribed a β-blocker, or the negation of cognitive benefit from a cholinesterase inhibitor when taken with an anticholinergic drug such as diphenhydramine or oxybutynin. Knowledge of a drug's therapeutic and adverse effects is essential to avoid unwanted pharmacodynamic drug interactions, such as additive or synergistic toxicities, or countertherapeutic effects.

Drug Interactions of Psychotropic Agents

Pharmacodynamic interactions between psychoactive drugs and drugs used to treat medical disorders are common and are discussed in the respective medical disorder chapters in this manual. Psychotropic drugs frequently contribute to or precipitate pharmacodynamic interactions. Excessive sedation or delirium frequently results from the combination of psychotropic drugs with sedating properties. Psychotropic polypharmacy can also precipitate severe adverse reactions, such as serotonin syndrome or cardiac arrhythmias due to prolonged QT interval (see Chapter 2, "Severe Drug Reactions").

Any psychotropic drug can be the recipient of a pharmacokinetic interaction, but only a few psychotropic drugs commonly precipitate a pharmacokinetic interaction. Fluoxetine, paroxetine, fluvoxamine, duloxetine, bupropion, modafinil, armodafinil, and atomoxetine significantly inhibit one or more CYP isozymes. The MAOIs block metabolism of some sympathomimetics and several triptan antimigraine medications. The mood stabilizer anticonvulsants carbamazepine and valproate induce one or more CYP isozymes (see Appendix A to this chapter). Valproate also inhibits Phase II metabolism via UGT. Preference should be given to psychotropic medications with little ability to precipitate a pharmacokinetic interaction (Table 1–4), especially when used in a polypharmacy situation. However, even though many psychotropic agents do not precipitate pharmacokinetic interactions, they can still be the subject of a pharmacokinetic interaction. For example, neither ziprasidone nor aripiprazole affects the pharmacokinetics of other drugs, but carbamazepine reduces the AUC of ziprasidone by 35% and aripiprazole by 70%.

Key Points

- Maintaining drug levels within the therapeutic range maximizes beneficial effects and minimizes adverse effects. Drug pharmacokinetics must be considered when developing a dosage regimen to achieve drug levels within this therapeutic range.

Table 1–4.   Psychotropic drugs that cause few or no known pharmacokinetic interactions

Antidepressants

SSRIs and SNRIs

   Citalopram

   Desvenlafaxine

   Escitalopram

   Levomilnacipran

   Sertraline (CYP2D6 inhibition at >200 mg/day)

   Venlafaxine

TCAs

   Amitriptyline

   Clomipramine (slight CYP2D6 inhibition)

   Desipramine (slight CYP2D6 inhibition)

   Doxepin

   Imipramine

   Maprotiline

   Nortriptyline

   Protriptyline

   Trimipramine

Mixed serotonin agents

   Trazodone

   Vilazodone

   Vortioxetine

Novel action agents

   Amoxapine

   Mirtazapine

Table 1–4.　Psychotropic drugs that cause few or no known pharmacokinetic interactions *(continued)*

Antipsychotics

All antipsychotics

Agents for drug-induced extrapyramidal symptoms

Benztropine

Biperiden

Ethopropazine

Trihexyphenidyl

Anxiolytics and sedative-hypnotics

All benzodiazepines

Nonbenzodiazepines

　Buspirone

　Eszopiclone

　Zaleplon

　Zolpidem

　Zopiclone

Cognitive enhancers

Donepezil

Galantamine

Memantine

Rivastigmine

Opioid analgesics

All opioid analgesics

Psychostimulants

Amphetamine

Dextroamphetamine

Lisdexamfetamine

Table 1–4.   Psychotropic drugs that cause few or no known pharmacokinetic interactions *(continued)*

Psychostimulants *(continued)*

Methamphetamine

Methylphenidate

Note.   CYP2D6=cytochrome P450 2D6 isoenzyme; SNRIs=serotonin-norepinephrine reuptake inhibitors; SSRIs=selective serotonin reuptake inhibitors; TCAs=tricyclic antidepressants.

- When the clinician is prescribing in a polypharmacy environment, it is best to minimize use of medications that significantly inhibit or induce cytochrome P450 enzymes and to prefer those eliminated by multiple pathways and with a wide safety margin.

- Over-the-counter drugs, herbal and complementary medicines, and certain foods can all affect drug pharmacokinetics.

- For a drug administered on an acute basis, the magnitude of the therapeutic effect is a function of peak drug levels, which are determined mainly by dose and the rate of drug absorption.

- For a drug administered chronically, the therapeutic effect is a function of the extent of absorption, not the speed of absorption. Rapid absorption is likely to cause transient, concentration-dependent adverse effects.

- For patients with medical conditions that alter levels of plasma proteins, therapeutic drug monitoring should use methods selective for free (unbound) drug, particularly for drugs that are highly bound to proteins (e.g., tricyclic antidepressants, valproate) and have potential for toxicity.

- Drug-drug interaction databases should be used to determine the clinical significance of interactions when the clinician is prescribing in a polypharmacy environment.

References

Al-Quteimat O, Laila A: Valproate interaction with carbapenems: review and recommendations. Hosp Pharm 55(3):181–187, 2020 32508355

American Geriatrics Society 2019 Beers Criteria® Update Expert Panel: American Geriatrics Society 2019 updated Beers criteria® for potentially inappropriate medication use in older adults. J Am Geriatr Soc 67(4):674–694, 2019 30693946

Armstrong SC, Cozza KL: Triptans. Psychosomatics 43(6):502–504, 2002 12444236

Balayssac D, Authier N, Cayre A, et al: Does inhibition of P-glycoprotein lead to drug-drug interactions? Toxicol Lett 156(3):319–329, 2005 15763631

Belle DJ, Singh H: Genetic factors in drug metabolism. Am Fam Physician 77(11):1553–1560, 2008 18581835

Benet LZ, Hoener BA: Changes in plasma protein binding have little clinical relevance. Clin Pharmacol Ther 71(3):115–121, 2002 11907485

Charlier B, Coglianese A, De Rosa F, et al: The effect of plasma protein binding on the therapeutic monitoring of antiseizure medications. Pharmaceutics 13(8):1208, 2021 34452168

Clarke G, O'Mahony SM, Cryan JF, et al: Verapamil in treatment resistant depression: a role for the P-glycoprotein transporter? Hum Psychopharmacol 24(3):217–223, 2009 19212940

Cozza KL, Armstrong SC, Oesterheld JR: Concise Guide to Drug Interaction Principles for Medical Practice: Cytochrome P450s, UGTs, P-Glycoproteins. Washington, DC, American Psychiatric Publishing, 2003

Dasgupta A: Usefulness of monitoring free (unbound) concentrations of therapeutic drugs in patient management. Clin Chim Acta 377(1–2):1–13, 2007 17026974

Debinski HS, Lee CS, Danks JA, et al: Localization of uridine 5'-diphosphate-glucuronosyltransferase in human liver injury. Gastroenterology 108(5):1464–1469, 1995 7729639

di Masi A, Trezza V, Leboffe L, et al: Human plasma lipocalins and serum albumin: plasma alternative carriers? J Control Release 228:191–205, 2016 26951925

Douros A, Grabowski K, Stahlmann R: Drug-drug interactions and safety of linezolid, tedizolid, and other oxazolidinones. Expert Opin Drug Metab Toxicol 11(12):1849–1859, 2015 26457865

Durán CE, Azermai M, Vander Stichele RH: Systematic review of anticholinergic risk scales in older adults. Eur J Clin Pharmacol 69(7):1485–1496, 2013 23529548

Eadie MJ: Clinically significant drug interactions with agents specific for migraine attacks. CNS Drugs 15(2):105–118, 2001 11460889

Ebert U, Thong NQ, Oertel R, et al: Effects of rifampicin and cimetidine on pharmacokinetics and pharmacodynamics of lamotrigine in healthy subjects. Eur J Clin Pharmacol 56(4):299–304, 2000 10954343

Egberts A, Moreno-Gonzalez R, Alan H, et al: Anticholinergic drug burden and delirium: a systematic review. J Am Med Dir Assoc 22(1):65.e4–73.e4, 2021 32703688

Eli Lilly: Strattera (atomoxetine) prescribing information. April 6, 2015. Available at: https://pi.lilly.com/us/strattera-pi.pdf. Accessed April 11, 2016.

English BA, Dortch M, Ereshefsky L, et al: Clinically significant psychotropic drug-drug interactions in the primary care setting. Curr Psychiatry Rep 14(4):376–390, 2012 22707017

Faber MS, Fuhr U: Time response of cytochrome P450 1A2 activity on cessation of heavy smoking. Clin Pharmacol Ther 76(2):178–184, 2004 15289794

Fiedorowicz JG, Swartz KL: The role of monoamine oxidase inhibitors in current psychiatric practice. J Psychiatr Pract 10(4):239–248, 2004 15552546

Finley PR: Drug interactions with lithium: an update. Clin Pharmacokinet 55(8):925–941, 2016 26936045

Fisher MB, Paine MF, Strelevitz TJ, et al: The role of hepatic and extrahepatic UDP-glucuronosyltransferases in human drug metabolism. Drug Metab Rev 33(3–4):273–297, 2001 11768770

Flanagan S, Bartizal K, Minassian SL, et al: In vitro, in vivo, and clinical studies of tedizolid to assess the potential for peripheral or central monoamine oxidase interactions. Antimicrob Agents Chemother 57(7):3060–3066, 2013 23612197

Freudenthaler S, Meineke I, Schreeb KH, et al: Influence of urine pH and urinary flow on the renal excretion of memantine. Br J Clin Pharmacol 46(6):541–546, 1998 9862242

Gardner DM, Shulman KI, Walker SE, et al: The making of a user friendly MAOI diet. J Clin Psychiatry 57(3):99–104, 1996 8617704

Gatti M, Raschi E, De Ponti F: Serotonin syndrome by drug interactions with linezolid: clues from pharmacovigilance-pharmacokinetic/pharmacodynamic analysis. Eur J Clin Pharmacol 77(2):233–239, 2021 32901348

Gillman PK: Monoamine oxidase inhibitors, opioid analgesics and serotonin toxicity. Br J Anaesth 95(4):434–441, 2005 16051647

Goode DL, Newton DW, Ueda CT, et al: Effect of antacid on the bioavailability of lithium carbonate. Clin Pharm 3(3):284–287, 1984 6428800

Greenblatt DJ, von Moltke LL: Interaction of warfarin with drugs, natural substances, and foods. J Clin Pharmacol 45(2):127–132, 2005 15647404

Guédon-Moreau L, Ducrocq D, Duc MF, et al: Absolute contraindications in relation to potential drug interactions in outpatient prescriptions: analysis of the first five million prescriptions in 1999. Eur J Clin Pharmacol 59(8–9):689–695, 2003 14557905

Hicks JK, Bishop JR, Sangkuhl K, et al: Clinical Pharmacogenetics Implementation Consortium (CPIC) guideline for CYP2D6 and CYP2C19 genotypes and dosing of selective serotonin reuptake inhibitors. Clin Pharmacol Ther 98(2):127–134, 2015 25974703

Hicks JK, Sangkuhl K, Swen JJ, et al: Clinical Pharmacogenetics Implementation Consortium guideline (CPIC) for CYP2D6 and CYP2C19 genotypes and dosing of tricyclic antidepressants: 2016 update. Clin Pharmacol Ther 102(1):37–44, 2017 27997040

Hiemke C, Bergemann N, Clement HW, et al: Consensus guidelines for therapeutic drug monitoring in neuropsychopharmacology: update 2017. Pharmacopsychiatry 51(1–02):9–62, 2018 28910830

Israili ZH, Dayton PG: Human alpha-1-glycoprotein and its interactions with drugs. Drug Metab Rev 33(2):161–235, 2001 11495502

Kharasch ED, Hoffer C, Altuntas TG, et al: Quinidine as a probe for the role of p-glycoprotein in the intestinal absorption and clinical effects of fentanyl. J Clin Pharmacol 44(3):224–233, 2004 14973303

Kiang TK, Ensom MH, Chang TK: UDP-glucuronosyltransferases and clinical drug-drug interactions. Pharmacol Ther 106(1):97–132, 2005 15781124

Knadler MP, Lobo E, Chappell J, et al: Duloxetine: clinical pharmacokinetics and drug interactions. Clin Pharmacokinet 50(5):281–294, 2011 21366359

Lavrador M, Castel-Branco MM, Cabral AC, et al: Association between anticholinergic burden and anticholinergic adverse outcomes in the elderly: pharmacological basis of their predictive value for adverse outcomes. Pharmacol Res 163:105306, 2021 33248197

Levey AS, Coresh J, Greene T, et al: Using standardized serum creatinine values in the Modification of Diet in Renal Disease Study equation for estimating glomerular filtration rate. Ann Intern Med 145(4):247–254, 2006 16908915

Levey AS, Inker LA, Coresh J: GFR estimation: from physiology to public health. Am J Kidney Dis 63(5):820–834, 2014 24485147

Lexicomp Inc: Lexicomp online. 2015. Available at: https://online.lexi.com/lco/action/home. Accessed April 11, 2016.

Lowenstein M, Bamgbose O, Gleason N, et al: Psychiatric consultation at your fingertips: descriptive analysis of electronic consultation from primary care to psychiatry. J Med Internet Res 19(8):e279, 2017 28778852

Madan A, Donovan PJ, Risetto T, et al: Monitoring for valproate and phenytoin toxicity in hypoalbuminaemia: a retrospective cohort study. Br J Clin Pharmacol 87(11):4341–4353, 2021 33835518

McEvoy G (ed): American Hospital Formulary Service (AHFS) Drug Information 2015. Bethesda, MD, American Society of Health-System Pharmacists, 2015

Meech R, Hu DG, McKinnon RA, et al: The UDP-glycosyltransferase (UGT) superfamily: new members, new functions, and novel paradigms. Physiol Rev 99(2):1153–1222, 2019 30724669

Merrick C, Madden CA, Capurso NA: A case of blunted orally disintegrating olanzapine effect due to coadministered psyllium. J Clin Psychiatry 82(2):20cr13633, 2021 33988934

Meyer JM, Proctor G, Cummings MA, et al: Ciprofloxacin and clozapine: a potentially fatal but underappreciated interaction. Case Rep Psychiatry 2016:5606098, 2016 27872784

Michalets EL: Update: clinically significant cytochrome P-450 drug interactions. Pharmacotherapy 18(1):84–112, 1998 9469685

Molenaar-Kuijsten L, Van Balen DEM, Beijnen JH, et al: A review of CYP3A drug-drug interaction studies: practical guidelines for patients using targeted oral anticancer drugs. Front Pharmacol 12:670862, 2021 34526892

Moons T, de Roo M, Claes S, et al: Relationship between P-glycoprotein and second-generation antipsychotics. Pharmacogenomics 12(8):1193–1211, 2011 21843066

Morris RG, Black AB, Lam E, et al: Clinical study of lamotrigine and valproic acid in patients with epilepsy: using a drug interaction to advantage? Ther Drug Monit 22(6):656–660, 2000 11128232

Nadkarni A, Oldham M, Howard M, et al: Detrimental effects of divalproex on warfarin therapy following mechanical valve replacement. J Card Surg 26(5):492–494, 2011 21859435

National Institute of Diabetes and Digestive and Kidney Diseases: National Institutes of Health CKD and drug dosing: information for providers. March 2021. Available at: www.niddk.nih.gov/research-funding/research-programs/kidney-clinical-research-epidemiology/laboratory/ckd-drug-dosing-providers#limitations. Accessed January 14, 2022.

National Library of Medicine: DailyMed. Available at: https://dailymed.nlm.nih.gov/dailymed. Accessed December 1, 2021.

Neuvonen PJ, Kivistö KT: Enhancement of drug absorption by antacids: an unrecognised drug interaction. Clin Pharmacokinet 27(2):120–128, 1994 7955775

Nilsson MI, Widerlöv E, Meresaar U, et al: Effect of urinary pH on the disposition of methadone in man. Eur J Clin Pharmacol 22(4):337–342, 1982 6286317

O'Brien FE, O'Connor RM, Clarke G, et al: P-glycoprotein inhibition increases the brain distribution and antidepressant-like activity of escitalopram in rodents. Neuropsychopharmacology 38(11):2209–2219, 2013 23670590

Pal D, Mitra AK: MDR- and CYP3A4-mediated drug-drug interactions. J Neuroimmune Pharmacol 1(3):323–339, 2006 18040809

Papadakis MA, Arieff AI: Unpredictability of clinical evaluation of renal function in cirrhosis: prospective study. Am J Med 82(5):945–952, 1987 3578363

Patsalos PN, Spencer EP, Berry DJ: Therapeutic drug monitoring of antiepileptic drugs in epilepsy: a 2018 update. Ther Drug Monit 40(5):526–548, 2018 29957667

Pezzia C, Pugh JA, Lanham HJ, et al: Psychiatric consultation requests by inpatient medical teams: an observational study. BMC Health Serv Res 18(1):336, 2018 29739414

Pichette V, Leblond FA: Drug metabolism in chronic renal failure. Curr Drug Metab 4(2):91–103, 2003 12678690

Procyshyn RM, Bezchlibnyk-Butler KZ, Jeffries JJ: Clinical Handbook of Psychotropic Drugs, 21st Revised Edition. Ashland, OH, Hogrefe, 2015

Punyawudho B, Cloyd JC, Leppik IE, et al: Characterization of the time course of carbamazepine deinduction by an enzyme turnover model. Clin Pharmacokinet 48(5):313–320, 2009 19566114

Reitman ML, Chu X, Cai X, et al: Rifampin's acute inhibitory and chronic inductive drug interactions: experimental and model-based approaches to drug-drug interaction trial design. Clin Pharmacol Ther 89(2):234–242, 2011 21191377

Ricken R, Ulrich S, Schlattmann P, et al: Tranylcypromine in mind (part II): review of clinical pharmacology and meta-analysis of controlled studies in depression. Eur Neuropsychopharmacol 27(8):714–731, 2017 28579071

Rolan PE: Plasma protein binding displacement interactions—why are they still regarded as clinically important? Br J Clin Pharmacol 37(2):125–128, 1994 8186058

Salahudeen MS, Duffull SB, Nishtala PS: Anticholinergic burden quantified by anticholinergic risk scales and adverse outcomes in older people: a systematic review. BMC Geriatr 15:31, 2015 25879993

Shulman KI, Walker SE: Refining the MAOI diet: tyramine content of pizzas and soy products. J Clin Psychiatry 60(3):191–193, 1999 10192596

Sokoll LJ, Russell RM, Sadowski JA, et al: Establishment of creatinine clearance reference values for older women. Clin Chem 40(12):2276–2281, 1994 7988015

Solomon HV, Cates KW, Li KJ: Does obtaining CYP2D6 and CYP2C19 pharmacogenetic testing predict antidepressant response or adverse drug reactions? Psychiatry Res 271:604–613, 2019 30554109

Spray JW, Willett K, Chase D, et al: Dosage adjustment for hepatic dysfunction based on Child-Pugh scores. Am J Health Syst Pharm 64(7):690, 692–693, 2007 17384352

Thummel KE, Shen DD, Isoherranen N, et al: Appendix II, Design and optimization of dosage regimens: pharmacokinetic data, in Goodman and Gilman's The Pharmacological Basis of Therapeutics, 13th Edition. Edited by Shananhan JF, Lebowitz H. New York, McGraw Hill, 2018

Toutoungi M, Schulz P, Widmer J, et al: Probable interaction entre le psyllium et le lithium [Probable interaction of psyllium and lithium]. Therapie 45(4):358–360, 1990 2399524

Tsanaclis LM, Allen J, Perucca E, et al: Effect of valproate on free plasma phenytoin concentrations. Br J Clin Pharmacol 18(1):17–20, 1984 6430316

Ulldemolins M, Roberts JA, Rello J, et al: The effects of hypoalbuminaemia on optimizing antibacterial dosing in critically ill patients. Clin Pharmacokinet 50(2):99–110, 2011 21142293

Ulrich S, Ricken R, Adli M: Tranylcypromine in mind (part I): review of pharmacology. Eur Neuropsychopharmacol 27(8):697–713, 2017 28655495

U.S. Food and Drug Administration: Cytochrome P450 2C19. April 6, 2016. Available at: www.fda.gov/drugs/drug-interactions-labeling/cytochrome-p450-2c19. Accessed April 1, 2022.

U.S. Food and Drug Administration: FDA issues warning letter to genomics lab for illegally marketing genetic test that claims to predict patients' responses to specific medications (press release). April 4, 2019. Available at: https://www.fda.gov/news-events/press-announcements/fda-issues-warning-letter-genomics-lab-illegally-marketing-genetic-test-claims-predict-patients. Accessed April 1, 2023.

USP DI Editorial Board (ed): United States Pharmacopeia Dispensing Information, Volume 1: Drug Information for the Health Care Professional, 27th Edition. Greenwood Village, CO, Thomson Micromedex, 2007

Woytowish MR, Maynor LM: Clinical relevance of linezolid-associated serotonin toxicity. Ann Pharmacother 47(3):388–397, 2013 23424229

Yagi T, Naito T, Mino Y, et al: Impact of concomitant antacid administration on gabapentin plasma exposure and oral bioavailability in healthy adult subjects. Drug Metab Pharmacokinet 27(2):248–254, 2012 22240839

Yasui-Furukori N, Saito M, Niioka T, et al: Effect of itraconazole on pharmacokinetics of paroxetine: the role of gut transporters. Ther Drug Monit 29(1):45–48, 2007 17304149

Yoshida H, Takahashi M, Honda M, et al: Co-administration of magnesium oxide reduces the serum concentration of hydrophobic basic drugs in patients treated with antipsychotic drugs. Biol Pharm Bull 42(6):1025–1029, 2019 31155577

Zanger UM, Schwab M: Cytochrome P450 enzymes in drug metabolism: regulation of gene expression, enzyme activities, and impact of genetic variation. Pharmacol Ther 138(1):103–141, 2013 23333322

Zanger UM, Raimundo S, Eichelbaum M: Cytochrome P450 2D6: overview and update on pharmacology, genetics, biochemistry. Naunyn Schmiedebergs Arch Pharmacol 369(1):23–37, 2004 14618296

Zeier Z, Carpenter LL, Kalin NH, et al: Clinical implementation of pharmacogenetic decision support tools for antidepressant drug prescribing. Am J Psychiatry 175(9):873–886, 2018 29690793

Appendix A

Psychotropic Drugs With Clinically Significant
Pharmacokinetic Interactions

Drug	Cytochrome P450 isozyme				MAO-A	UGT	P-gp
	1A2	2C[a]	2D6	3A4			
Anticonvulsants and mood stabilizers							
Carbamazepine	I	I		S, I		S, I	S
Lamotrigine						S	S
Oxcarbazepine		X		I			
Phenytoin	I	S, I		I		I	S
Valproate		I				S, X	
Antidepressants							
Amitriptyline	S	S	S	S			S, X
Brexanolone		X				S	
Bupropion			X	S			
Citalopram		S					
Clomipramine	S	S	S, X	S			
Desipramine			S, X				X
Desvenlafaxine						S	
Doxepin			S				
Duloxetine	S		S, X				
Escitalopram		S					S
Esketamine[b]		S		S			
Fluoxetine	X	X	S, X	Metabolite S, X			

Drug	Cytochrome P450 isozyme				MAO-A	UGT	P-gp
	1A2	2Cᵃ	2D6	3A4	MAO-A	UGT	P-gp
Antidepressants *(continued)*							
Fluvoxamine	S, X	X		X			S
Gepirone				S			
Imipramine	S	S	S	S			S, X
Levomilnacipran				S			
Maprotiline			S				X
Milnacipran							
Mirtazapine			S	S			
Moclobemide		S	X		X		
Nefazodone				S, X			
Nortriptyline			S				S
Paroxetine			S, X				S, X
Phenelzine					X		
Sertraline							X
Tranylcypromine		X			X		
Trazodone			S	S			I
Trimipramine			S				
Venlafaxine			S	S			S
Vilazodone				S			
Vortioxetine			S	S			
Antiparkinsonian agents							
Rasagiline	S						
Selegiline					X		
Antipsychotics							
Aripiprazole			S	S			S

Drug	Cytochrome P450 isozyme				MAO-A	UGT	P-gp
	1A2	2C[a]	2D6	3A4			
Antipsychotics *(continued)*							
Asenapine	S					S	
Brexpiprazole			S	S			
Cariprazine			S	S			
Chlorpromazine	S		S				X
Clozapine	S		S	S			
Fluphenazine			S				X
Haloperidol	S		S, X				X
Iloperidone			S	S			
Lumateperone	S	S		S		S	
Lurasidone				S			
Molindone			S				
Olanzapine	S		S			S	S
Perphenazine			S				
Pimavanserin				S			
Pimozide				S			X
Quetiapine				S			S
Risperidone			S				S, X
Thioridazine	S	S	S				
Trifluoperazine							X
Ziprasidone				S			
Anxiolytics and sedative-hypnotics							
Alprazolam				S			
Bromazepam				S			
Buspirone				S			

Drug	Cytochrome P450 isozyme				MAO-A	UGT	P-gp
	1A2	2C[a]	2D6	3A4			
Anxiolytics and sedative-hypnotics *(continued)*							
Clonazepam				S			
Diazepam		S		S			
Lemborexant				S			
Lorazepam						S	
Midazolam				S			X
Oxazepam						S	
Phenobarbital	I	I		I			
Ramelteon	S						
Suvorexant				S			
Tasimelteon	S						
Temazepam						S	
Triazolam				S			
β-Blockers							
Metoprolol			S				
Propranolol	S	S	S, X				X
Opioids							
Alfentanil				S			
Buprenorphine				S			
Codeine			S	S		S	
Fentanyl				S			X
Hydrocodone			S				
Meperidine			S				
Methadone			S	S			X

Drug	Cytochrome P450 isozyme				MAO-A	UGT	P-gp
	1A2	2C[a]	2D6	3A4			
Opioids *(continued)*							
Morphine						S	S
Oxycodone			S				
Tramadol			S				
Opioid antagonists							
Samidorphan		S		S			
Psychostimulants							
Armodafinil	I	X		S, I			
Atomoxetine			S, X				
Modafinil	I	X		S, I			
Viloxazine	X		S			S	
VMAT-2 inhibitors							
Deutetrabenazine			S				
Tetrabenazine			S				
Valbenazine			S	S	S		

Note.   Pharmacokinetic drug interactions: I = inducer; S = substrate; X = inhibitor. Only significant interactions are listed. MAO-A = monoamine oxidase A; P-gp = P-glycoprotein efflux transporter; UGT = uridine 5′-diphosphate glucuronosyltransferase; VMAT-2 = vesicular monoamine transporter 2.

[a]Combined properties on 2C8/9/10 and 2C19 cytochrome P450 isozymes.
[b]Esketamine is also a CYP2B6 substrate.

Source.   Compiled in part from Armstrong and Cozza 2002; Balayssac et al. 2005; Cozza et al. 2003; Eli Lilly 2015; English et al. 2012; Fiedorowicz and Swartz 2004; Flanagan et al. 2013; Gillman 2005; Guédon-Moreau et al. 2003; Hiemke et al. 2018; Kiang et al. 2005; Lexicomp Inc 2015; McEvoy 2015; Michalets 1998; Molenaar-Kuijsten et al. 2021; National Library of Medicine 2021; Pal and Mitra 2006; Procyshyn et al. 2015; Thummel et al. 2018; U.S. Food and Drug Administration 2019.

Appendix B

Select List of Medications, Foods, and Herbals
With Clinically Significant Pharmacokinetic Interactions

Drug	Cytochrome P450 isozyme						
	1A2	2C[a]	2D6	3A4	MAO-A	UGT	P-gp
Antiarrhythmics							
Amiodarone	X	S, X	X	S, X			X
Antifungals							
Fluconazole		X		X			
Itraconazole				X			X
Ketoconazole	X			S, X			X
Posaconazole				X		S	S
Antineoplastics							
Cobimetinib				S			
Everolimus				S			S
Procarbazine					X		
Antibiotics							
Ciprofloxacin	X			X			S
Clarithromycin				X			X
Erythromycin				X			X
Linezolid					X		
Rifabutin				I			
Rifampin (rifampicin)	I	I		S, I		I	S, I
Sulfamethoxazole-trimethoprim		X					
Tedizolid					X		

Drug	Cytochrome P450 isozyme				MAO-A	UGT	P-gp
	1A2	2C[a]	2D6	3A4			
Antimigraine drugs							
Almotriptan				S	S		
Rizatriptan					S		
Sumatriptan					S		
Zolmitriptan	S				S		
Antiretrovirals							
Atazanavir		X		S, X		X	X
Cobicistat				S, X			
Delavirdine		X		S, X			
Etravirine		S, X		S, I			X
Indinavir				S, X			S
Nelfinavir				S, X			S, X
Ritonavir	I	X	X	S, X			S, X
Saquinavir				S, X			S, X
Histamine H$_2$-receptor antagonists							
Cimetidine	X	X	X	X			S
Foods, substances, and herbal medicines							
Caffeine	S			S			
Cannabinoids		S		S, X			
Cruciferous vegetables[b]	I						
Grapefruit juice				X			X
Smoking (e.g., tobacco)	I				S		

Drug	Cytochrome P450 isozyme				MAO-A	UGT	P-gp
	1A2	2C[a]	2D6	3A4			
Foods, substances, and herbal medicines *(continued)*							
St. John's wort				I			I
Tyramine-containing foods[c]					S		

Note.   Pharmacokinetic drug interactions: I=inducer; S=substrate; X=inhibitor. Only significant interactions are listed. MAO-A=monoamine oxidase A; P-gp=P-glycoprotein efflux transporter; UGT=uridine 5'-diphosphate glucuronosyltransferase.
[a]Combined properties on 2C8/9/10 and 2C19 cytochrome P450 isozymes.
[b]Cruciferous vegetables include cabbage, cauliflower, broccoli, brussels sprouts, and kale.
[c]Tyramine-containing foods include banana peel, beer (all tap, "self-brew," and nonalcoholic), broad bean pods (not beans), fava beans, aged cheese (tyramine content increases with age), red wines, sauerkraut, sausage (fermented or dry), soy sauce and soy condiments, pickled herring, and concentrated yeast extract (Marmite); 6 mg of tyramine is considered to be the cutoff for safe consumption (Shulman and Walker 1999).

Appendix C

Some Websites With Drug-Drug Interaction Checking Software

Epocrates	www.epocrates.com
Micromedex	www.micromedexsolutions.com
Lexicomp	www.uptodate.com (Wolters Kluwer)
Indiana University School of Medicine, Department of Medicine: Drug Interactions	https://drug-interactions.medicine.iu.edu
University of Liverpool HIV drug interactions	www.hiv-druginteractions.org/checker

Note.   Many of these require a username or subscription to use.

2

Severe Drug Reactions

E. Cabrina Campbell, M.D.

Stanley N. Caroff, M.D.

Stephan C. Mann, M.D.

Robert M. Weinrieb, M.D., FACLP

Rosalind M. Berkowitz, M.D.

Kimberly N. Olson, CRNP

This chapter diverges from other chapters by reviewing not how psychotropic drugs are used in treating patients with medical illnesses but, conversely, how psychotropic drugs occasionally cause medical disorders. Although many important common side effects are associated with psychotropic drugs, we limit the discussion in this chapter to selected rare, severe, and potentially life-threatening drug reactions that occur within therapeutic doses and may require emergency medical treatment. Mirroring the book as a whole, the discussion is organized by specific organ systems. Severe drug-induced dermatological reactions are covered in Chapter 13, "Dermatological Disorders."

In reading this chapter, clinicians should keep in mind that psychotropic drugs, when indicated and used properly, are potentially beneficial for the majority of patients and should not be withheld because of the risk of these rare reactions. Instead, the best defense against adverse reactions consists of careful monitoring of patients, informed by familiarity with adverse signs and symptoms to allow prompt recognition, rapid drug discontinuation or modification, and supportive treatment.

Central Nervous System Drug Reactions

Although psychotropic drugs are developed for therapeutic effects on specific neurotransmitter pathways or neuronal circuits in the brain, severe and life-threatening drug reactions may result from a toxic or idiosyncratic exaggeration of the pharmacological effect on neurotransmitter systems (e.g., neuroleptic malignant syndrome) or from unexpected actions on systemic or other CNS mechanisms that affect brain function (e.g., seizures) (Table 2–1).

Neuroleptic Malignant Syndrome

Neuroleptic malignant syndrome (NMS) has been the subject of numerous reviews (Caroff 2003a; Caroff and Mann 1993; Strawn et al. 2007). Large database studies confirm the incidence of NMS as being in the range of 1:1,000 to 1:5,000 (0.10%–0.02%) patients treated with antipsychotic drugs (Lao et al. 2020; Schneider et al. 2020). Although newer (second- or third-generation) antipsychotics have been implicated, NMS is found in most studies to be at least two to three times more likely to occur with older, high-potency antipsychotics (Anzai et al. 2019; Belvederi Murri et al. 2015; Guinart et al. 2021a; Lao et al. 2020; Schneider et al. 2020; Su et al. 2014). Newer antipsychotics, especially clozapine, may result in milder symptoms with a better prognosis (Belvederi Murri et al. 2015; Nakamura et al. 2012; Picard et al. 2008; Sarkar and Gupta 2017). NMS may also result from treatment with other dopamine-blocking drugs (promethazine, prochlorperazine, metoclopramide) used in medical settings and could be an added risk when dopamine-depleting drugs are used concurrently for tardive dyskinesia (Caroff 2020). Long-acting injectable forms of newer antipsychotics may not be associated with greater risk

Table 2–1. Central nervous system drug reactions

Disorder	Implicated drugs	Risk factors	Signs and symptoms	Diagnostic studies[a]	Management[b]
Neuroleptic malignant syndrome	Dopamine receptor antagonists (antipsychotics, antiemetics)	Dehydration, exhaustion, agitation, catatonia, previous episodes, polypharmacy, dose, and parenteral route	Hyperthermia, rigidity, mental status changes, dysautonomia	Enzyme elevations (CK), ↑WBCs, acidosis, ↓iron, hypoxia	Drug discontinuation Supportive care Specific agents (lorazepam, dopamine agonists, dantrolene, ECT)?
Parkinsonism-hyperpyrexia syndrome	Withdrawal of dopaminergic therapies	Parkinson's disease Deep brain stimulation Reduced CSF HVA levels	Hyperthermia, rigidity, mental status changes, dysautonomia	Enzyme elevations (CK), ↑WBCs	Reinstitution of dopaminergic therapy
Dyskinesia-hyperpyrexia syndrome	Dopaminergic therapy	Parkinson's disease Ambient heat	Severe dyskinesias, hyperthermia, mental status changes, rhabdomyolysis	Enzyme elevations (CK)	Reduce dopaminergic therapy

Table 2–1.   Central nervous system drug reactions *(continued)*

Disorder	Implicated drugs	Risk factors	Signs and symptoms	Diagnostic studies[a]	Management[b]
Antipsychotic hypersensitivity syndrome	Dopamine receptor antagonists (antipsychotics)	Lewy body dementia, Parkinson's disease	Confusion, immobility, rigidity, postural instability, falls, fixed-flexion posture, poor oral intake		Drug discontinuation
Lithium-antipsychotic encephalopathy	Antipsychotics plus lithium	Same as for NMS plus lithium toxicity	Same as for NMS plus lithium toxicity (ataxia, dysarthria, myoclonus, seizures)	Lithium level	Drug discontinuation

Table 2–1. Central nervous system drug reactions *(continued)*

Disorder	Implicated drugs	Risk factors	Signs and symptoms	Diagnostic studies[a]	Management[b]
Serotonin syndrome	Antidepressants (TCAs, MAOIs, SSRIs, SNRIs) Triptans Linezolid Methylene blue Some opiates (meperidine, tramadol, dextromethorphan, fentanyl) Herbals (St. John's wort) Drugs of abuse (MDMA)	Overdose, polypharmacy	Behavioral (delirium, agitation, restlessness) Neuromotor (tremor, myoclonus, hyperreflexia, ataxia, rigidity, shivering) Dysautonomia (tachycardia, tachypnea, hyperthermia, mydriasis, blood pressure lability) Gastrointestinal (diarrhea, nausea, vomiting, incontinence)		Drug discontinuation Supportive care Specific agents (cyproheptadine, benzodiazepines)?
Mortality in dementia-related psychosis	Antipsychotics	Dementia-related psychosis or behavior disorders in elderly patients	Cerebrovascular events Cardiovascular (heart failure, sudden death) Infections (pneumonia)		Drug discontinuation Alternative drugs (e.g., cholinesterase inhibitors, pimavanserin in Parkinson's disease) and supportive care

Table 2–1.   Central nervous system drug reactions (continued)

Disorder	Implicated drugs	Risk factors	Signs and symptoms	Diagnostic studies[a]	Management[b]
Seizures	Antipsychotics (clozapine, chlorpromazine) Antidepressants (clomipramine, bupropion) Lithium (toxicity) Withdrawal of benzodiazepines, anticonvulsants Flumazenil	Epilepsy, substance abuse, brain damage, overdose, drug interactions, dose, and rate of titration	Generalized or partial seizures	Electroencephalography Drug plasma levels	Drug discontinuation, reinstitution (anticonvulsants), or detoxification (benzodiazepines) Supportive care

Note.   CK=creatine kinase; CSF HVA=cerebrospinal fluid homovanillic acid; ECT=electroconvulsive therapy; MAOIs=monoamine oxidase inhibitors; MDMA=3,4-methylenedioxymethamphetamine; NMS=neuroleptic malignant syndrome; SNRIs=serotonin-norepinephrine reuptake inhibitors; SSRIs=selective serotonin reuptake inhibitors; TCAs=tricyclic antidepressants; WBC=white blood cell count.

[a]Standard imaging and laboratory studies to rule out other conditions in the differential diagnosis or complications are assumed. Only studies associated with or specific to each reaction are listed.

[b]Mainstay of management in all reactions includes careful monitoring, prompt recognition, rapid cessation or modification of the offending drug, and supportive medical care. Specific therapies that have been reported are listed. A question mark indicates lack of evidence of safety and efficacy.

of NMS (Guinart et al. 2021a; Kane et al. 2019; Misawa et al. 2021; Su et al. 2014). Risk factors include dehydration, exhaustion, agitation, catatonia, encephalitis, previous episodes, multiple antipsychotics, and higher doses of high-potency drugs given parenterally at a rapid rate of titration. The effect of concurrent drugs, including benzodiazepines, lithium, selective serotonin reuptake inhibitors (SSRIs), and serotonin-norepinephrine reuptake inhibitors (SNRIs), on the risk of NMS also has been reported (Guinart et al. 2021a; Schneider et al. 2020; Su et al. 2014).

NMS is an idiosyncratic drug reaction that occurs within therapeutic doses and may develop within hours but usually evolves over days. About two-thirds of cases occur during the first 1–2 weeks after drug initiation. Classic signs are elevated temperatures (from minimal to life-threatening hyperthermia), generalized rigidity with tremors, altered consciousness with catatonia, and autonomic instability (Caroff and Mann 1993; Gurrera et al. 2011). Laboratory findings are not specific or pathognomonic but commonly include muscle enzyme elevations (e.g., creatine kinase [CK]), myoglobinuria, leukocytosis, metabolic acidosis, hypoxia, elevated serum catecholamine levels, and low serum iron levels. Neuroimaging findings in NMS are nonspecific, except for generalized slowing reported on the electroencephalogram (EEG). However, case reports have described reduced striatal dopamine transporter binding on SPECT and reversible splenial lesions of the corpus callosum in patients with NMS (Gasparini et al. 2018; Martino et al. 2015).

Gurrera et al. (2011) developed expert consensus diagnostic criteria and a priority point score system that could be used to confirm the likelihood of diagnosing NMS. In a subsequent validation study, a threshold score of 74 points achieved the highest agreement with DSM-IV-TR (American Psychiatric Association 2000) and consultant diagnoses with sensitivity of 69.6% and specificity of 90.7% (Gurrera et al. 2017).

The differential diagnosis of NMS is complex, including disorders in which patients present with elevated temperatures and encephalopathy, such as malignant catatonia due to psychosis (Mann et al. 1986); CNS infections and autoimmune disorders (Caroff and Campbell 2015; Caroff et al. 2001a); benign extrapyramidal side effects; agitated delirium of diverse causes; heatstroke; serotonin syndrome; malignant hyperthermia associated with anesthesia (Caroff et al. 2001b); and withdrawal from dopamine agonists, sedatives, or alcohol. Although no laboratory test is diagnostic for NMS, a thorough laboratory assessment and neuroimaging studies are essential for excluding other serious medical conditions. Evidence strongly implicates drug-induced dopamine blockade as the primary triggering mechanism in NMS (Mann et al. 2000). Efforts at identifying underlying genetic vulnerabilities, focusing on mutations in neurotransmitter, ryanodine receptor, and cytochrome enzyme genes, are preliminary and inconclusive to date.

Once dopamine-blocking drugs are withheld, two-thirds of NMS cases resolve within 1–2 weeks, with an average duration of 7–10 days (Caroff 2003a). Recent data suggest that mortality may not necessarily differ significantly between oral and long-acting injectable formulations, but the outcome of NMS with ultra-long-acting antipsychotics deserves further study (Guinart et al. 2021a, 2021b). Occasionally, patients are left with a residual catatonic and parkinsonian state that may be responsive to electroconvulsive therapy (ECT) (Caroff et al. 2000). Despite advances in recognition and treatment, NMS is still potentially fatal in approximately 5%–10% of cases because of renal failure, cardiorespiratory arrest, disseminated intravascular coagulation, pulmonary emboli, sepsis, or aspiration pneumonia (Guinart et al. 2021a; Lao et al. 2020; Modi et al. 2016; Nakamura et al. 2012). Older age, cardiorespiratory disease, and higher severity of hyperthermia may increase adverse outcomes (Guinart et al. 2021b). Recurrence of NMS on rechallenge with antipsychotics is possible, but the risk may be minimized by conservative management (Guinart et al. 2021a; Strawn et al. 2007).

The mainstay of treatment consists of early diagnosis, discontinuation of dopamine antagonists, and supportive medical care. Benzodiazepines, dopamine agonists, dantrolene, and ECT have been advocated in clinical reports, but randomized controlled trials of these agents may not be feasible because NMS is rare, often self-limited after drug discontinuation, and heterogeneous in presentation, course, and outcome. These agents may be considered in individual cases on the basis of symptoms, severity, and duration of the episode (Strawn et al. 2007). A systematic analysis of case reports found that mortality and duration of NMS were not significantly lower with dantrolene, bromocriptine, or ECT compared with symptomatic therapy. However, mortality was lower for patients with severe symptoms in a subgroup analysis (Kuhlwilm et al. 2020). This finding, in addition to our experience that specific treatments are most often reserved for severe or refractory symptoms, underscores the need to consider confounding effects of severity in studies of NMS treatment outcomes.

Parkinsonism-Hyperpyrexia Syndromes

Patients with Parkinson's disease or Lewy body dementia are at risk for severe exacerbations of motor symptoms progressing to akinetic crises following drug-induced changes in dopamine activity (Huddleston and Factor 2021). In Parkinson's disease, reports of NMS attributable to antipsychotics are often compounded by concomitant withdrawal of dopamine agonists or addition of cholinesterase inhibitors. However, following discontinuation or loss of efficacy of dopaminergic drugs, during spontaneous "off" episodes, or because of malfunctioning deep brain stimulation devices, patients with Parkinson's disease may develop a parkinsonism-hyperpyrexia syndrome (PHS) that is indistinguishable from NMS, providing evidence of the pivotal role of acute dopamine deficiency in the pathophysiology of both disorders. Further support for hypodopaminergia is provided by Ueda et al. (2001), who showed that patients with Parkinson's disease who had low concentrations of homovanillic acid in cerebrospinal fluid were more likely to develop the syndrome after drug withdrawal.

Reports suggest an incidence of PHS of about 2%–3% among patients treated for Parkinson's disease, including several deaths (Factor and Santiago 2005; Serrano-Dueñas 2003). More patients who develop PHS are male, with a duration of preexisting Parkinson's disease ranging from 2 to 16 years. Other risk factors for the syndrome include more severe parkinsonism, higher daily doses of levodopa, and the presence of motor fluctuations, psychosis, or dehydration.

The clinical features of PHS resemble NMS and range in onset from 18 hours to 7 days after changes in dopaminergic therapy. Initial rigidity and tremor may rapidly progress over a few days to immobility, altered mental status, dysautonomia, and elevated temperatures accompanied by leukocytosis and CK elevations (Huddleston and Factor 2021). However, Serrano-Dueñas (2003) reported that compared with NMS, PHS developed more slowly, resulted in less robust laboratory abnormalities, resolved more quickly, and had a better prognosis. Nevertheless, PHS can be lethal (mortality rate of 4%–23%), and patients may also experience medical consequences (infection, renal or cardiorespiratory failure, coagulopathies) or sustain worsened symptoms of Parkinson's disease (Huddleston and Factor 2021).

PHS is a neurological emergency. The mainstay of treatment is early recognition and rapid reintroduction of dopaminergic medications, or correction of deep brain stimulation devices, as well as aggressive medical support, with reversal of symptoms occurring in 10 hours to 7 days. Sato et al. (2003) reported that the addition of methylprednisolone to a combination of levodopa, bromocriptine, and dantrolene significantly reduced the severity and duration of symptoms compared with placebo in patients with PHS.

Two other drug-related neurological emergencies among patients with Lewy body disorders are a dyskinesia-hyperpyrexia syndrome and an antipsychotic sensitivity syndrome. Increased dopamine activity in the striatum associated with dopaminergic therapy can lead to severe, continuous dyskinesias with elevated temperatures, rhabdomyolysis, and altered mental status (Huddleston and Factor 2021). Risk factors may include longer duration of illness, motor fluctuations, dose changes, infections, dehydration, trauma, and ambient heat. Treatment includes supportive care and reduced dopaminergic therapy.

Antipsychotic sensitivity syndrome (neuroleptic sensitivity syndrome) is a potentially fatal complication of treatment with antipsychotic drugs originally reported to affect 50% or more of patients with Lewy body dementia (McKeith et al. 1992). McKeith et al. (1992) reported that 4 of 14 patients (29%) receiving antipsychotics showed mild extrapyramidal symptoms, but 8 (57%) showed severe symptoms, with half the survival of untreated patients. Although antipsychotic sensitivity is known as a distinguishing feature of Lewy body dementia, the diagnostic value of antipsychotic sensitivity has been reduced to suggestive only in revised criteria after studies showed few cases of sensitivity in small series of early-stage Lewy body dementia cases in which the patients received treatment with second-generation antipsychotics (Pyun et al. 2020; Tampi et al. 2019). Antipsychotic sensitivity is characterized by the acute onset or exacerbation of parkinsonism and impaired consciousness, with sedation, agitation, or delirium, followed by rigidity, postural instability, and falls. Rapid deterioration with increased confusion, immobility, rigidity, fixed-flexion posture, and decreased food and fluid intake is not reversed by anticholinergic medications. Aarsland et al. (2005) reported that patients with Lewy body dementia, Parkinson's disease dementia, or Parkinson's disease alone all had high frequencies of severe antipsychotic sensitivity (53%, 39%, and 27%, respectively), which distinguishes them from patients with Alzheimer's disease. Death results usually from complications of immobility and/or reduced food and fluid intake and may occur within days to weeks. As a substitute for antipsychotics, cholinesterase inhibitors have been recommended as the first-line treatment for neuropsychiatric symptoms in Lewy body dementia (despite occasional reports of crises in patients with Parkinson's disease), but if they are ineffective, clozapine or quetiapine may be used cautiously, with patients carefully monitored for worsening motor symptoms and mental status changes (Tampi et al. 2019; Weintraub and Hurtig 2007) (see also Chapter 9, "Central Nervous System Disorders").

Lithium-Antipsychotic Encephalopathy

In 1974, a severe encephalopathic syndrome, characterized by neuromuscular symptoms, hyperthermia, and impairment of consciousness, was reported in four patients treated with lithium and haloperidol, suggesting synergistic toxic effects between these two drugs (Cohen and Cohen 1974). This report was both alarming and highly controversial and was met with disbelief as to the iatrogenic nature of the syndrome, but similar cases continued to be reported. For example, Miller and Menninger (1987) reported neurotoxicity consisting of delirium, extrapyramidal symptoms, and ataxia in 8 of 41 patients (19.5%) receiving concurrent treatment with lithium and antipsychotics. Similar cases, most often associated with haloperidol and lithium but implicating newer antipsychotics as well, have continued to be reported (Caroff 2003b). A recent review (Netto et al. 2019) of neurotoxicity due to lithium in combination with second-generation antipsychotics identified 8 reports involving 11 cases; 5 cases were associated with clozapine, and 2 each with quetiapine, risperidone, and aripiprazole. Eight cases were fully reversible, although 3 resulted in lasting movement disorders, cognitive deficits, and cerebellar signs.

The manifestations of neurotoxicity in these cases may include stupor, delirium, catatonia, rigidity, ataxia, dysarthria, myoclonus, seizures, and fever. Electroencephalographic findings of diffuse slowing or triphasic waves have been suggested as a useful method in these cases for differentiating lithium-associated toxic encephalopathy from purely psychiatric changes in mental status and from nonconvulsive status (Kaplan and Birbeck 2006).

Spring and Frankel (1981) proposed two types of combined lithium–antipsychotic drug toxicity: an NMS-like reaction associated with haloperidol and other high-potency antipsychotics and a separate reaction associated with phenothiazines, especially thioridazine, resulting in lithium toxicity. Goldman (1996) reviewed 237 cases of neurotoxicity ascribed to lithium with or without antipsychotics and found support for Spring and Frankel's bipartite concept. However, the heterogeneity of cases led Goldman to suggest that adverse reactions to combination therapy form a continuum ranging from predominantly antipsychotic induced (NMS) to largely lithium induced. The mechanism for possible toxic synergy remains unknown.

Lithium-antipsychotic encephalopathy is extremely rare and does not outweigh the potential benefit and tolerance of this drug combination in the vast majority of patients presenting with mania and psychosis. Rather, the clinician is obligated to carefully monitor the response to treatment, including lithium levels, and to promptly recognize this reaction in order to rapidly discontinue medications and institute supportive medical care.

Serotonin Syndrome

Serotonin syndrome generally results when two or more serotonergic drugs are taken concurrently, but it also occurs following overdose and during single-drug exposure. Nearly all serotonergic drugs have been implicated in the syndrome, the occurrence of which appears to be primarily dose related or result from toxic levels of serotonin in the brain. Medications associated with severe or fatal cases typically include monoamine oxidase inhibitors (MAOIs) when combined with other antidepressants or with certain opioids that potentiate serotonergic activity (meperidine, tramadol, dextromethorphan, or fentanyl) (Boyer and Shannon 2005). Morphine has not been implicated in this interaction and is a reasonable choice for pain control in the context of concurrent serotonergic treatment, provided an allowance is made for possible potentiation of its depressive narcotic effect (Browne and Linter 1987). Nonpsychiatric medications that increase serotonergic activity also have been implicated in serotonin syndrome. Although antimigrainous triptans have been implicated in serotonin syndrome, this association has been challenged (Orlova et al. 2018). Certain drugs used in medical settings (e.g., linezolid, methylene blue) (Gillman 2011) or derived from herbal products (e.g., St. John's wort) have clandestine MAOI activity and may produce severe instances of serotonin syndrome when used inadvertently in combination with serotonergic drugs. Use of illicit drugs (e.g., cocaine, methamphetamines) has been associated with hyperthermic states (Hohmann et al. 2014), and serotonergic mechanisms have been specifically implicated in toxic reactions following abuse of 3,4-methylenedioxymethamphetamine (MDMA; "molly," "ecstasy") (Armenian et al. 2013). Furthermore, over the past decade, hundreds of new psychoactive substances known as designer or synthetic drugs have emerged on the illicit drug market (Scherbaum et al. 2017; Shafi et al. 2020). Many new psychoactive substances have significant serotonergic activity and can be associated with serotonin syndrome (Schifano et al. 2021). These include synthetic cathinones (e.g., bath salts), selected synthetic cannabinoids, psychedelic phenethylamines, synthetic tryptamines, and bupropion misused at high dosages ("welbys," "dubs," or "barnies"), among numerous other agents.

The incidence of serotonin syndrome among patients receiving SSRI monotherapy has been estimated in the range of 0.5–0.9 cases per 1,000 patient-months of treatment (Mackay et al. 1999), and serotonin syndrome occurs in about 14%–16% of persons who overdose on SSRIs (Boyer and Shannon 2005). In analyses of both a Department of Veterans Affairs database and a commercial insurance database, Nguyen et al. (2015) reported that the incidence of reported claims for serotonin syndrome in 2012 among patients prescribed serotonergic agents was 0.07% and 0.09%, respectively, and that the incidence had declined by about half since 2009. In addition, they found that the highest RR for developing the syndrome was observed in patients prescribed MAOIs in combination with other agents and in patients prescribed five or more non-MAOI serotonergic agents. Abadie et al. (2015) reviewed cases of serotonin syndrome reported to a pharmacovigilance database between the years 1985 and 2013 and found 125 cases that met standard criteria. The syndrome was caused by a single serotonergic drug in 40.8% of these cases, most often at therapeutic doses, whereas 59.2% resulted from combined use of a serotonin reuptake inhibitor with either an opioid or an MAOI. Although 86.9% of patients recovered without sequelae, 6 cases were fatal, and the more severe cases were associated with use of a serotonin reuptake inhibitor in combination with an MAOI.

Although serotonin syndrome has been known for decades (Oates and Sjoerdsma 1960), Sternbach (1991) is credited with developing operational diagnostic criteria on the basis of a triad of cognitive-behavioral, neuromuscular, and autonomic abnormalities. These criteria were later revised by Radomski et al. (2000). The onset of symptoms is usually abrupt, and clinical manifestations range from mild to fatal. Presentation of serotonin syndrome reflects a spectrum of concentration-dependent toxicity, ranging in severity from a transient agitated delirium to a full-blown hypermetabolic syndrome that is indistinguishable from NMS.

Behavioral symptoms of serotonin syndrome include alterations in consciousness and mood and restlessness and agitation. Autonomic disturbances include tachycardia, labile blood pressure, diaphoresis, shivering, tachypnea, mydriasis, sialorrhea, and hyperthermia. Neuromuscular signs include tremor, myoclonus, ankle clonus, hyperreflexia, ataxia, incoordination, and muscular rigidity. Gastrointestinal symptoms, including diarrhea, incontinence, nausea, and vomiting, may also occur. In a review of cases of overdose on SSRIs alone, Dunkley et al. (2003) derived the Hunter serotonin toxicity criteria. They proposed that these criteria are simpler and more sensitive and specific for serotonin toxicity than Sternbach's criteria and involve the use of only a few well-defined clinical features (clonus, agitation, diaphoresis, tremor, hyperreflexia, hypertonia, and elevated temperature).

The differential diagnosis of serotonin syndrome includes anticholinergic toxicity, heatstroke, carcinoid syndrome, infection, drug or alcohol withdrawal, lithium toxicity, and SSRI withdrawal. In more severe cases, it may be difficult to differentiate serotonin syndrome from NMS, especially in patients receiving serotonergic drugs in combination with antipsychotics. This latter conundrum prompted inclusion of warnings in product labeling of serotonergic antidepressants, cautioning against precipitation of NMS-like reactions when these two drug classes are prescribed simultaneously.

Management of serotonin syndrome entails recognition of the syndrome, cessation of serotonergic medications, and provision of supportive care. Serotonin syndrome is usually self-limited and resolves rapidly, but it can be sustained and fatal in severe cases of hyperthermia, associated most often with the use of MAOIs (Abadie et al. 2015). Sedation with benzodiazepines may be useful for controlling agitation and for correcting mild increases in heart rate and blood pressure. On the basis of anecdotal clinical reports, moderate cases appear to benefit from administration of serotonin type 2A receptor (5-HT_{2A}) antagonists such as cyproheptadine (Boyer and Shannon 2005). Antipsychotics with serotonergic antagonist properties have been suggested as well, but they may add the confounding autonomic, neurological, and thermoregulatory effects of dopamine blockade. Dantrolene has been used in cases of serotonin syndrome with extreme hyperthermia.

Cerebrovascular Events and Mortality Associated With Antipsychotics in Elderly Patients With Dementia-Related Psychosis

In 2003, the U.S. FDA issued an advisory that the incidence of cerebrovascular adverse events, including fatalities, was significantly higher in elderly patients with dementia-related psychosis treated with second-generation antipsychotics. Collectively, 11 risperidone and olanzapine trials indicated that 2.2% of drug-treated subjects experienced cerebrovascular adverse events compared with 0.8% of those taking placebo, indicating an RR of 2.8 versus placebo but an absolute risk of only 1.4% when these drugs are prescribed (Jeste et al. 2008). Subsequent database studies and meta-analyses of the risk of stroke have varied in definitions of dementia, study designs, and methodologies. Evidence is limited and inconsistent, but recent studies support an increased risk in patients with dementia receiving antipsychotics, especially during the first few weeks after initiation (Koponen et al. 2022; Prior et al. 2014; Zivkovic et al. 2019). Although vascular dementia may confer a higher risk of stroke, recent studies have not shown differences in risk by dementia type (Koponen et al. 2022). Results from studies comparing antipsychotics have been inconsistent, with studies finding greater risk with either newer or older antipsychotics or no significant difference in risk of stroke (Koponen et al. 2022; Prior et al. 2014; Zivkovic et al. 2019). Risk of cerebrovascular events is not limited to antipsychotics; recent evidence indicates a significant association between SSRIs and cerebral vasoconstriction and ischemic or hemorrhagic stroke (adjusted $OR = ~1.2–2.7$) (Biffi et al. 2017; Hung et al. 2013; Shin et al. 2014).

In 2005, the FDA analyzed 17 placebo-controlled trials and followed with a black box warning of increased mortality ($RR = 1.6–1.7$ vs. placebo), primarily due to cardiovascular (heart failure, sudden death) or infectious (pneumonia) causes, associated with newer antipsychotic drugs in the treatment of behavioral disorders in elderly patients with dementia (U.S. Food and Drug Administration 2005). A similar FDA alert for higher mortality with older first-generation antipsychotics followed in 2008 (U.S. Food and Drug Administration 2008). Multiple subsequent analyses have consistently replicated the risk of mortality associated with antipsychotic drugs when used for the treatment of behavioral disorders in elderly patients who have dementia (Kales et al. 2012; Maust et al. 2015; Rochon et al. 2008; Yunusa et al. 2021). The drug-related risk of mortality has also been extended to elderly patients with Parkinson's disease and coronavirus SARS-CoV-2 disease (COVID-19) (Austria et al. 2021; Weintraub et al. 2016).

Although evidence is inconclusive regarding the risk-benefit ratio of antipsychotics in elderly patients (Schneider et al. 2006; Sultzer et al. 2008; Yunusa et al. 2021), their off-label use is likely to remain standard practice, given the limited efficacy and safety of other agents or psychosocial treatments in this age group (Jeste et al. 2008). Informed discussion with patients and caregivers of the benefits, risks, and alternatives and careful clinical monitoring are essential.

Mechanisms for antipsychotic-associated cerebrovascular adverse events and death may include cardiac conduction disturbances, sedation leading to venous stasis or aspiration pneumonia, metabolic disturbances, orthostatic hypotension, tachycardia, and increased platelet aggregation. These risk factors underscore the need for thorough medical evaluation and ongoing monitoring of elderly patients receiving antipsychotics.

Seizures

The risk of drug-induced seizures is difficult to estimate because of predisposing factors, such as epilepsy, drug interactions, or substance abuse, which are infrequently cited in clinical trials (Alper et al. 2007; Montgomery 2005). Thus, if a seizure occurs in a given patient, a thorough history and neurological investigation are necessary to identify underlying risk factors. Patients with epilepsy are at risk for drug-induced seizures; however, psychotropic drugs are not contraindicated in the setting of adequate anticonvulsant therapy. In fact, effective psychopharmacotherapy has been shown to improve seizure control once psychiatric symptoms are controlled (Alper et al. 2007). As a rule, seizures correlate with drug dose and rate of titration and are more likely to be observed after an overdose.

Clozapine is associated with the highest rate of seizures among antipsychotics, followed by chlorpromazine (Wong and Delva 2007). Olanzapine and quetiapine may have proconvulsant effects compared with other atypical drugs (Alper et al. 2007). Because clozapine is most often indicated and most effective for treatment-refractory schizophrenia patients, lowering the dose or adding valproic acid may be worthwhile prior to switching to a different antipsychotic if a seizure occurs.

Among antidepressants, tricyclic drugs at therapeutic doses were associated with an incidence of seizures of about 0.4%–2.0% and are particularly hazardous in overdose (Montgomery 2005). Clomipramine and the tetracyclic agents amoxapine and maprotiline (Tallian 2018) are considered most likely to be associated with seizures. MAOIs are considered to have low risk for seizures. Bupropion has a 10-fold increase in seizure risk in dosages greater than 600 mg/day relative to patients taking 450 mg/day or less, and it is relatively contraindicated in patients with epilepsy or severe eating disorders, or at least requires careful documentation and monitoring in these patients (Alper et al. 2007). The SSRIs and SNRIs have a low risk of seizures, except in large overdoses, and have been associated with reduction in seizure frequency compared with placebo (Alper et al. 2007; Cardamone et al. 2013). However, some SSRIs and SNRIs can increase plasma levels of other drugs, with potential for secondarily increasing seizure activity.

Among mood stabilizers, lithium is associated with seizures only during intoxication. Carbamazepine has been associated with seizures after overdose and can increase the risk of seizures during withdrawal; as a rule, the risk of withdrawal seizures can be minimized by not abruptly stopping carbamazepine, valproic acid, or any anticonvulsant and by slowly tapering the drug over a 2-week period. Recent studies suggest that stimulants and other drugs used to treat ADHD are not associated with increased seizure risk, even in patients with epilepsy, providing seizures are well controlled (Andrade 2020). Short- and intermediate-acting benzodiazepines, especially alprazolam, have been associated with withdrawal seizures. Finally, seizure induction is a serious complication of the benzodiazepine receptor antagonist flumazenil, with fatal cases of status epilepticus having been reported.

Cardiovascular Drug Reactions

Severe adverse cardiovascular reactions are the most unexpected and often catastrophic reactions to psychotropic drugs (Table 2–2). Cardiac reactions are observed primarily with antipsychotic drugs, especially clozapine, and with tricyclic antidepressants, whereas hypertensive crises are associated with nonselective and irreversible MAOIs.

Table 2–2.   Cardiovascular drug reactions

Disorders	Implicated drugs	Risk factors	Signs and symptoms	Diagnostic studies[a]	Management[b]
Ventricular arrhythmias and sudden death					
QTc interval prolongation and torsades de pointes	Antipsychotics (clozapine, chlorpromazine, haloperidol, droperidol, pimozide, sulpiride, ziprasidone) Methadone	Long QT syndrome; cardiac, renal, or hepatic disease; family history; syncope; drug history; electrolytes; drug interactions; abnormal ECG; QTc > 500 ms	Palpitations, syncope, chest pain	ECG monitoring in at-risk patients	
Brugada syndrome	Antipsychotics Antidepressants Mood stabilizers	Genetic predisposition, overdose, drug combinations	ECG (RBBB, ST elevations)	ECG monitoring in at-risk patients	
Heart block	TCAs	Intraventricular conduction defects	Heart block	ECG monitoring in at-risk patients	

Table 2–2. Cardiovascular drug reactions *(continued)*

Disorders	Implicated drugs	Risk factors	Signs and symptoms	Diagnostic studies[a]	Management[b]
Hypertensive crisis	MAOIs	Tyramine-containing food Sympathomimetic drugs	Hypertension, stiff neck, nausea, palpitations, diaphoresis, confusion, seizures, arrhythmias, headache, stroke	Blood pressure monitoring	Phentolamine intravenously; nifedipine by mouth for headache
Myocarditis, pericarditis, and cardiomyopathy	Antipsychotics (clozapine)	Cardiovascular disease, pulmonary disease	Fever, dyspnea, flulike symptoms, chest pain, fatigue	Echocardiography (reduced ejection fraction, ventricular dysfunction), ECG (T wave changes), leukocytosis, eosinophilia, cardiac enzyme elevations	

Note. ECG=electrocardiogram; MAOIs=monoamine oxidase inhibitors; RBBB=right bundle branch block; TCAs=tricyclic antidepressants.
[a]Standard imaging and laboratory studies to rule out other conditions in the differential diagnosis or complications are assumed. Only studies associated with or specific for each reaction are listed.
[b]Mainstay of management in all reactions includes careful monitoring, prompt recognition, rapid cessation or modification of the offending drug, and supportive medical care. Only specific therapies that have been reported are listed.

Ventricular Arrhythmias and Sudden Cardiac Death

Sudden unexpected deaths are a major contributor to increased mortality in schizophrenia, 15%–40% of which are attributed to sudden cardiac death (Li et al. 2018). Reports of sudden cardiac death have been associated with exposure to both first- and second-generation antipsychotics, perhaps based in part on genetic predisposition. Several studies have confirmed a two- to fivefold increased risk of sudden cardiac death in patients receiving antipsychotics (Hennessy et al. 2002; Liperoti et al. 2005; Reilly et al. 2002; Straus et al. 2004). The risk is dose related and is heightened by preexisting cardiovascular disease.

The increased risk of arrhythmias leading to sudden death has been attributed to specific drug effects on cardiac conduction (Glassman and Bigger 2001; Sicouri and Antzelevitch 2008). QTc interval prolongation predicts risk of lethal ventricular arrhythmias such as torsades de pointes or ventricular fibrillation, syncope, and death. Although QTc interval is the best available predictor, it is imperfect: the threshold for increased risk is usually set at 500 ms, but other risk factors (see below) may determine occurrence of torsades (Glassman and Bigger 2001); it can be difficult to interpret in the presence of underlying conduction blocks or implanted cardiac devices (Beach et al. 2018); and finally, the automatic calculation by electrocardiograph machines is accurate only for normal heart rates, with the true QTc interval higher in patients with bradycardia and lower in patients with tachycardia (Funk et al. 2020).

Antipsychotic drugs, particularly those with propensity for blockade of the delayed potassium rectifier current, have the highest potential for QTc interval prolongation and resulting arrhythmias. The prevalence of drug-induced long QT interval (>500 ms) in schizophrenia patients taking antipsychotics was reported as between 0.9% and 2.6% (Vohra 2020). In general, first-generation antipsychotics, primarily phenothiazines, have a greater risk of prolonging the QTc interval, but differences in risk of ventricular arrhythmias, torsades, or sudden cardiac death are less clear. Although haloperidol, primarily intravenously, has been associated with QTc interval prolongation, ventricular arrhythmias, and sudden death, these risks are confounded by the frequent use of haloperidol for patients with medical comorbidities in intensive care settings (Marra et al. 2021). Among second-generation antipsychotics, clozapine, ziprasidone, and iloperidone are considered to have a higher risk and aripiprazole a lower risk of prolonging the QTc interval (Beach et al. 2018). As prescribing of newer antipsychotics (cariprazine, lurasidone, quetiapine, olanzapine/fluoxetine) for depression becomes more common, especially in older patients and those with preexisting cardiovascular disease, the frequency of adverse cardiac events may increase dramatically.

A second mechanism for sudden cardiac death may be Brugada syndrome, which is characterized by right bundle branch block and ST elevation in right precordial leads but relatively normal QTc intervals (Rastogi et al. 2020). Clinical manifestations may also include atrial fibrillation, atrioventricular block, and syncope. A Brugada pattern on the electrocardiogram (ECG) is more prevalent among schizophrenia patients than in the general population. Brugada syndrome is a channelopathy with multiple known genetic variants that may overlap with genetic predisposition to schizophrenia. It is well documented that certain tricyclic antidepressants (amitriptyline, clomipramine, desipramine, nortriptyline), antipsychotics (loxapine, trifluoperazine), mood stabilizers (lithium, oxcarbazepine), and other medications that modulate sodium and calcium potentiation may induce or unmask Brugada electrocardiographic patterns and lead to malignant arrhythmias and sudden cardiac death independent of prolonged QTc interval in predisposed patients (Rastogi et al. 2020).

Early concerns over cardiac effects of tricyclic antidepressants derived primarily from the occurrence of heart block and arrhythmias observed after drug overdoses. However, subsequent studies suggested that risk of conduction disturbances also existed when therapeutic doses were used (Roose et al. 1989). QTc interval prolongation and torsades de pointes have been reported with tricyclics, but far less often than with antipsychotics (Sala et al. 2006). QTc interval prolongation with tricyclics is primarily due to prolonged QRS conduction, which, along with increased PR intervals, reflects delays in the intraventricular His-Purkinje conduction system involved in depolarization. Tricyclics proved to be effective type 1A quinidine-like antiarrhythmics, capable of suppressing ventricular ectopy. Although tricyclic-induced suppression of conduction at therapeutic doses is of no consequence in patients with normal hearts, there is a 10-fold risk of significant atrioventricular block in patients with preexisting intraventricular conduction defects (Roose et al. 1989). In general, tricyclics are associated with increased risk of acute heart disease (Biffi et al. 2017).

Although there have been isolated reports of torsades following SSRI over-dose (Tarabar et al. 2008), SSRIs have lower rates of adverse cardiac events compared with tricyclic antidepressants, MAOIs, and SNRIs. As a result, SSRIs are the first-line treatment choice in older adults or in patients with cardiovas-cular disease, with sertraline particularly favorable for cardiac patients (Beach et al. 2018; Behlke et al. 2020). Although FDA warnings in 2011 and 2012 not to exceed daily doses of citalopram of 40 mg (20 mg in patients older than 65) were supported by clinical studies confirming age- and dose-related po-tential for QTc interval prolongation compared with other SSRIs, the clinical significance of this effect remains uncertain (Beach et al. 2018). Subsequent studies found that high-dose citalopram did not differ from other agents in terms of arrhythmias, sudden cardiac death, or total mortality. Nevertheless, the FDA warning led to reduced dosages and frequency of prescriptions of citalopram and escitalopram, often compromising effective antidepressant treatment (Beach et al. 2018). Venlafaxine may increase QT interval prolon-gation, but the risk for arrhythmias remains low. Similarly, evidence of sig-nificant adverse cardiac effects is limited for other antidepressants, including bupropion, mirtazapine, duloxetine, milnacipran, levomilnacipran, vilazo-done, vortioxetine, moclobemide, ketamine/esketamine, and agomelatine, which remain safe alternatives for symptoms that do not respond to SSRIs (Beach et al. 2018; Behlke et al. 2020).

Methadone is an inhibitor of the cardiac ion channel KCNH2 and causes QT interval prolongation in a dose-dependent manner. Methadone has been reported to cause torsades de pointes, particularly with predisposing factors such as hypokalemia, hypomagnesemia, and concomitant treatment with metabolic inhibitors or other QTc interval–prolonging agents (Mujtaba et al. 2013).

Patients who are considered for antipsychotic and antidepressant treat-ment should be screened for heart disease, congenital long QT and Brugada syndromes, family history of sudden death, syncope, drug history of adverse cardiac effects, electrolyte imbalance (especially hypokalemia, hypocalcemia, and hypomagnesemia), and renal or hepatic disease. Drugs implicated in QTc interval prolongation and torsades de pointes when used concurrently can be divided into drugs that directly prolong QTc interval, including antiarrhyth-mics (quinidine, procainamide, sotalol, amiodarone), antihistamines (diphen-hydramine), antibiotics (azithromycin, clarithromycin, erythromycin), and others (cisapride, loperamide, methadone); drugs that interfere with metabolism of agents associated with torsades, including antifungals (ketoconazole), antivirals (indinavir, ritonavir), calcium channel blockers (diltiazem, verapamil), and antibiotics (erythromycin, clarithromycin), as well as grapefruit juice; and drugs that may affect electrolytes or other risk factors (diuretics) (Kao and Furbee 2005). An ECG should be obtained at baseline and after drug administration in patients with any of these risk factors. Conservative doses of psychotropic drugs should be prescribed and polypharmacy minimized, with close clinical monitoring and warnings for patients to report promptly any new symptoms such as palpitations or syncope as well as the prescription of new medications. Cessation and change of medication should be considered if the ECG shows significant prolongation of the QTc interval, a QTc interval greater than 500 ms, new T wave abnormalities, marked bradycardia, or a Brugada phenotype.

Hypertensive Crises Due to Monoamine Oxidase Inhibitors

Hypertension is a known side effect of several psychotropic drugs, including venlafaxine, bupropion, and stimulants (Smith et al. 2008). This condition is usually mild and can be detected by routine blood pressure measurements. In contrast, drug and food interactions with MAOIs may produce a potentially fatal hypertensive crisis. Symptoms include throbbing headaches with marked blood pressure elevations, nausea, neck stiffness, palpitations, diaphoresis, and confusion, sometimes complicated by seizures, cardiac arrhythmias, myocardial infarction, intracerebral hemorrhage, or death. Episodes follow ingestion of indirect-acting sympathomimetic drugs or foods containing high concentrations of tyramine (Rapaport 2007). Prior to recognition of the need for dietary restrictions, rates of hypertensive reactions were estimated to range from 2% to 25% (Krishnan 2007; Ricken et al. 2017). Previous MAOI diets were probably overly conservative; more recent dietary restrictions are less daunting and still have reduced the incidence of hypertensive reactions to near zero (Gardner et al. 1996; Ricken et al. 2017).

Monoamine oxidase (MAO) is the principal enzyme responsible for the oxidative deamination of monoamines. There are two subtypes of MAO isozymes: MAO-A and MAO-B. MAO-A occurs primarily in the brain, where its primary substrates are epinephrine, norepinephrine, dopamine, and serotonin, and in the intestine and liver, where it plays a critical role in the catabolism of dietary tyramine. Inhibition of MAO-A by MAOIs permits absorption of tyramine into the systemic circulation, triggering a significant release of norepinephrine from sympathetic nerve terminals, with resultant hypertensive crisis. MAO-B also occurs in the brain and has phenylethylamine and dopamine as substrates.

Extreme blood pressure elevations constitute a medical emergency and incur the risk of intracranial hemorrhage or myocardial infarction unless treated quickly with α-adrenergic antagonists. Intravenous phentolamine is the preferred treatment to reverse the acute rise in blood pressure in hypertensive crisis. In the event of a severe headache that may reflect elevated blood pressures, patients may be provided with nifedipine to take by mouth until they can be seen by a clinician.

Although MAOIs have been eclipsed in practice by SSRIs and other new agents, they remain an effective alternative class of antidepressants for treatment-resistant, bipolar, and atypical depression. Several relatively selective inhibitors of one or the other isoform that may not require strict dietary restrictions have been developed (Flockhart 2012). Selective but reversible MAO-A inhibition by moclobemide leaves sufficient MAO activity in liver and gut without substantial impairment of the margin necessary for safe ingestion of tyramine in food (Flockhart 2012). Selegiline, a selective but irreversible inhibitor of primarily MAO-B at oral dosages used to increase dopaminergic activity in Parkinson's disease, becomes an inhibitor of both MAO-A and MAO-B at higher dosages needed to treat depression; rare cases of hypertensive reactions have been reported, so dietary precautions should be taken (Tábi et al. 2020). A transdermal delivery system is available that allows selegiline to be directly absorbed into the systemic circulation, bypassing MAO-A inhibition in the gastrointestinal tract and minimizing the need for dietary restrictions (see Chapter 3, "Alternative Routes of Drug Administration"). However, dietary restrictions are still required at higher dosages. Several authorities have argued that transdermal selegiline has been markedly underused in treatment-resistant depression (Asnis and Henderson 2014; Culpepper 2013). Rasagiline is another orally administered selective but irreversible inhibitor of MAO-B. However, it contains the tyramine warning even at the recommended dosages of 0.5 mg/day or 1 mg/day and loses enzyme selectivity at higher doses.

Myocarditis, Cardiomyopathy, and Pericarditis

Disorders of the myocardium and pericardium are associated primarily with clozapine (Alawami et al. 2014; Merrill et al. 2005; Siskind et al. 2020). Clozapine exposure has been associated with a myocarditis event rate of 7 per 1,000 people and a case fatality rate of 12.7% (Siskind et al. 2020). The median age of affected patients is 30–36 years. Myocarditis occurs at therapeutic doses, usually within 2 months after initiation of treatment. Symptoms can be diverse and nonspecific, such as fever, dyspnea, flulike illness, chest discomfort, and fatigue. Diagnostic studies may detect ventricular dysfunction and reduced ejection fraction on echocardiography; ECG abnormalities, particularly T wave changes; leukocytosis and eosinophilia; and elevations in cardiac enzymes. Symptoms may improve following discontinuation of clozapine, but several recurrences on rechallenge have been reported. The exact pathophysiology has yet to be determined but is thought to reflect an acute hypersensitivity reaction.

Dilated or congestive cardiomyopathy characterized by ventricular dilatation, contractile dysfunction, and congestive heart failure also has been associated with clozapine (Alawami et al. 2014; Merrill et al. 2005; Siskind et al. 2020). Symptoms reflective of heart failure include dyspnea, palpitations or tachycardia, pedal edema, chest pain, and fatigue. Nonspecific ECG changes may occur, but reduced ejection fraction on echocardiography can confirm the diagnosis. The incidence of clozapine-induced cardiomyopathy has been estimated at 6 per 1,000 people. As with myocarditis, the median age of patients with clozapine-related cardiomyopathy is in the 30s, and it does not appear to be dose related; doses among reported cases ranged from 125 to 700 mg. The duration of treatment with clozapine before cardiomyopathy onset ranges from weeks to years, with a median duration of 6–9 months. Improvement after clozapine discontinuation has been described depending on severity; patients with ejection fractions below 25% have a poorer prognosis. Rechallenge is discouraged. The case fatality rate has been estimated at 7.8% (Siskind et al. 2020). Cardiomyopathy could represent a direct cardiotoxic effect of clozapine, but more likely it evolves from clozapine-induced myocarditis.

Pericarditis and polyserositis (involving the pleura as well) also have been described in association with clozapine (Merrill et al. 2005; Wehmeier et al.

2005). These inflammatory disorders occur within the first few weeks after drug initiation and appear to resolve after drug discontinuation.

Clozapine should be used cautiously in patients with cardiovascular and pulmonary disease. Patients and families should be informed of symptoms and questioned for any signs of cardiac dysfunction. A baseline ECG should be obtained prior to starting clozapine and repeated 2–4 weeks afterward. The value of repeat ECGs, echocardiography, MRI, and monitoring of serum cardiac enzymes and eosinophilia has not been substantiated, but these should be considered together with cardiology consultation if new symptoms of cardiovascular disease develop. In elderly patients, an echocardiogram is recommended every 6 months to monitor for myocarditis (Gareri et al. 2008). If myocarditis, pericarditis, or cardiomyopathy is suspected, clozapine should be discontinued immediately and should not be reinstituted if the diagnosis is confirmed.

Gastrointestinal Drug Reactions

Although mild gastrointestinal upset is not uncommon as a side effect associated with several psychotropic drug classes (e.g., SSRIs, lithium), severe hepatic and pancreatic toxicity may occur rarely (Table 2–3). The goal of this section is to provide the reader with a summary of the current literature regarding the association between psychiatric medications and drug-induced liver and pancreatic injury.

Drug-Induced Liver Injury

Prescribers of psychotropic medications must be mindful of the potential for idiosyncratic drug-induced liver injury (DILI), which, in a worst-case scenario, can cause chronic liver injury or death or require liver transplantation. Although the symptoms and signs of hepatotoxicity are nonspecific when considered individually, a clustering of symptoms that includes some or all of the following should assist the clinician in a diagnostic formulation: weakness, anorexia, fever, lethargy, jaundice, nausea, vomiting, hemorrhages, confusion, asterixis, seizures, and facial edema. Furthermore, liver chemistry results are variable; for example, elevations of transaminases and bilirubin can range from mild to extreme and do not reliably predict progression to fatal hepatotoxicity. Thus, regular clinical monitoring for prodromal symptoms is essen-

Table 2–3.   Gastrointestinal drug reactions

Disorder	Implicated drugs	Risk factors	Signs and symptoms	Diagnostic studies[a]	Management[b]
Hepatotoxicity	Anticonvulsants (valproic acid, carbamazepine, lamotrigine, topiramate) Antipsychotics (chlorpromazine) Antidepressants	Child, multiple anticonvulsants	Lethargy, jaundice, nausea, vomiting, anorexia, hemorrhages, seizures, fever, facial edema	Transaminitis, hyperbilirubinemia	Acetyl-L-Carnitine (for valproate toxicity?)
Hyperammonemic encephalopathy	Valproic acid		Decreased consciousness, focal deficits, impaired cognition, lethargy, vomiting, seizures	Serum ammonia, electroencephalography	Acetyl-L-Carnitine (for valproate toxicity?)
Acute pancreatitis	Valproic acid	Child, multiple anticonvulsants	Abdominal pain, nausea, vomiting, anorexia, fever	Serum amylase, lipase	

[a]Standard imaging and laboratory studies to rule out other conditions in the differential diagnosis or complications are assumed. Only studies associated with or specific to each reaction are listed.

[b]Mainstay of management in all reactions includes careful monitoring, prompt recognition, rapid cessation of the offending drug, and supportive medical care. Only specific therapies that have been reported are listed. A question mark indicates lack of evidence of safety and efficacy.

tial, followed by withholding of the suspected drug if symptoms emerge or enzymes are elevated.

The best available evidence from population-based studies indicates that the annual incidence of idiosyncratic, all-cause DILI in the general population is between approximately 14 and 19 events per 100,000 (Björnsson et al. 2013; Sgro et al. 2002). Varying degrees of liver injury will occur in up to 27% of cases of DILI, and of those, nearly 1 in 5 will develop chronic liver injury within 6 months and 1 in 10 will die or require liver transplantation to survive (Fontana et al. 2014).

In terms of the histopathology of liver injury associated with the psychotropic drugs, Voican et al. (2014) classified DILI as either hepatocellular, cholestatic, or mixed, depending on the presence or absence of an underlying liver injury. Hepatocellular injury was identified as having abnormally high serum alanine transaminase (ALT) levels with small or no increase in titers of alkaline phosphatase (ALP). If bilirubin levels are also elevated, this suggests that severe hepatocellular damage has occurred and is a marker of a poor prognosis. Cholestatic injury to the liver is characterized by high serum ALP levels with only slightly elevated levels of ALT and sometimes with elevated levels of bilirubin. In mixed injuries, both ALT and ALP titers are high. The authors reported that because serum transaminase levels less than three times the upper limit of normal (ULN) were found in 1%–5% of the general population, ALT levels greater than three times the ULN or ALP titers greater than two times the ULN are strongly suggestive of DILI.

Drug-Induced Liver Injury and Antiepileptic Drugs

The Drug-Induced Liver Injury Network (DILIN), funded by the National Institutes of Health, is a prospective multisite observational study of DILI in children and adults in the United States for which data collection began in 2004. In the DILIN's latest report of DILI from antiepileptic drugs (AEDs) from 2004 to 2020, academic centers from all over the United States reported on 1,711 participants with definite, highly likely, or probable DILI (Chalasani et al. 2021). Sixty-six participants (3.9%) had AED-associated DILI, and we report here on only the AEDs most relevant to the treatment of psychiatric illness; lamotrigine ($n=18$), carbamazepine ($n=11$), valproate ($n=10$), and gabapentin ($n=4$). The frequency of AED-associated liver injury was reported to significantly decrease during the study, from 8.5% of cases during 2004–2007 to 2.6% during 2015–2020. This may reflect greater use of safer second-generation AEDs. The study also found that compared with patients in the 2004–2007 cohort, patients in the 2015–2020 group at greatest risk were younger (mean age of 38.5 years vs. 50.1 years) and more likely to be African American (27% vs. 12%). It was found that a drug rash with eosinophilia and systemic symptoms was likely when liver injury was caused by lamotrigine or carbamazepine but not valproate or gabapentin. Liver injury was moderate to severe in most study participants, among whom five died and three required liver transplantation.

Another recent article on DILI associated with AEDs described data from the U.S. FDA Adverse Event Reporting System (Kamitaki et al. 2021). The purpose of this study was to quantify reports of DILI attributable to both older- and newer-generation AEDs. The authors analyzed data from 2.6 million adverse event reports from July 2018 to March 2020. Of the 2,175 DILI cases, 97.2% involved what were considered to be serious reactions, including death. AEDs with highest to lowest likelihood of causing a serious DILI (represented as reported odds ratios [RORs]) were carbamazepine (2.92), oxcarbazepine (2.58), valproate (2.22), lamotrigine (2.06), levetiracetam (1.56), and diazepam (1.53). Increased RORs for the development of serious DILI were not seen for clonazepam, pregabalin, cannabidiol, topiramate, and gabapentin.

Carbamazepine is associated with liver injury in all age groups but with no gender specificity (Devarbhavi and Andrade 2014). The clinical picture can range from an asymptomatic rise in liver chemistries to acute liver failure. Carbamazepine can also cause isolated asymptomatic γ-glutamyltransferase (GGT) elevations. These GGT elevations do not warrant stopping the medication, as long as bilirubin levels do not increase as well. This is also true for mild elevations in transaminases. When bilirubin levels do increase, carbamazepine must be stopped immediately because mortality or the need for liver transplantation has been estimated to be as high as 17% in such cases, especially in children younger than 10 years or when the patient has developed hepatocellular injury and DILI after several weeks of drug exposure. The typical latency period is 6–12 weeks.

Results from the DILIN study indicate that valproic acid is the most frequently implicated AED associated with drug-induced hepatotoxicity, affecting an age range of 2–47 years (median=27 years) (Devarbhavi and Andrade 2014). Valproic acid typically causes one of two types of liver injury. The more common type is characterized by a reversible relatively mild elevation in transaminases (ALT, ALP) and usually manifests without clinical symptoms. This reaction is dose dependent, typically occurs during initiation of treatment, and can occur in up to 44% of patients (Lopez and Hendrickson 2014). The second type of DILI associated with valproic acid is less common, but it is irreversible, idiosyncratic, and potentially fatal. Children younger than 2 years taking multiple AEDs are at greatest risk, but fatal outcomes in adults may be underestimated. The incidence is estimated to be 1 per 550 patients if valproic acid is used with other antiepileptic medications and 1 per 8,000 if it is used as a single agent (Lopez and Hendrickson 2014).

The putative mechanism for hepatotoxicity from valproic acid is related to its inhibition of fatty acid transport and mitochondrial β-oxidation (Devarbhavi and Andrade 2014). A deficiency in coenzyme A is thought to impair the mitochondrial enzymes responsible for breaking down fatty acids, which then results in a shift of the metabolism to a different type of oxidation reaction, thus generating hepatotoxic metabolites (Voican et al. 2014).

One such hepatotoxic metabolite is called 4-en-valproic acid, which can elevate serum ammonia levels by inhibiting urea production. Although hyperammonemia occurs in nearly 50% of patients receiving valproic acid, it remains asymptomatic in most cases (Lheureux et al. 2005). Rarely, patients taking valproic acid develop a severe form of hyperammonemic encephalopathy characterized by decreased consciousness, focal neurological deficits, asterixis, cognitive slowing, vomiting, lethargy, and increased seizure frequency (Segura-Bruna et al. 2006). These symptoms should prompt immediate discontinuation of the drug and screening for serum ammonia levels, which can be elevated despite normal liver chemistry results. Signs of severe hyperammonemic encephalopathy, which are evident on EEGs, can be reversed once valproic acid is discontinued. Another proposed mechanism for hyperammonemia is that valproic acid decreases serum levels and body stores of carnitine, an amino acid derivative that facilitates mitochondrial metabolism of ammonia. A deficiency of carnitine can therefore result in the accumulation of ammonia (Lheureux et al. 2005).

Elevations in levels of ammonia have been implicated more broadly in the development of hepatic encephalopathy due to hepatic failure in general. A review by Malaguarnera (2013) described the results of six randomized controlled studies of acetyl-L-carnitine (ALC) in the treatment of hepatic encephalopathy associated with hyperammonemia. In this review, Malaguarnera provided evidence suggesting that supplementation with 4 g daily of ALC improved physical and mental fatigue in patients who developed mild to moderate hepatic encephalopathy and significantly improved electroencephalographic parameters, cognitive and memory functions, and visual scanning and tracking in patients with severe hyperammonemic encephalopathy. Lopez and Hendrickson (2014) also reported that ALC benefited patients whose serum ammonia levels were greater than 450 mg/mL by facilitating fatty acid transport and regulating the ratio of coenzyme A into mitochondria. When serum ammonia levels were between 850 and 1,000 mg/mL in patients who also had hemodynamic instability or significant metabolic derangements or were in a coma, hemodialysis was shown to be beneficial.

Hepatotoxicity from lamotrigine is typically seen in the setting of rash and severe hypersensitivity reactions (Devarbhavi and Andrade 2014). Most symptoms will subside with discontinuation of the drug, but some cases will progress to Stevens-Johnson syndrome and toxic epidermal necrolysis. Younger age and rapid titration of the medicine can increase the risk of a DILI, and because valproic acid increases the serum lamotrigine concentration by more than 200%, giving both drugs simultaneously should be avoided whenever possible.

Drug-Induced Liver Injury and Antidepressant Drugs

A review of DILI and antidepressants reported that mild liver chemistry elevations were found in 0.5%–1% of patients treated with second-generation antidepressants such as SSRIs and SNRIs and in up to 3% of patients taking MAOIs, tricyclics, or tetracyclic antidepressants (Voican et al. 2014). The overall incidence of antidepressant-induced liver injury resulting in hospitalization is between 1.28 and 4 cases per 100,000 patient-years; however, the incidence is much higher with nefazodone (estimated to be 29 cases per 100,000 patient-years).

The mechanism of antidepressant-associated hepatic injury is usually hepatocellular and is thought to be metabolic or immune-allergic (Voican et al. 2014). As with the AEDs, patients with antidepressant-associated hepatic injury can present with a hypersensitivity syndrome of fever, rash, eosinophilia, autoantibodies, and a short latency period of between 1 and 6 weeks. When the latency period is longer (1 month to 1 year), the metabolic mechanism of hepatotoxicity is more likely to be idiosyncratic. Furthermore, Chen et al. (2013) found that high daily doses and high lipophilicity of an antidepressant are more predictive of liver injury. Interestingly, preexisting liver disease is not usually associated with a greater risk of antidepressant-associated DILI. However, duloxetine may pose some risk of DILI in people at risk for liver disease or in those with cirrhosis or chronic liver disease (Lin et al. 2015). Cases of acute liver failure leading to liver transplantation or death have been reported for the following antidepressants: phenelzine, imipramine, amitriptyline, venlafaxine, sertraline, bupropion, trazodone, and, in Europe, agomelatine (Voican et al. 2014).

Drug-Induced Liver Injury and Antipsychotic Drugs

Marwick et al. (2012) reviewed the literature concerning the association between regular antipsychotic use and abnormal liver function in adults and found that a median of 32% (5%–78%) of patients had abnormal liver chemistries while taking antipsychotics, and 4% (0%–15%) had clinically significant elevations in liver chemistries. Transaminases were the most likely liver enzymes to be elevated. Most cases were asymptomatic, arose within 6 weeks of starting the drug, and either resolved with ongoing treatment or stably persisted (Marwick et al. 2012).

Although there are case reports of multiple different antipsychotics associated with fatalities due to drug-induced hepatotoxicity, Marwick et al. (2012) found that chlorpromazine was the antipsychotic most commonly associated with acute liver injury. Liver injury associated with chlorpromazine use is thought to be due to the drug or its metabolites causing impairment of bile secretions, leading to cholestasis via immune-mediated mechanisms. A primary care database study in the United Kingdom was referenced that reported an incidence rate of chlorpromazine-associated liver injury of approximately 1.3 per 1,000 patients, with such injury being more likely to affect patients older than 70 years. Marwick et al. (2012) advised that patients with preexisting liver disease not be prescribed chlorpromazine. They also noted that because of the potential for patients with serious mental illness to develop antipsychotic-associated metabolic syndrome, patients taking antipsychotics long term may also be at increased risk for the development of nonalcoholic steatohepatitis, which can eventually lead to cirrhosis.

Valproic Acid and Acute Pancreatitis

Acute pancreatitis has been reported as an idiosyncratic reaction to therapeutic dosages of valproic acid in 1 per 40,000 treated patients (Gerstner et al. 2007). When valproic acid–induced pancreatitis does occur, it is most common in children, especially if they are being treated with multiple anticonvulsants. The onset is variable and ranges from drug initiation to several years after treatment initiation. The causative mechanisms are currently unknown. Diagnosis is based on the presence of abdominal pain, nausea, vomiting, anorexia, and fever and is associated with elevations in amylase and lipase. Mortality can reach 15%–20%, and treatment is supportive after discontinuation of valproic acid. Transient asymptomatic hyperamylasemia occurs in 20% of adult patients taking valproate but is unrelated to risk of pancreatitis (Gerstner et al. 2007). Drug-induced pancreatitis has been reported less often with other anticonvulsants (carbamazepine, lamotrigine, topiramate, levetiracetam, vigabatrin) (Zaccara et al. 2007), antipsychotics (clozapine, olanzapine, risperidone, haloperidol) (Koller et al. 2003), and antidepressants (mirtazapine, bupropion, venlafaxine, SSRIs) (Hussain and Burke 2008; Spigset et al. 2003). Alcohol use disorder increases the risk for drug-induced pancreatitis. Following recovery, the offending drug should not be reinstated; use of a drug from a different class is preferred (Dhir et al. 2007).

Renal Drug Reactions

Severe renal toxicity, including renal insufficiency and nephrogenic diabetes insipidus (NDI), has been associated primarily with lithium administration (Table 2–4). However, the syndrome of inappropriate antidiuretic hormone secretion (SIADH) leading to hyponatremia has been associated with several drug classes. These disorders necessitate careful clinical and laboratory monitoring to prevent irreversible kidney damage.

Chronic Renal Insufficiency

Lithium has been implicated in several disorders of kidney function, including renal tubular acidosis, interstitial nephritis, proteinuria with nephrotic syndrome, acute renal failure after intoxication, NDI, and chronic renal in-

Table 2–4. Renal drug reactions

Disorder	Implicated drugs	Risk factors	Signs and symptoms	Diagnostic studies[a]	Management[b]
Chronic renal insufficiency	Lithium	Elderly, duration of treatment, concomitant drugs (NSAIDs), lithium toxicity		Creatinine, creatinine clearance (at least every 3–6 months)	
Nephrogenic diabetes insipidus	Lithium, pimozide, alcohol		Excessive urine volume → dehydration, encephalopathy, lithium toxicity	Water deprivation Serum vasopressin Response to exogenous vasopressin	Monitor urinary output Specific agents (amiloride, thiazides, NSAIDs)?

Table 2–4.   Renal drug reactions *(continued)*

Disorder	Implicated drugs	Risk factors	Signs and symptoms	Diagnostic studies[a]	Management[b]
Acute hyponatremia (SIADH)	Antipsychotics Antidepressants (tricyclics, SSRIs, SNRIs) Opiates		Nausea, vomiting, anorexia, dysgeusia, disorientation, confusion, fatigue, headaches, weakness, irritability, lethargy, muscle cramps → delirium, hallucinations, diminished consciousness, seizures, coma, respiratory arrest	Hyponatremia Elevated urine, reduced plasma osmolality	Hyponatremic encephalopathy: hypertonic fluids[c]
Chronic hyponatremia (SIADH)	Antipsychotics Antidepressants (tricyclics, SSRIs, SNRIs) Opiates		Impaired cognition, falls, mood changes		Fluid restriction[c] Specific agents (clozapine, demeclocycline, conivaptan, tolvaptan)?

Note.   NSAIDs=nonsteroidal anti-inflammatory drugs; SIADH=syndrome of inappropriate antidiuretic hormone secretion; SNRIs=serotonin-norepinephrine reuptake inhibitors; SSRIs=selective serotonin reuptake inhibitors.

[a]Standard imaging and laboratory studies to rule out other conditions in the differential diagnosis or complications are assumed. Only studies associated with or specific to each reaction are listed.

[b]Mainstay of management in all reactions includes careful monitoring, prompt recognition, rapid cessation of the offending drug, and supportive medical care. Only specific therapies that have been reported are listed. A question mark indicates lack of evidence of safety and efficacy.

[c]Risk of central pontine or extrapontine myelinolysis (mood changes, lethargy, mutism, dysarthria, pseudobulbar palsy, and quadriplegia) if serum sodium corrected by >8 mmol/L over 24-hour period.

sufficiency progressing to end-stage renal disease (Oliveira et al. 2010; Raedler and Wiedemann 2007). Histopathological studies indicate that approximately 10%–20% of the patients receiving long-term lithium therapy demonstrate changes, including tubular atrophy, interstitial fibrosis, cysts, and glomerular sclerosis.

Evidence supports an association between long-term lithium treatment and progressive renal insufficiency (Raedler and Wiedemann 2007). Studies have shown that about 15%–20% of patients show evidence of reduced renal function after 10 years of taking lithium. Abnormalities may develop as early as 1 year after beginning treatment. Kidney dysfunction is related to duration of lithium treatment and is progressive, even after lithium is discontinued in some cases. The rate of progression is variable; although many patients show a decreased filtration rate, few develop renal insufficiency, and frank renal failure is rare. In a study among dialysis patients, 0.22% had lithium-induced nephropathy (Presne et al. 2003). Fogo and associates (2017) estimated that end-stage renal disease occurs in 1.5% of long-term lithium users, although more recent studies suggest lower rates (Van Alphen et al. 2021). No reliable risk factors predict renal failure, but decreased renal function has been associated with duration of treatment, age, concomitant medications (e.g., nonsteroidal anti-inflammatory drugs [NSAIDs], especially indomethacin), and episodes of lithium toxicity.

Management focuses on prevention by screening patients for underlying kidney disease, discussing risks and benefits of treatment, using lowest effective doses, avoiding lithium intoxication, carefully monitoring lithium levels, measuring kidney function every 3–6 months or as indicated by the patient's condition, and reassessing risks of continuing lithium if renal function declines. Useful measures to follow include serum level of creatinine, glomerular filtration rate, and urinalyses (Jefferson 2010). Imaging studies of the kidneys, especially MRI, have been helpful in determining whether renal dysfunction is related to lithium by detecting the presence of characteristic renal microcysts (Ali and El-Mallakh 2021; Karaosmanoglu et al. 2013). Withdrawal of lithium after prolonged treatment may not result in reversal of kidney dysfunction; rather, kidney function may continue to decline and, conversely, may increase the risk of psychiatric relapse with associated risk of suicide (Rej et al. 2012; Werneke et al. 2012).

Nephrogenic Diabetes Insipidus

In early studies, impairment in urine concentration with resulting polyuria, which was observed in 20%–30% of patients receiving lithium, was considered benign (Khanna 2006). However, some patients went on to develop acquired NDI, a condition whose most common cause is lithium. NDI is defined as the inability of the kidneys to concentrate urine, resulting in excessive volumes of dilute urine caused by the insensitivity of the distal nephron to the antidiuretic hormone, vasopressin. Although mild cases, which may occur within a few weeks of initiating treatment, can be compensated by increased fluid intake, severe cases can result in dehydration, hypernatremia, neurological symptoms, encephalopathy, and lithium intoxication. NDI can be congenital or acquired from drugs, including pimozide and alcohol in addition to lithium (Moeller et al. 2013).

The diagnosis of NDI can be confirmed and distinguished from primary psychogenic polydipsia by comparing urine and plasma osmolality during a water deprivation or dehydration test (Garofeanu et al. 2005; Khanna 2006; Moeller et al. 2013). In psychogenic polydipsia, patients will show concentration of urine (osmolality >500 mOsmol/kg with plasma osmolality >295 mOsmol/kg) after water deprivation, whereas patients with NDI will continue to show dilute urine (<300 mOsmol/kg). To distinguish NDI from central diabetes insipidus, plasma vasopressin is measured after dehydration. In NDI, plasma vasopressin exceeds 5 ng/L, whereas in central diabetes insipidus, vasopressin will be reduced or negligible. After exogenous vasopressin, patients with central diabetes insipidus will increase urine osmolality, whereas patients with NDI will experience little or no change (Khanna 2006).

Although the mechanism of lithium-induced NDI has been attributed to the effects of lithium on aquaporin-2, probably through interference in the adenylate cyclase system, more recent evidence suggests multifactorial effects on signaling pathways and cellular organization of the tubular system (Khanna 2006; Moeller et al. 2013). Aquaporin-2 is the primary target for vasopressin regulation of collecting duct water permeability. Downregulation of aquaporin-2 expression is only partially reversed after lithium discontinuation, which is consistent with findings suggesting that NDI can become irreversible even after lithium discontinuation, depending on the duration of treatment. Although impaired concentration is usually reversible within 1–2 years of treatment, concentrating capacity may not improve at all after 10–20 years of lithium treatment (Garofeanu et al. 2005).

Management of NDI consists of regular monitoring of urinary symptoms and output, with testing of urine osmolality and electrolytes as necessary, followed by discontinuation of lithium. Current evidence supports the use of amiloride as treatment for NDI, but thiazide diuretics and NSAIDs have been suggested as well, although close monitoring of lithium levels, which can be raised by these agents, is required (Moeller et al. 2013; Rej et al. 2012).

Syndrome of Inappropriate Antidiuretic Hormone Secretion

The converse of diabetes insipidus is the retention of water resulting in hyponatremia. Hyponatremia may occur in 5%–15% of chronic psychiatric patients (Siegel 2008; Sterns 2015). In such patients, both psychogenic polydipsia and the psychotropic drug–induced SIADH represent prominent causes of hyponatremia, with SIADH the leading cause (Ellison and Berl 2007; see Chapter 5, "Renal and Urological Disorders"). The severity of symptoms is related to the rate of onset as well as the absolute serum level of sodium. In acute-onset hyponatremia, patients may first develop nausea, vomiting, anorexia, dysgeusia, disorientation, headache, fatigue, weakness, irritability, lethargy, confusion, and muscle cramps, with progression to hypotonic encephalopathy characterized by impaired responsiveness, delirium, and hallucinations. If the condition is not corrected, the resulting cerebral edema may result in seizures, coma, and death from cerebral herniation, brain stem compression, and respiratory arrest (Ellison and Berl 2007; Siegel 2008). Patients with slow-onset or chronic hyponatremia may be asymptomatic or may present with impaired cognition, frequent falls, anxiety, and depression, after an adaptive response to hypotonicity restores brain volume.

SIADH is diagnosed in patients with normal renal, thyroid, and adrenal function who develop hyponatremia (serum sodium concentration <135 mmol/L) with reduced plasma osmolality, reduced renal excretion of sodium, absence of volume depletion or overload, and elevated urine osmolality despite plasma hypotonicity. Phenothiazines, tricyclics, anticonvulsants (carbamazepine, valproic acid, and oxcarbazepine), atypical antipsychotics (except for clozapine, which has shown positive results, correcting idiopathic hyponatremia in schizophrenia patients; Canuso and Goldman 1999), opiates, and SSRIs and SNRIs have been implicated in causing SIADH from stimulating release of or enhancing renal sensitivity to vasopressin. The incidence of hyponatremia with SSRIs has been reported to range from 0.5% to 32% of patients, with elderly patients at highest risk (Siegel 2008). Use of NSAIDs in those with SIADH increases the risk and severity of developing hyponatremia. SIADH associated with psychotropic drugs usually has a slow onset and reverses within 24–48 hours after the drugs are discontinued. However, if the hyponatremia is asymptomatic and undetected, sodium levels can decrease to dangerous levels (<125 mmol/L), resulting in acute encephalopathy.

Treatment depends on the severity and duration of the hyponatremia and neuropsychiatric symptoms (Woodward et al. 2018). Definitive treatment consists of discontinuing the causative drug. Acute, symptomatic, life-threatening hyponatremic encephalopathy is a medical emergency, dictating the need for treatment with hypertonic solutions to reverse cerebral edema. Management of patients with chronic hyponatremia of uncertain onset or with absence of symptoms is less clear. With a lower risk of neurological sequelae of hyponatremia, patients with longer durations of hyponatremia are paradoxically at higher risk for osmotic demyelination if the serum sodium level is corrected by more than 8 mmol/L over a 24-hour period (Ellison and Berl 2007; Sterns 2015). Osmotic demyelination, resulting in central pontine or extrapontine myelinolysis, begins with affective changes and lethargy, progressing to mutism, dysarthria, spastic quadriplegia, and pseudobulbar palsy. For patients with chronic hyponatremia, fluid restriction can be an effective critical intervention but can be burdensome and difficult to enforce and monitor. Use of saline infusions or salt tablets has limited evidence (Woodward et al. 2018). Several medications have been tried as well (e.g., demeclocycline, which inhibits vasopressin), but recently developed vasopressin-receptor antagonists or vaptans (e.g., tolvaptan) offer a promising treatment for chronic hypervolemic or euvolemic hyponatremia resulting from drug-induced SIADH in patients with sodium levels lower than 125 mmol/L or in patients with hyponatremia and sodium levels greater than 125 mmol/L with symptoms. Vaptans can increase serum sodium concentrations by increasing electrolyte-free water excretion (Benoit et al. 2018; Josiassen et al. 2008; Woodward et al. 2018). However, the effects of vasopressin antagonists on serum sodium levels are delayed, such that these agents are not useful in patients who have acute CNS symptoms. Because of the risk of osmotic demyelination, effects on sodium should be frequently monitored. The use of vasopressin antagonists in patients with chronic hyponatremia, who may require maintenance treatment with antipsychotics, for example, has yet to be established.

Hematological Drug Reactions

Essentially all classes of psychotropic drugs have been associated with blood dyscrasias (Table 2–5) (Flanagan and Dunk 2008). Serious hematological toxicity is rare, with an annual incidence of only 1–2 per 100,000 population. The white blood cells are affected most commonly, resulting in neutropenia (absolute neutrophil count < 1,500/mm^3) or agranulocytosis (neutrophils < 500/mm^3). Blood dyscrasias may result from a direct toxic effect on the bone marrow, peripheral destruction, or formation of antibodies that target the hematopoietic cells or their precursors. Antipsychotics are most likely to cause neutropenia or agranulocytosis (Nooijen et al. 2011). Among patients beginning therapy with clozapine, 3% may develop neutropenia and 0.8% may develop agranulocytosis, usually in the first year of treatment (Alvir et al. 1993). This was confirmed by a more recent meta-analysis that included 108 studies and found that the incidence of clozapine-associated neutropenia was 3.8%, and the incidence of agranulocytosis was 0.9% (Myles et al. 2018). The development of neutropenia (< 1,500/mm^3) was associated with a fatality rate of 0.013%, whereas the development of agranulocytosis (< 500/mm^3) was associated with a fatality rate of 2.1%. Another consideration when prescribing clozapine is treatment of gastroesophageal reflux disease, a common side effect, with proton pump inhibitors. Using a proton pump inhibitor in combination with clozapine has been shown to increase the risk of neutropenia and agranulocytosis (Wiciński et al. 2017).

The risk of neutropenia in patients taking phenothiazines may be 1 per 10,000, and for patients taking chlorpromazine, the risk of agranulocytosis is 0.13% (Flanagan and Dunk 2008). Tohen et al. (1995) reported that 2.1% of 977 patients given carbamazepine developed mild (3,000–4,000/mm^3) or moderate (< 3,000/mm^3) neutropenia, about six to seven times higher in rate than with valproic acid or antidepressants.

Clinically, drug-induced neutropenia will become evident after 1–2 weeks of therapy; the degree of the neutropenia is related to the dose and duration of exposure. Recovery can be expected within 3–4 weeks after stopping the caus-

Table 2–5. Hematological drug reactions

Disorders	Implicated drugs	Risk factors	Signs and symptoms	Diagnostic studies[a]	Management[b]
Neutropenia and agranulocytosis	Antipsychotics (clozapine, chlorpromazine) Anticonvulsants (carbamazepine)	Older age, Asian ethnicity, concurrent proton pump inhibitors	Fever, infection	CBC with differential	G-CSF and GM-CSF have been shown to reduce duration
Thrombocytopenia	Antipsychotics Antidepressants (SSRI effects on platelet function) Benzodiazepines	Existing coagulopathies, high dosages	Hemorrhages	Platelet count	Dose reduction, rather than discontinuation, may suffice
Anemia	Antipsychotics (chlorpromazine, clozapine, risperidone) Antidepressants (MAOIs, SSRIs) Anticonvulsants (valproic acid, oxcarbazepine) Benzodiazepines		Weakness, fatigue	CBC	

Note. CBC = complete blood count; G-CSF = granulocyte colony-stimulating factor; GM-CSF = granulocyte-macrophage colony-stimulating factor; MAOIs = monoamine oxidase inhibitors; SSRIs = selective serotonin reuptake inhibitors.

[a]Standard imaging and laboratory studies to rule out other conditions in the differential diagnosis or complications are assumed. Only studies associated with or specific to each reaction are listed.

[b]Mainstay of management in all reactions includes careful monitoring, prompt recognition, rapid cessation of the offending drug, and supportive medical care. Only specific therapies that have been reported are listed.

ative drug. Agranulocytosis can take longer to appear, up to 3–4 weeks after starting treatment. With clozapine, the risk of agranulocytosis is greatest during the first 18 weeks of treatment; it is rare to see it develop beyond 6 months. After the first year, the risk of clozapine-induced agranulocytosis is estimated at 0.39 per 1,000 patients per year (Mijovic and MacCabe 2020). There is an increased risk of clozapine-induced agranulocytosis in elderly people, and the risk in Asian populations has been reported to be 2.4 times higher than in Caucasians (Mijovic and MacCabe 2020). A report by Alvir et al. (1993) that the risk of agranulocytosis was greater in female patients was not confirmed by subsequent studies. After 6 months of treatment, the risk with clozapine may be similar to the risk with other antipsychotic medications (Nooijen et al. 2011).

In the United States, clozapine therapy should be discontinued if the absolute neutrophil count declines to less than $1,000/mm^3$. The only exception would be in a Black patient previously diagnosed with benign essential neutropenia, in which case discontinuation of clozapine would occur at a neutrophil count lower than $500/mm^3$ (Mijovic and MacCabe 2020).

For patients taking drugs known to cause neutropenia or agranulocytosis, proper management involves obtaining a complete blood count (CBC) with differential initially and periodically. A strict protocol of monitoring in patients taking clozapine, along with treatment including broad-spectrum antibiotics, supportive care, and agents to stimulate the production of granulocytes, has resulted in a decrease in the mortality from clozapine-induced agranulocytosis from 3%–4% to 0.01% (Meltzer et al. 2002; Nooijen et al. 2011). Granulocyte colony-stimulating factor (G-CSF) and granulocyte-macrophage colony-stimulating factor (GM-CSF) have been shown to be well tolerated and may reduce the duration of clozapine-induced agranulocytosis (Lally et al. 2017). Fever or infection, particularly pharyngitis, may be the only symptom of neutropenia or agranulocytosis and is an indication for withholding the drugs until a CBC with differential can be performed.

Although they occur less frequently than problems with white blood cells, platelet abnormalities have been associated with psychotropic drugs. SSRIs decrease platelet serotonin, which may cause a decrease in platelet function and prolongation of bleeding time. Patients with known coagulation disorders or von Willebrand disease and those taking NSAIDs and coumarin should be monitored if SSRIs are prescribed (Halperin and Reber 2007). Some evidence indicates that serotonergic antidepressants and antipsychotics may be associated with increased risk of hospitalization for bleeding, especially in new users of the drugs, probably as a result of decreased platelet aggregation (Verdel et al. 2011). Previous work by this same group showed an association between serotonergic antidepressant drugs and the need for perioperative blood transfusion in orthopedic surgery, whereas nonserotonergic drugs showed no such association (Movig et al. 2003). Clinicians and patients should be aware of the potential for bleeding during procedures.

Most of the typical and atypical antipsychotics have been reported to cause thrombocytopenia. Clozapine has also been reported to cause thrombocytosis, and there are case reports of quetiapine-induced thrombotic thrombocytopenic purpura (Husnain et al. 2017). Valproate monotherapy has been associated with thrombocytopenia and rare bleeding complications, with potential risk factors being increasing serum levels, female sex, and lower baseline platelet count (Nasreddine and Beydoun 2008). A review by Buoli et al. (2018) found the incidence of thrombocytopenia in patients taking valproic acid to be 12%–18%. Risk factors were again found to be female sex, advanced age, and dosage in excess of 1 g/day or serum valproate level greater than 100 μg/mL (Acharya and Bussel 2000). A decrease in dose, rather than discontinuation, in those patients who developed thrombocytopenia was sufficient to return platelet counts to a normal range. Caution is advised when prescribing valproic acid to elderly women, especially at dosages greater than 1 g/day. In addition, patients taking valproic acid should have a hematological evaluation, including platelet function studies, prior to surgical procedures (Kumar et al. 2019). Thrombocytopenia also has been reported with tricyclic antidepressants, MAOIs, and benzodiazepines.

Chlorpromazine, clozapine, risperidone, and sertraline have also been associated with anemia. There are case reports of valproic acid causing pure red cell aplasia, which resolves when the drug is discontinued (Bartakke et al. 2008). Oxcarbazepine was reported to cause hemolytic anemia in an elderly man, which resolved after discontinuation of the drug (Chaudhry et al. 2008). Lithium has been well known to cause leukocytosis and thrombocytosis. Pancytopenia has been reported with fluphenazine and lamotrigine.

Discontinuation of the offending drug is usually followed by hematological recovery. If the patient cannot be prescribed a different class of drug, hematology consultation should be obtained regarding appropriate monitoring of hematological parameters.

Metabolic Drug Reactions and Body as a Whole

Antipsychotic-Induced Heatstroke

Patients with serious mental illness have an increased risk of heatstroke (Bark 1998; Page et al. 2012), related to behavioral and environmental factors. For example, Page et al. (2012), in a primary care cohort study, found that patients with psychosis, dementia, or substance abuse and those prescribed sedatives or antipsychotics had more than twice the risk of heat-related mortality compared with control subjects. Furthermore, climate change is triggering an increased number of days with dangerously elevated temperatures and more frequent heat waves, both of which disproportionately affect the mentally ill (Rublee et al. 2021). Thermal effects of climate change are magnified in large cities, where psychiatric patients often reside. Antipsychotic drugs can promote heatstroke by impairing heat loss (Mann and Boger 1978) (Table 2–6). Substantial evidence supports a key role for dopamine in preoptic-anterior hypothalamic thermoregulatory heat loss mechanisms (Lee et al. 1985). All typical antipsychotics promote hyperthermia by blocking dopamine receptors. The role of atypical antipsychotics in suppressing heat loss appears less clear. Although atypical antipsychotics block dopamine receptors, they also block 5-HT_{2C} and postsynaptic 5-HT_{1A} receptors, which participate in heat loss mechanisms, suggesting that atypical antipsychotics could further promote hyperthermia in a hot environment (Mann 2003).

In most cases, anticholinergic-induced inhibition of sweating appears to contribute significantly to the development of antipsychotic-induced heatstroke. Low-potency typical antipsychotic drugs having marked anticholinergic activity are frequent offenders, whereas heatstroke associated with high-potency typical antipsychotic drugs often involves concurrent treatment with anticholinergic drugs (Clark and Lipton 1984). In addition, some atypical antipsychotics (clozapine, quetiapine, and olanzapine) possess anticholinergic activity. Comorbid medical illnesses—especially cardiovascular disease, which necessitates treatment with drugs such as diuretics that may also impair thermoregulation—and substance abuse further increase the risk of heatstroke.

Clark and Lipton (1984) reviewed 45 cases of antipsychotic-induced heatstroke and concluded that the majority of cases resembled classic environmental heatstroke. Classic heatstroke is characterized by body temperature greater than 40.6°C, anhidrosis, and profound CNS dysfunction, typically

Table 2–6. Metabolic drug reactions and body as a whole

Disorder	Implicated drugs	Risk factors	Signs and symptoms	Diagnostic studies[a]	Management[b]
Drug-induced heatstroke					
Classic heatstroke	Antipsychotics Anticholinergics	Heat waves, systemic illness, older age	Hyperthermia, anhidrosis, confusion → multiorgan failure, delirium, coma, seizures		Rapid cooling measures
Exertional heatstroke	Antipsychotics Anticholinergics	Exertion, heat waves	Hyperthermia, rhabdomyolysis, confusion, metabolic acidosis → multiorgan failure, delirium, coma, seizures		Rapid cooling measures
Diabetic ketoacidosis	Antipsychotics (clozapine, olanzapine)	African American, younger age	Anorexia, nausea, vomiting, polydipsia, polyuria → altered mental status, coma	Urine ketones	

Table 2–6. Metabolic drug reactions and body as a whole *(continued)*

Disorder	Implicated drugs	Risk factors	Signs and symptoms	Diagnostic studies[a]	Management[b]
Rhabdomyolysis	Antipsychotics Alcohol Stimulants Hallucinogens	Agitation, trauma, substance abuse, injections, restraints, dystonia	Weakness, myalgias, edema, dark urine → compartment syndromes, DIC, renal failure, hyperkalemia, arrhythmias	Serum CK (>5 times normal), other muscle enzymes, myoglobin, electrolytes (potassium), urinalysis	Fluid repletion, alkalinization of urine, correction of electrolytes

Note. CK=creatine kinase; DIC=disseminated intravascular coagulation.

[a]Standard imaging and laboratory studies to rule out other conditions in the differential diagnosis or complications are assumed. Only studies associated with or specific to each reaction are listed.

[b]Mainstay of management in all reactions includes careful monitoring, prompt recognition, rapid cessation of the offending drug, and supportive medical care. Only specific therapies that have been reported are listed.

occurring during summer heat waves in elderly and medically compromised patients. Other cases associated with antipsychotics, however, resembled exertional heatstroke, which occurs primarily in young, healthy people with normal thermoregulatory capacity in whom muscular work in a hot environment exceeds the body's capacity for heat loss. Both forms of heatstroke may result in multiorgan failure, with lactic acidosis, rhabdomyolysis, coagulopathy, and renal failure occurring more commonly in exertional heatstroke. CNS manifestations include delirium, stupor, coma, seizures, pupillary dysfunction, and cerebellar symptoms.

Antipsychotic-induced heatstroke is a preventable condition. During summer heat waves, psychiatric patients must be warned to avoid excessive heat, sunlight, and exertion and should be urged to drink fluids. Air-conditioning probably represents the most effective way of preventing heatstroke, with even an hour a day helpful. Heatstroke is a medical emergency and may be fatal in up to 50% of cases. All forms of treatment aim at rapid cooling, fluid and electrolyte support, and management of seizures.

Diabetic Ketoacidosis

A serious life-threatening complication of diabetes is diabetic ketoacidosis (DKA). The rate of type 2 diabetes in patients with schizophrenia is two to five times that in the general population (Suvisaari et al. 2016). Schizophrenia and diabetes may share overlapping susceptibility genes, and there is added risk with antipsychotic medications (Vuk et al. 2017b). Weight gain and hyperglycemia, hallmarks of diabetes, are two of the most frequent side effects of second-generation antipsychotics, even at therapeutic doses. First-generation antipsychotics—chlorpromazine in particular—also increase the risk of weight gain (Solmi et al. 2017; Vancampfort et al. 2015). Given the risk of diabetes and the lethality of DKA, there is a black box warning for monitoring weight, fasting glucose, and lipids while prescribing antipsychotics (American Diabetes Association et al. 2004).

DKA occurs in patients requiring exogenous insulin. DKA most often happens in type 1 diabetes, but it can occur in type 2 diabetes mellitus (Vuk et al. 2017b). DKA results from persistent hyperglycemia, increased concentration of ketones, and metabolic acidosis. It arises when patients have insulinopenia and glucose cannot be transported into the cells. Hence, fatty acids are broken down for energy, creating an acidotic state. The clinical manifestations are anorexia, nausea, vomiting, polydipsia, polyuria, hyperglycemia, ketoacidosis, and ketonuria. One of the first-line laboratory assessments to determine DKA is to test urine for ketones. If DKA is untreated, altered mental status ensues and eventually coma or death.

Epidemiological studies show that DKA-related hospitalizations have been higher over the past 20 years, reaching rates of 32.4 per 1,000 among adults younger than 45 years, 3.3 between ages 45 and 64, and 1.4 in those age 65 or older (Benoit et al. 2018; Vuk et al. 2017b). Underlying infections are a leading risk factor for DKA that needs to be assessed and treated. Psychological stress, pancreatitis, surgery, or myocardial ischemia may precipitate DKA (Polcwiartek et al. 2016). Of note, these stressful and physiological conditions are less likely a factor in drug-induced DKA (Ely et al. 2013).

DKA occurs 10 times more often in patients with schizophrenia and at a younger age when antipsychotic medications are added (Correll et al. 2015; Lahijani and Harris 2017; Ramaswamy et al. 2007). Second-generation antipsychotics are also used for bipolar disorder and augmentation for depression (Solmi et al. 2017). Thus, monitoring these patients for adverse side effects is also warranted. The rate of DKA in patients taking antipsychotics with a diagnosis of diabetes is 30 times higher than the rate in those without an established diagnosis of diabetes (Lipscombe et al. 2014; Vuk et al. 2017b). DKA has occurred in patients with schizophrenia as the presenting complication of antipsychotic-induced diabetes. DKA can occur throughout the course of treatment with antipsychotic medications, most often in the first 6 months, even in patients without substantial weight gain, and the risk is not dose dependent. In a Department of Veterans Affairs study (Leslie and Rosenheck 2004), 0.2% of all patients taking antipsychotic medications required hospitalization for DKA. Hazard ratios for DKA were significant only for clozapine and olanzapine. Among second-generation antipsychotics, quetiapine and risperidone had less risk of causing DKA, whereas ziprasidone and aripiprazole were infrequently associated with DKA, although all required a class black box warning (Guo et al. 2006). Taking multiple antipsychotic medications concurrently compounds the occurrence of DKA (Correll et al. 2007). The mortality rate of antipsychotic-associated DKA is approximately 13% (Vuk et al. 2017b).

Recognition of DKA is imperative along with lifesaving management in patients receiving antipsychotic medications. Patients need education about recognizing symptoms that herald DKA, such as reduction in appetite, nausea and vomiting, frequent urination, dry mouth, and weakness. When managing DKA, the clinician should first discontinue antipsychotics. DKA should be treated with intravenous insulin, volume repletion, electrolyte replacement, and carbohydrate-controlled diet. Any underlying conditions, such as infections, acute pancreatitis, and cardiac ischemia, should be identified and treated (Newton and Raskin 2004). Vuk et al. (2017a) found that when the offending antipsychotic was discontinued, acute treatment with insulin and fluid repletion most often led to resolution of antipsychotic-associated DKA.

Because patients may continue to need treatment with antipsychotics after DKA, it is prudent to change to a metabolically neutral or lower-propensity agent that may reverse glucose elevation. Reinitiating the offending agent, especially clozapine and olanzapine, is most likely to result in diabetes or DKA. Adding medications for treatment of diabetes is critical, and careful titration and glucose monitoring are required. Blood glucose levels should be carefully monitored and hypoglycemic agents adjusted accordingly when changing antipsychotic agents in patients with diabetes. If not contraindicated, metformin is the medication of choice for treatment because it is unlikely to cause hypoglycemia. Based on a review of case reports, Guenette et al. (2013) found that most patients who developed antipsychotic-associated DKA were subsequently treated with a different second-generation antipsychotic in combination with insulin or oral antidiabetic agents.

Prior to starting treatment with antipsychotic medications, the clinician should ascertain individual and family histories of diabetes. Antipsychotic medication that has less propensity to cause weight gain and diabetes should be used unless a clear reason exists to select a different agent because of efficacy. Polypharmacy should be avoided. Patients should receive education about medication side effects, and body mass index, fasting glucose level, and fasting lipid levels should be monitored according to guidelines (American Diabetes Association et al. 2004).

Rhabdomyolysis

Rhabdomyolysis results from injury to skeletal muscle cells, with leakage of myoglobin, aldolase, potassium, lactate dehydrogenase, transaminases, CK, and phosphate into the extracellular space and general circulation (Cervellin et al. 2010; Khan 2009). The classic triad of clinical symptoms consists of weakness; muscle pain; and dark, cola-colored urine if myoglobinuria occurs. However, rhabdomyolysis may be detected coincidentally on laboratory examination in patients who are otherwise asymptomatic (Masi et al. 2014). Serious complications include compartment syndromes; arrhythmias from hyperkalemia; disseminated intravascular coagulation; and acute tubular necrosis with renal failure, which occurs in up to 16.5% of patients with myoglobinuria (David 2000). The estimated risk of mortality associated with rhabdomyolysis is 8% (Cervellin et al. 2010).

Diagnosis of rhabdomyolysis can be confirmed by the CK level, which is the most sensitive indicator of muscle damage and correlates with degree of muscle necrosis. Most authorities agree that at least a fivefold increase in CK (>1,000 U/L) is consistent with the diagnostic threshold (Walter and Catenacci 2008). Other muscle enzymes may be elevated as well (aldolase, transaminase, aspartate transaminase/ALT). Myoglobin is released and cleared earlier than CK and is therefore less reliable in diagnosing muscle breakdown, and it is not predicted by a specific CK level. Patients with unexplained elevations of muscle enzymes should be referred for thorough diagnostic evaluation, which includes workup for underlying neuromuscular genetic diseases, infections, hypothyroidism, and trauma (Cervellin et al. 2010; Khan 2009).

Elevations of CK are often observed in psychiatric patients, who are at risk for several reasons, such as agitation, physical trauma, use of restraints, intramuscular injections, prolonged immobility, and dystonia (Melkersson 2006; Meltzer et al. 1996). Elevations in CK levels may occur in association with other disorders (e.g., NMS, heatstroke, serotonin syndrome, seizures) but may be observed independently.

CK level elevations and rhabdomyolysis leading to kidney failure are commonly associated with abuse of substances (especially alcohol, cocaine, amphetamines, hallucinogens, and phencyclidine), some of which (ketamine, 3,4-methylenedioxymethamphetamine) are receiving potential approval for therapeutic indications (Schifano et al. 2016). But antipsychotics are most associated with increases in CK levels, occasionally resulting in frank rhabdomyolysis (Li et al. 2020). For example, Star et al. (2012) found 26 cases of rhabdomyolysis in children and adolescents treated with antipsychotics among reports of adverse reactions in a World Health Organization database; 6 of these cases were associated with NMS, but the other 20 occurred without evidence of NMS. Most symptomatic patients presented with muscle and abdominal pain and dark urine, which usually developed within 2 months of drug initiation or dosage changes (Star et al. 2012). A review of published cases (Laoutidis and Kioulos 2014) reported a prevalence of significant CK level elevations in 2%–7% of antipsychotic-treated patients. Meltzer et al. (1996) found significant increases in CK levels in 11 of 121 patients (9%) who received antipsychotic drugs. Peak levels ranged from 1,591 to 177,363 IU/L (median = 11,004 IU/L), with only 1 patient developing myoglobinuria. Onset ranged from 5 days to 2 years after initiation of drug treatment, and elevations lasted from 4 to 28 days. Most patients were asymptomatic without complications. CK level elevations were more common with atypical antipsychotics. Similarly, Melkersson (2006) studied 49 patients receiving clozapine (median = 66 IU/L; range = 30–299 IU/L), olanzapine (median = 81 IU/L; range = 30–713 IU/L), or typical antipsychotics (median = 48 IU/L; range = 17–102 IU/L) and found that CK levels were higher and more often elevated in patients receiving the atypical drugs, although reported increases were minimal in comparison with the findings of Meltzer et al. (1996). Laoutidis et al. (2015) found four cases of patients treated with amisulpride in a pharmacovigilance database who developed myalgias and elevated CK concentrations ranging from 1,498 to 21,018 IU/L. The reasons for overrepresentation of atypical drugs is unclear, but it may be an artifact of increased recognition and reporting in the years since introduction of these drugs (Laoutidis and Kioulos 2014).

Management of rhabdomyolysis rests on monitoring to detect clinical signs, including assessment of CK levels and myoglobinuria in symptomatic patients. Discontinuation of suspected drugs with correction of any predisposing risk factors and prevention of complications are essential. It is important to remember that prescription drugs apart from psychotropics (e.g., statins, antiretrovirals) are also associated with rhabdomyolysis (Klopstock 2008). General supportive measures include aggressive volume and fluid repletion, correction of electrolyte abnormalities, and use of mannitol or alkalinization of the urine to prevent renal failure; hemodialysis may become necessary in some cases. In contrast, the clinical significance of mild or asymptomatic CK level elevations during pharmacotherapy is unclear (Masi et al. 2014). A careful differential diagnosis of CK level elevations should be considered. Although patients with pronounced elevations should be followed up and managed to prevent progression to rhabdomyolysis and renal failure and risk factors should be identified and corrected (by holding or switching suspected drugs such as antipsychotics), only limited data suggest that mild asymptomatic CK level elevations correlate with risk of developing NMS or other acute or chronic complications (Hermesh et al. 2002a, 2002b). In most asymptomatic cases of CK level elevation, close monitoring alone or stopping or switching the antipsychotic drug may be sufficient. Laoutidis and Kioulos (2014) proposed a reasonable management algorithm for detecting, diagnosing, and treating patients who have CK level elevations.

Key Points

- Severe psychotropic drug reactions are best managed by careful monitoring, familiarity with adverse symptoms, prompt recognition, rapid drug discontinuation or modification, and supportive treatment.

- Adverse CNS syndromes are diverse and are associated mostly with antipsychotic and antidepressant drugs.

- Antipsychotic and antidepressant drugs have been associated with arrhythmias and sudden death.

- Severe hepatic toxicity is mostly associated with antiepileptic drugs.

- Severe renal syndromes are primarily associated with lithium, but the syndrome of inappropriate antidiuretic hormone secretion is associated with several drug classes.

- Several psychotropic drug classes are associated with hematological toxicity.

- Lives can be saved by maintaining awareness of and a high index of suspicion for potentially lethal iatrogenic drug reactions.

- Severe drug reactions provide evidence for the importance of careful postmarketing surveillance measures to detect rare and serious drug reactions.

References

Aarsland D, Perry R, Larsen JP, et al: Neuroleptic sensitivity in Parkinson's disease and parkinsonian dementias. J Clin Psychiatry 66(5):633–637, 2005 15889951

Abadie D, Rousseau V, Logerot S, et al: Serotonin syndrome: analysis of cases registered in the French Pharmacovigilance Database. J Clin Psychopharmacol 35(4):382–388, 2015 26082973

Acharya S, Bussel JB: Hematologic toxicity of sodium valproate. J Pediatr Hematol Oncol 22(1):62–65, 2000 10695824

Alawami M, Wasywich C, Cicovic A, et al: A systematic review of clozapine induced cardiomyopathy. Int J Cardiol 176(2):315–320, 2014 25131906

Ali ZA, El-Mallakh RS: Lithium and kidney disease: understand the risks. Curr Psychiatry 20(6):34–50, 2021

Alper K, Schwartz KA, Kolts RL, et al: Seizure incidence in psychopharmacological clinical trials: an analysis of Food and Drug Administration (FDA) Summary Basis of Approval reports. Biol Psychiatry 62(4):345–354, 2007 17223086

Alvir JM, Lieberman JA, Safferman AZ, et al: Clozapine-induced agranulocytosis: incidence and risk factors in the United States. N Engl J Med 329(3):162–167, 1993 8515788

American Diabetes Association; American Psychiatric Association; American Association of Clinical Endocrinologists; North American Association for the Study of Obesity: Consensus development conference on antipsychotic drugs and obesity and diabetes. J Clin Psychiatry 65(2):267–272, 2004 15003083

American Psychiatric Association: Diagnostic and Statistical Manual of Mental Disorders, 4th Edition, Text Revision. Washington, DC, American Psychiatric Association, 2000

Andrade C: Methylphenidate and the risk of new-onset seizures. J Clin Psychiatry 81(4):20f13586, 2020 32726522

Anzai T, Takahashi K, Watanabe M: Adverse reaction reports of neuroleptic malignant syndrome induced by atypical antipsychotic agents in the Japanese Adverse Drug Event Report (JADER) database. Psychiatry Clin Neurosci 73(1):27–33, 2019 30375086

Armenian P, Mamantov TM, Tsutaoka BT, et al: Multiple MDMA (Ecstasy) overdoses at a rave event: a case series. J Intensive Care Med 28(4):252–258, 2013 22640978

Asnis GM, Henderson MA: EMSAM (deprenyl patch): how a promising antidepressant was underutilized. Neuropsychiatr Dis Treat 10:1911–1923, 2014 25336957

Austria B, Haque R, Mittal S, et al: Mortality in association with antipsychotic medication use and clinical outcomes among geriatric psychiatry outpatients with COVID-19. PLoS One 16(10):e0258916, 2021 34673821

Bark N: Deaths of psychiatric patients during heat waves. Psychiatr Serv 49(8):1088–1090, 1998 9712220

Bartakke S, Abdelhaleem M, Carcao M: Valproate-induced pure red cell aplasia and megakaryocyte dysplasia. Br J Haematol 141(2):133, 2008 18353161

Beach SR, Celano CM, Sugrue AM, et al: QT prolongation, torsades de pointes, and psychotropic medications: a 5-year update. Psychosomatics 59(2):105–122, 2018 29275963

Behlke LM, Lenze EJ, Carney RM: The cardiovascular effects of newer antidepressants in older adults and those with or at high risk for cardiovascular diseases. CNS Drugs 34(11):1133–1147, 2020 33064291

Belvederi Murri M, Guaglianone A, Bugliani M, et al: Second-generation antipsychotics and neuroleptic malignant syndrome: systematic review and case report analysis. Drugs R D 15(1):45–62, 2015 25578944

Benoit SR, Zhang Y, Geiss LS, et al: Trends in diabetic ketoacidosis hospitalizations and in-hospital mortality — United States, 2000–2014. MMWR Morb Mortal Wkly Rep 67(12):362–365, 2018 29596400

Berl T: Vasopressin antagonists. N Engl J Med 372(23):2207–2216, 2015 26039601

Biffi A, Scotti L, Corrao G: Use of antidepressants and the risk of cardiovascular and cerebrovascular disease: a meta-analysis of observational studies. Eur J Clin Pharmacol 73(4):487–497, 2017 28070601

Björnsson ES, Bergmann OM, Björnsson HK, et al: Incidence, presentation, and outcomes in patients with drug-induced liver injury in the general population of Iceland. Gastroenterology 144(7):1419–1425, 1425.e1–1425.e3, quiz e19–e20, 2013 23419359

Boyer EW, Shannon M: The serotonin syndrome. N Engl J Med 352(11):1112–1120, 2005 15784664

Browne B, Linter S: Monoamine oxidase inhibitors and narcotic analgesics: a critical review of the implications for treatment. Br J Psychiatry 151:210–212, 1987 2891392

Buoli M, Serati M, Botturi A, et al: The risk of thrombocytopenia during valproic acid therapy: a critical summary of available clinical data. Drugs R D 18(1):1–5, 2018 29260458

Canuso CM, Goldman MB: Clozapine restores water balance in schizophrenic patients with polydipsia-hyponatremia syndrome. J Neuropsychiatry Clin Neurosci 11(1):86–90, 1999 9990561

Cardamone L, Salzberg MR, O'Brien TJ, et al: Antidepressant therapy in epilepsy: can treating the comorbidities affect the underlying disorder? Br J Pharmacol 168(7):1531–1554, 2013 23146067

Caroff SN: Neuroleptic malignant syndrome, in Neuroleptic Malignant Syndrome and Related Conditions, 2nd Edition. Edited by Mann SC, Caroff SN, Keck PE Jr, Lazarus A. Washington, DC, American Psychiatric Publishing, 2003a, pp 1–44

Caroff SN: Hyperthermia associated with other neuropsychiatric drugs, in Neuroleptic Malignant Syndrome and Related Conditions, 2nd Edition. Edited by Mann S, Caroff S, Keck PE Jr, Lazarus A. Washington, DC, American Psychiatric Publishing, 2003b, pp 93–120

Caroff SN: Risk of neuroleptic malignant syndrome with vesicular monoamine transporter inhibitors. Clin Psychopharmacol Neurosci 18(2):322–326, 2020 32329312

Caroff SN, Campbell EC: Risk of neuroleptic malignant syndrome in patients with NMDAR encephalitis. Neurol Sci 36(3):479–480, 2015 25480349

Caroff SN, Mann SC: Neuroleptic malignant syndrome. Med Clin North Am 77(1):185–202, 1993 8093494

Caroff SN, Mann SC, Keck PE Jr, et al: Residual catatonic state following neuroleptic malignant syndrome. J Clin Psychopharmacol 20(2):257–259, 2000 10770467

Caroff SN, Mann SC, Gliatto MF, et al: Psychiatric manifestations of acute viral encephalitis. Psychiatr Ann 31:193–204, 2001a

Caroff SN, Rosenberg H, Mann SC, et al: Neuroleptic malignant syndrome in the perioperative setting. Am J Anesthesiol 28:387–393, 2001b

Cervellin G, Comelli I, Lippi G: Rhabdomyolysis: historical background, clinical, diagnostic and therapeutic features. Clin Chem Lab Med 48(6):749–756, 2010 20298139

Chalasani NP, Maddur H, Russo MW, et al: ACG clinical guideline: diagnosis and management of idiosyncratic drug-induced liver injury. Am J Gastroenterol 116(5):878–898, 2021 33929376

Chaudhry MM, Abrar M, Mutahir K, et al: Oxcarbazepine-induced hemolytic anemia in a geriatric patient. Am J Ther 15(2):187–189, 2008 18356642

Chen M, Borlak J, Tong W: High lipophilicity and high daily dose of oral medications are associated with significant risk for drug-induced liver injury. Hepatology 58(1):388–396, 2013 23258593

Clark WG, Lipton JM: Drug-related heatstroke. Pharmacol Ther 26(3):345–388, 1984 6152566

Cohen WJ, Cohen NH: Lithium carbonate, haloperidol, and irreversible brain damage. JAMA 230(9):1283–1287, 1974 4479505

Correll CU, Frederickson AM, Kane JM, et al: Does antipsychotic polypharmacy increase the risk for metabolic syndrome? Schizophr Res 89(1–3):91–100, 2007 17070017

Correll CU, Detraux J, De Lepeleire J, et al: Effects of antipsychotics, antidepressants and mood stabilizers on risk for physical diseases in people with schizophrenia, depression and bipolar disorder. World Psychiatry 14(2):119–136, 2015 26043321

Culpepper L: Reducing the burden of difficult-to-treat major depressive disorder: revisiting monoamine oxidase inhibitor therapy. Prim Care Companion CNS Disord 15(5):PCC13r01515, 2013 24511450

David WS: Myoglobinuria. Neurol Clin 18(1):215–243, 2000 10658177

Devarbhavi H, Andrade RJ: Drug-induced liver injury due to antimicrobials, central nervous system agents, and nonsteroidal anti-inflammatory drugs. Semin Liver Dis 34(2):145–161, 2014 24879980

Dhir R, Brown DK, Olden KW: Drug-induced pancreatitis: a practical review. Drugs Today (Barc) 43(7):499–507, 2007 17728850

Dunkley EJ, Isbister GK, Sibbritt D, et al: The Hunter Serotonin Toxicity Criteria: simple and accurate diagnostic decision rules for serotonin toxicity. QJM 96(9):635–642, 2003 12925718

Ellison DH, Berl T: Clinical practice: the syndrome of inappropriate antidiuresis. N Engl J Med 356(20):2064–2072, 2007 17507705

Ely SF, Neitzel AR, Gill JR: Fatal diabetic ketoacidosis and antipsychotic medication. J Forensic Sci 58(2):398–403, 2013 23278567

Factor SA, Santiago A: Parkinsonism-hyperpyrexia syndrome in Parkinson's disease, in Movement Disorder Emergencies: Diagnosis and Treatment. Edited by Frucht SJ, Fahn S. Totowa, NJ, Humana Press, 2005, pp 29–40

Flanagan RJ, Dunk L: Haematological toxicity of drugs used in psychiatry. Hum Psychopharmacol 23(Suppl 1):27–41, 2008 18098216

Flockhart DA: Dietary restrictions and drug interactions with monoamine oxidase inhibitors: an update. J Clin Psychiatry 73(Suppl 1):17–24, 2012 22951238

Fogo AB, Lusco MA, Andeen NK, et al: AJKD atlas of renal pathology: lithium nephrotoxicity. Am J Kidney Dis 69(1):e1–e2, 2017 28007195

Fontana RJ, Hayashi PH, Gu J, et al: Idiosyncratic drug-induced liver injury is associated with substantial morbidity and mortality within 6 months from onset. Gastroenterology 147(1):96.e4–108.e4, 2014 24681128

Funk MC, Beach SR, Bostwick JR, et al: QTc prolongation and psychotropic medications. Am J Psychiatry 177(3):273–274, 2020 32114782

Gardner DM, Shulman KI, Walker SE, et al: The making of a user friendly MAOI diet. J Clin Psychiatry 57(3):99–104, 1996 8617704

Gareri P, De Fazio P, Russo E, et al: The safety of clozapine in the elderly. Expert Opin Drug Saf 7(5):525–538, 2008 18759705

Garofeanu CG, Weir M, Rosas-Arellano MP, et al: Causes of reversible nephrogenic diabetes insipidus: a systematic review. Am J Kidney Dis 45(4):626–637, 2005 15806465

Gasparini A, Poloni N, Caselli I, et al: Reversible splenial lesion in neuroleptic malignant syndrome. Panminerva Med 60(3):134–135, 2018 29696960

Gerstner T, Büsing D, Bell N, et al: Valproic acid-induced pancreatitis: 16 new cases and a review of the literature. J Gastroenterol 42(1):39–48, 2007 17322992

Gillman PK: CNS toxicity involving methylene blue: the exemplar for understanding and predicting drug interactions that precipitate serotonin toxicity. J Psychopharmacol 25(3):429–436, 2011 20142303

Glassman AH, Bigger JT Jr: Antipsychotic drugs: prolonged QTc interval, torsade de pointes, and sudden death. Am J Psychiatry 158(11):1774–1782, 2001 11691681

Goldman SA: Lithium and neuroleptics in combination: the spectrum of neurotoxicity [corrected]. Psychopharmacol Bull 32(3):299–309, 1996 8961772

Guenette MD, Hahn M, Cohn TA, et al: Atypical antipsychotics and diabetic ketoacidosis: a review. Psychopharmacology (Berl) 226(1):1–12, 2013 23344556

Guinart D, Taipale H, Rubio JM, et al: Risk factors, incidence, and outcomes of neuroleptic malignant syndrome on long-acting injectable vs oral antipsychotics in a nationwide schizophrenia cohort. Schizophr Bull 47(6):1621–1630, 2021a 34013325

Guinart D, Misawa F, Rubio JM, et al: A systematic review and pooled, patient-level analysis of predictors of mortality in neuroleptic malignant syndrome. Acta Psychiatr Scand 144(4):329–341, 2021b 34358327

Guo JJ, Keck PE Jr, Corey-Lisle PK, et al: Risk of diabetes mellitus associated with atypical antipsychotic use among patients with bipolar disorder: a retrospective, population-based, case-control study. J Clin Psychiatry 67(7):1055–1061, 2006 16889448

Gurrera RJ, Caroff SN, Cohen A, et al: An international consensus study of neuroleptic malignant syndrome diagnostic criteria using the Delphi method. J Clin Psychiatry 72(9):1222–1228, 2011 21733489

Gurrera RJ, Mortillaro G, Velamoor V, et al: A validation study of the international consensus diagnostic criteria for neuroleptic malignant syndrome. J Clin Psychopharmacol 37(1):67–71, 2017 28027111

Halperin D, Reber G: Influence of antidepressants on hemostasis. Dialogues Clin Neurosci 9(1):47–59, 2007 17506225

Hennessy S, Bilker WB, Knauss JS, et al: Cardiac arrest and ventricular arrhythmia in patients taking antipsychotic drugs: cohort study using administrative data. BMJ 325(7372):1070, 2002 12424166

Hermesh H, Manor I, Shiloh R, et al: High serum creatinine kinase level: possible risk factor for neuroleptic malignant syndrome. J Clin Psychopharmacol 22(3):252–256, 2002a 12006894

Hermesh H, Stein D, Manor I, et al: Serum creatine kinase levels in untreated hospitalized adolescents during acute psychosis. J Am Acad Child Adolesc Psychiatry 41(9):1045–1053, 2002b 12218425

Hohmann N, Mikus G, Czock D: Effects and risks associated with novel psychoactive substances: mislabeling and sale as bath salts, spice, and research chemicals. Dtsch Arztebl Int 111(9):139–147, 2014 24661585

Huddleston DE, Factor SA: Parkinsonism-hyperpyrexia syndrome in Parkinson's disease, in Movement Disorder Emergencies: Diagnosis and Treatment, 3rd Edition. Edited by Frucht SJ. Cham, Switzerland, Springer Nature Switzerland AG, 2021, pp 77–93

Hung CC, Lin CH, Lan TH, et al: The association of selective serotonin reuptake inhibitors use and stroke in geriatric population. Am J Geriatr Psychiatry 21(8):811–815, 2013 23567390

Husnain M, Gondal F, Raina AI, et al: Quetiapine associated thrombotic thrombocytopenic purpura: a case report and literature review. Am J Ther 24(5):e615–e616, 2017 27340908

Hussain A, Burke J: Mirtazapine associated with recurrent pancreatitis—a case report. J Psychopharmacol 22(3):336–337, 2008 18208920

Jefferson JW: A clinician's guide to monitoring kidney function in lithium-treated patients. J Clin Psychiatry 71(9):1153–1157, 2010 20923621

Jeste DV, Blazer D, Casey D, et al: ACNP White Paper: update on use of antipsychotic drugs in elderly persons with dementia. Neuropsychopharmacology 33(5):957–970, 2008 17637610

Josiassen RC, Goldman M, Jessani M, et al: Double-blind, placebo-controlled, multicenter trial of a vasopressin V2-receptor antagonist in patients with schizophrenia and hyponatremia. Biol Psychiatry 64(12):1097–1100, 2008 18692175

Kales HC, Kim HM, Zivin K, et al: Risk of mortality among individual antipsychotics in patients with dementia. Am J Psychiatry 169(1):71–79, 2012 22193526

Kamitaki BK, Minacapelli CD, Zhang P, et al: Drug-induced liver injury associated with antiseizure medications from the FDA Adverse Event Reporting System (FAERS). Epilepsy Behav 117:107832, 2021 33626490

Kane JM, Correll CU, Delva N, et al: Low incidence of neuroleptic malignant syndrome associated with paliperidone palmitate long-acting injectable: a database report and case study. J Clin Psychopharmacol 39(2):180–182, 2019 30811377

Kao LW, Furbee RB: Drug-induced Q-T prolongation. Med Clin North Am 89(6):1125–1144, x, 2005 16227057

Kaplan PW, Birbeck G: Lithium-induced confusional states: nonconvulsive status epilepticus or triphasic encephalopathy? Epilepsia 47(12):2071–2074, 2006 17201705

Karaosmanoglu AD, Butros SR, Arellano R: Imaging findings of renal toxicity in patients on chronic lithium therapy. Diagn Interv Radiol 19(4):299–303, 2013 23439253

Khan FY: Rhabdomyolysis: a review of the literature. Neth J Med 67(9):272–283, 2009 19841484

Khanna A: Acquired nephrogenic diabetes insipidus. Semin Nephrol 26(3):244–248, 2006 16713497

Klopstock T: Drug-induced myopathies. Curr Opin Neurol 21(5):590–595, 2008 18769254

Koller EA, Cross JT, Doraiswamy PM, et al: Pancreatitis associated with atypical antipsychotics: from the Food and Drug Administration's MedWatch surveillance system and published reports. Pharmacotherapy 23(9):1123–1130, 2003 14524644

Koponen M, Rajamaki B, Lavikainen P, et al: Antipsychotic use and risk of stroke among community-dwelling people with Alzheimer's disease. J Am Med Dir Assoc 23(6):1059.e4–1065.e4, 2022 34717887

Krishnan KR: Revisiting monoamine oxidase inhibitors. J Clin Psychiatry 68(Suppl 8):35–41, 2007 17640156

Kuhlwilm L, Schönfeldt-Lecuona C, Gahr M, et al: The neuroleptic malignant syndrome—a systematic case series analysis focusing on therapy regimes and outcome. Acta Psychiatr Scand 142(3):233–241, 2020 32659853

Kumar R, Vidaurre J, Gedela S: Valproic acid-induced coagulopathy. Pediatr Neurol 98:25–30, 2019 31201069

Lahijani SC, Harris KA: Medical complications of psychiatric treatment: an update. Crit Care Clin 33(3):713–734, 2017 28601142

Lally J, Malik S, Whiskey E, et al: Clozapine-associated agranulocytosis treatment with granulocyte colony-stimulating factor/granulocyte-macrophage colony-stimulating factor: a systematic review. J Clin Psychopharmacol 37(4):441–446, 2017 28437295

Lao KSJ, Zhao J, Blais JE, et al: Antipsychotics and risk of neuroleptic malignant syndrome: a population-based cohort and case-crossover study. CNS Drugs 34(11):1165–1175, 2020 33010024

Laoutidis ZG, Kioulos KT: Antipsychotic-induced elevation of creatine kinase: a systematic review of the literature and recommendations for the clinical practice. Psychopharmacology (Berl) 231(22):4255–4270, 2014 25319963

Laoutidis ZG, Konstantinidis A, Grohmann R, et al: Reversible amisulpride-induced elevation of creatine kinase (CK): a case series from the German AMSP Pharmacovigilance Project. Pharmacopsychiatry 48(4–5):178–181, 2015 25984709

Lee TF, Mora F, Myers RD: Dopamine and thermoregulation: an evaluation with special reference to dopaminergic pathways. Neurosci Biobehav Rev 9(4):589–598, 1985 3001601

Leslie DL, Rosenheck RA: Incidence of newly diagnosed diabetes attributable to atypical antipsychotic medications. Am J Psychiatry 161(9):1709–1711, 2004 15337666

Lheureux PE, Penaloza A, Zahir S, et al: Science review: carnitine in the treatment of valproic acid-induced toxicity—what is the evidence? Crit Care 9(5):431–440, 2005 16277730

Li KJ, Greenstein AP, Delisi LE: Sudden death in schizophrenia. Curr Opin Psychiatry 31(3):169–175, 2018 29517519

Li T, Wang Y, Li W, et al: Quetiapine-associated rhabdomyolysis: a case report and literature review. J Clin Psychopharmacol 40(6):619–624, 2020 33060431

Lin ND, Norman H, Regev A, et al: Hepatic outcomes among adults taking duloxetine: a retrospective cohort study in a US health care claims database. BMC Gastroenterol 15:134, 2015 26467777

Liperoti R, Gambassi G, Lapane KL, et al: Conventional and atypical antipsychotics and the risk of hospitalization for ventricular arrhythmias or cardiac arrest. Arch Intern Med 165(6):696–701, 2005 15795349

Lipscombe LL, Austin PC, Alessi-Severini S, et al: Atypical antipsychotics and hyperglycemic emergencies: multicentre, retrospective cohort study of administrative data. Schizophr Res 154(1–3):54–60, 2014 24581419

Lopez AM, Hendrickson RG: Toxin-induced hepatic injury. Emerg Med Clin North Am 32(1):103–125, 2014 24275171

Mackay FJ, Dunn NR, Mann RD: Antidepressants and the serotonin syndrome in general practice. Br J Gen Pract 49(448):871–874, 1999 10818650

Malaguarnera M: Acetyl-L-carnitine in hepatic encephalopathy. Metab Brain Dis 28(2):193–199, 2013 23389620

Mann SC: Thermoregulatory mechanisms and antipsychotic drug–related heatstroke, in Neuroleptic Malignant Syndrome and Related Conditions, 2nd Edition. Edited by Mann SC, Caroff SN, Keck PE Jr, Lazarus A. Washington, DC, American Psychiatric Publishing, 2003, pp 45–74

Mann SC, Boger WP: Psychotropic drugs, summer heat and humidity, and hyperpyrexia: a danger restated. Am J Psychiatry 135(9):1097–1100, 1978 29501

Mann SC, Caroff SN, Bleier HR, et al: Lethal catatonia. Am J Psychiatry 143(11):1374–1381, 1986 3777225

Mann SC, Caroff SN, Fricchione G, et al: Central dopamine hypoactivity and the pathogenesis of neuroleptic malignant syndrome. Psychiatr Ann 30:363–374, 2000

Marra A, Vargas M, Buonanno P, et al: Haloperidol for preventing delirium in ICU patients: a systematic review and meta-analysis. Eur Rev Med Pharmacol Sci 25(3):1582–1591, 2021 33629327

Martino G, Capasso M, Nasuti M, et al: Dopamine transporter single-photon emission computerized tomography supports diagnosis of akinetic crisis of parkinsonism and of neuroleptic malignant syndrome. Medicine (Baltimore) 94(13):e649, 2015 25837755

Marwick KF, Taylor M, Walker SW: Antipsychotics and abnormal liver function tests: systematic review. Clin Neuropharmacol 35(5):244–253, 2012 22986798

Masi G, Milone A, Viglione V, et al: Massive asymptomatic creatine kinase elevation in youth during antipsychotic drug treatment: case reports and critical review of the literature. J Child Adolesc Psychopharmacol 24(10):536–542, 2014 25387323

Maust DT, Kim HM, Seyfried LS, et al: Antipsychotics, other psychotropics, and the risk of death in patients with dementia: number needed to harm. JAMA Psychiatry 72(5):438–445, 2015 25786075

McKeith IG, Perry RH, Fairbairn AF, et al: Operational criteria for senile dementia of Lewy body type (SDLT). Psychol Med 22(4):911–922, 1992 1362617

Melkersson K: Serum creatine kinase levels in chronic psychosis patients—a comparison between atypical and conventional antipsychotics. Prog Neuropsychopharmacol Biol Psychiatry 30(7):1277–1282, 2006 16806625

Meltzer HY, Cola PA, Parsa M: Marked elevations of serum creatine kinase activity associated with antipsychotic drug treatment. Neuropsychopharmacology 15(4):395–405, 1996 8887994

Meltzer HY, Davidson M, Glassman AH, et al: Assessing cardiovascular risks versus clinical benefits of atypical antipsychotic drug treatment. J Clin Psychiatry 63(Suppl 9):25–29, 2002 12088173

Merrill DB, Dec GW, Goff DC: Adverse cardiac effects associated with clozapine. J Clin Psychopharmacol 25(1):32–41, 2005 15643098

Mijovic A, MacCabe JH: Clozapine-induced agranulocytosis. Ann Hematol 99(11):2477–2482, 2020 32815018

Miller F, Menninger J: Correlation of neuroleptic dose and neurotoxicity in patients given lithium and a neuroleptic. Hosp Community Psychiatry 38(11):1219–1221, 1987 2889659

Misawa F, Okumura Y, Takeuchi Y, et al: Neuroleptic malignant syndrome associated with long-acting injectable versus oral second-generation antipsychotics: analyses based on a spontaneous reporting system database in Japan. Schizophr Res 231:42–46, 2021 33752105

Modi S, Dharaiya D, Schultz L, et al: Neuroleptic malignant syndrome: complications, outcomes, and mortality. Neurocrit Care 24(1):97–103, 2016 26223336

Moeller HB, Rittig S, Fenton RA: Nephrogenic diabetes insipidus: essential insights into the molecular background and potential therapies for treatment. Endocr Rev 34(2):278–301, 2013 23360744

Montgomery SA: Antidepressants and seizures: emphasis on newer agents and clinical implications. Int J Clin Pract 59(12):1435–1440, 2005 16351676

Movig KL, Janssen MW, de Waal Malefijt J, et al: Relationship of serotonergic antidepressants and need for blood transfusion in orthopedic surgical patients. Arch Intern Med 163(19):2354–2358, 2003 14581256

Mujtaba S, Romero J, Taub CC: Methadone, QTc prolongation and torsades de pointes: current concepts, management and a hidden twist in the tale? J Cardiovasc Dis Res 4(4):229–235, 2013 24653586

Myles N, Myles H, Xia S, et al: Meta-analysis examining the epidemiology of clozapine-associated neutropenia. Acta Psychiatr Scand 138(2):101–109, 2018 29786829

Nakamura M, Yasunaga H, Miyata H, et al: Mortality of neuroleptic malignant syndrome induced by typical and atypical antipsychotic drugs: a propensity-matched analysis from the Japanese Diagnosis Procedure Combination database. J Clin Psychiatry 73(4):427–430, 2012 22154901

Nasreddine W, Beydoun A: Valproate-induced thrombocytopenia: a prospective monotherapy study. Epilepsia 49(3):438–445, 2008 18031547

Netto I, Phutane VH, Ravindran B: Lithium neurotoxicity due to second-generation antipsychotics combined with lithium: a systematic review. Prim Care Companion CNS Disord 21(3):17r02225, 2019 31237432

Newton CA, Raskin P: Diabetic ketoacidosis in type 1 and type 2 diabetes mellitus: clinical and biochemical differences. Arch Intern Med 164(17):1925–1931, 2004 15451769

Nguyen C, Xie L, Alley S, et al: Epidemiology and economic burden of serotonin syndrome with concomitant use of serotonergic agents in the U.S. clinical practice. Poster presented at the annual meeting of the American Society of Clinical Psychopharmacology, Miami, FL, June 22–25, 2015

Nooijen PM, Carvalho F, Flanagan RJ: Haematological toxicity of clozapine and some other drugs used in psychiatry. Hum Psychopharmacol 26(2):112–119, 2011 21416507

Oates JA, Sjoerdsma A: Neurologic effects of tryptophan in patients receiving a monoamine oxidase inhibitor. Neurology 10:1076–1078, 1960 13730138

Oliveira JL, Silva Júnior GB, Abreu KL, et al: Lithium nephrotoxicity. Rev Assoc Med Bras (1992) 56(5):600–606, 2010 21152836

Orlova Y, Rizzoli P, Loder E: Association of coprescription of triptan antimigraine drugs and selective serotonin reuptake inhibitor or selective norepinephrine reuptake inhibitor antidepressants with serotonin syndrome. JAMA Neurol 75(5):566–572, 2018 29482205

Page LA, Hajat S, Kovats RS, et al: Temperature-related deaths in people with psychosis, dementia and substance misuse. Br J Psychiatry 200(6):485–490, 2012 22661680

Picard LS, Lindsay S, Strawn JR, et al: Atypical neuroleptic malignant syndrome: diagnostic controversies and considerations. Pharmacotherapy 28(4):530–535, 2008 18363536

Polcwiartek C, Vang T, Bruhn CH, et al: Diabetic ketoacidosis in patients exposed to antipsychotics: a systematic literature review and analysis of Danish adverse drug event reports. Psychopharmacology (Berl) 233(21–22):3663–3672, 2016 27592232

Presne C, Fakhouri F, Noël LH, et al: Lithium-induced nephropathy: rate of progression and prognostic factors. Kidney Int 64(2):585–592, 2003 12846754

Prior A, Laursen TM, Larsen KK, et al: Post-stroke mortality, stroke severity, and preadmission antipsychotic medicine use—a population-based cohort study. PLoS One 9(1):e84103, 2014 24416196

Pyun JM, Park YH, Yang J, et al: Hypersensitivity to atypical antipsychotics in dementia with Lewy bodies: is it common or rare? Parkinsonism Relat Disord 76:44–45, 2020 32563050

Radomski JW, Dursun SM, Reveley MA, et al: An exploratory approach to the serotonin syndrome: an update of clinical phenomenology and revised diagnostic criteria. Med Hypotheses 55(3):218–224, 2000 10985912

Raedler TJ, Wiedemann K: Lithium-induced nephropathies. Psychopharmacol Bull 40(2):134–149, 2007 17514192

Ramaswamy K, Kozma CM, Nasrallah H: Risk of diabetic ketoacidosis after exposure to risperidone or olanzapine. Drug Saf 30(7):589–599, 2007 17604410

Rapaport MH: Dietary restrictions and drug interactions with monoamine oxidase inhibitors: the state of the art. J Clin Psychiatry 68(Suppl 8):42–46, 2007 17640157

Rastogi A, Viani-Walsh D, Akbari S, et al: Pathogenesis and management of Brugada syndrome in schizophrenia: a scoping review. Gen Hosp Psychiatry 67:83–91, 2020 33065406

Reilly JG, Ayis SA, Ferrier IN, et al: Thioridazine and sudden unexplained death in psychiatric in-patients. Br J Psychiatry 180:515–522, 2002 12042230

Rej S, Herrmann N, Shulman K: The effects of lithium on renal function in older adults—a systematic review. J Geriatr Psychiatry Neurol 25(1):51–61, 2012 22467847

Ricken R, Ulrich S, Schlattmann P, et al: Tranylcypromine in mind (part II): review of clinical pharmacology and meta-analysis of controlled studies in depression. Eur Neuropsychopharmacol 27(8):714–731, 2017 28579071

Rochon PA, Normand SL, Gomes T, et al: Antipsychotic therapy and short-term serious events in older adults with dementia. Arch Intern Med 168(10):1090–1096, 2008 18504337

Roose SP, Glassman AH, Dalack GW: Depression, heart disease, and tricyclic antidepressants. J Clin Psychiatry 50(Suppl):12–16, discussion 17, 1989 2661547

Rublee C, Dresser C, Giudice C, et al: Evidence-based heatstroke management in the emergency department. West J Emerg Med 22(2):186–195, 2021 33856299

Sala M, Coppa F, Cappucciati C, et al: Antidepressants: their effects on cardiac channels, QT prolongation and torsade de pointes. Curr Opin Investig Drugs 7(3):256–263, 2006 16555686

Sarkar S, Gupta N: Drug information update: atypical antipsychotics and neuroleptic malignant syndrome: nuances and pragmatics of the association. BJPsych Bull 41(4):211–216, 2017 28811916

Sato Y, Asoh T, Metoki N, et al: Efficacy of methylprednisolone pulse therapy on neuroleptic malignant syndrome in Parkinson's disease. J Neurol Neurosurg Psychiatry 74(5):574–576, 2003 12700295

Scherbaum N, Schifano F, Bonnet U: New psychoactive substances (NPS): a challenge for the addiction treatment services. Pharmacopsychiatry 50(3):116–122, 2017 28444659

Schifano F, Papanti GD, Orsolini L, et al: Novel psychoactive substances: the pharmacology of stimulants and hallucinogens. Expert Rev Clin Pharmacol 9(7):943–954, 2016 26985969

Schifano F, Chiappini S, Miuli A, et al: New psychoactive substances (NPS) and serotonin syndrome onset: a systematic review. Exp Neurol 339(5):113638, 2021 33571533

Schneider LS, Tariot PN, Dagerman KS, et al: Effectiveness of atypical antipsychotic drugs in patients with Alzheimer's disease. N Engl J Med 355(15):1525–1538, 2006 17035647

Schneider M, Regente J, Greiner T, et al: Neuroleptic malignant syndrome: evaluation of drug safety data from the AMSP program during 1993–2015. Eur Arch Psychiatry Clin Neurosci 270(1):23–33, 2020 30506147

Segura-Bruna N, Rodriguez-Campello A, Puente V, et al: Valproate-induced hyperammonemic encephalopathy. Acta Neurol Scand 114(1):1–7, 2006 16774619

Serrano-Dueñas M: Neuroleptic malignant syndrome-like, or—dopaminergic malignant syndrome—due to levodopa therapy withdrawal: clinical features in 11 patients. Parkinsonism Relat Disord 9(3):175–178, 2003 12573874

Sgro C, Clinard F, Ouazir K, et al: Incidence of drug-induced hepatic injuries: a French population-based study. Hepatology 36(2):451–455, 2002 12143055

Shafi A, Berry AJ, Sumnall H, et al: New psychoactive substances: a review and updates. Ther Adv Psychopharmacol 10(12):1–21, 2020 33414905

Shin D, Oh YH, Eom CS, et al: Use of selective serotonin reuptake inhibitors and risk of stroke: a systematic review and meta-analysis. J Neurol 261(4):686–695, 2014 24477492

Sicouri S, Antzelevitch C: Sudden cardiac death secondary to antidepressant and antipsychotic drugs. Expert Opin Drug Saf 7(2):181–194, 2008 18324881

Siegel AJ: Hyponatremia in psychiatric patients: update on evaluation and management. Harv Rev Psychiatry 16(1):13–24, 2008 18306096

Siskind D, Sidhu A, Cross J, et al: Systematic review and meta-analysis of rates of clozapine-associated myocarditis and cardiomyopathy. Aust N Z J Psychiatry 54(5):467–481, 2020 31957459

Smith FA, Wittmann CW, Stern TA: Medical complications of psychiatric treatment. Crit Care Clin 24(4):635–656, vii, 2008 18929938

Solmi M, Murru A, Pacchiarotti I, et al: Safety, tolerability, and risks associated with first- and second-generation antipsychotics: a state-of-the-art clinical review. Ther Clin Risk Manag 13:757–777, 2017 28721057

Spigset O, Hägg S, Bate A: Hepatic injury and pancreatitis during treatment with serotonin reuptake inhibitors: data from the World Health Organization (WHO) database of adverse drug reactions. Int Clin Psychopharmacol 18(3):157–161, 2003 12702895

Spring G, Frankel M: New data on lithium and haloperidol incompatibility. Am J Psychiatry 138(6):818–821, 1981 6113770

Star K, Iessa N, Almandil NB, et al: Rhabdomyolysis reported for children and adolescents treated with antipsychotic medicines: a case series analysis. J Child Adolesc Psychopharmacol 22(6):440–451, 2012 23234587

Sternbach H: The serotonin syndrome. Am J Psychiatry 148(6):705–713, 1991 2035713

Sterns RH: Disorders of plasma sodium—causes, consequences, and correction. N Engl J Med 372(1):55–65, 2015 25551526

Straus SM, Bleumink GS, Dieleman JP, et al: Antipsychotics and the risk of sudden cardiac death. Arch Intern Med 164(12):1293–1297, 2004 15226162

Strawn JR, Keck PE Jr, Caroff SN: Neuroleptic malignant syndrome. Am J Psychiatry 164(6):870–876, 2007 17541044

Su YP, Chang CK, Hayes RD, et al: Retrospective chart review on exposure to psychotropic medications associated with neuroleptic malignant syndrome. Acta Psychiatr Scand 130(1):52–60, 2014 24237642

Sultzer DL, Davis SM, Tariot PN, et al: Clinical symptom responses to atypical antipsychotic medications in Alzheimer's disease: phase 1 outcomes from the CATIE-AD effectiveness trial. Am J Psychiatry 165(7):844–854, 2008 18519523

Suvisaari, J, Keinänen J, Eskelinen S, et al: Diabetes and schizophrenia. Curr Diab Rep 16(2):16, 2016 26803652

Tábi T, Vécsei L, Youdim MB, et al: Selegiline: a molecule with innovative potential. J Neural Transm (Vienna) 127(5):831–842, 2020 31562557

Tallian K: Three clinical pearls in the treatment of patients with seizures and comorbid psychiatric disorders. Ment Health Clin 7(6):235–245, 2018 29955529

Tampi RR, Young JJ, Tampi D: Behavioral symptomatology and psychopharmacology of Lewy body dementia. Handb Clin Neurol 165:59–70, 2019 31727230

Tarabar AF, Hoffman RS, Nelson L: Citalopram overdose: late presentation of torsades de pointes (TdP) with cardiac arrest. J Med Toxicol 4(2):101–105, 2008 18570170

Tohen M, Castillo J, Baldessarini RJ, et al: Blood dyscrasias with carbamazepine and valproate: a pharmacoepidemiological study of 2,228 patients at risk. Am J Psychiatry 152(3):413–418, 1995 7864268

Ueda M, Hamamoto M, Nagayama H, et al: Biochemical alterations during medication withdrawal in Parkinson's disease with and without neuroleptic malignant-like syndrome. J Neurol Neurosurg Psychiatry 71(1):111–113, 2001 11413275

U.S. Food and Drug Administration: Public health advisory: deaths with antipsychotics in elderly patients with behavioral disturbances. April 11, 2005. Available at: https://psychrights.org/drugs/FDAatypicalswarning4elderly.pdf. Accessed March 30, 2016.

U.S. Food and Drug Administration: FDA expands mortality warnings on antipsychotic drugs. June 17, 2008. Available at: https://www.fdanews.com/articles/107752-fda-expands-mortality-warnings-on-antipsychotic-drugs. Accessed March 13, 2023.

Van Alphen AM, Bosch TM, Kupka RW, et al: Chronic kidney disease in lithium-treated patients, incidence and rate of decline. Int J Bipolar Disord 9(1):1, 2021 33392830

Vancampfort D, Stubbs B, Mitchell AJ, et al: Risk of metabolic syndrome and its components in people with schizophrenia and related psychotic disorders, bipolar disorder and major depressive disorder: a systematic review and meta-analysis. World Psychiatry 14(3):339–347, 2015 26407790

Verdel BM, Souverein PC, Meenks SD, et al: Use of serotonergic drugs and the risk of bleeding. Clin Pharmacol Ther 89(1):89–96, 2011 21107313

Vohra J: Sudden cardiac death in schizophrenia: a review. Heart Lung Circ 29(10):1427–1432, 2020 32800442

Voican CS, Corruble E, Naveau S, et al: Antidepressant-induced liver injury: a review for clinicians. Am J Psychiatry 171(4):404–415, 2014 24362450

Vuk A, Baretic M, Osvatic MM, et al: Treatment of diabetic ketoacidosis associated with antipsychotic medication: literature review. J Clin Psychopharmacol 37(5):584–589, 2017a 28816925

Vuk A, Kuzman M, Baretic M, et al: Diabetic ketoacidosis associated with antipsychotic drugs: case reports and a review of literature. Psychiatr Danub 29(2):121–135, 2017b 28636569

Walter LA, Catenacci MH: Rhabdomyolysis. Hosp Physician 44:25–31, 2008

Wehmeier PM, Heiser P, Remschmidt H: Myocarditis, pericarditis and cardiomyopathy in patients treated with clozapine. J Clin Pharm Ther 30(1):91–96, 2005 15659009

Weintraub D, Hurtig HI: Presentation and management of psychosis in Parkinson's disease and dementia with Lewy bodies. Am J Psychiatry 164(10):1491–1498, 2007 17898337

Weintraub D, Chiang C, Kim HM, et al: Association of antipsychotic use with mortality risk in patients with Parkinson disease. JAMA Neurol 73(5):535–541, 2016 26999262

Werneke U, Ott M, Renberg ES, et al: A decision analysis of long-term lithium treatment and the risk of renal failure. Acta Psychiatr Scand 126(3):186–197, 2012 22404233

Wiciński M, Węclewicz MM, Miętkiewicz M, et al: Potential mechanisms of hematological adverse drug reactions in patients receiving clozapine in combination with proton pump inhibitors. J Psychiatr Pract 23(2):114–120, 2017 28291036

Wong J, Delva N: Clozapine-induced seizures: recognition and treatment. Can J Psychiatry 52(7):457–463, 2007 17688010

Woodward M, Gonski P, Grossmann M, et al: Diagnosis and management of hyponatraemia in the older patient. Intern Med J 48(Suppl 1):5–12, 2018 29318728

Yunusa I, Rashid N, Abler V, et al: Comparative efficacy, safety, tolerability, and effectiveness of antipsychotics in the treatment of dementia-related psychosis (DRP): a systematic literature review. J Prev Alzheimers Dis 8(4):520–533, 2021 34585228

Zaccara G, Franciotta D, Perucca E: Idiosyncratic adverse reactions to antiepileptic drugs. Epilepsia 48(7):1223–1244, 2007 17386054

Zivkovic S, Koh CH, Kaza N, et al: Antipsychotic drug use and risk of stroke and myocardial infarction: a systematic review and meta-analysis. BMC Psychiatry 19(1):189, 2019 31221107

3

Alternative Routes of Drug Administration

Ericka L. Crouse, Pharm.D.

Jonathan G. Leung, Pharm.D.

Katie S. Adams, Pharm.D.

James L. Levenson, M.D.

Psychotropic medications are usually delivered orally, but this administration route may not be ideal or even be possible for many patients. Oral administration of medications may be difficult in patients who are medically

The authors acknowledge James A. Owen, Ph.D., for his original authorship of this chapter. We also thank Michael Kemp, B.Sc. (pharm), Pharm.D., a psychiatric pharmacist and clinical researcher who practices in Canada, and Stacy Eon, Pharm.D., BCPP, Senior Content Management Consultant at Wolters Kluwer, for their contributions to the chapter.

compromised, including patients with severe nausea or vomiting, dysphagia, or severe malabsorption; unconscious patients; and patients who are unable or unwilling to take medications by mouth (Table 3–1). In such situations, a non-oral route is preferred or necessary.

Medication administration can be problematic with patients who are cognitively impaired or experiencing acute psychosis. When an alternative delivery route is used, adherence may be more easily verified. Non-oral routes of administration relevant to psychotropic medication include intravenous, intramuscular, subcutaneous, sublingual, buccal, rectal, topical or transdermal, inhalation, and intranasal.

In this chapter, we review the availability of non-oral formulations of anxiolytics and sedative-hypnotics, antidepressants, antipsychotics, mood stabilizers, psychostimulants, and medications approved for dementia and opioid use disorder. Many formulations discussed are commercially available, although not necessarily in the United States or Canada (Table 3–2). We also report formulations for a few agents that may be available through extemporaneous compounding by a pharmacist. Caution is indicated when using a formulation for unapproved purposes and for which adequate studies of safety and efficacy are lacking. The need for such vigilance is due to possible alterations in absorption when a medication is administered via a route by which it has not been evaluated.

Properties of Specific Routes of Administration

Intravenous Administration

Intravenous administration delivers drug directly into the patient's circulation and avoids first-pass metabolism. It provides rapid drug distribution with 100% bioavailability. The rate of drug delivery can be controlled from very rapid to slow infusion. Potential complications include difficulty with venous access, infiltration, and infection. Intravenous forms of several benzodiazepines (in the United States and Canada) and valproate (in the United States) are available. Intravenous ketamine has been used off label for treatment of depression. Intravenous brexanolone is approved for postpartum depression. Off-label intravenous administration of short-acting intramuscular haloperidol is a common clinical practice, while the off-label use of intravenous olan-

Table 3–1.   Situations potentially requiring alternative routes of drug administration

Severe nausea and vomiting

Cancer chemotherapy

Severe gastroparesis

Gastric outlet obstruction

Intestinal obstruction

Cyclical vomiting/cannabis hyperemesis syndrome

Esophageal disorders

Severe gastroesophageal reflux disease

Carcinoma

Eosinophilic esophagitis

Severe malabsorption

Short gut syndrome

Inflammatory bowel disease

Pancreatic insufficiency

Gastrointestinal discontinuity

Neurological dysphagia

Poststroke period

Parkinson's disease

Amyotrophic lateral sclerosis

Delirium, stupor, or coma

Patient's refusal of oral medication

NPO (nothing by mouth) orders in effect

Facial trauma

Perioperative period

Intraabdominal abscesses or fistulae

Table 3–2. Alternative preparations of psychotropic medications

Medication	Route of administration						
	IV	IM	Sublingual/buccal	Rectal	Transdermal	Intranasal	Oral inhalation
Anxiolytics							
Alprazolam			n				
Clonazepam			n	n			
Diazepam	US, C, O	US, C[a]	n	US, C, O		US	
Lorazepam	US, C	US, C	C	n		n	
Midazolam	US, C	US, C	n, O	n		US	
Prazepam			n				
Triazolam			n	n			
Hypnotics							
Zolpidem			US				US

Table 3–2.   Alternative preparations of psychotropic medications *(continued)*

Medication	IV	IM	Sublingual/ buccal	Rectal	Transdermal	Intranasal	Oral inhalation
Antidepressants							
Amitriptyline		O		n			
Citalopram	O						
Brexanolone	US						
Clomipramine	O			n			
Doxepin	n, O			n			
Esketamine						US	
Fluoxetine				n			
Imipramine		O		n			
Ketamine	US[b]					n	
Maprotiline	O						

Table 3–2.   Alternative preparations of psychotropic medications *(continued)*

Medication	IV	IM	Sublingual/buccal	Rectal	Transdermal	Intranasal	Oral inhalation
Antidepressants *(continued)*							
Selegiline			US[c]		US		
Trazodone	O			n			
Viloxazine[d]	O						
Antipsychotics, atypical							
Amisulpride	US,[e] O						
Aripiprazole		O Depot: US, C					
Aripiprazole lauroxil		Depot: US					
Asenapine			US		US		
Olanzapine	n	US, C Depot: US					
Paliperidone		Depot: US					

Table 3–2. Alternative preparations of psychotropic medications *(continued)*

Medication	IV	IM	Sublingual/ buccal	Rectal	Transdermal	Intranasal	Oral inhalation
Antipsychotics, atypical *(continued)*							
Quetiapine				n			
Risperidone		Depot: US, C SubQ Depot: US					
Ziprasidone	n	US					
Antipsychotics, typical							
Chlorpromazine		US, C					
Droperidol	US, C	US, C					
Flupenthixol		Depot: C					
Fluphenazine		US, C^f SubQ Depot: C^f Depot: US, C^e					
Haloperidol		US, C Depot: US, C					n

Table 3–2. Alternative preparations of psychotropic medications *(continued)*

Medication	IV	IM	Sublingual/buccal	Rectal	Transdermal	Intranasal	Oral inhalation
Antipsychotics, typical *(continued)*							
Loxapine		C					US
Methotrimeprazine		C					
Prochlorperazine		US, C		US, C			
Promazine	O	C, O					
Sulpiride		O					
Zuclopenthixol		C Depot: C					
Mood stabilizers							
Carbamazepine				n			
Lamotrigine				n			
Topiramate				n			
Valproate	US			n			

Table 3–2. Alternative preparations of psychotropic medications *(continued)*

	Route of administration						
Medication	IV	IM	Sublingual/ buccal	Rectal	Transdermal	Intranasal	Oral inhalation
Psychostimulants							
Dextroamphetamine				n	US		
Methamphetamine						n	
Methylphenidate					US		
Medications for opioid use disorders							
Buprenorphine[g]	US	SubQ Depot: US	US, C		US		
Naloxone	US, C	US, C				US, C	
Naltrexone		Depot: US					
Medications for dementia							
Aducanumab	US						
Donepezil					US		
Galantamine						n	
Lecanemab	US						

Table 3–2.   Alternative preparations of psychotropic medications *(continued)*

			Route of administration				
Medication	**IV**	**IM**	**Sublingual/ buccal**	**Rectal**	**Transdermal**	**Intranasal**	**Oral inhalation**
Medications for dementia (continued)							
Rivastigmine					US, C		

Note.   Depot=long-acting depot formulation; IM=intramuscular; IV=intravenous; n=noncommercial formulation; SubQ=subcutaneous. Approved formulations; C=Canada; O=country other than United States or Canada; US=United States. Noncommercial formulations may be available in Europe but not in the United States. For these formulations, intranasal and sublingual formulations may be administered from injectable formulations; sublingual formulation may also be a tablet administered sublingually; rectal dosage forms are often compounded.

[a]But not advised because of erratic absorption.

[b]Commercially available as an anesthetic agent; off label for use in depression.

[c]Buccal administration. (See text for details.)

[d]Viloxazine is available in the United States as an oral formulation for ADHD.

[e]Amisulpride is available parenterally in the United States as an antiemetic.

[f]Fluphenazine decanoate is currently considered to have dormant status in Canada.

[g]Only sublingual, buccal, and subcutaneous formulations are approved for opioid use disorder. Also available as an implant. The intravenous and transdermal formulations are for pain/analgesia.

Source.   Compiled in part from Boddu and Kumari 2020; Bou Khalil 2011; DrugBank Online (https://go.drugbank.com); Gallagher 2022; Gopalakrishna et al. 2013; Government of Canada 2022; Kaminsky et al. 2015; Kasper and Müller-Spahn 2002; Lexicomp online (https://online.lexi.com/lco/action/home); Lexi-Drugs/MNC online database (https://online.lexi.com); Thompson and DiMartini 1999.

zapine (Khorassani and Saad 2019) and ziprasidone (Girard et al. 2018) is accumulating evidence to support their safety and effectiveness. Intravenous administration of atypical antipsychotics should be used cautiously and patients monitored for hypotension, respiratory status, and electrocardiographic changes.

Intramuscular Administration

Fast absorption and avoidance of first-pass metabolism are advantages of intramuscular administration, but bioavailability is often less than 100% because of drug retention or metabolism by local tissues. Intramuscular injections should be avoided in the setting of infection at injection site, suspected myocardial infarction, severe thrombocytopenia, hypovolemic shock, myopathies, and significant muscular atrophy. Repeated injections of some drugs may cause muscle irritation, necrosis, elevated creatine kinase levels, indurations, or abscesses (Polania Gutierrez and Munakomi 2023).

Subcutaneous Administration

Subcutaneous administration of medications to manage medical illnesses (e.g., subcutaneous insulin for diabetes or low-molecular-weight heparins for venous thromboembolism prophylaxis) is routinely used in medical settings.

Subcutaneous administration of psychotropics is generally reserved for chronic administration of long-acting injections. The typical antipsychotic fluphenazine decanoate can be administered subcutaneously, and a monthly formulation of risperidone is available for subcutaneous administration. Buprenorphine for opioid use disorder is also available for monthly subcutaneous administration. Pain at injection site has been reported with subcutaneous administration. Additionally, inadvertent intradermal administration of a subcutaneous injection may result in skin necrosis (Crouse et al. 2022).

Subcutaneous administration of haloperidol, methotrimeprazine (available in Canada and Europe), and fluphenazine (Health Canada–approved for subcutaneous administration) can be used to manage terminal restlessness and nausea or vomiting in palliative care patients (Fonzo-Christe et al. 2005).

Midazolam has been administered off-label subcutaneously for insomnia and to wean pediatric patients off intravenous sedation (Kaneishi et al. 2015; Tobias 1999).

Sublingual or Buccal Administration

The rapid sublingual absorption and good bioavailability of small lipid–soluble drugs suggest that many psychotropic medications could be administered sublingually. Drugs absorbed sublingually avoid first-pass metabolism and gastric degradation and may have fewer gastrointestinal adverse effects. Sublingual delivery can be used in patients who are fasting, have difficulty swallowing, or are unable to absorb medication from the gastrointestinal tract. Sublingual administration may not be practical in patients with severe nausea or those who cannot tolerate the taste of some medications.

A few psychotropics are available in a sublingual or buccal form, including the anxiolytic lorazepam (in Canada), the hypnotic zolpidem, the monoamine oxidase B (MAO-B) inhibitor selegiline, and the atypical antipsychotic asenapine.

Midazolam solution for injection has been administered sublingually and buccally. Changes on the electroencephalogram were seen as early as 5–10 minutes after buccal administration of midazolam. If the solution is swallowed, it is less effective.

Buprenorphine is available in sublingual and buccal formulations (tablets, films) as a monoproduct or a combination product with naloxone for the treatment of opioid use disorder. Buprenorphine has very low oral bioavailability (Coe et al. 2019). The addition of naloxone is to deter the misuse of buprenorphine via intravenous or intranasal routes, as it has poor oral or sublingual bioavailability (approximately 3%) (Coe et al. 2019).

Orally Disintegrating Tablets

Many antipsychotics are available in orally disintegrating tablets (ODTs), which disintegrate quickly when exposed to saliva. The saliva containing medication should be swallowed, and absorption occurs in the esophageal and gastric mucosa (Nordstrom and Allen 2013). This dosage form is thought to improve compliance by reducing the ability to "cheek" medications and may be beneficial in patients with dysphagia. The antipsychotics aripiprazole, clozapine, olanzapine, and risperidone; the antidepressant mirtazapine; the mood stabilizer lamotrigine; the stimulants amphetamine and methylphenidate; the anxiolytics clonazepam and alprazolam; and the antidementia medication donepezil are available as ODTs. In Canada, an ODT formulation of escitalopram is also available. ODTs should not be administered to patients with phenylketonuria because many ODTs contain phenylalanine.

Although ODTs dissolve in the mouth, time to peak plasma concentrations (T_{max}) is similar to that of standard tablet formulations (U.S. Food and Drug Administration 1999). However, absorption may occur earlier within the gastrointestinal tract (i.e., pharynx or esophagus). A small study of 19 participants suggested that 79% of patients who took olanzapine ODTs had a measurable concentration versus 0% of patients who took the standard tablets at 15 minutes (San et al. 2008). When olanzapine ODTs were administered buccally, there were no measurable concentrations at 5 minutes (U.S. Food and Drug Administration 1999). Conversely, a small study in 11 healthy volunteers found that both sublingual administration (held under tongue for 15 minutes) and oral administration of olanzapine ODTs resulted in earlier plasma concentrations (15 minutes) than regular tablets administered orally (30 minutes) and quicker T_{max} (Markowitz et al. 2006). It is unknown if most ODTs have significant buccal or sublingual absorption.

Rectal Administration

Rectal administration of medications can be used in patients with severe nausea, in those who cannot tolerate any gastric stimulation (including sublingual administration), and in those taking drugs for which a parenteral form is unavailable or not tolerated. Drug absorption is often erratic because the rectal mucosa lacks the extensive microvilli and surface area of the small intestine. However, the rectum is highly vascular, and absorption can also be influenced by the properties of a medication (lipophilicity, particle size) and drug placement within the rectal vault. With this in mind, any oral dosage form can be administered rectally. These ideally would be immediate-release or oral solutions. The lack of data is the largest barrier to confidently knowing the potential absorption or lack thereof. Because a substantial portion of rectal venous drainage bypasses the portal circulation, first-pass metabolism is about 50% of that reported for oral administration. This can have potential dosing consequences. One study of extemporaneously compounded quetiapine suppositories demonstrated close to a twofold increase in area under the curve (AUC) compared with an equal dose of oral quetiapine (Leung et al. 2016). Bioavailability increases when enema volume is increased because the mucosa surface in contact with drug expands; however, increasing the enema volume may cause discomfort, with difficulty ensuring drug retention in the rectum. Suppositories may be preferred to enemas.

Diazepam and prochlorperazine are the only psychotropic drugs available in rectal forms. However, rectal administration of many drugs, including lorazepam, dextroamphetamine, anticonvulsants, and antidepressants (e.g., tricyclic antidepressants, sertraline, and trazodone), has been reported (Leung et al. 2017). Parenteral formulations and oral solutions have been administered as enemas, and rectal insertion of oral capsules has delivered acceptable bioavailability. Suppositories may be compounded from tablets or capsules. When possible, therapeutic serum level monitoring is recommended. Rectal administration should be avoided in the setting of severe neutropenia, severe bleeding risk, active diarrhea, anorectal disease, and previous abdominoperineal resection.

Topical or Transdermal Administration

Continuous drug delivery from a transdermal patch reduces the peak-to-trough fluctuation of drug levels produced by oral dosing and provides near-constant plasma drug levels, even for drugs with a short half-life, over longer dosing intervals. Transdermal drug delivery bypasses the gut, avoids first-pass metabolism, reduces gastrointestinal adverse effects, and is unaffected by food intake. Local irritation can be avoided by varying the administration site. Transdermal preparations of psychotropics are now approved for depression (selegiline), ADHD (methylphenidate, dextroamphetamine), schizophrenia (asenapine), and Alzheimer's disease (rivastigmine, donepezil). A topical cream is available for doxepin; however, this medication is indicated for pruritus and not for management of depression. Some compounding pharmacies make an off-label topical formulation of quetiapine for use in agitation, but it does not appear to be absorbed well transdermally (Kayhart et al. 2018).

Intranasal Administration

Intranasal administration has been suggested as the best alternative to parenteral injection for rapid systemic drug delivery.

Esketamine for depression was the first psychotropic medication to be approved in a commercial intranasal formulation (Bozymski et al. 2020). Prior to this, racemic ketamine had been compounded into an intranasal formulation. Intranasal diazepam and midazolam are also commercially available for acute treatment of seizures. The time to peak for intranasal diazepam was comparable to that for rectal gel under "ideal" conditions; however, there was more variability in peak concentrations and AUC with rectal diazepam, especially in higher-weight patients (Hogan et al. 2020). Intranasal naloxone is used to treat opioid overdoses in the community setting.

Other custom intranasal formulations are reported for anxiolytics (midazolam and lorazepam), psychostimulants (methamphetamine), antipsychotics (haloperidol), and cognitive enhancers (galantamine). Intranasal midazolam has a faster onset of action than midazolam by the sublingual route, but time of onset with intranasal administration is similar to that for intramuscular administration (Nordstrom and Allen 2013; Preethy and Somasundaram 2021). Several devices to atomize drug solutions for intranasal delivery are available (Wolfe and Bernstone 2004).

Oral Inhalation

Administration by oral inhalation has been suggested to be less invasive than intramuscular injection. Zolpidem and loxapine are the only two psychotropic medications available via oral inhalation. Loxapine is used for acute agitation and is contraindicated in persons with pulmonary disorders such as asthma or chronic obstructive pulmonary disease.

Administration via Tube

Many patients in a critical care setting receive medications via nasogastric (NG) tube or percutaneous endoscopic gastrostomy (PEG) tube. Medications available in a liquid form provide easy administration via NG or PEG tube. The antidepressants citalopram, doxepin, escitalopram, fluoxetine, nortriptyline, paroxetine, and sertraline are available as oral liquids. The antipsychotics aripiprazole, chlorpromazine, clozapine, fluphenazine, haloperidol, risperidone, and ziprasidone are available as oral liquids. The mood stabilizers carbamazepine, lithium, and valproic acid are available as oral liquids. Amphetamine and methylphenidate are available as an oral suspension. Some tablet forms may be crushed and administered via NG or PEG tube. Some ODT formulations may be dispersed in water or another suitable beverage prior to NG or PEG tube administration. Olanzapine ODTs can be dispersed in water, juice, milk, or coffee.

Tablets that come as extended-release or sustained-release formulations (e.g., bupropion XL) should not be crushed. Many capsules, such as those for duloxetine or levomilnacipran, should not be opened (Bostwick and Demehri

2014) and may result in clogging of the tube. Duloxetine is now commercially available as a sprinkle capsule specifically designed to be opened and either sprinkled on food or administered via NG tube (Dailymed 2021).

Psychotropic Medications

Anxiolytics and Sedative-Hypnotics

Internationally, many benzodiazepines are available in intravenous, intramuscular, rectal, sublingual, and intranasal preparations. Injectable forms of diazepam, lorazepam, and midazolam are marketed in the United States and Canada; diazepam rectal gel is also available in both countries; and intranasal forms for diazepam and midazolam are available in the United States for seizures. Clonazepam and alprazolam are available as ODTs in the United States. Sublingual lorazepam is available in Canada. Lorazepam for injection and midazolam for injection have been used off-label sublingually. Chloral hydrate has been given off-label rectally to achieve sedation in young children (Nie et al. 2021). Buspirone and the nonbenzodiazepine hypnotics eszopiclone, zopiclone, zaleplon, melatonin, and ramelteon are available only in oral forms. A sublingual preparation and an oral inhalation preparation of zolpidem are available in the United States.

Intravenous benzodiazepines are commonly used to treat status epilepticus and severe alcohol or sedative withdrawal and to calm severely agitated patients. Intravenous lorazepam is preferred because of its more favorable and predictable pharmacokinetics. Because intravenous lorazepam redistributes more slowly from the CNS to peripheral tissues than does diazepam or midazolam, it has a longer duration of effect after a single dose. Midazolam is a rapid-acting short-duration benzodiazepine frequently used in preoperative sedation, induction and maintenance of anesthesia, and treatment of status epilepticus. The effects of intravenous midazolam begin within minutes but last for less than 2 hours unless in the setting of renal impairment, which can significantly delay clearance (Bauer et al. 1995; Rey et al. 1999). Because severe respiratory depression may accompany intravenous benzodiazepine administration, facilities for respiratory resuscitation should always be available when using this route.

Injectable forms of lorazepam, midazolam, and diazepam are available for intramuscular delivery. For behavioral emergencies, lorazepam is preferred because it is readily absorbed and has no active metabolites. Midazolam is also rapidly absorbed after intramuscular administration, with an onset of action between 5 and 15 minutes. Intramuscular diazepam is not recommended because of its erratic absorption (Rey et al. 1999; Weintraub 2017).

Rectal administration of benzodiazepines is useful for the acute management of seizures in children. Diazepam is available as a rectal gel for use when other delivery routes are not readily available. A pharmacokinetic study of a parenteral solution of lorazepam administered rectally to healthy adults found average bioavailability of 80% but with considerable variation in the rate and extent of absorption. Peak concentrations were considerably lower and achieved later than those with the equivalent intravenous dose. The authors suggested that to achieve rapid therapeutic effect, rectal doses may need to be two to four times the intravenous dose, but cautioned that these higher doses may cause prolonged toxicity (Graves et al. 1987). Other benzodiazepines, such as clonazepam, triazolam, and midazolam (Aydintug et al. 2004; Leppik and Patel 2015), have also been administered rectally. Although rectal benzodiazepine absorption is rapid, it is not always reliable because rectal bioavailability is highly variable, and the onset of action is delayed (Hogan et al. 2020; Rey et al. 1999).

Sublingual benzodiazepines are often used to control anxiety in patients undergoing dental procedures. Only lorazepam in Canada is marketed in a sublingual form, although many benzodiazepines, including alprazolam, clonazepam, diazepam, flunitrazepam, lormetazepam, midazolam, prazepam, temazepam, and triazolam, have been administered sublingually using commercial nonsublingual formulations or custom preparations. Pharmacokinetic studies comparing sublingual administration of oral tablets against intramuscular administration suggested slightly slower sublingual drug absorption but similar bioavailability (Greenblatt et al. 1982).

The pharmacokinetics of a sublingual form of lorazepam has been compared with that of an intramuscular injection or a sublingual dosage of an oral tablet in 10 fasting subjects. Lorazepam blood levels peaked more rapidly with intramuscular injection (1.15 hours postdose) than with sublingual oral tablets (2.35 hours) or the sublingual lozenge (2.25 hours), but these differences were not significant. Bioavailability for all preparations was indistinguishable from 100% (Greenblatt et al. 1982). Midazolam administered buccally for seizures was found to be at least as effective (75% seizure control) as rectal diazepam (59% seizure control) in a case series of 28 children (Sánchez Fernández and Loddenkemper 2015). Diazepam buccal films are currently undergoing investigation for acute treatment of seizures (Rogawski and Heller 2019). Midazolam is available in Europe as an oromucosal solution available for buccal administration (Boddu and Kumari 2020).

The pharmacokinetics of alprazolam oral tablets administered either sublingually or orally has been studied in 13 fasting volunteers. Although not significantly different, plasma drug levels peaked faster and higher following sublingual administration (Scavone et al. 1987). Whereas sublingual alprazolam administration postprandially may delay peak by 1 hour, other kinetic variables were not considered significantly different (Scavone et al. 1992). Sublingual alprazolam has been successfully used in two small studies as premedication for upper gastrointestinal endoscopy (Sebghatollahi et al. 2017; Shavakhi et al. 2014). Sublingual administration of oral tablets may be an alternative for patients with panic disorder or preprocedure anxiety who are unable to swallow tablets.

Diazepam and midazolam are available in FDA-approved intranasal formulations (Boddu and Kumari 2020). Intranasal diazepam had a rapid onset of action (around 5 minutes) but achieved peak plasma levels later (>60 minutes) than rectal diazepam (10–45 minutes). Bioavailability of intranasal diazepam was 97%, better than that of diazepam administered rectally or intramuscularly (Boddu and Kumari 2020). Intranasal midazolam is approximately 44% bioavailable; its onset of effects occurs within 10 minutes, and effects peak within 30–120 minutes. Peak plasma levels occurred at 17.3 minutes (Schrier et al. 2017; UCB Group 2023). In a prospective study of 92 children, seizure cessation with intranasal midazolam was achieved in a mean of 3 minutes versus 4.3 minutes with rectal diazepam (Sánchez Fernández and Loddenkemper 2015). Intranasal lorazepam also has been reported to be effective (Anderson and Saneto 2012). The bioavailability of intranasal lorazepam is similar (78%) to that of intramuscular (100%) or oral (93%) lorazepam, but intranasal administration has more rapid absorption (0.5 hours) than the intramuscular route (3 hours) (Wermeling et al. 2001).

Intrathecal administration of a buffered, preservative-free midazolam solution is a safe and effective adjunctive treatment for postoperative pain in a variety of settings (Duncan et al. 2007).

A sublingual formulation of zolpidem, a nonbenzodiazepine hypnotic, is available in the United States. In a clinical study, the sublingual form produced a significantly earlier sleep initiation than the oral preparation (Staner et al. 2009). Standard dosages are taken at bedtime to improve sleep latency, and lower dosages (1.75 and 3.5 mg) are available for middle-of-the-night awakening (Pergolizzi et al. 2014).

Antidepressants

The monoamine oxidase inhibitor selegiline is available as a transdermal patch, approved for depression in the United States. The antidepressant dosage of oral selegiline requires dietary tyramine restriction because of clinically significant inhibition of intestinal MAO-A. By avoiding intestinal exposure to selegiline, transdermal administration reduces intestinal MAO-A inhibition and the need for dietary tyramine restrictions at dosages of 6 mg/day or less, as well as circumventing first-pass metabolism to provide higher plasma levels and reduced metabolite formation. Short-term (8-week; Feiger et al. 2006) and long-term (52-week; Amsterdam and Bodkin 2006) placebo-controlled, double-blind clinical trials have demonstrated antidepressant efficacy with adverse effects similar to those of placebo, except for application site reactions and insomnia. An ODT formulation of selegiline, designed for buccal absorption, is approved in the United States for Parkinson's disease (Tábi et al. 2013). There are no reports of its use for the treatment of depression.

Transdermal amitriptyline was reported to be well absorbed and effective in a case report (Scott et al. 1999) but to have no significant systemic absorption in a small open trial (Lynch et al. 2005). The variability may be due to different transdermal formulations. This product is not commercially available.

Transdermal delivery of the novel agents esketamine and brexanolone for the treatment of depression has been explored (Bhattaccharjee et al. 2020). Experimental techniques for transdermal delivery of these agents have been assessed, with variable success in achieving adequate percutaneous absorption. Viability of these dosage forms is unknown, and therefore they are not commercially available.

Injectable preparations of amitriptyline, citalopram, clomipramine, doxepin, imipramine, maprotiline, trazodone, and viloxazine are available in Europe and are sometimes used for the initial treatment of hospitalized, severely depressed patients. It has been suggested that antidepressants with extensive first-pass metabolism act more rapidly if given intravenously rather than orally, but superior efficacy has not been demonstrated (Moukaddam and Hirschfeld

2004). The safety and efficacy of intravenous antidepressants in medically ill patients are uncertain because studies to date have been performed only in medically healthy patients. These antidepressant agents are not available in injectable formulations in the United States or Canada.

Intravenous mirtazapine (15 mg/day) was well tolerated and effective in two small uncontrolled trials (Konstantinidis et al. 2002; Mühlbacher et al. 2006). Citalopram is the only selective serotonin reuptake inhibitor available in an intravenous formulation. To date, open and double-blind, controlled clinical studies have shown citalopram infusion followed by oral citalopram (Kasper and Müller-Spahn 2002) or escitalopram (Schmitt et al. 2006) to be effective and well tolerated for severe depression.

Brexanolone is a neuroactive steroid approved in an injectable formulation for the treatment of postpartum depression in adults (Sage Therapeutics 2019). It is administered intravenously as a continuous infusion over 60 hours with a goal of titrating to 90 µg/kg/hour. Brexanolone requires an associated Risk Evaluation and Mitigation Strategy because of the risk of excessive sedation and loss of consciousness (Sage Therapeutics 2019).

Off-label use of ketamine intranasally, intravenously, and orally has gained attention for treatment of depression, with response described as early as day 1. Intravenous dosing typically begins at 0.5 mg/kg over a 40-minute infusion (Corriger and Pickering 2019). Administration should occur in a supervised setting with staff available to monitor vital signs and observe for symptoms of dissociation.

Esketamine is commercially available as a nasal spray and is approved in the United States for treatment-resistant depression and for major depressive disorder with acute suicidality (Bozymski et al. 2020; Janssen Pharmaceuticals 2020). Esketamine is the *S*-enantiomer of racemic ketamine. The mean bioavailability when esketamine is administered intranasally is estimated at 54% with the 56-mg dose and 51% with the 84-mg dose (Perez-Ruixo et al. 2021). Case reports have also described oral and intravenous administration of esketamine for treatment-resistant depression (Smith-Apeldoorn et al. 2021; Zhang et al. 2022).

Several antidepressants, including amitriptyline, clomipramine, imipramine, and trazodone, have been compounded as rectal suppositories, with anecdotal reports of success in depression (Koelle and Dimsdale 1998; Mirassou 1998). Therapeutic serum levels of doxepin were produced in three of four cancer patients following rectal insertion of oral capsules (Storey and Trumble 1992). The bioavailability of fluoxetine oral capsules administered rectally was only 15% that of oral administration, but rectal administration of oral capsules was reasonably well tolerated in seven healthy subjects (Teter et al. 2005). With an appropriate dosage adjustment, rectal administration of antidepressants may be feasible in patients who cannot take oral medications. Serum drug levels (if available) and clinical response should guide dosage.

Sublingual administration of fluoxetine oral solution has been studied in two medically compromised patients with depression. After 4 weeks of 20-mg/day dosing, plasma levels of fluoxetine plus norfluoxetine were in the low therapeutic range, and depressive symptoms had improved in both patients (Pakyurek and Pasol 1999).

Mirtazapine is available in an ODT for gastrointestinal absorption, but the extent of sublingual or buccal absorption from this formulation is unknown. Given its serotonin type 3 receptor (5-HT$_3$) antagonist properties, and lack of nausea as an adverse effect, mirtazapine ODTs may be a useful alternative in patients with severe nausea or vomiting.

Antipsychotics

The atypical antipsychotics olanzapine and ziprasidone, as well as many typical agents, are available as short-acting intramuscular preparations. The short-acting preparation of aripiprazole is no longer commercially available in the United States but it is still available in Europe. Long-acting intramuscular depot formulations of aripiprazole, risperidone, paliperidone, olanzapine, fluphenazine, and haloperidol are available in the United States (Gopalakrishna et al. 2013). In Canada, long-acting intramuscular depot formulations of aripiprazole, risperidone, fluphenazine, haloperidol, flupenthixol, and zuclopenthixol are approved. The olanzapine pamoate long-acting injection requires additional monitoring postinjection to evaluate for postinjection delirium sedation syndrome. Prior to administration of a long-acting injection in the inpatient setting, the date of last administration should be confirmed.

The short-acting injectable atypical antipsychotics olanzapine and ziprasidone have been approved for intramuscular administration. Short-acting intramuscular forms of atypical antipsychotics are less likely than haloperidol to cause acute dystonia and akathisia (Currier and Medori 2006; Zimbroff 2008), but there has been less experience using them in medically ill patients.

Haloperidol can be mixed with a benzodiazepine in the same syringe but should not be mixed with diphenhydramine. Ziprasidone was studied as monotherapy but can be administered in conjunction with an intramuscular benzodiazepine. Concurrent intramuscular olanzapine within 1 hour of a parenteral benzodiazepine is not recommended because of excessive sedation and cardiorespiratory depression (Wilson et al. 2012b). Intramuscular olanzapine should also be used cautiously in alcohol-intoxicated patients because it may reduce oxygen saturations (Wilson et al. 2012a). Secondary to its potential to cause QTc interval prolongation, intramuscular ziprasidone is contraindicated in patients with a recent acute myocardial infarction or uncompensated heart failure (Pfizer 2015). Intramuscular ziprasidone should be used cautiously in patients with renal impairment because it contains cyclodextrin, a renally cleared excipient (Patel et al. 2021). A retrospective review of intramuscular olanzapine and ziprasidone in medically ill patients found that they were frequently used when contraindicated (olanzapine 27%, ziprasidone 9.5%). The rate of hypotension was higher with olanzapine (23% vs. 7%). Patients with a baseline higher QTc interval were more likely to receive olanzapine; however, QTc interval prolongation was seen in both groups, and 71% of patients were taking concurrent QTc interval–prolonging medications. No reports of torsades de pointes occurred (Patel et al. 2021).

Antipsychotic agents are not approved by the U.S. FDA or Health Canada for intravenous use in psychiatric conditions. Intravenous administration of olanzapine and ziprasidone has been reported in clinical trials (Girard et al. 2018; Wang et al. 2022). The clinical use of intravenous olanzapine is emerging as a potential option in emergency department and critical care settings but requires further investigation to confirm safety (Khorassani and Saad 2019). Similar to intramuscular use, there have been recommendations to separate the administration of intravenous olanzapine and a parenteral benzodiazepine by 30–60 minutes because of the potential risk of severe hypotension and respiratory depression (Naso 2008). Typical antipsychotics, primarily haloperidol, are often administered off-label intravenously in medical inpatient settings, especially for delirium. Caution should be exercised when administering haloperidol and ziprasidone intravenously, because this route of administration and higher than recommended doses are considered risk factors for prolonging the QTc interval. Evidence-based monitoring recommendations suggest electrocardiographic monitoring when doses exceed 5 mg of intravenous haloperidol and telemetry for high-risk patients receiving cumulative doses of 100 mg or with a QTc interval greater than 500 ms (Beach et al. 2020). Intravenous chlorpromazine has been used for agitation in the critically ill. However, it should be noted that because of the risk of orthostatic hypotension, it is recommended that the chlorpromazine be diluted and delivered via intravenous piggyback and infused at a rate of 1 mg/min. Therefore, a 50-mg dose will take close to 1 hour to administer (Choi et al. 2020). Amisulpride, used as an antipsychotic in other countries, is available in the United States as an intravenous antiemetic in substantially lower doses (2.5 mg/mL) than those used to treat psychosis.

Intravenous droperidol has been used for rapid tranquilization even though it is approved only as an anesthetic adjunct and antiemetic. Droperidol causes dose-dependent prolongation of the QTc interval and has been associated with torsades de pointes, although this association is controversial (Nuttall et al. 2007). As a result, droperidol was withdrawn from the United Kingdom and has a black box warning in North America. More recent studies continue to reevaluate the QTc risk of droperidol, refuting the need for electrocardiographic or telemetry monitoring with intravenous or intramuscular doses less than 2.5 mg and suggesting that the safety profile of intramuscular doses up to 10 mg is similar to that of other agents used for sedation or agitation (Cole et al. 2020; Gaw et al. 2020; Perkins et al. 2015). A small randomized controlled trial ($n=115$) comparing intramuscular droperidol (5 mg), intramuscular ziprasidone (10 and 20 mg), and intramuscular lorazepam (2 mg) found similar QTc interval durations across all groups (Martel et al. 2021). A large retrospective review identified one case of torsades de pointes out of 16,546 patients who received droperidol in the emergency department (rate of 0.006%; 95% CI=0.00015%–0.03367%) (Cole et al. 2020).

Subcutaneous administration of haloperidol, methotrimeprazine, or fluphenazine has been used to manage terminal restlessness and nausea or vomiting in palliative care patients (Fonzo-Christe et al. 2005). Most other phenothiazines are too irritating for subcutaneous injection. Risperidone is available as a long-acting monthly subcutaneous injection. This drug should not be administered acutely.

Intranasal delivery of antipsychotics is the subject of patent applications, and reports of intranasal quetiapine abuse suggest the feasibility of antipsychotic delivery by this route (Morin 2007). In a small trial, an intranasal haloperidol preparation was more rapidly absorbed and had greater bioavailability than the intramuscular form (Miller et al. 2008). More recently, absorption of an intranasal preparation of olanzapine in healthy subjects was comparable to that of olanzapine administered intramuscularly or as an ODT (Shrewsbury et al. 2020).

Asenapine is the only antipsychotic approved in a transdermal form. Maximum serum concentrations are reached 12–24 hours after application, and thus the transdermal formulation is not beneficial for acute agitation. Prochlorperazine is the only phenothiazine currently available in the United States and Canada as a rectal suppository; chlorpromazine suppositories were discontinued in 2002. A lack of absorption has been demonstrated with off-label topical formulations of quetiapine and chlorpromazine, which have been used in the long-term-care setting for agitation (Weiland et al. 2013). Topical gel haloperidol has been used for chemotherapy-induced nausea and vomiting, and research aimed at enhancing transdermal delivery of haloperidol has been conducted (Bleicher et al. 2008; Fahmy et al. 2019).

Asenapine is the first and only antipsychotic available in a sublingual preparation. Asenapine is available only sublingually and transdermally because its bioavailability when administered orally is less than 2%.

ODTs, designed to facilitate preintestinal absorption, are available for many atypical agents. There are limited and conflicting data on sublingual absorption of olanzapine ODTs (see subsection "Orally Disintegrating Tablets" earlier in this chapter). Sublingual or buccal absorption of ODTs for other antipsychotics has not been reported.

Mood Stabilizers

Lithium is marketed in the United States and Canada in an oral form only, but intravenous, intraperitoneal, and sublingual forms of lithium administration have been reported. Non-oral administration of lithium is not approved by the FDA, and insufficient clinical experience or data are available to recommend non-oral routes. Because lithium is not metabolized, parenteral administration has fewer pharmacokinetic advantages than for other psychotropic drugs.

Intravenous valproic acid has been available in Europe for more than 18 years and in the United States since 1997. (It was discontinued in Canada in 2004.) Valproate is the only mood stabilizer, apart from several atypical antipsychotics, with an approved parenteral formulation for which case reports and small open-label clinical trials exist describing its effective use in bipolar disorder (Fontana et al. 2020). The infusion does not require cardiac monitoring and causes no significant orthostatic hypotension.

Rapid systemic loading of valproate with the intravenous formulation has been proposed to accelerate its antimanic effect, but two small case series found no such advantage over orally administered valproate (Jagadheesan et al. 2003; Phrolov et al. 2004). A small study ($n = 90$) comparing an initial dose of oral loading (20 mg/kg) with intravenous loading (20 mg/kg) or traditional dosing found that oral and intravenous loading led to more efficient improvement compared with traditional dosing; similar improvement was seen with oral versus intravenous loading (Ghaleiha et al. 2014).

Findings from several studies indicate that rectal administration of carbamazepine, lamotrigine, and topiramate provides acceptable bioavailability and tolerability. Carbamazepine has been rectally administered as a solution (Leppik and Patel 2015; Neuvonen and Tokola 1987; Patel et al. 2014) and as a crushed tablet in a gelatin capsule (Storey and Trumble 1992), attaining therapeutic blood levels in some but not all patients. Rectal forms of lamotrigine and topiramate have been prepared from oral formulations. Compared with oral dosing, rectal lamotrigine had reduced bioavailability (approximately 50%), leading to lower drug levels and slower absorption (Birnbaum et al. 2001), whereas blood levels were identical after rectal and oral administration of topiramate (Conway et al. 2003). Provided relative bioavailability is considered, rectal administration of an aqueous suspension of these tablets may be acceptable.

Rectal absorption of other anticonvulsants, including felbamate, gabapentin, oxcarbazepine, and phenytoin, is not reliable (Clemens et al. 2007; Leppik and Patel 2015). Oxcarbazepine is available as an oral suspension, but its rectal administration achieved only 10% of the oral bioavailability for the parent drug or active metabolite (Clemens et al. 2007). Thus, rectal delivery is not an appropriate route for oxcarbazepine.

Psychostimulants

Transdermal methylphenidate was approved for ADHD in children in 2006 in the United States. The patch is worn for 9 hours but provides therapeutic effect through 12 hours. Several patch doses are available, and the duration of effect can be modified by early removal of the patch (Manos et al. 2007). It is indicated for hip application only. Application site reactions may occur. Cases of chemical leukoderma have been reported with transdermal methylphenidate (Cheng et al. 2017). No trials of transdermal methylphenidate have been reported in patients with serious medical illness.

Transdermal dextroamphetamine was approved in 2022 for both children 6 years or older and adults with ADHD. Similarly, the patch is designed to be worn for 9 hours. It offers various application sites including the hip, upper arm, chest, upper back, or flank (Transdermal dextroamphetamine [Xelstrym] for ADHD 2023).

Both methylphenidate and dextroamphetamine transdermal formulations should be applied 2 hours before desired effect.

Although no other non-oral forms of psychostimulants are available, custom preparations are described. Dextroamphetamine has been administered intravenously to human participants in research but not clinically (Ernst and Goldberg 2002). There is one published case report of 5-mg dextroamphetamine suppositories compounded by a pharmacy that significantly improved depressed mood in a woman who had gastrointestinal obstruction (Holmes et al. 1994).

Medications for Dementia

Two cholinesterase inhibitors are available in a non-oral formulation as transdermal patches. The rivastigmine patch is dosed daily and provides less fluctuating plasma levels than the twice-daily oral capsules or solution. The patch provides greater bioavailability but with slower absorption, which reduces peak drug levels by 20%. This more consistent drug exposure might improve efficacy, but this possibility remains to be investigated. The incidence of nausea and vomiting declined from 33% with the oral form to 20% with the patch (Lefèvre et al. 2008). A once-weekly transdermal formulation of donepezil received FDA approval in 2022. It is designed to produce less fluctuation in concentration and reduce gastrointestinal adverse effects (Gallagher 2022). Donepezil is also available as an ODT.

Aducanumab was controversially FDA approved for Alzheimer's disease in 2021. This is only available in a 1-hour intravenous infusion administered once every 4 weeks. A second agent, lecanemab, was approved in 2023 and is also available as a 1-hour infusion but dosed every 2 weeks (Eisai 2023). Both products' use may be limited by cost and risks of adverse effects (Aducanumab

[Aduhelm] for Alzheimer's disease 2021; Rabinovici 2021; Walsh et al. 2022). Other antiamyloid agents are currently under investigation for Alzheimer's disease (Tolar et al. 2020).

Conclusion

Non-oral formulations are now approved in the United States for at least one agent in each psychotropic drug class, and several others are routinely prepared by compounding pharmacies. There is no single best administration route for all patients. In addition to the availability of dosing forms, administrative and pharmacokinetic concerns govern formulation choice. In this regard, non-oral routes of drug delivery have several advantages over oral administration. Medication adherence may improve if the delivery route is perceived as more convenient, and compliance is more easily verified with certain routes. Preparations can be selected to provide rapid drug delivery for acute treatment or more continuous drug absorption for chronic therapy. By decreasing the variation in plasma drug levels, continuous drug delivery reduces adverse effects, improves tolerability and patient adherence, and enhances therapeutic effect. Drugs delivered by a non-oral route at least partly bypass the gastrointestinal tract and avoid first-pass metabolism. Bioavailability is often improved, and metabolite formation, a potential source of adverse effects, is reduced. Also, because the high gut concentration of drug following oral administration is avoided, gastrointestinal adverse effects are lessened.

The trend in continued development of alternative dosage formulations of psychotropic drug delivery systems recognizes many of these advantages of non-oral preparations. However, there remains a need for drug forms that are easier, less expensive, and less invasive to administer, especially in situations where medical resources are limited.

Key Points

- Drug delivery by non-oral routes may improve medication administration in patients with severe nausea or vomiting, dysphagia, or severe malabsorption; unconscious or uncooperative patients; and patients unable or unwilling to take medications by mouth.

- In comparison with drugs taken orally, drugs delivered by a non-oral route may have fewer gastrointestinal adverse effects.

- Bioavailability of medications can vary considerably between different routes of administration. Literature recommendations, therapeutic drug monitoring, and clinical response should be used to guide dosing.

- Short-acting injectable atypical antipsychotics are recommended to be administered only intramuscularly.

- Transdermal drug delivery reduces the peak-to-trough fluctuation of drug levels produced by oral dosing and provides near-constant plasma drug levels, even for short-half-life drugs, over longer dosing intervals.

- Transdermal formulations are available for antidepressant, cognitive enhancement, and psychostimulant medications.

- Sublingual or buccal formulations are available for antipsychotic (asenapine), anxiolytic (lorazepam; Canada only), and hypnotic medications. The monoamine oxidase B inhibitor selegiline is available in a sublingual preparation for use in Parkinson's disease.

- Intravenous administration and intranasal administration of approved agents to manage depression require delivery and monitoring in a health care facility.

References

Aducanumab (Aduhelm) for Alzheimer's disease. Med Lett Drugs Ther 63(1628):105–106, 2021 34543258

Amsterdam JD, Bodkin JA: Selegiline transdermal system in the prevention of relapse of major depressive disorder: a 52-week, double-blind, placebo-substitution, parallel-group clinical trial. J Clin Psychopharmacol 26(6):579–586, 2006 17110814

Anderson GD, Saneto RP: Current oral and non-oral routes of antiepileptic drug delivery. Adv Drug Deliv Rev 64(10):911–918, 2012 22326840

Aydintug YS, Okcu KM, Guner Y, et al: Evaluation of oral or rectal midazolam as conscious sedation for pediatric patients in oral surgery. Mil Med 169(4):270–273, 2004 15132227

Bauer TM, Ritz R, Haberthür C, et al: Prolonged sedation due to accumulation of conjugated metabolites of midazolam. Lancet 346(8968):145–147, 1995 7603229

Beach SR, Gross AF, Hartney KE, et al: Intravenous haloperidol: a systematic review of side effects and recommendations for clinical use. Gen Hosp Psychiatry 67:42–51, 2020 32979582

Bhattaccharjee SA, Murnane KS, Banga AK: Transdermal delivery of breakthrough therapeutics for the management of treatment-resistant and post-partum depression. Int J Pharm 591:120007, 2020 33191204

Birnbaum AK, Kriel RL, Im Y, et al: Relative bioavailability of lamotrigine chewable dispersible tablets administered rectally. Pharmacotherapy 21(2):158–162, 2001 11213851

Bleicher J, Bhaskara A, Huyck T, et al: Lorazepam, diphenhydramine, and haloperidol transdermal gel for rescue from chemotherapy-induced nausea/vomiting: results of two pilot trials. J Support Oncol 6(1):27–32, 2008 18257398

Boddu SHS, Kumari S: A short review on the intranasal deliver of diazepam for treating acute repetitive seizures. Pharmaceutics 12(12):1167, 2020 33265963

Bostwick JR, Demehri A: Pills to powder: a clinician's reference for crushable psychotropic medications. Curr Psychiatr 13(5):e1–e34, 2014

Bou Khalil R: Intravenous mirtazapine (letter). Clin Neuropharmacol 34(3):134, 2011 21586922

Bozymski KM, Crouse EL, Titus-Lay EN, et al: Esketamine: a novel option for treatment-resistant depression. Ann Pharmacother 54(6):567–576, 2020 31795735

Cheng C, La Grenade L, Diak I-L, et al: Chemical leukoderma associated with methylphenidate transdermal system: data from the US Food and Drug Administration Adverse Event Reporting System. J Pediatr 180:241–246, 2017 27745746

Choi M, Barra ME, Newman K, et al: Safety and effectiveness of intravenous chlorpromazine for agitation in critically ill patients. J Intensive Care Med 35(10):1118–1122, 2020 30558470

Clemens PL, Cloyd JC, Kriel RL, et al: Relative bioavailability, metabolism and tolerability of rectally administered oxcarbazepine suspension. Clin Drug Investig 27(4):243–250, 2007 17358096

Coe MA, Lofwall MR, Walsh SL: Buprenorphine pharmacology review: update on transmucosal and long-acting formulations. J Addict Med 13(2):93–103, 2019 30531584

Cole JB, Lee SC, Martel ML, et al: The incidence of QT prolongation and torsades des pointes in patients receiving droperidol in an urban emergency department. West J Emerg Med 21(4):728–736, 2020 32726229

Conway JM, Birnbaum AK, Kriel RL, et al: Relative bioavailability of topiramate administered rectally. Epilepsy Res 54(2–3):91–96, 2003 12837560

Corriger A, Pickering G: Ketamine and depression: a narrative review. Drug Des Devel Ther 13:3051–3067, 2019 31695324

Crouse E, Haught J, Tobarran N, et al: Skin necrosis following inadvertent dermal injection of extended-release buprenorphine. J Addict Med 16(2):242–245, 2022 33795578

Currier GW, Medori R: Orally versus intramuscularly administered antipsychotic drugs in psychiatric emergencies. J Psychiatr Pract 12(1):30–40, 2006 16432443

Dailymed: Drizalma sprinkle: duloxetine capsule, delayed release. July 28, 2021. Available at: https://dailymed.nlm.nih.gov/dailymed/lookup.cfm?setid=b41423b8-dfec-4d79-ba3c-e43a87803d85. Accessed March 21, 2023.

Duncan MA, Savage J, Tucker AP: Prospective audit comparing intrathecal analgesia (incorporating midazolam) with epidural and intravenous analgesia after major open abdominal surgery. Anaesth Intensive Care 35(4):558–562, 2007 18020075

Eisai: Full prescribing information for LEQEMBI. Nutley, NJ, Eisai, January 2023. Available at: https://www.accessdata.fda.gov/drugsatfda_docs/label/2023/761269s000lbl.pdf. Accessed March 21, 2023.

Ernst CL, Goldberg JF: The reproductive safety profile of mood stabilizers, atypical antipsychotics, and broad-spectrum psychotropics. J Clin Psychiatry 63(Suppl 4):42–55, 2002 11913676

Fahmy AM, El-Setouhy DA, Habib BA, et al: Enhancement of transdermal delivery of haloperidol via spanlastic dispersions: entrapment efficiency vs. particle size. AAPS PharmSciTech 20(3):95, 2019 30694404

Feiger AD, Rickels K, Rynn MA, et al: Selegiline transdermal system for the treatment of major depressive disorder: an 8-week, double-blind, placebo-controlled, flexible-dose titration trial. J Clin Psychiatry 67(9):1354–1361, 2006 17017821

Fontana E, Mandolini GM, Delvecchio G, et al: Intravenous valproate in the treatment of acute manic episode in bipolar disorder: a review. J Affect Disord 260:738–743, 2020 31581039

Fonzo-Christe C, Vukasovic C, Wasilewski-Rasca AF, et al: Subcutaneous administration of drugs in the elderly: survey of practice and systematic literature review. Palliat Med 19(3):208–219, 2005 15920935

Gallagher A: FDA approves donepezil transdermal patch for treatment of Alzheimer disease. Pharmacy Times, March 16, 2022. Available at: https://www.pharmacytimes.com/view/fda-approves-donepezil-transdermal-patch-for-treatment-of-alzheimer-disease. Accessed March 21, 2023.

Gaw CM, Cabrera D, Bellolio F, et al: Effectiveness and safety of droperidol in a United States emergency department. Am J Emerg Med 38(7):1310–1314, 2020 31831345

Ghaleiha A, Haghighi M, Sharifmehr M, et al: Oral loading of sodium valproate compared to intravenous loading and oral maintenance in acutely manic bipolar patients. Neuropsychobiology 70(1):29–35, 2014 25171133

Girard TD, Exline MC, Carson SS, et al: Haloperidol and ziprasidone for treatment of delirium in critical illness. N Engl J Med 379(26):2506–2516, 2018 30346242

Gopalakrishna G, Aggarwal A, Lauriello J: Long-acting injectable aripiprazole: how might it fit in our tool box? Clin Schizophr Relat Psychoses 7(2):87–92, 2013 23644169

Government of Canada: Drug product database. 2022. Available at: www.canada.ca/en/health-canada/services/drugs-health-products/drug-products/drug-product-database.html. Accessed March 24, 2022.

Graves NM, Kriel RL, Jones-Saete C: Bioavailability of rectally administered lorazepam. Clin Neuropharmacol 10(6):555–559, 1987 3427562

Greenblatt DJ, Divoll M, Harmatz JS, et al: Pharmacokinetic comparison of sublingual lorazepam with intravenous, intramuscular, and oral lorazepam. J Pharm Sci 71(2):248–252, 1982 6121043

Hogan RE, Gidal BE, Koplowitz B, et al: Bioavailability and safety of diazepam intranasal solution compared to oral and rectal diazepam in healthy volunteers. Epilepsia 61(3):455–464, 2020 32065672

Holmes TF, Sabaawi M, Fragala MR: Psychostimulant suppository treatment for depression in the gravely ill. J Clin Psychiatry 55(6):265–266, 1994 8071285

Jagadheesan K, Duggal H, Gupta S, et al: Acute antimanic efficacy and safety of intravenous valproate loading therapy: an open-label study. Neuropsychobiology 47(2):90–93, 2003 12707491

Janssen Pharmaceuticals: Spravato (esketamine) prescribing information. June 2020. Available at: www.janssenlabels.com/package-insert/product-monograph/prescribing-information/SPRAVATO-pi.pdf. Accessed September 15, 2022.

Kaminsky BM, Bostwick JR, Guthrie SK: Alternate routes of administration of antidepressant and antipsychotic medications. Ann Pharmacother 49(7):808–817, 2015 25907529

Kaneishi K, Kawabata M, Morita T: Single-dose subcutaneous benzodiazepines for insomnia in patients with advanced cancer. J Pain Symptom Manage 49(6):e1–e2, 2015 25827855

Kasper S, Müller-Spahn F: Intravenous antidepressant treatment: focus on citalopram. Eur Arch Psychiatry Clin Neurosci 252(3):105–109, 2002 12192466

Kayhart B, Lapid MI, Nelson S, et al: A lack of systemic absorption following the repeated application of topical quetiapine in healthy adults. Am J Hosp Palliat Care 35(8):1076–1080, 2018 29343085

Khorassani F, Saad M: Intravenous olanzapine for the management of agitation: review of the literature. Ann Pharmacother 53(8):853–859, 2019 30758221

Koelle JS, Dimsdale JE: Antidepressants for the virtually eviscerated patient: options instead of oral dosing. Psychosom Med 60(6):723–725, 1998 9847031

Konstantinidis A, Stastny J, Ptak-Butta J, et al: Intravenous mirtazapine in the treatment of depressed inpatients. Eur Neuropsychopharmacol 12(1):57–60, 2002 11788241

Lefèvre G, Pommier F, Sedek G, et al: Pharmacokinetics and bioavailability of the novel rivastigmine transdermal patch versus rivastigmine oral solution in healthy elderly subjects. J Clin Pharmacol 48(2):246–252, 2008 18199897

Leppik IE, Patel SI: Intramuscular and rectal therapies of acute seizures. Epilepsy Behav 49:307–312, 2015 26071998

Leung JG, Nelson S, Cunningham JL, et al: A single-dose crossover pharmacokinetic comparison study of oral, rectal and topical quetiapine in healthy adults. Clin Pharmacokinet 55(8):971–976, 2016 26873228

Leung JG, Philbrick KL, Loomis EA, et al: Rectal bioavailability of sertraline tablets in a critically ill patient with bowel compromise. J Clin Psychopharmacol 37(3):372–373, 2017 28277400

Lynch ME, Clark AJ, Sawynok J, et al: Topical amitriptyline and ketamine in neuropathic pain syndromes: an open-label study. J Pain 6(10):644–649, 2005 16202956

Manos MJ, Tom-Revzon C, Bukstein OG, et al: Changes and challenges: managing ADHD in a fast-paced world. J Manag Care Pharm 13(9 Suppl B):S2–S13, quiz S14–S16, 2007 18062734

Markowitz JS, DeVane CL, Malcolm RJ, et al: Pharmacokinetics of olanzapine after single-dose oral administration of standard tablet versus normal and sublingual administration of an orally disintegrating tablet in normal volunteers. J Clin Pharmacol 46(2):164–171, 2006 16432268

Martel ML, Driver BE, Miner JR, et al: Randomized double-blind trial of intramuscular droperidol, ziprasidone, and lorazepam for acute undifferentiated agitation in the emergency department. Acad Emerg Med 28(4):421–434, 2021 32888340

Miller JL, Ashford JW, Archer SM, et al: Comparison of intranasal administration of haloperidol with intravenous and intramuscular administration: a pilot pharmacokinetic study. Pharmacotherapy 28(7):875–882, 2008 18576902

Mirassou MM: Rectal antidepressant medication in the treatment of depression (letter). J Clin Psychiatry 59(1):29, 1998 9491063

Morin AK: Possible intranasal quetiapine misuse. Am J Health Syst Pharm 64(7):723–725, 2007 17384357

Moukaddam NJ, Hirschfeld RM: Intravenous antidepressants: a review. Depress Anxiety 19(1):1–9, 2004 14978779

Mühlbacher M, Konstantinidis A, Kasper S, et al: Intravenous mirtazapine is safe and effective in the treatment of depressed inpatients. Neuropsychobiology 53(2):83–87, 2006 16511339

Naso AR: Optimizing patient safety by preventing combined use of intramuscular olanzapine and parenteral benzodiazepines. Am J Health Syst Pharm 65(12):1180–1183, 2008 18541690

Neuvonen PJ, Tokola O: Bioavailability of rectally administered carbamazepine mixture. Br J Clin Pharmacol 24(6):839–841, 1987 3440107

Nie Q, Hui P, Ding H, et al: Rectal chloral hydrate sedation for computed tomography in young children with head trauma. Medicine (Baltimore) 100(9):e25033, 2021 33655976

Nordstrom K, Allen MH: Alternative delivery systems for agents to treat acute agitation: progress to date. Drugs 73(16):1783–1792, 2013 24151084

Nuttall GA, Eckerman KM, Jacob KA, et al: Does low-dose droperidol administration increase the risk of drug-induced QT prolongation and torsade de pointes in the general surgical population? Anesthesiology 107(4):531–536, 2007 17893447

Pakyurek M, Pasol E: Sublingually administered fluoxetine for major depression in medically compromised patients. Am J Psychiatry 156(11):1833–1834, 1999 10553754

Patel SM, Crouse EL, Levenson JL: Evaluation of intramuscular olanzapine and ziprasidone in the medically ill. Ment Health Clin 11(1):6–11, 2021 33505819

Patel V, Cordato DJ, Malkan A, et al: Rectal carbamazepine as effective long-acting treatment after cluster seizures and status epilepticus. Epilepsy Behav 31:31–33, 2014 24333499

Perez-Ruixo C, Rossenu S, Zannikos P, et al: Population pharmacokinetics of esketamine nasal spray and its metabolite noresketamine in healthy subjects and patients with treatment-resistant depression. Clin Pharmacokinet 60(4):501–516, 2021 33128208

Pergolizzi JV Jr, Taylor R Jr, Raffa RB, et al: Fast-acting sublingual zolpidem for middle-of-the-night wakefulness. Sleep Disord 2014:527109, 2014 24649369

Perkins J, Ho JD, Vilke GM, et al: American Academy of Emergency Medicine position statement: safety of droperidol use in the emergency department. J Emerg Med 49(1):91–97, 2015 25837231

Pfizer: Ziprasidone prescribing information. 2015. Available at: https:// labeling.pfizer.com/ShowLabeling.aspx?id=584. Accessed April 11, 2016.

Phrolov K, Applebaum J, Levine J, et al: Single-dose intravenous valproate in acute mania. J Clin Psychiatry 65(1):68–70, 2004 14744171

Polania Gutierrez JJ, Munakomi S: Intramuscular injection, in StatPearls. Treasure Island, FL, StatPearls Publishing, Updated February 12, 2023. Available at: www.ncbi.nlm.nih.gov/books/NBK556121. Accessed March 21, 2023.

Preethy NA, Somasundaram S: Sedative and behavioral effects of intranasal midazolam in comparison with other administrative routes in children undergoing dental treatment: a systematic review. Contemp Clin Dent 12(2):105–120, 2021 34220149

Rabinovici GD: Controversy and progress in Alzheimer's disease: FDA approval of aducanumab. N Engl J Med 385(9):771–774, 2021 34320284

Rey E, Tréluyer JM, Pons G: Pharmacokinetic optimization of benzodiazepine therapy for acute seizures: focus on delivery routes. Clin Pharmacokinet 36(6):409–424, 1999 10427466

Rogawski MA, Heller AH: Diazepam buccal film for the treatment of acute seizures. Epilepsy Behav 101(Pt B):106537, 2019 31699662

Sage Therapeutics: Zulresso prescribing information. June 2019. Available at: www.zulressohcp.com/about-zulresso?gclid= Cj0KCQjwmouZBhDSARIsALYcoupGVmo2S54IWPUtM-PQp1XubLifc39yjU09Px0dzkACxJGp2jhch3QaAjo0EALw_wcB&gclsrc= aw.ds. Accessed September 15, 2022.

San L, Casillas M, Ciudad A, et al: Olanzapine orally disintegrating tablet: a review of efficacy and compliance. CNS Neurosci Ther 14(3):203–214, 2008 18801113

Sánchez Fernández I, Loddenkemper T: Therapeutic choices in convulsive status epilepticus. Expert Opin Pharmacother 16(4):487–500, 2015 25626010

Scavone JM, Greenblatt DJ, Shader RI: Alprazolam kinetics following sublingual and oral administration. J Clin Psychopharmacol 7(5):332–334, 1987 3680603

Scavone JM, Greenblatt DJ, Goddard JE, et al: The pharmacokinetics and pharmacodynamics of sublingual and oral alprazolam in the post-prandial state. Eur J Clin Pharmacol 42(4):439–443, 1992 1516609

Schmitt L, Tonnoir B, Arbus C: Safety and efficacy of oral escitalopram as continuation treatment of intravenous citalopram in patients with major depressive disorder. Neuropsychobiology 54(4):201–207, 2006 17337913

Schrier L, Zuiker R, Merkus FWHM, et al: Pharmacokinetics and pharmacodynamics of a new highly concentrated intranasal midazolam formulation for conscious sedation. Br J Clin Pharmacol 83(4):721–731, 2017 27780297

Scott MA, Letrent KJ, Hager KL, et al: Use of transdermal amitriptyline gel in a patient with chronic pain and depression. Pharmacotherapy 19(2):236–239, 1999 10030776

Sebghatollahi V, Tabesh E, Gholamrezaei A, et al: Premedication with benzodiazepines for upper gastrointestinal endoscopy: comparison between oral midazolam and sublingual alprazolam. J Res Med Sci 22:133, 2017 29387120

Shavakhi A, Soleiman S, Gholamrezaei A, et al: Premedication with sublingual or oral alprazolam in adults undergoing diagnostic upper gastrointestinal endoscopy. Endoscopy 46(8):633–639, 2014 24977401

Shrewsbury SB, Hocevar-Trnka J, Satterly KH, et al: The SNAP 101 double-blind, placebo/active-controlled, safety, pharmacokinetic, and pharmacodynamic study of INP105 (nasal olanzapine) in healthy adults. J Clin Psychiatry 81(4):19m13086, 2020 32609960

Smith-Apeldoorn SY, Veraart JKE, Ruhé HG, et al: Repeated, low-dose oral esketamine in patients with treatment-resistant depression: pilot study. BJPsych Open 8(1):e4, 2021 34865676

Staner L, Eriksson M, Cornette F, et al: Sublingual zolpidem is more effective than oral zolpidem in initiating early onset of sleep in the post-nap model of transient insomnia: a polysomnographic study. Sleep Med 10(6):616–620, 2009 18996742

Storey P, Trumble M: Rectal doxepin and carbamazepine therapy in patients with cancer. N Engl J Med 327(18):1318–1319, 1992 1406828

Tábi T, Szökő E, Vécsei L, et al: The pharmacokinetic evaluation of selegiline ODT for the treatment of Parkinson's disease. Expert Opin Drug Metab Toxicol 9(5):629–636, 2013 23506388

Teter CJ, Phan KL, Cameron OG, et al: Relative rectal bioavailability of fluoxetine in normal volunteers. J Clin Psychopharmacol 25(1):74–78, 2005 15643102

Thompson D, DiMartini A: Nonenteral routes of administration for psychiatric medications: a literature review. Psychosomatics 40(3):185–192, 1999 10341530

Tobias JD: Subcutaneous administration of fentanyl and midazolam to prevent withdrawal after prolonged sedation in children. Crit Care Med 27(10):2262–2265, 1999 10548218

Tolar M, Abushakra S, Hey JA, et al: Aducanumab, gantenerumab, BAN2401, and ALZ-801—the first wave of amyloid-targeting drugs for Alzheimer's disease with potential for near term approval. Alzheimers Res Ther 12(1):95, 2020 32787971

Transdermal dextroamphetamine (Xelstrym) for ADHD. Med Lett Drugs Ther 65(1669):22–24, 2023 36757350

UCB Group: Nayzilam (midazolam) nasal spray prescribing information. January 2023. Available at: www.ucb-usa.com/nayzilam-prescribing-information.pdf. Accessed March 21, 2023.

U.S. Food and Drug Administration: Clinical pharmacology and biopharmaceutics review for olanzapine (Zyprexa Zydis). Center for Drug Evaluation and Research, 1999. Available at: www.accessdata.fda.gov/drugsatfda_docs/nda/2000/21-086_Zyprexa%20Zydis_biopharmr.pdf. Accessed August 6, 2015.

Walsh S, Merrick R, Richard E, et al: Lecanemab for Alzheimer's disease. BMJ 379:o3010, 2022 36535691

Wang M, Yankama TT, Abdallah GT, et al: A retrospective comparison of the effectiveness and safety of intravenous olanzapine versus intravenous haloperidol for agitation in adult intensive care unit patients. J Intensive Care Med 37(2):222–230, 2022 33426981

Weiland AM, Protus BM, Kimbrel J, et al: Chlorpromazine bioavailability from a topical gel formulation in volunteers. J Support Oncol 11(3):144–148, 2013 24400394

Weintraub SJ: Diazepam in the treatment of moderate to severe alcohol withdrawal. CNS Drugs 31(2):87–95, 2017 28101764

Wermeling DP, Miller JL, Archer SM, et al: Bioavailability and pharmacokinetics of lorazepam after intranasal, intravenous, and intramuscular administration. J Clin Pharmacol 41(11):1225–1231, 2001 11697755

Wilson MP, Chen N, Vilke GM, et al: Olanzapine in ED patients: differential effects on oxygenation in patients with alcohol intoxication. Am J Emerg Med 30(7):1196–1201, 2012a 22633728

Wilson MP, MacDonald K, Vilke GM, et al: A comparison of the safety of olanzapine and haloperidol in combination with benzodiazepines in emergency department patients with acute agitation. J Emerg Med 43(5):790–797, 2012b 21601409

Wolfe TR, Bernstone T: Intranasal drug delivery: an alternative to intravenous administration in selected emergency cases. J Emerg Nurs 30(2):141–147, 2004 15039670

Zhang K, Yang Y, Yuan X, et al: Efficacy and safety of repeated esketamine intravenous infusion in the treatment of treatment-resistant depression: a case series. Asian J Psychiatr 68:102976, 2022 34971937

Zimbroff DL: Pharmacological control of acute agitation: focus on intramuscular preparations. CNS Drugs 22(3):199–212, 2008 18278976

PART 2

Psychopharmacology in Organ System Disorders and Specialty Areas

4

Gastrointestinal Disorders

Catherine C. Crone, M.D.

Jacqueline Posada, M.D.

Cullen Truett, D.O.

Michael Marcangelo, M.D.

Diseases of the gastrointestinal (GI) system are prevalent and often associated with distress and psychiatric disorders, which may cause, exacerbate, or be a reaction to these disorders (Holtmann et al. 2017; Peery et al. 2019; Van Oudenhove et al. 2016). In this chapter, we review the use of psychotropic medications in the treatment of GI disorder symptoms and comorbid psychopathology, potential interactions between GI medications and psychotropic agents, risks of prescribing psychiatric medications in the presence of particular GI disorders, and alterations in the pharmacokinetics of psychotropic drugs induced by GI disorders (e.g., hepatic failure, short bowel syndrome). The chapter is organized first by organ system and then by specific GI disorders.

Oropharyngeal Disorders

Burning Mouth Syndrome

Burning mouth syndrome (BMS) is a clinical syndrome characterized by persistent and fluctuating levels of burning, numbness, stinging, or pain in the intraoral region without evidence of mucosal changes. Symptoms recurring daily for more than 2 hours per day over more than a 3-month period fulfill diagnostic criteria established by the International Headache Society (2020). Onset is often spontaneous and occurs primarily in perimenopausal and postmenopausal women (Klein et al. 2020). The anterior tip of the tongue, the lips, and the hard palate are typically involved, although it can affect any part of the oral cavity (Feller et al. 2017; Klein et al. 2020). Xerostomia and taste disturbances often accompany the clinical presentation (Feller et al. 2017).

BMS is primarily a diagnosis of exclusion, because it is not linked to local or systemic causative factors such as oral candidiasis, medications, nutritional deficiencies, or Sjögren's syndrome (Bender 2018). Although the pathophysiology remains unclear, there is evidence of peripheral and central nervous system involvement, particularly peripheral small fiber neuropathy, subclinical trigeminal nerve neuropathy, and dopaminergic deficiencies within central inhibitory pain pathways (Bender 2018; Jääskeläinen 2018; Ritchie and Kramer 2018). Psychiatric comorbidity is common, particularly anxiety, depression, and somatization (de Souza et al. 2012).

Treatment of BMS is challenging because of a lack of a clear understanding of its pathophysiology, and management focuses on symptom reduction and improved quality of life. Evidence from clinical trials is limited by differences in diagnostic criteria, small sample sizes, short treatment periods, lack of long-term follow-up, and differences in study design. However, results from placebo-controlled randomized trials consistently support use of topical and systemic clonazepam and, to a lesser degree, capsaicin (Cui et al. 2016; Kisely et al. 2016; Ślebioda et al. 2020). Capsaicin has been used systemically and as an oral rinse in trials, but tolerability has been an issue contributing to dropouts (Ślebioda et al. 2020). α-Lipoic acid, a mitochondrial coenzyme with antioxidant and neuroprotective properties, has had mixed results (Kisely et al. 2016; Ślebioda et al. 2020). Although earlier case reports and lower-quality studies suggested potential benefits from antidepressants such as sertraline, duloxetine, and paroxetine, recent systematic reviews have noted that the evidence base is inadequate (Reyad et al. 2020). However, a recent randomized open-label trial involving 150 patients compared fixed-dosage vortioxetine with other antidepressants and noted a significantly higher rate of clinical response at 6 months and clinical remission at 12 months with vortioxetine than with the other agents (Adamo et al. 2021).

Xerostomia

Xerostomia is a subjective complaint of dry mouth that may be accompanied by decreased saliva production (Villa et al. 2014). Adequate saliva production is necessary for swallowing, speech, dental health, and the protection of mucous membranes in the upper GI tract. Xerostomia may be caused by a number of conditions, including connective tissue disorders, radiation therapy, anxiety, and depression (Han et al. 2015; Villa et al. 2014). Psychotropic agents are a common contributor to xerostomia. Almost all antidepressants, typical and atypical antipsychotic agents, lithium, sodium valproate, gabapentin, nonbenzodiazepine sedative-hypnotics, and several stimulants have shown evidence of causing xerostomia (Cappetta et al. 2018; Cockburn et al. 2017; Tan et al. 2018; Wolff et al. 2017). This may be particularly problematic for medically ill or older patients who are also taking other medications that produce xerostomia (e.g., antihypertensives, diuretics, opioids, anticholinergics). Management of symptoms may require medication changes or dosage reductions, avoidance of caffeine and alcohol, frequent sips of water, sugarless gum or candies, xylitol-containing lozenges, saliva substitutes, topical fluoride, and cholinergic agents such as pilocarpine or cevimeline (Han et al. 2015; Villa et al. 2014; Wolff et al. 2017).

Dysphagia

Dysphagia, difficulty in swallowing, is a highly prevalent problem, affecting up to 50% of adults older than 50 and 50% of patients with neurological disorders (Clavé and Shaker 2015). Malnutrition, dehydration, acute asphyxia, and aspiration pneumonia are serious complications of dysphagia (Panebianco et al. 2020). Neurological disorders such as cerebrovascular accidents, multiple sclerosis, Alzheimer's disease, and Parkinson's disease often produce incoordination of swallowing efforts. Psychotropic medications often cause or aggravate dysphagia, especially in geriatric populations and patients with severe, persistent mental illness (Clavé and Shaker 2015; Kulkarni et al. 2017).

This is especially true with typical and atypical antipsychotics (e.g., haloperidol, trifluoperazine, clozapine, risperidone, aripiprazole, quetiapine) secondary to acute dystonia, parkinsonism, or tardive dyskinesia or dystonia, often occurring in the absence of other movement disorder symptoms (Cicala et al. 2019; Miarons Font and Rofes Salsench 2017; Nieves et al. 2007). Xerostomia, sialorrhea, and sedation are also causative factors for dysphagia associated with antipsychotics, and dysphagia also may occur with other psychotropic medications such as antidepressants, benzodiazepines, cholinesterase inhibitors, and mood stabilizers (Cicala et al. 2019; Spieker 2000). Finally, dysphagia can manifest as part of the clinical presentation of neuroleptic malignant syndrome and rarely in serotonin syndrome (Passmore et al. 2004; Shamash et al. 1994).

Acute dystonia responds to intravenous diphenhydramine or benztropine. However, dysphagia due to drug-induced parkinsonism may not respond to an anticholinergic agent or amantadine, although it may respond to dosage reduction of the antipsychotic, changes in agents, swallowing therapy, or discontinuation of pharmacotherapy (Cicala et al. 2019; Kulkarni et al. 2017; Nieves et al. 2007). Dysphagia associated with tardive dyskinesia or dystonia may respond to similar measures, with case reports also suggesting potential benefits from clonazepam and the vesicular monoamine transporter 2 inhibitor tetrabenazine (Cicala et al. 2019; Kulkarni et al. 2017; Nieves et al. 2007). For discussion of patients whose dysphagia prevents swallowing medications, see Chapter 3, "Alternative Routes of Drug Administration."

Esophageal and Gastric Disorders

Nomenclature and treatment options for esophageal disorders have become increasingly complex. Terms include gastroesophageal reflux disease (GERD), nonerosive reflux disease (NERD), heartburn, esophageal chest pain, esophageal dysmotility, esophageal hypersensitivity, noncardiac chest pain (NCCP), and functional heartburn.

In functional GI illnesses, several common physiological elements have been identified. They include dysmotility, visceral hypersensitivity, disturbed central perception of peripheral visceral events, and a tendency for symptoms to worsen under stress (Quigley and Lacy 2013). Patients also may share demographic similarities, including female sex, comorbid anxiety and depression, and decreased quality of life (Quigley and Lacy 2013). Finally, treatment strategies can be quite similar. As one reviews the literature, the overlap between illnesses is striking.

Reflux Disease and Noncardiac Chest Pain

Presenting symptoms of "chest pain" are a significant burden both on patients and on the medical system. Of approximately 6 million patients who present annually to U.S. emergency departments with chest pain, it is estimated that up to 90% of the complaints may be noncardiac in origin (Burgstaller et al. 2014). NCCP may be caused by esophageal pathology in 30%–50% of cases (Coss-Adame et al. 2014; Nguyen and Eslick 2012). *GERD* is a label routinely used by clinicians and patients alike to define the "heartburn" sensation accompanying reentry of stomach contents into the esophagus. Symptomatic reflux continues to be a significant health problem in Western countries, where more than 20% of people report reflux symptoms (Bashashati et al. 2014; Weijenborg et al. 2015).

For patients who have endoscopically identified cellular changes in their esophagus, the label *GERD* is appropriate. For patients who have no cellular changes noted (more than 70% of patients with GERD symptoms), the label *NERD* has been adopted (Quigley and Lacy 2013). These patients may experience physical sensations similar to those of patients with GERD, although they are considered to have lower risk of developing Barrett's esophagus or adenocarcinoma. Notably, reflux is a normal occurrence, so it is a decrease in lower esophageal sphincter (LES) pressure or an increase in the number of LES relaxations (transient LES relaxations) that is thought to contribute to patient symptoms (Nwokediuko 2012). GERD-related NCCP is commonly treated with histamine H_2-receptor antagonists (H_2 blockers) and proton pump inhibitor (PPI) medications (Hershcovici et al. 2012). Dysmotility NCCP can be treated with smooth muscle relaxants, including nitrates, nitric oxide donors, phosphodiesterase type 5 inhibitors, anticholinergics, and calcium channel blockers (Hershcovici et al. 2012).

It is thought that visceral hypersensitivity plays a role in GERD, NCCP, and other functional GI disorders (Weijenborg et al. 2015). Some authors postulate that up to 80% of patients with unexplained NCCP have lower esophageal sensory thresholds compared with peer control subjects (Bashashati et al. 2014; Remes-Troche 2010). NCCP related to esophageal hypersensitivity may be best addressed with antidepressants, as well as cognitive-behavioral therapy, biofeedback, and hypnotherapy (Coss-Adame et al. 2014; Hershcovici et al. 2012; Nwokediuko 2012; Remes-Troche 2010). In studies focusing on NCCP or esophageal sensitivity, various antidepressant classes such as selective serotonin reuptake inhibitors (SSRIs), tricyclic antidepressants (TCAs), trazodone, and serotonin-norepinephrine reuptake inhibitors (SNRIs) were found to reduce patients' perceptions of the frequency and intensity of chest pain in certain subgroups (Coss-Adame et al. 2014; Nguyen and Eslick 2012; Nwokediuko 2012; Viazis et al. 2012; Weijenborg et al. 2015). However, another meta-analysis focusing on NCCP that excluded patients with comorbid psychiatric illness found no improvement of chest pain with SSRI treatment relative to placebo (Atluri et al. 2015). Consequently, although a modest treatment response of NCCP to antidepressant treatment is possible, further investigation is warranted.

Psychological symptoms such as anxiety, depression, and neurosis are common in more than one-third of patients with GERD, and psychological stress may worsen GERD in more than half of all cases (Ciovica et al. 2009). Positive effects of antidepressants for patients with GERD or NCCP have been noted despite a lack of appreciable improvement in anxiety or depression scores, suggesting a possible mechanism responsible for improvement aside from amelioration of underlying psychiatric disorders (Bashashati et al. 2014; Nguyen and Eslick 2012; Weijenborg et al. 2015).

Although TCAs and SSRIs may show benefits for esophageal nociception and NCCP, multiple studies indicate that clinicians should avoid prescribing highly anticholinergic medications. Anticholinergic medications are thought to decrease LES pressure, leading to an increase in the number of reflux episodes (Bashashati et al. 2014; Martín-Merino et al. 2010). These medications also may prolong orocecal transit time, increasing the time that gastric contents remain in the stomach and thus the opportunity for reflux to occur (van Veggel et al. 2013; Weijenborg et al. 2015). They also may inhibit esophageal peristalsis and salivary secretions, which are needed to clear refluxed material. Indeed, some research has found that depressed patients taking TCAs had a higher risk of being diagnosed with GERD than those who were not taking TCAs (Martín-Merino et al. 2010). Similar research on patients taking antipsychotics found that patients given clozapine had a higher rate of reflux than patients taking other atypical antipsychotics, presumably because of the robust anticholinergic properties of clozapine (van Veggel et al. 2013). Benzodiazepines also are associated with GERD exacerbation, possibly related to their muscle-relaxing effect on the LES (Balon and Starcevic 2020; Martín-Merino et al. 2010). This, in addition to addiction potential, should lead clinicians to exercise caution in using benzodiazepines for these patients, despite some positive case reports in the past.

Nonulcer (Functional) Dyspepsia

Between 10% and 20% of Western patients who report reflux symptoms may meet criteria for functional heartburn (Weijenborg et al. 2015). Functional esophageal disorders are "disorders presenting with symptoms assumed to originate from the esophagus without a structural or anatomic explanation" (Weijenborg et al. 2015, p. 251). According to the Rome III diagnostic criteria, there are four key functional esophageal disorders: functional heartburn, functional chest pain of presumed esophageal origin, functional dysphagia, and globus (Viazis et al. 2012; Weijenborg et al. 2015).

Functional dyspepsia is thought to affect fewer people than reflux disease, although it still accounts for annual costs of nearly $1 billion in the United States (Camilleri and Stanghellini 2013). It is estimated that of all patients with dyspepsia, up to 80% may have no identified cause for their symptoms and thus will be considered to have functional dyspepsia (Ford et al. 2020). The four core symptoms of functional dyspepsia are bloating (or postprandial fullness), early satiety, epigastric pain, and epigastric burning, and symptoms may be worsened by food (Camilleri and Stanghellini 2013; Oustamanolakis and Tack 2012).

Patients with functional dyspepsia have high rates of comorbid psychopathology, including neuroticism, anxiety, depression, hostility, tension, PTSD, and somatization (Faramarzi et al. 2014; Levy et al. 2006; Oustamanolakis and Tack 2012; Piacentino et al. 2011). A history of physical, sexual, and emotional abuse also may be more prevalent in patients with functional GI disorders. However, psychological factors may not be underlying causes of functional dyspepsia or other functional GI issues, but rather psychological factors may influence how GI illnesses are experienced and expressed (Piacentino et al. 2011). Traditional treatment often includes PPIs, H$_2$ blockers, and prokinetic agents (Oustamanolakis and Tack 2012; Quigley and Lacy 2013).

As in GERD, psychotropic medications are also used in functional dyspepsia. Antidepressants and anxiolytics may have particular effects on pain reduction in functional dyspepsia (Overland 2014). Although antidepressants may offer symptomatic relief and analgesia, more data support use of TCAs (such as amitriptyline) than SSRIs (Ford et al. 2020; Lacy et al. 2018; Overland 2014). In particular, TCAs have demonstrated evidence for specific symptoms such as early satiety and dysmotility (Lu et al. 2016; Luo et al. 2019). After a relatively weak performance of venlafaxine in a placebo-controlled trial in patients with functional dyspepsia, investigators recommended against the SNRI class (Camilleri and Stanghellini 2013; Oustamanolakis and Tack 2012). The evidence for use of SSRIs, including paroxetine and escitalopram, is limited, although studies of SSRIs continue (Camilleri and Stanghellini 2013). Notably, buspirone, a serotonin type 1A receptor (5-HT_{1A}) agonist, seemed to have appreciable benefit for patients with functional dyspepsia when compared with placebo in a double-blind, randomized, controlled, crossover trial (Camilleri and Stanghellini 2013; Overland 2014; Tack et al. 2012). Patients took buspirone 15 minutes before meals and noted overall reduction in functional dyspepsia symptoms (with accompanying increased gastric accommodation but not altered gastric emptying time) (Overland 2014; Tack et al. 2012). A double-blind, placebo-controlled trial used a combination of an antispasmodic agent, clidinium, with a benzodiazepine, chlordiazepoxide, as add-on therapy for patients with functional dyspepsia for whom PPI had treatment failed. Those receiving this combination experienced significant reduction in dyspepsia symptoms and improved quality of life compared with those in the placebo group (Puasripun et al. 2020).

Peptic Ulcer Disease

Found in both the stomach and the duodenum, peptic ulcers have been commonly linked to infection with *Helicobacter pylori* and chronic use of anti-inflammatory medications. Patients report a gnawing sensation in the abdomen, and this sensation often improves with food, as opposed to functional dyspepsia, which may worsen with food. In addition to *H. pylori* and nonsteroidal anti-inflammatory drugs (NSAIDs), alternative etiologies may include other infections (cytomegalovirus, herpes simplex virus, tuberculosis, syphilis) and substances (potassium chloride, bisphosphonates, crack cocaine, and amphetamine) (Jones 2006). Peptic ulcer disease has long been regarded as a "psychosomatic disease" (Faramarzi et al. 2014). One prospective study based in Denmark noted that a high stress index more than doubled the chances of developing an ulcer (Levenstein et al. 2015). Two recent studies confirmed the association of psychological vulnerability such as depression or anxiety with the development of peptic ulcer disease in groups with idiopathic peptic ulcer disease and those colonized with *H. pylori* or exposed to NSAIDs (Levenstein et al. 2017; Paik et al. 2020).

Patients with peptic ulcer disease are often started on multiple medications, including antibiotics, antacids, PPIs, and H_2 blockers in varying therapeutic regimens (den Hollander and Kuipers 2012). Several small randomized controlled trials in the 1980s demonstrated benefits of TCAs (doxepin, trimipramine) in the treatment and prevention of duodenal ulcers, perhaps via antihistaminic and anticholinergic effects (Mackay et al. 1984; Shrivastava et al. 1985). It is now known that SSRIs have been associated with a hemorrhagic tendency resulting from their effects on platelet aggregation, particularly with respect to GI bleeding (Oka et al. 2014), and some investigators have wondered whether SSRI medications could be directly ulcerogenic (Dall et al. 2010). This possibility may prompt clinicians to use alternative medications, rather than SSRIs, in this population. Interestingly, melatonin and its precursor, L-tryptophan, may enhance healing in patients with gastroduodenal ulcers and thus may be worthwhile additions to current treatment regimens for these patients (Celinski et al. 2011).

Gastroparesis

GI motility and functional disorders account for a large percentage of referrals to gastroenterologists. Gastroparesis is characterized by abnormal gastric motility and delayed gastric emptying without identifiable obstruction (Fonseca Mora et al. 2021; Lacy et al. 2022). Symptoms include abdominal pain, nausea and vomiting, bloating, and early satiety (Fonseca Mora et al. 2021; Lacy et al. 2022). Common etiologies of gastroparesis are diabetes mellitus, post–gastric surgery syndrome, neurological disease, autoimmune disorders, iatrogenic causes such as medication side effects (e.g., from opioids), and idiopathic causes (Camilleri et al. 2018; Fonseca Mora et al. 2021). Idiopathic gastroparesis is increasingly recognized and was identified in more than 50% of patients enrolled in the National Institutes of Health Gastroparesis Clinical Research Consortium study (Grover et al. 2019). Anxiety, depression, and somatization are common, although it is difficult to tell whether they are precursors to or sequelae of gastroparesis. Other complications of gastroparesis include esophagitis, Mallory-Weiss tears, and severe peptic ulcer disease (Enweluzo and Aziz 2013).

Advising patients to eat multiple small-particle, low-fat small meals; encouraging more liquids than solids; and ensuring tight glucose control by patients with diabetes are dietary changes that can be helpful and are primary approaches for managing gastroparesis (Camilleri and Sanders 2022; Fonseca Mora et al. 2021; Limketkai et al. 2020). A nonpharmacological approach, gastric electrical stimulation, has shown variable success, with authors recommending it for patients who have intractable nausea and vomiting not responsive to standard treatment and who are not taking opioids (Fonseca Mora et al. 2021). Per oral endoscopic myotomy is a newer approach for refractory gastroparesis (Fonseca Mora et al. 2021; Lacy et al. 2022). Pharmacological options include the prokinetic medicines metoclopramide and erythromycin, with studies under way for other agents, including $5\text{-}HT_4$ and ghrelin agonists, as well as neurokinin 1 antagonists (Camilleri and Sanders 2022). Metoclopramide, a dopamine D_2 receptor–blocking antiemetic agent, can produce extrapyramidal symptoms, somnolence, depression, anxiety, and decreased mental acuity, as well as tardive dyskinesia with chronic use.

Antidepressants (e.g., TCAs) may be another treatment option, although it remains unclear whether they confer prokinetic effects, reduce pain or nausea and vomiting, or simply alleviate distress due to gastroparesis. Evidence remains limited to a small 2013 placebo-controlled trial evaluating use of nortriptyline in idiopathic gastroparesis, but it failed to show improvement in overall symptoms (Parkman et al. 2013). Mirtazapine has been advocated by some as another option. In a small open-label study of 30 patients with gastroparesis refractory to other treatments, mirtazapine significantly improved nausea, vomiting, and appetite (Malamood et al. 2017). Mirtazapine may act via its effects on serotonin and norepinephrine, along with its ability to block $5\text{-}HT_3$ receptors. Although other psychotropic drugs (e.g., phenothiazines, benzodiazepines) were previously used for their antiemetic properties, these seem to have fallen out of favor in recent years. As noted in the earlier subsection "Reflux Disease and Noncardiac Chest Pain," anticholinergic psychiatric drugs can worsen GI symptoms, including gastroparesis, and should be avoided.

Nausea and Vomiting

Vomiting of unknown origin was traditionally attributed to psychological stress (so-called psychogenic vomiting), particularly anxiety and panic (Kirkcaldy et al. 2004). Physical or sexual abuse history is common in patients with idiopathic nausea and vomiting. Specific syndromes of nausea and vomiting include cyclic vomiting syndrome, hyperemesis gravidarum, cancer-related nausea and vomiting, and cannabinoid hyperemesis syndrome. In patients without evident cause of vomiting, disordered eating behaviors should not be overlooked.

Cyclic vomiting syndrome is commonly reported in children but increasingly recognized in adults, with a large population-based survey reporting a 2% prevalence among adults in the United States (Aziz et al. 2019). This syndrome is characterized by episodes of vomiting, separated by prolonged periods without vomiting. These episodes may have triggers (e.g., migraine headaches, seizures, menstrual cycles, stress) or may be unrelated to specific triggers or environmental cues (Bhandari et al. 2018; Herlihy et al. 2019; Kovacic and Li 2021). Some authors have reported that among pediatric and adult populations, migraine, anxiety, depression, and irritable bowel syndrome (IBS) are common personal and family comorbidities (Herlihy et al. 2019). Treatment involves avoiding known triggers (e.g., cannabis use, certain foods, sleep deprivation) and taking prophylactic medications, particularly TCAs for those with moderate to severe cyclic vomiting syndrome (Bhandari et al. 2018; Herlihy et al. 2019; Kovacic and Li 2021; Venkatesan et al. 2019b). Amitriptyline has been studied the most and is the most commonly prescribed agent for cyclic vomiting syndrome, with dosages starting at 10 mg at bedtime and gradual adjustment up to 250 mg nightly if necessary (Kovacic and Li 2021; Venkatesan et al. 2019b). Second-line agents include zonisamide, levetiracetam, and aprepitant (Kovacic and Li 2021). For patients with cyclic vomiting syndrome with a migraine component, propranolol, cyproheptadine, or topiramate may also be added (Kovacic and Li 2021). Because it is a functional GI syndrome, meditation, relaxation, and biofeedback therapies also should be considered as part of the treatment (Venkatesan et al. 2019b).

More than 80% of women experience transient nausea and vomiting in the early stages of pregnancy, but most cases resolve after the first trimester (Abramowitz et al. 2017; Austin et al. 2019). Hyperemesis gravidarum is a condition involving persistent and excessive vomiting that can lead to nutritional problems, fluid and electrolyte imbalance, weight loss, and esophageal tear (London et al. 2017). Although clear diagnostic criteria are lacking, hyperemesis gravidarum affects 0.3%–3% of pregnant women and is one of the most common causes of hospitalization during the first 20 weeks of pregnancy

(Abramowitz et al. 2017; Austin et al. 2019; London et al. 2017). Risk factors include being young, primiparous, or of Black or Asian ethnicity or having type 1 diabetes, history of hyperemesis gravidarum, or multiple gestations. The etiology of hyperemesis gravidarum remains unknown and is considered to probably be multifactorial (London et al. 2017). The belief that hyperemesis gravidarum is a physical manifestation of psychological symptoms largely has been discredited, with authors noting that psychological distress is a result, not a cause, of hyperemesis gravidarum (Kjeldgaard et al. 2017; Tan et al. 2010); clinicians should screen patients with hyperemesis gravidarum to ensure that incident depression or anxiety is not missed.

Numerous medications have been proposed and used for the treatment of hyperemesis gravidarum, including GI medications (e.g., metoclopramide, ondansetron, promethazine), antihistamines, and corticosteroids, as well as nontraditional treatments (e.g., acupuncture, pyridoxine [vitamin B_6], ginger root) (Abramowitz et al. 2017; Austin et al. 2019; London et al. 2017). Limited clinical trials have shown potential benefits with transdermal clonidine and gabapentin, although more studies are needed (Austin et al. 2019). Mirtazapine has also been found helpful in hyperemesis gravidarum, although clinicians should be aware of the risk of serotonin syndrome (Abramowitz et al. 2017). Data suggest a lack of increased risk of major birth defects with mirtazapine (Abramowitz et al. 2017; London et al. 2017). Despite the relative safety of hyperemesis gravidarum medications in pregnancy, clinicians should remain vigilant for adverse effects, particularly extrapyramidal symptoms (acute dystonia, akathisia), if using dopamine antagonists. A 2018 Cochrane review concluded that little high-quality or consistent evidence is available to guide the treatment of hyperemesis gravidarum, so providers must complete a risk-benefit analysis considering side-effect profiles, safety, comorbidities, and economic costs when choosing an intervention (Boelig et al. 2018).

Patients with cancer experience nausea and vomiting for many reasons, including the cancer itself and its complications (e.g., tumor location and metastases, medication effects, metabolic problems, pain, anxiety, impaired gastric emptying), as well as its treatment with chemotherapy and radiation (Hardy and Davis 2021; Navari 2020). These symptoms have negative effects on patients' overall function and quality of life and may deter some patients from continuing treatment (Badar et al. 2015; Jordan et al. 2014). The prevalence of chemotherapy-induced nausea and vomiting has improved with use of corticosteroids plus 5-HT$_3$ receptor blockers, with further progress being made by neurokinin 1 receptor antagonists, including aprepitant, casopitant, fosaprepitant, netupitant, and rolapitant (Badar et al. 2015; Bošnjak et al. 2017; Jordan et al. 2014). Classes of medications used to treat cancer-related nausea and vomiting include typical and atypical antipsychotics (especially olanzapine), 5-HT$_3$ receptor antagonists, neurokinin receptor antagonists, anticholinergics, antihistamines, cannabinoids, and corticosteroids (Bošnjak et al. 2017; Hardy and Davis 2021; Jordan et al. 2014; Navari 2020). Benzodiazepines have been cited as helpful in refractory or breakthrough symptoms as well as anticipatory nausea and vomiting that may develop as a conditioned response to chemotherapy (Cangemi and Kuo 2019; Jordan et al. 2014). Mirtazapine, as noted earlier, has robust antiemetic properties (Cao et al. 2020); it has been found helpful for both depression and nausea in patients with cancer (Cao et al. 2020; Economos et al. 2020; Maleki et al. 2020). When added to standard antiemetic therapies used during chemotherapy, olanzapine increases the likelihood of experiencing no nausea or vomiting during chemotherapy from 25% to 50%; adverse effects include fatigue and somnolence, and it is unclear if the 5-mg dose is as beneficial as 10 mg (Sutherland et al. 2018).

An increasingly recognized clinical entity is cannabinoid hyperemesis syndrome (Perisetti et al. 2020; Sorensen et al. 2017; Venkatesan et al. 2019a). This syndrome is sometimes mistaken for cyclic vomiting syndrome, and inaccurate diagnosis can delay appropriate treatment and clinical recommendations. Traditionally, cannabinoids have been thought of as beneficial for GI upset, because they are used in conditions such as chemotherapy-induced nausea and vomiting (Hardy and Davis 2021). However, in cases of regular heavy use, there appears to be paradoxical activity of the endogenous cannabinoid system. Extreme nausea and vomiting (more than five times per hour), as well as abdominal pain, are often accompanied by repeated hot baths or showers in an effort to relieve the nausea and vomiting (Perisetti et al. 2020; Sorensen et al. 2017; Venkatesan et al. 2019a). Use of standard antiemetics alone may be ineffective for cannabinoid hyperemesis syndrome, and alternative agents such as haloperidol, benzodiazepines, and topical capsaicin applied to the abdomen have been used with variable effectiveness (McConachie et al. 2019; Richards 2018). Cessation of cannabis use leads to resolution of GI symptoms. Patients may resist the suggestion of cannabinoid abstinence, but in numerous case reports, abstinence resulted in complete cessation of symptoms. Although there is no consensus regarding psychopharmacology recommendations for cannabinoid hyperemesis syndrome, referral to appropriate chemical dependency services probably is the most appropriate and effective treatment strategy.

Intestinal Disorders

Bariatric Surgery

Bariatric surgery, including restrictive procedures such as gastric banding and malabsorptive procedures such as the Roux-en-Y gastric bypass, has become a first-line therapy for morbid obesity. Accumulating evidence indicates that in addition to the beneficial effects on metabolism and endocrine function, bariatric surgery reduces depression in obese patients (Fu et al. 2022). The procedures have the potential to significantly reduce the absorption of medications by decreasing the time they are subject to gastric breakdown and decreasing the area across which they are absorbed by the mucosal walls of the intestine (Padwal et al. 2010). This may be of particular importance for medications that are encapsulated for extended release, in that there may not be sufficient time in the postbypass gastrum for the capsule to break down. A comparison of serum levels of extended-release venlafaxine before and after gastric bypass surgery did not find a significant difference (Krieger et al. 2017), however, which suggests that a combination of clinical evaluation and serum level monitoring may be the best approach for the individual patient.

After surgery, patients are at risk for developing dumping syndrome. Nausea, vomiting, diarrhea, palpitations, and flushing can all manifest as part of dumping syndrome, which is most commonly caused by rapid gastric emptying (Scarpellini et al. 2020). Medications that pass quickly through the stomach and small intestine and thus are not absorbed will be ineffective. Alternative delivery methods of medications, such as long-acting intramuscular formulations of antipsychotics (Brietzke and Lafer 2011), or liquid formulations, such as those available for several SSRIs, may be necessary in the setting of dumping syndrome. Orally disintegrating formulations of psychiatric medications (i.e., risperidone, olanzapine, aripiprazole, clozapine, mirtazapine, asenapine) may provide more reliable serum levels.

Some medications may actually have higher levels of absorption after bariatric surgery. Medications that undergo cytochrome P450 3A (CYP3A) metabolism may be more highly absorbed after bariatric surgery because CYP3A is present in the proximal small bowel, which is shortened by the surgical procedure, thus leading to some of the drug being metabolized before absorption (Canaparo et al. 2007). The liver may increase CYP3A activity over time to compensate for the loss of function in the gut (Tandra et al. 2013), so checking serum levels of medications that undergo CYP3A metabolism may be advisable after bariatric surgery.

Studies comparing serum levels of antidepressants, including sertraline, citalopram, and duloxetine, consistently find lower serum levels after bariatric surgery than before (Kingma et al. 2021). Levels may continue to decline even a year after surgery, and therapeutic drug monitoring is recommended for patients experiencing loss of medication efficacy after surgery. One case of lithium toxicity after gastric bypass surgery was thought to be caused primarily by dehydration (Tripp 2011), although evidence shows that lithium levels tend to increase after gastric bypass surgery (Seaman et al. 2005). There are numerous other case reports of lithium toxicity after bariatric surgery (Alam et al. 2016; Jamison and Aheron 2020). Overall, it is difficult to predict what will happen to serum levels of psychotropic medications after bariatric surgery because of significant interindividual differences and limited data. Most medications appear to have unchanged or reduced absorption after gastric bypass surgery when compared with absorption in control subjects, with the exceptions of bupropion and lithium, which may have elevated serum levels (Table 4–1) (Roerig et al. 2013; Seaman et al. 2005).

Celiac Disease and Microscopic Colitis

Celiac disease is an autoimmune process that impairs intestinal absorption of nutrients. Classic symptoms, such as diarrhea and weight loss, are less common than nonspecific presentations, which can include chronic fatigue, headache, and bloating (Lebwohl et al. 2018). Gluten, found in wheat, rye, barley, and oats, worsens the disease; withdrawal of these grains improves symptoms. Mild impairment in cognition ("brain fog") is often reported by patients with untreated celiac disease and can affect performance of daily tasks. Cognitive performance improves with adherence to a gluten-free diet (Lichtwark et al. 2014).

Microscopic colitis, a common cause of chronic diarrhea in older adults, is found histologically in 33% of patients with celiac disease (Pardi 2014). Although genetic and infectious etiologies have been proposed for microscopic

Table 4–1.   Medication absorption after Roux-en-Y gastric bypass surgery

Greater after surgery	Unchanged after surgery	Reduced after surgery
Bupropion	Buspirone	Amitriptyline
Lithium	Citalopram	Clonazepam
	Diazepam	Clozapine
	Haloperidol	Fluoxetine
	Lorazepam	Olanzapine
	Methylphenidate	Paroxetine
	Oxcarbazepine	Quetiapine
	Trazodone	Risperidone
	Venlafaxine	Sertraline
	Zolpidem	Ziprasidone

Source.   Roerig et al. 2013; Seaman et al. 2005.

colitis, medication effects have also occasionally been implicated in the disorder. SSRIs have been linked in numerous case-control studies to the development of microscopic colitis (Burke et al. 2021; Lucendo 2017; Salter and Williams 2017). Other medications, including duloxetine, clozapine, and carbamazepine, have been linked to the condition in case studies (Bahin et al. 2013; Rask et al. 2020; Tuqan et al. 2018). In patients with chronic diarrhea who are taking psychotropic medications, especially those with celiac disease, consideration should be given to microscopic colitis, and the potential offending agents should be discontinued. Another consideration for patients with celiac disease is the potential presence of gluten or gluten-containing excipients and binders in prescription medications (Cruz et al. 2015; Shah et al. 2018). Patients may need to consult with their local pharmacist or their prescription delivery company to determine whether their medications are gluten-free.

Inflammatory Bowel Disease

The inflammatory bowel diseases (IBDs) include Crohn's disease and ulcerative colitis. Crohn's disease can affect both the large and the small intestine and is characterized by transmural inflammation, a tendency to form fistulae, and strictures. Ulcerative colitis typically begins in the rectum and extends caudally, affecting only the mucosal layer of the bowel. Patients with IBD have rates of anxiety greater than 20% and a rate of depression greater than 15%, with psychiatric disorders more common in Crohn's disease and in patients with active disease (Neuendorf et al. 2016). Depression may be a risk factor for nonresponse to treatment with infliximab, an antibody against tumor necrosis factor-α, and has been shown to decrease adherence to therapy (Dolovich et al. 2021).

Antidepressants have been used in IBD both to treat depression that is co-morbid with the disease and to treat symptoms of IBD itself. A 2017 systematic review of 15 studies found that antidepressants may have a beneficial effect on the course of IBD, but only one study was a randomized controlled trial (Macer et al. 2017). Duloxetine was shown to improve both depressive symptoms and clinical disease indexes in patients who had IBD (Daghaghzadeh et al. 2015). In a large cohort study, antidepressants were observed to lower disease activity in both Crohn's disease and ulcerative colitis (Kristensen et al. 2019). There are case reports of disease remission with bupropion and phenelzine (Kast 1998; Kast and Altschuler 2001). Possible mechanisms include phenelzine reducing gut permeability, thereby limiting the passage of antigens that activate inflammation (Kast 1998), and bupropion decreasing levels of tumor necrosis factor-α (Kast and Altschuler 2001). Antidepressants may exert their beneficial effects by reducing inflammation as measured by cytokine levels (Mikocka-Walus et al. 2020). Conversely, anti-inflammatory therapy has been found to improve depressive and anxiety symptoms in patients with IBD over a 5-year period (Siebenhüner et al. 2021).

Irritable Bowel Syndrome

IBS is the most common functional GI disorder, with prevalence estimates ranging from 2% to 6% under the most recent diagnostic criteria (Sperber et al. 2021). Symptoms include abdominal pain or discomfort that is relieved by defecation and is associated with altered stool frequency or form. Depression and anxiety are two to three times as common in patients with IBS as in the general population (Zamani et al. 2019). Genomewide association studies suggest that shared genetic risk factors are the most likely reason for the rate of comorbidity (Eijsbouts et al. 2021). GI infection, food, and stress are all recognized as triggers for IBS (Videlock and Chang 2021). ADHD, adjustment disorders, somatic symptom disorders, and substance use, particularly with opioids, are also more common in patients with IBS than in the general population (Whitehead et al. 2007).

A large body of evidence supports the efficacy of antidepressants for IBS (Ford et al. 2019; Ruepert et al. 2011; Törnblom and Drossman 2021). TCAs have been shown to have efficacy in patients with predominant abdominal pain (Black et al. 2020), and SNRIs have been shown to have benefit in patients with comorbid pain syndromes and depression (Drossman et al. 2018). SSRIs are efficacious when patients have significant anxiety and depression but are not found to be as helpful for abdominal pain itself (Törnblom and Drossman 2021). The underlying mechanism responsible for these benefits remains unknown; however, TCAs have often been chosen for patients with IBS and predominant diarrhea and abdominal spasm because of their anticholinergic effects. At dosages lower than those typically prescribed for treatment of anxiety and depression, TCAs have shown benefits among patients studied in randomized placebo-controlled trials (Ford et al. 2014).

Alosetron, a 5-HT$_3$ antagonist, was approved for the treatment of IBS but was later withdrawn because of rare cases of ischemic colitis and severe constipation (Palsson and Drossman 2005). It is now available under a risk management plan that requires close supervision by the prescriber. Mirtazapine, which is also a 5-HT$_3$ antagonist, may have similar features and a better safety profile; case reports support its use in IBS (Spiegel and Kolb 2011), and trials have shown its efficacy for patients with diarrhea (Khalilian et al. 2021). Atypical antipsychotics, particularly quetiapine and olanzapine, are second-line agents for IBS (Pae et al. 2013) and have been shown to decrease abdominal pain when used at low doses. Pregabalin has been shown to decrease abdominal pain in IBS (Saito et al. 2019) and may also decrease visceral hypersensitivity, a phenomenon found in about 40% of patients with IBS, more effectively than placebo (Houghton et al. 2007). Practically speaking, available data suggest that patients with constipation-predominant IBS may benefit from SSRIs, whereas patients with diarrhea-predominant IBS should take TCAs or mirtazapine.

Incontinence

Fecal incontinence occurs in 0.7%–10% of noninstitutionalized American adults, with higher rates found in women, older adults, and those with medical comorbidities (Whitehead et al. 2009). People residing in nursing homes may have rates approaching 50% (Whitehead et al. 2001). Incontinence adversely affects quality of life and occupational and social functioning. Numerous reports of incontinence in patients taking antipsychotic medications have been published (Arasteh et al. 2021). A workshop paper found that loperamide and diphenoxylate (which are both opioid agonists), fiber supplements for bulking, and amitriptyline were all recommended for incontinence (Whitehead et al. 2015). Amitriptyline at low dosages (20 mg/day) decreased incontinence in 80% of patients and decreased the strength and frequency of rectal motor discharges (Santoro et al. 2000).

Diarrhea

Functional diarrhea can be part of IBS or a stand-alone, painless syndrome. In addition to loperamide and centrally acting opioids, desipramine has been recommended at dosages of 25–200 mg/day (Dellon and Ringel 2006). Fecal microbiota transplantation has been shown to improve both diarrhea and psychiatric symptoms for patients with functional diarrhea or IBS and comorbid depression or anxiety (Kurokawa et al. 2018).

Constipation

Constipation can result from diet, metabolic diseases such as diabetes or hypothyroidism, neurological disease, and medications, including many psychotropics (Wald 2007) (see discussion in the section "Gastrointestinal Side Effects of Psychiatric Drugs" later in this chapter). Behavioral interventions include increased fiber and fluid intake, physical activity, and use of bulking agents. Stool softeners and osmotic laxatives (e.g., polyethylene glycol, nonabsorbable sugars) also may be considered. Evidence for the use of antidepressants is not as strong for functional constipation as in IBS (Ford et al. 2014).

Liver Disorders

General Pharmacokinetics in Liver Disease

Impaired hepatic function affects many critical aspects of pharmacokinetics, from absorption, through first-pass metabolism and hepatic biotransformation, to the production of drug-binding proteins and overall fluid status, which will determine the volume of drug distribution. *Bioavailability* describes the rate and extent (proportion of the dose) of drug delivered to the systemic circulation. For oral dosing, bioavailability is influenced mainly by gut function and first-pass metabolism (see Chapter 1, "Pharmacokinetics, Pharmacodynamics, and Principles of Drug-Drug Interactions," for a discussion of pharmacokinetics).

The small intestine is the major site of absorption for most orally administered psychotropic drugs. Some patients with liver disease may have gastroparesis or impaired GI motility, resulting in delayed drug delivery to the intestine. Absorption also may be slowed by vascular congestion, which may exist in cirrhotic patients with portal hypertension or portal hypertensive gastropathy. In hepatic insufficiency, both first-pass metabolism before the drug reaches the systemic circulation and hepatic biotransformation may be slowed, resulting in higher plasma concentrations. Cirrhotic patients may have portosystemic shunting that circumvents first-pass metabolism and results in higher systemic drug levels. Although liver disease reduces the amounts of plasma proteins produced and alters protein binding, compensatory changes in metabolism and excretion result in only transient and generally clinically insignificant changes in free drug levels (Adedoyin and Branch 1996; Blaschke 1977). However, disease-related changes in metabolism, excretion, and volume of distribution do alter plasma drug levels, often in complex ways. Ascites and peripheral edema increase the volume of distribution of water-soluble drugs and reduce their plasma concentration. In contrast, hepatic disease may impair P450-mediated drug metabolism, reducing drug clearance and increasing drug levels. Disruption of P450 oxidative metabolism likely results from reduced sinusoidal capillarization that reduces both oxygen and drug exposure to hepatocytes during cirrhosis (McLean and Morgan 1991). Because most psychotropic drugs are highly protein bound (often 80% or more), less albumin and α_1-acid glycoprotein result in a larger proportion being free and pharmacologically active. Although more free drug in circulation increases the risks of side effects and intoxication (e.g., increased sedation with benzodiazepines) (Greenblatt and Koch-Weser 1974), it also makes more drug available for enzymatic metabolism.

Drug-Specific Issues and Dosing

The clinician prescribing psychotropic medications for a patient with liver disease should assess the severity of the liver disease, the medication being considered, the margin between therapeutic and toxic plasma levels, and whether hepatic encephalopathy is present or likely to occur. Clinical response and signs of toxicity should guide dosage. Therapeutic drug monitoring may be of value, but results must be interpreted with caution because changes in protein binding may lead to falsely low estimates of active drug levels. Ideally, therapeutic drug monitoring methods selective for unbound drug should be used. In general, drugs with a small therapeutic window (e.g., lithium) should be used with caution or avoided.

Patients with hepatic encephalopathy may have additional psychiatric disorders that warrant treatment. An initial assessment is necessary to establish whether affective symptoms represent an underlying mood disorder or an affective dysregulation associated with encephalopathy. In some cases, treatment of encephalopathy addresses mood symptoms. If additional psychotropic medication is needed, drugs that can worsen encephalopathy (i.e., sedatives, tranquilizers, anticholinergic medications) should be avoided.

Whereas the creatinine clearance rate can be used to adjust the dosages of drugs that are primarily excreted by the kidneys, there is no biochemical marker or measure to estimate hepatic clearance of drugs or specifically the decrement in drug metabolism in liver disease. However, one measure of hepatic functioning, the Child-Pugh score (CPS) (Table 4–2), often has been used to estimate the degree of cirrhosis, thereby providing some guidance on hepatic clearance. The CPS reflects the severity of cirrhosis (rated as mild, moderate, or severe), not hepatic clearance or drug kinetics (Albers et al. 1989). Nevertheless, the degree of cirrhosis as measured by the CPS has been used as a proxy for the potential decrease in drug metabolism, and some of the clinical variables used to calculate the CPS reflect aspects of liver disease important to drug dosing considerations (i.e., albumin, ascites, and encephalopathy).

The safest strategy is to begin with lower initial dosages and perhaps longer dosing intervals and then gradually titrate up the dosage because it may take longer for medications to reach steady state (Table 4–3). From our clinical experience, we have found that patients rated with CPS-A (mild) liver failure are early in the disease process and can usually tolerate 75%–100% of a standard initial dose. More cautious doses should be used in those with CPS-B (moderate) disease. A 50%–75% reduction in the normal starting dose is prudent. Prolongation of the elimination half-life will delay drug levels from reaching steady state, so smaller incremental dosing increases are recommended.

Table 4–2.   Grading the severity of liver disease by the Child-Pugh score

	1 point	2 points	3 points
Albumin (g/dL)	>3.5	2.8–3.5	<2.8
Ascites	None	Mild	Moderate
Bilirubin (mg/dL)	<2.0	2–3	>3.0
Encephalopathy	None	Mild to moderate (grade 1–2)	Severe (grade 3–4)
International normalized ratio	<1.7	1.7–2.3	>2.3

Note.   Child-Pugh score is calculated by adding the number of points from each of the five clinical categories, yielding a CPS grade: A=5–6 points; B=7–9 points; C=10–15 points.
Source.   Adapted from Albers et al. 1989.

Patients with CPS-B cirrhosis can often be successfully treated with 50% of a typical psychotropic dose. Patients with CPS-C (severe) cirrhosis commonly have some degree of hepatic encephalopathy, and medications must be cautiously monitored to avoid toxicity or worsening of the encephalopathy. Some patients need dosage reductions as their liver function deteriorates over time. Certain drugs warrant more careful consideration than others. Adjusting the dosage of drugs that require multistep biotransformation or those that are metabolized into active metabolites (e.g., amitriptyline, imipramine, venlafaxine, bupropion) may be more complex than for those that undergo only one-step biotransformation or are converted to inactive drug with the first biotransformation step (e.g., most SSRIs). Drugs with long half-lives, such as fluoxetine, usually should be avoided. Extended- or slow-release drug formulations usually should be avoided because their pharmacokinetics are less predictable in liver insufficiency. Benzodiazepines should be avoided in patients at risk for hepatic encephalopathy, but when they are needed (e.g., for delirium tremens), a benzodiazepine requiring only Phase II glucuronidation and not oxidative metabolism should be prescribed, specifically lorazepam, temazepam, or oxazepam. Glucuronidation is generally preserved in cirrhosis (Pacifici et al. 1990). Although olanzapine undergoes significant first-pass metabolism, it is metabolized primarily by Phase II glucuronidation, suggesting less susceptibility to hepatic impairment (Telles-Correia et al. 2017). Valproate is generally contraindicated for patients with known hepatic impairment or advanced

Table 4–3.   Psychotropic medication dosing in hepatic insufficiency (HI)

Medication	Dosing information
Antidepressants	
MAOIs	Potentially hepatotoxic. No dosing guidelines.
SSRIs	Extensively metabolized; decreased clearance and prolonged half-life. Initial dose should be reduced by 50%, with potentially longer dosing intervals between subsequent doses. Target doses are typically substantially lower than usual.
TCAs	Extensively metabolized. Potentially serious hepatic effects. No dosing guidelines.
Brexanolone	Extensively metabolized. No dosage adjustment necessary in HI.
Bupropion	Extensively metabolized; decreased clearance. In even mild cirrhosis, use at reduced dosage or frequency. In severe cirrhosis, do not exceed 75 mg/day for conventional tablets or 100 mg/day for sustained-release formulations.
Desvenlafaxine	Metabolized primarily by conjugation. No adjustment in starting dose needed in HI. Do not exceed 100 mg/day in severe HI.
Duloxetine	Extensively metabolized; reduced metabolism and elimination. Do not use for patients with any HI.
Esketamine	Metabolized by liver. For moderate HI, monitor for adverse reactions for a longer period of time because exposure may be higher and elimination half-life may be prolonged. Not recommended in severe HI.
Mirtazapine	Extensively metabolized; decreased clearance. No dosing guidelines.
Nefazodone	May cause hepatic failure. Avoid use in patients with active liver disease.
Selegiline	Extensively metabolized; use caution in HI. No dosing guidelines.
Trazodone	Extensively metabolized. No dosing guidelines.
Venlafaxine	Decreased clearance of venlafaxine and its active metabolite, *O*-desmethylvenlafaxine. Reduce dosage by 50% in mild to moderate HI, per manufacturer.
Vortioxetine	Extensively metabolized. No dosage adjustments recommended by manufacturer.

Table 4–3.   Psychotropic medication dosing in hepatic
insufficiency (HI) *(continued)*

Medication	Dosing information
Atypical antipsychotics	
Amisulpride	Renally excreted, not appreciably metabolized. No dosage adjustments needed.
Aripiprazole	Extensively metabolized. No dosage adjustment needed in mild to severe HI, per manufacturer.
Aripiprazole lauroxil	Metabolized by liver. No dosage adjustments needed.
Asenapine transdermal	Extensively metabolized. Contraindicated in severe HI; no dosage adjustment in mild or moderate HI.
Brexpiprazole	Extensively metabolized. Dosage reduction for moderate HI.
Cariprazine	Extensively metabolized. No dosage adjustments in mild or moderate HI. Not recommended in severe HI, per manufacturer.
Clozapine	Extensively metabolized. Discontinue in patients with marked transaminase elevations or jaundice. No dosing guidelines.
Iloperidone	Extensively metabolized. Unknown pharmacokinetics in mild or moderate HI. Not recommended for patients with HI, per manufacturer.
Lumateperone	Extensive hepatic metabolism. Not recommended for patients with moderate to severe HI.
Lurasidone	Metabolized by liver, primarily CYP3A4. For moderate HI, initial dosing should start at 20 mg/day, and daily dose should not exceed 80 mg. With severe HI, initial dosing should start at 20 mg/day, and daily dose should not exceed 40 mg.
Olanzapine	Extensively metabolized. Periodic assessment of transaminases recommended. No dosage adjustment needed, per manufacturer.
Olanzapine/ samidorphan	No dosage adjustment necessary.
Paliperidone	Primarily renally excreted. No dosage adjustment needed in mild to moderate HI. No dosing guidelines in severe HI.
Pimavanserin	Primarily renally excreted. No hepatic dosage adjustments necessary.

Table 4–3. Psychotropic medication dosing in hepatic insufficiency (HI) *(continued)*

Medication	Dosing information
Atypical antipsychotics *(continued)*	
Quetiapine	Extensively metabolized; clearance decreased 30%. Start at 25 mg/day; increase by 25–50 mg/day.
Risperidone	Extensively metabolized; free fraction increased 35%. Starting dosage and dose increments not to exceed 0.5 mg twice daily. Increases of > 1.5 mg twice daily should be made at intervals of ≥1 week.
Ziprasidone	Extensively metabolized; increased half-life and serum level in mild to moderate HI. However, manufacturer recommends no dosage adjustment.
Conventional antipsychotics	
Haloperidol, etc.	All metabolized in liver. No specific dosing recommendations. Avoid phenothiazines (e.g., thioridazine, trifluoperazine). If nonphenothiazines are used, reduce dosage and titrate more slowly than usual.
Anxiolytic and sedative-hypnotic drugs	
Alprazolam	Decreased metabolism and increased half-life. Reduce dosage by 50%. Avoid use in patients with cirrhosis.
Buspirone	Extensively metabolized; half-life may be prolonged. Reduce dosage and frequency in mild to moderate cirrhosis. Do not use in patients with severe impairment.
Chlordiazepoxide, clonazepam, diazepam, flurazepam, and triazolam	Extensively metabolized; reduced clearance and prolonged half-life. Avoid use if possible.
Lemborexant	Metabolized by liver, primarily CYP3A4. No dosage adjustment in mild HI but may have increased risk of somnolence. Initial and maximum dosage in moderate HI is 5 mg qhs. Not recommended in severe HI.
Lorazepam, oxazepam, and temazepam	Metabolized by conjugation; clearance not affected. No dosage adjustment needed. Lorazepam preferred choice.

Table 4–3.   Psychotropic medication dosing in hepatic insufficiency (HI) *(continued)*

Medication	Dosing information
Anxiolytic and sedative-hypnotic drugs *(continued)*	
Ramelteon	Extensively metabolized. Exposure to ramelteon increased 4-fold in mild HI and 10-fold in moderate HI. Use with caution in patients with moderate HI. Not recommended in severe HI.
Suvorexant	Metabolized by liver, primarily CYP3A4. No dosage adjustments needed in mild to moderate HI but not recommended for use in severe HI.
Tasimelteon	Extensively metabolized. Contraindicated in severe HI; no dosage adjustment in mild or moderate HI.
Zaleplon and zolpidem	Metabolized in liver. Reduced clearance. Usual ceiling dose 5 mg. Not recommended in severe HI.
Zopiclone and eszopiclone	Metabolized in liver. No dosage adjustment needed for mild to moderate HI. Reduce dose by 50% in severe HI.
Mood stabilizers	
Carbamazepine	Extensively metabolized. Perform baseline liver function tests and periodic evaluations during therapy. Discontinue in patients with active liver disease or aggravation of liver dysfunction. No dosing guidelines.
Gabapentin	Renally excreted; not appreciably metabolized. May require dosage adjustment in cases of cirrhosis and fluid overload.
Lamotrigine	Initial, escalation, and maintenance dosages should be reduced by 50% in moderate HI (Child-Pugh B) and by 75% in severe HI (Child-Pugh C).
Lithium	Renally excreted; not metabolized. Adjust dosage on basis of fluid status.
Oxcarbazepine	No dosage adjustment needed in mild to moderate HI, per manufacturer.
Topiramate	Reduced clearance. No dosing guidelines.
Valproate	Extensively metabolized; reduced clearance and increased half-life. Reduce dosage; obtain liver function tests frequently, especially in first 6 months of therapy. Avoid in patients with substantial hepatic dysfunction. Caution in patients with history of hepatic disease.

Table 4–3. Psychotropic medication dosing in hepatic insufficiency (HI) *(continued)*

Medication	Dosing information
Cognitive enhancers and movement disorder drugs	
Aducanumab-avwa	Expected to be degraded into small peptides and amino acids via catabolic pathways in the same manner as endogenous immunoglobulin G. No specific recommendations available.
Amantadine	Primarily renally excreted. No hepatic dosing guidelines.
Deutetrabenazine	Extensive metabolism. Primarily renally excreted. Contraindicated in hepatic impairment because no dosage adjustments are available.
Donepezil	Mildly reduced clearance in cirrhosis. No specific recommendations for dosage adjustment.
Galantamine	Use with caution in mild to moderate HI. Dosage should not exceed 16 mg/day in moderate HI (Child-Pugh 7–9). Use not recommended in severe HI (Child-Pugh 10–15).
Memantine	Primarily renally eliminated. No dosage adjustment expected, per manufacturer.
Rivastigmine	Clearance reduced 60%–65% in mild to moderate HI, but dosage adjustment may not be necessary.
Valbenazine	Moderately metabolized. Dosage should not exceed 40 mg/day in moderate to severe HI.
Psychostimulants and agents for wakefulness	
Armodafinil, modafinil	Decreased clearance. Reduce dosage by 50% in severe HI.
Atomoxetine	Extensively metabolized. Reduce initial and target dosage by 50% in moderate HI and 75% in severe HI, per manufacturer.
Methylphenidate	Unclear association with hepatotoxicity, particularly when coadministered with other adrenergic drugs. No dosing guidelines.
Pitolisant	Metabolized by liver. No adjustments needed with mild HI. For moderate HI, initial dosing is 8.9 mg/day; increase after 14 days to maximum of 17.8 mg/day. Use contraindicated in severe HI.
Solriamfetol	Does not undergo significant metabolism in humans.
Viloxazine	Metabolized in liver; renal excretion. Not recommended for use in HI.

Table 4–3.   Psychotropic medication dosing in hepatic insufficiency (HI) *(continued)*

Medication	Dosing information
Substance use agents	
Acamprosate	Renally excreted; does not undergo hepatic metabolism. No specific recommendations with HI.
Buprenorphine	Extensive metabolism. No dosage adjustments needed in mild to moderate HI. Reduce initial incremental dosage during titration to one-half in severe HI.
Disulfiram	Metabolized in liver; 5%–20% is excreted unchanged. Use with caution in presence of HI or cirrhosis.
Lofexidine	Extensive metabolism. Dosing is 0.54 mg qid in mild HI, 0.36 mg qid in moderate HI, and 0.18 mg qid in severe HI.
Methadone	Metabolized in liver. Lower initial doses and slower dose titration recommended in HI.
Naltrexone	Metabolized in liver. Dose adjustment not needed in mild to moderate HI. Injectable form not studied yet in severe HI.
Varenicline	Does not undergo significant metabolism. No adjustment necessary in HI.

Note.   CYP = cytochrome P450; MAOIs = monoamine oxidase inhibitors; SSRIs = selective serotonin reuptake inhibitors; TCAs = tricyclic antidepressants. Child-Pugh score is calculated by adding the number of points from each of the five clinical categories, yielding a CPS grade: A = 5–6 points; B = 7–9 points; C = 10–15 points.
Source.   Compiled from manufacturers' product information and Crone et al. 2006; Jacobson 2002; Monti and Pandi-Perumal 2007.

hepatic disease. Hyperammonemia independent of its hepatotoxicity increases the risk of hepatic encephalopathy in compromised patients (Lewis et al. 2017).

Caution is warranted even for drugs not requiring hepatic metabolism. Drugs distributed in total body water (e.g., lithium) or drugs that require renal clearance of the parent drug or active metabolites (e.g., gabapentin) can be difficult to manage in cirrhotic patients with fluid overload. In addition, even patients with mild cirrhosis can have impaired renal function (due to hepatorenal syndrome or secondary hyperaldosteronism), including a reduced glomerular filtration rate. Possible abnormal renal hemodynamics, an increase in volume of distribution, and dramatic changes in fluid status may make maintaining stable therapeutic drug levels difficult, if not impossible. For example, rapid changes in fluid status may occur in the routine medical management of cirrhotic patients (e.g., paracentesis, adjustment of diuretics or aggressive diuresis, or fluid loss from diarrhea caused by medications used for the treatment of hepatic encephalopathy). In these situations, as the volume of total body fluid decreases, a previously therapeutic drug level could change dramatically or even become toxic. This may be due to the slow equilibration of the drug between intracellular and extracellular fluid compartments (Anderson et al. 1976).

Hepatitis C

Chronic infection with hepatitis C virus (HCV) is one of the leading causes of progressive liver disease in the United States and remains a common indication for liver transplantation. HCV liver disease is also the primary cause of hepatocellular carcinoma. The most common route of infection in the United States is intravenous drug use, which accounts for more than half of all cases of HCV. Psychiatric comorbidity is common among patients with HCV, and reciprocally, psychiatrically hospitalized patients are at greater risk for HCV compared with the U.S. general population (Rifai et al. 2010).

Before 2011, when direct-acting antiviral agents began to play a role, treatment of HCV was based on a combination of interferon (IFN) and ribavirin. Treatment with this regimen was challenging because of problems with side effects, including anemia, fatigue, flulike symptoms, anorexia, insomnia, cognitive impairment, irritability, and depression, as well as length of treatment (24–48 weeks) required. IFN-induced psychiatric adverse effects were reported in 77% of patients, and depression occurred in approximately 25%–30% of patients, tending to develop early and persist throughout the course of therapy, impairing quality of life and contributing to premature treatment discontinuation (Rifai et al. 2010; Sockalingam et al. 2013, 2015). Concerns about IFN-induced depression contributed to reluctance about treating HCV-infected patients with comorbid psychiatric or substance use disorders. However, collaborative treatment involving medical staff and mental health providers showed that successful treatment was possible. Although evidence showed that the presence of subthreshold depressive symptoms before treatment increased the risk of developing IFN-induced depression, clinical trials suggested that prophylactic treatment with SSRIs could reduce the incidence and severity of depression in patients with or without a history of mood disorder (Hou et al. 2013; Rifai et al. 2010). Rarely, there were also reports of IFN-induced mania, delirium, and psychosis (Cheng et al. 2009; Goh et al. 2011; Patten 2006).

Compared with IFN-based treatment, direct-acting antiviral regimens have offered marked improvements in treatment tolerability, length of therapy, and sustained viral response rates. These regimens have evolved over time, and currently five combinations are considered first-line treatment options: glecaprevir/pibrentasvir, ledipasvir/sofosbuvir, elbasvir/grazoprevir, sofosbuvir/velpatasvir, and sofosbuvir/velpatasvir sometimes combined with a third agent, voxilaprevir (American Association for the Study of Liver Diseases 2021; European Association for the Study of the Liver et al. 2020). Side effects are usually mild and consist mainly of fatigue, headache, nausea, insomnia, and irritability. Among these combination agents, there appears to be less potential for adverse drug-drug interactions with psychotropic agents compared with earlier antiviral combinations that involved agents such as ritonavir and dasabuvir. Most of the current antiviral combinations should not be combined with carbamazepine, oxcarbazepine, or St. John's wort because of CYP3A4 and P-glycoprotein induction causing reduced plasma antiviral levels and reduced clinical efficacy. Because of CYP3A4 inhibition from ledipasvir/sofosbuvir and elbasvir/grazoprevir, combined use with pimozide should be avoided, particularly with ledipasvir/sofosbuvir (Roncero et al. 2018).

Gastrointestinal Side Effects of Psychiatric Drugs

Psychopharmacological agents cause a range of GI side effects, from mild to moderate and transient to severe. Persistent and more severe effects are covered here and in Chapter 2, "Severe Drug Reactions," and are summarized in Table 4–4.

Nausea and Vomiting

Many psychiatric medications, including SSRIs, mood stabilizers, psychostimulants, and cognitive enhancers, have nausea as an early side effect. In fact, GI distress is arguably the leading cause of acute discontinuation of drugs by patients starting treatment with SSRIs and SNRIs. Lithium may cause nau-

Table 4–4. Gastrointestinal (GI) adverse effects of psychiatric medications

Medication	GI adverse effects
Anxiolytics and sedative-hypnotics	
Buspirone	Nausea
Eszopiclone and zopiclone	Bitter taste, dry mouth, nausea
Suvorexant	Diarrhea, dry mouth
Tasimelteon	Alanine transaminase elevated
Zolpidem	Nausea, dyspepsia
Antidepressants	
SSRIs	
General	Nausea, diarrhea
Brexanolone	Dry mouth, pain in throat or mouth, dyspepsia, diarrhea
Esketamine	Nausea, vomiting, diarrhea
Paroxetine	Nausea, diarrhea, constipation
Vilazodone	Nausea, abdominal pain, diarrhea, flatulence
Vortioxetine	Nausea, vomiting, constipation
SNRIs and novel action agents	
Bupropion, desvenlafaxine, duloxetine, and venlafaxine	Nausea, constipation, dry mouth
Levomilnacipran	Nausea, vomiting, constipation
Mirtazapine	Dry mouth, constipation, increased appetite
Nefazodone	Dry mouth, nausea, constipation, hepatotoxicity
TCAs	Dry mouth, constipation; more severe GI adverse effects with tertiary-amine TCAs (e.g., amitriptyline, imipramine, doxepin, clomipramine) than with secondary-amine agents (e.g., desipramine, nortriptyline)

Table 4–4.   Gastrointestinal (GI) adverse effects of psychiatric medications *(continued)*

Medication	GI adverse effects
Antidepressants *(continued)*	
MAOIs	
Selegiline (transdermal)	Diarrhea, dyspepsia, dry mouth
Substance use agents	
Acamprosate	Nausea, dry mouth, diarrhea
Buprenorphine	Abdominal pain, nausea, constipation, oral hypoesthesia
Disulfiram	Elevated liver enzymes, hepatitis, liver failure
Lofexidine	Dry mouth
Methadone	Nausea, vomiting, constipation, hepatotoxicity
Naltrexone	Abdominal pain, nausea, vomiting, diarrhea, anorexia
Varenicline	Nausea, vomiting, flatulence, constipation
Antipsychotics	
Atypical agents	
General	Constipation, nausea, dyspepsia
Aripiprazole lauroxil	Pancreatitis
Aripiprazole with sensor (MyCite)	Nausea, vomiting, constipation, dyspepsia
Brexpiprazole	Dyspepsia, constipation, diarrhea
Cariprazine	Dyspepsia, vomiting
Clozapine	Hypersalivation, constipation
Lumateperone	Dry mouth, nausea
Lurasidone	Nausea, vomiting, diarrhea
Olanzapine/ samidorphan	Nausea, dry mouth, constipation
Low-potency typical agents	Dry mouth, constipation, reversible cholestatic hepatotoxicity (especially with chlorpromazine)

Table 4–4. Gastrointestinal (GI) adverse effects of psychiatric medications *(continued)*

Medication	GI adverse effects
Medications for EPS, tardive dyskinesia, and Parkinson's disease	
Amantadine ER capsules or tablets	Nausea, dry mouth, constipation
Benztropine, biperiden, diphenhydramine, and trihexyphenidyl	Dry mouth, constipation
Deutetrabenazine/ valbenazine	Dry mouth, vomiting, diarrhea
Istradefylline	Nausea, constipation
Mood stabilizers	
Carbamazepine	Nausea, vomiting, dyspepsia, diarrhea, hepatotoxicity
Lamotrigine	Nausea, vomiting, dyspepsia, diarrhea
Lithium	Nausea, vomiting, diarrhea, decreased appetite
Oxcarbazepine	Nausea, vomiting, dyspepsia, diarrhea (less than with carbamazepine)
Valproate	Nausea, vomiting, dyspepsia, diarrhea, hyperammonemia, hepatotoxicity
Cholinesterase inhibitors, aducanumab-avwa, and memantine	
Aducanumab-avwa	Diarrhea
Cholinesterase inhibitors	Nausea, vomiting, diarrhea, anorexia; most common with rivastigmine
Memantine	Constipation
Psychostimulants and agents for wakefulness	
Amphetamines and methylphenidate	Stomachache, appetite suppression
Armodafinil and modafinil	Nausea, dry mouth, anorexia
Atomoxetine	Nausea, dry mouth, constipation, decreased appetite, abdominal pain

Table 4–4.   Gastrointestinal (GI) adverse effects of psychiatric
medications *(continued)*

Medication	GI adverse effects
Psychostimulants and agents for wakefulness *(continued)*	
Pitolisant	Nausea
Solriamfetol	Nausea, decreased appetite
Viloxazine	Nausea, dry mouth, constipation, decreased appetite, abdominal pain

Note.   EPS=extrapyramidal side effects; ER=extended-release; MAOIs=monoamine oxidase inhibitors; SNRIs=serotonin-norepinephrine reuptake inhibitors; SSRIs=selective serotonin reuptake inhibitors; TCAs=tricyclic antidepressants.

sea or vomiting, but changing the formulation to lithium citrate often helps. Providing divided doses of carbamazepine throughout the day may be helpful, as may changing sodium valproate to valproic acid. Furthermore, the presence of nausea, vomiting, and diarrhea may herald psychiatric medication toxicity, such as early signs of lithium toxicity or serotonin syndrome. For patients whose nausea and vomiting prevent adequate intake of psychiatric medication, alternative routes of administration must be considered (see Chapter 3, "Alternative Routes of Drug Administration").

Diarrhea

Diarrhea occurs as a side effect of lithium treatment and may be an early sign of lithium toxicity. A cross-sectional population-based study found that 33% of patients taking lithium reported diarrhea (Fosnes et al. 2011). Slow-release formulations of lithium can decrease the likelihood of diarrhea as a side effect. Paradoxically, lithium has also been used to treat chronic unexplained diarrhea, perhaps by modulating cyclic adenosine monophosphate activity in the gut (Owyang 1984). Diarrhea occurred in 25% of patients taking carbamazepine in the same population-based study. A comparison of colonic transit times that included venlafaxine, paroxetine, and buspirone found no difference between medications and placebo (Fosnes et al. 2011). Clinically, valproate, cholinesterase inhibitors, and SSRIs can also cause diarrhea (Chial et al. 2003; McCain et al. 2007).

Constipation

Constipation is often caused by psychotropic medications, particularly agents with significant anticholinergic activity (e.g., TCAs, paroxetine, low-potency antipsychotics, olanzapine, benztropine). Even among somewhat newer agents, such as venlafaxine, bupropion, and mirtazapine, constipation can be a problematic side effect. If dietary and medication-oriented remedies described earlier (section "Intestinal Disorders," subsection "Constipation") are ineffective, switching to medications with less risk of constipation should be considered. Constipation can be particularly problematic with second-generation antipsychotics, particularly clozapine, which has led to serious complications, as noted later in this chapter (see " ").

Psychotropic Drug–Induced Gastrointestinal Complications

Selective Serotonin Reuptake Inhibitors and Upper Gastrointestinal Bleeding

Over the past several years, concerns have been raised about SSRIs causing an increased risk for upper GI bleeding. Although results from individual cohort and case-control studies have yielded conflicting findings, the overall data suggest an elevated risk. For example, a meta-analysis of 42 observational studies representing about 1.4 million patients found a 55% elevated risk (OR = 1.55; 95% CI = 1.32–1.81) of upper GI bleeding (Laporte et al. 2017). Similarly, a meta-analysis of 22 case-control and cohort studies found a 55% elevated risk (OR = 1.55; 95% CI = 1.35–1.78; $P < 0.0001$) of upper GI bleeding and calculated the number needed to harm with SSRI use as 791 per year (Jiang et al. 2015). Other meta-analyses have produced comparable results, showing a 1.55- to 2.36-fold elevated risk for upper GI bleeding among SSRI users (Bixby et al. 2019; Nochaiwong et al. 2022). This elevated risk should be tempered by the knowledge that the baseline incidence of upper GI bleeds among the general population is 23 per 10,000 patients (Bixby et al. 2019). In a different context, Laporte et al. (2017) estimated a crude incidence of 1 upper GI bleeding event per 8,000 SSRI prescriptions. The underlying mechanism behind the increased risk of bleeding is thought to be inhibition of serotonin uptake by platelets leading to reduced platelet serotonin levels and inhibition of platelet aggregation and hemostasis. Alternatively, SSRIs increase gastric acidity, which may increase the risk of peptic ulcer disease and GI bleeding (Andrade and Sharma 2016; Anglin et al. 2014). SNRIs also affect platelet serotonin levels and thus should affect platelet aggregation, but risk data are lacking (Bixby et al. 2019; Spina et al. 2020). Although some authors have suggested use of mirtazapine or bupropion for patients at higher risk for GI bleeds, a meta-analysis of available data showed an elevated risk with mirtazapine and inadequate data to recommend bupropion (Na et al. 2018).

Whatever mechanism is responsible for the increased risk for bleeding with SSRIs, evidence has shown that concurrent use with NSAIDs significantly increases the risk of upper GI bleeding, particularly among those considered at higher risk (e.g., older adults, history of GI bleed or peptic ulcer disease, cirrhosis, chronic renal disease, left ventricular assist device) (Bixby et al. 2019; C. G. Guo et al. 2019; Iwagami et al. 2018; Mawardi et al. 2020). Notably, the addition of PPIs appears to lower this risk (Jiang et al. 2015). Recent meta-analyses of combined use of SSRIs with warfarin (Wang et al. 2021) and SSRIs with newer anticoagulants (e.g., apixaban, rivaroxaban) (Lee et al. 2020) found about the same magnitude of risk for GI bleeding as for SSRIs alone. There have been no case reports of GI bleeds with SSRIs combined with newer anticoagulants. Overall, although current information suggests that the risk of upper GI bleeding with SSRIs is low among healthy adults, risks and benefits should be weighed for those at higher risk for upper GI bleeding.

Psychotropic Drug–Induced Hepatitis and Hepatic Dysfunction or Failure

Most psychotropic medication–induced liver injury is of the idiosyncratic type and as such cannot be predicted from specific risk factors or drug dosages (DeSanty and Amabile 2007; Telles-Correia et al. 2017). Drug-induced liver injury occurs in fewer than 1 in 1,000 to 1 in 100,000 treated patients and is usually not caused by overdose (DeSanty and Amabile 2007; Telles-Correia et al. 2017). Although almost all antidepressants have been implicated in cases of drug-induced hepatotoxicity, only nefazodone and duloxetine have received additional scrutiny. With duloxetine, 1% of patients developed a threefold increase in alanine transaminase, compared with 0.2% receiving placebo. The findings suggest a higher risk of duloxetine-mediated hepatotoxicity in patients with preexisting chronic liver disease and in those who consume large amounts of alcohol (DeSanty and Amabile 2007). In an independent study funded by Eli Lilly that included matched comparator groups of venlafaxine, other antidepressant, and no antidepressant use, duloxetine use was associated with a four- to fivefold greater incidence of less severe hepatic outcomes (e.g., liver enzyme elevations) but not hepatic-related death or potential acute hepatic failure (Xue et al. 2011). In addition, patients taking duloxetine who developed severe hepatic injuries were found to have a greater prevalence of baseline hepatic risk factors (e.g., hepatic insufficiency or cirrhosis), and patients with baseline hepatic risk factors had earlier onset of hepatic events (Xue et al. 2011). Because of a significant number of nefazodone-induced liver injury cases (1 case of death or transplantation per 250,000–300,000 patient-years of treatment), Bristol-Myers Squibb stopped manufacturing it in 2004, although generic nefazodone is still available (DeSanty and Amabile 2007). Subsequent studies have found similar risk with antidepressant-induced liver toxicity necessitating hospitalization (1.28–4 cases per 100,000 patient-years), and the incidence of hospitalization for nefazodone-associated liver toxicity was estimated at 29 cases per 100,000 patient-years (Voican et al. 2014).

Valproate is associated with an overall 1 in 20,000 incidence of liver toxicity, although the frequency can be as high as 1 in 600 in certain groups (i.e., infants younger than 2 years, patients receiving anticonvulsant polytherapy) (Jones et al. 2015). The risk of carbamazepine-induced hepatotoxicity is estimated at 16 cases per 100,000 patient-years, and 20 cases of severe lamotrigine-induced liver toxicity have been reported (Jones et al. 2015). Chlorpromazine, and less commonly other phenothiazines, may cause reversible cholestatic hepatotoxicity in up to 2% of patients, typically within the first 4 weeks of therapy. Because this reaction is believed to be due to impaired sulfoxidation, patients with primary biliary cirrhosis, who often have impaired sulfoxidation, should not be given these drugs (Leipzig 1990; Telles-Correia et al. 2017). Most other antipsychotics, including the atypical antipsychotics, have been implicated in cases of drug-induced elevations in liver transaminases, with clozapine most associated with elevated aminotransferases (Marwick et al. 2012; Telles-Correia et al. 2017). Benzodiazepine-induced liver damage remains rare and has been limited to a few case reports detailing cholestatic patterns of injury (Telles-Correia et al. 2017). In most cases, transaminase elevations were asymptomatic and arose within the first 6 weeks of treatment (Marwick et al. 2012). Acute drug-induced liver toxicity that results in hepatic failure and liver transplantation is very rare. Most of these cases of acute toxicity were due to acetaminophen (mostly in overdose); only 3% were due to phenytoin, 3% valproate, and less than 1% nefazodone (Hussaini and Farrington 2014). Thus, even severe drug-induced liver injury is usually reversible and rarely results in fatality if the drug is discontinued.

Despite the potential risk of liver injury, there is no justification for routinely monitoring liver enzymes with most psychotropic drugs (with the exception of valproate) because hepatic adverse effects are unpredictable and occur abruptly at varying times after drug initiation (Russo and Watkins 2004). Routine laboratory monitoring of hepatic enzymes and liver functions may be indicated before starting treatment to establish baseline liver enzymes, for high-risk patients, for patients with impaired ability to communicate, or in the presence of early symptoms or prodromal signs of a possible adverse reaction (Zaccara et al. 2007). Although most episodes are asymptomatic, patients can be instructed on the signs and symptoms of liver injury (e.g., right upper quadrant pain, dark urine, itching, jaundice, nausea, and anorexia) when prescribed a medication that may cause such an adverse effect. Additionally, prescribers must recognize the more chronic risk of nonalcoholic fatty liver disease associated with metabolic syndrome caused by atypical antipsychotics (Telles-Correia et al. 2017).

Because there are no specific biomarkers and the clinical presentation of drug-induced liver injury can mimic many other hepatological disorders, the diagnosis is essentially one of clinical suspicion after exclusion of common causes of liver disease (e.g., alcohol, viruses) (Gerstner et al. 2007). Instances of idiosyncratic hepatocellular jaundice are almost always associated with minor and asymptomatic aminotransferase elevations, exceeding three times the upper limit of normal in up to 15% of patients treated with drugs capable of causing these reactions (H.L. Guo et al. 2019). Inexplicably, aminotransferase elevations, which reflect liver injury, often reverse even if drug therapy is continued, although a minority of patients develop progressive liver injury (Gerstner et al. 2007; H.L. Guo et al. 2019; Hussaini and Farrington 2014). Nevertheless, because it is impossible to predict the smaller subset of patients who are susceptible to progressive injury from the drug, therapy should be discontinued for patients who develop aminotransferase elevations two to three times the upper limit of normal. In most cases, the liver injury spontaneously resolves on drug discontinuation, although in some cases the enzymes continue to rise for several days. Therefore, clinical symptoms and liver enzymes should be followed closely after the drug is discontinued. However, the combination of high aminotransferase levels (representing hepatocellular injury) and jaundice has been associated with a mortality rate of 10%–15%, and any patient with drug-induced injury and jaundice should be carefully monitored for signs of acute hepatic failure, particularly coagulopathy or encephalopathy (Gerstner et al. 2007). In the case of valproate-induced hepatotoxicity, carnitine and antioxidant supplementation have shown some benefit in improving outcomes (Ali et al. 2021).

It is unclear whether patients with preexisting liver disease are more susceptible to idiosyncratic drug-induced liver injury, although the manufacturer of duloxetine has recommended avoiding its use for patients with hepatic dysfunction; the manufacturer's database analysis supports the theory that those with preexisting liver disease are at higher risk (Nitsche et al. 2010). Conventional wisdom has usually held that these idiosyncratic drug reactions are based on other factors (i.e., genetics) and are not dose- or clearance-dependent (H.L. Guo et al. 2019). Nevertheless, caution is recommended because these patients may be less able to handle the additional loss of hepatic function caused by drug-induced injury. Another consideration is the challenge of interpreting elevations in hepatic enzyme levels in patients with preexisting liver dysfunction. If a drug-induced injury occurs in a patient with significant cirrhosis, the resulting elevation in aminotransferases may understate the true severity of the insult (H.L. Guo et al. 2019).

Drug-Induced Pancreatitis

Drug-induced pancreatitis is a rare cause of acute pancreatitis, representing only 0.1%–2% of cases (Roquin et al. 2010). Although most cases are mild to moderate, prompt recognition is necessary to reduce the risk of serious complications, including systemic inflammation, chronic pancreatitis, multiple organ failure, and death (Franco et al. 2015; Vaidyanathan et al. 2019). Accurate diagnosis is challenging because the clinical presentation is not readily distinguishable from those of other causes of acute pancreatitis (Alastal et al. 2016; Roquin et al. 2010). Time of onset is variable, often occurring within a few weeks to months after a particular drug is started. There is also no dose-response relationship for drug-induced pancreatitis, because it can develop over a wide range of drug dosages. Efforts to connect a specific drug to acute pancreatitis have been hampered by its infrequent occurrence and case reports failing to clearly rule out other causes of pancreatitis or include a causality assessment (Lally et al. 2018). However, certain patients may be at greater risk for drug-induced pancreatitis, including women, children, older adults, and those with advanced HIV infection or IBD (Nitsche et al. 2010).

Valproic acid is the psychotropic agent with the greatest number of reported cases of drug-induced pancreatitis, the majority involving children (Gerstner et al. 2007). The true incidence is considered to be 1 in 40,000, with patients typically presenting with abdominal pain, nausea, vomiting, diarrhea, and anorexia. Transient asymptomatic hyperamylasemia occurs in 20% of adults taking valproic acid, but this does not correlate with a greater risk for pancreatitis (Zaccara et al. 2007). Infrequent case reports have linked other anticonvulsants to drug-induced pancreatitis, including carbamazepine, lamotrigine, and levetiracetam (Ali et al. 2021; Roquin et al. 2010; Zaccara et al. 2007).

Numerous cases of antipsychotic-induced pancreatitis have been reported, most involving olanzapine, clozapine, quetiapine, or risperidone (Alastal et al. 2016; Franco et al. 2015; Lally et al. 2018; Vaidyanathan et al. 2019). Rarely, ziprasidone and aripiprazole have also been implicated. A case series including 41 cases of pancreatitis noted that olanzapine, clozapine, and quetiapine were implicated in 80% of the reported cases (Silva et al. 2016). Overall, most cases developed within 2 months after the antipsychotic agent was started and resolved after it was discontinued; notably, most patients were concurrently taking other drugs linked to pancreatitis (Silva et al. 2016). The underlying mechanism behind antipsychotic-related pancreatitis is unclear but is suspected to be similar to that for valproate-related pancreatitis, being idiosyncratic and involving the buildup of cytotoxic metabolites (Simons-Linares et al. 2019).

Among antidepressants, mirtazapine has been implicated in several cases of drug-induced pancreatitis; some involved the development of marked hypertriglyceridemia, a risk factor for pancreatitis (Bowers et al. 2019; Simons-Linares et al. 2019). There are also rare reports involving sertraline, venlafaxine, and bupropion (Jones et al. 2015; Simons-Linares et al. 2019). Rechallenge with the offending drug after an episode of pancreatitis is not recommended, even if a lower dose or different route of administration is used, because of the risk of recurrence. However, substitution with another drug of the same class is reportedly considered an acceptable option (Dhir et al. 2007).

Intestinal or Colonic Toxicity

Psychotropic drugs, particularly antipsychotic medications, often cause constipation, yet clinical attention to this side effect is often lacking. The prevalence of antipsychotic-induced constipation ranges from approximately 30% to 60%, with higher rates with clozapine (Chen and Hsieh 2018). Infrequently, antipsychotic-induced GI hypomotility leads to serious complications, including paralytic ileus, bowel ischemia, toxic megacolon, bowel perforation, and death (Every-Palmer and Ellis 2017; Nielsen and Meyer 2012). The main mechanism for this hypomotility appears to be the anticholinergic effects on intestinal smooth muscle contractions, producing delayed transit times and constipation. Additionally, antiserotonergic properties of antipsychotics contribute to alterations in gut motility and sensitivity to bowel distension (Nielsen and Meyer 2012; West et al. 2017). Most of the focus has been on clozapine because a significant number of hypomotility cases have been reported with serious complications. Notably, a review of 104 cases found a 38% mortality rate (West et al. 2017), a meta-analysis of clozapine-treated patients identified a 44% mortality rate (Cohen 2017), and a pharmacovigilance study reported a case fatality rate of 18% among 160 patients who had serious hypomotility (Every-Palmer and Ellis 2017). Risk factors for death were linked to older age and male sex (Liu et al. 2020; West et al. 2017). A study found that inpatients taking clozapine had colonic transit times four times longer than those of patients taking other antipsychotics (Every-Palmer et al. 2016). However, self-reported constipation was a poor predictor for the presence of GI hypomotility (Every-Palmer et al. 2020). These findings led the authors to recommend use of prophylactic laxatives for patients taking clozapine. Another potentially serious complication related to antipsychotic-induced constipation is ischemic colitis, which is most often associated with clozapine or phenothiazines (Bielefeldt 2016; Shah and Anderson 2013; Upala et al. 2015). A small number of case reports have included other agents, such as olanzapine and quetiapine (Arkfeld et al. 2018; de Beaurepaire et al. 2015; Fernandes et al. 2016; Park et al. 2012).

Psychiatric Side Effects of Gastrointestinal Medications

In addition to psychiatric medications causing GI disorders, GI medications can have psychiatric side effects. Although much has been written about IFN, psychiatrists need to be alert to the potential effects of other GI medications because they may alter a patient's clinical presentation and necessitate medication adjustments. Potential psychiatric adverse effects of GI medications are listed in Table 4–5.

Drug-Drug Interactions

Potential interactions between GI and psychotropic medications are summarized in Tables 4–6 and 4–7. Drug interactions for antibiotics used for *H. pylori* regimens (e.g., metronidazole, tetracycline, clarithromycin, amoxicillin) are reviewed in Chapter 12, "Infectious Diseases." Additional information on corticosteroids is presented in Chapter 10, "Endocrine and Metabolic Disorders." See Chapter 1, "Pharmacokinetics, Pharmacodynamics, and Principles of Drug-Drug Interactions," for a discussion of pharmacokinetics, pharmacodynamics, and principles of drug-drug interactions.

Conclusion

GI disorders include a wide range of physiological and functional disturbances that span multiple organ systems, from the mouth to the colorectal region. Often, psychological stress or comorbid psychopathology appears to influence the level of GI symptoms that a patient experiences. Psychopharmacological treatment can be beneficial in improving quality of life, reducing physical discomfort, and controlling anxiety and depression. However, the selection of pharmacological agent requires consideration of potential undesirable side effects (e.g., dysphagia, xerostomia, nausea, and vomiting), tolerability, and safety.

Table 4–5. Psychiatric adverse effects of gastrointestinal medications

Medication	Psychiatric adverse effects
Agents for constipation	
Naldemedine/naloxegol	Possible opioid withdrawal
Prucalopride	Suicidal ideation or suicide attempt, self-injurious ideation, depression, insomnia, headache, dizziness
Antidiarrheal agents	
Diphenoxylate	Sedation, lethargy, insomnia, depression, euphoria, confusion
Loperamide	Dizziness
Antiemetics	
Amisulpride	Confusional state, insomnia, somnolence
Aprepitant	Dizziness
Corticosteroids (e.g., dexamethasone)	Mania, anxiety, irritability, psychosis (acute), depression (chronic)
Dimenhydrinate	Drowsiness, ataxia, disorientation, convulsions, stupor
Diphenhydramine	Drowsiness, dizziness, confusion, cognitive impairment
Dolasetron	Headache, fatigue, dizziness
Domperidone	Acute dystonic reactions (rare)
Dronabinol and nabilone	Dizziness, euphoria, paranoid reaction, abnormal thinking, somnolence, confusion
Droperidol	EPS
Fosnetupitant/ palonosetron/ netupitant	Headache, asthenia, fatigue
Granisetron	Headache, asthenia, somnolence
Metoclopramide	Restlessness, drowsiness, fatigue, dystonic reactions, dyskinesia
Palonosetron	Anxiety
Prochlorperazine	Drowsiness, dizziness, headache (common), EPS, seizures, confusion, insomnia, neuroleptic malignant syndrome

Table 4–5.   Psychiatric adverse effects of gastrointestinal medications *(continued)*

Medication	Psychiatric adverse effects
Antiemetics *(continued)*	
Promethazine	Drowsiness, confusion, hyperexcitability, EPS, seizures, confusion, neuroleptic malignant syndrome
Rolapitant	Dizziness, decreased appetite
Trimethobenzamide	Drowsiness, dizziness, disorientation, depression, seizures, EPS
Hepatitis C treatment and liver disease	
Elbasvir/grazoprevir (Zepatier)	Headache, fatigue, irritability, depression
Glecaprevir/pibrentasvir (Mavyret)	Headache, fatigue
Ledipasvir/sofosbuvir (Harvoni)	Fatigue, headache, insomnia
Obeticholic acid	Fatigue, dizziness, palpitations
Ombitasvir/ paritaprevir/ritonavir copackaged with dasabuvir (Viekira Pak)	Fatigue, insomnia, asthenia
Sofosbuvir/velpatasvir/ voxilaprevir (Vosevi)	Headache, fatigue, asthenia, insomnia
Histamine H_2-receptor antagonists	
Cimetidine	Headache, dizziness
Nizatidine	Dizziness, somnolence, anxiety, nervousness
Ranitidine	Headache, malaise, dizziness
Irritable bowel drugs	
Alosetron	Headache
Antispasmodics (dicyclomine, glycopyrrolate, and methscopolamine)	Dizziness, blurred vision, drowsiness, weakness, confusion, excitement (especially in older adults)

Table 4–5. Psychiatric adverse effects of gastrointestinal medications *(continued)*

Medication	Psychiatric adverse effects
Irritable bowel drugs *(continued)*	
Eluxadoline	Euphoric mood, confusion, dizziness, fatigue, sedation, somnolence
Lubiprostone	Headache
Renzapride	Headache, dizziness
Sulfasalazine	Headache, anorexia
Tegaserod	Headache, dizziness
Inflammatory bowel drugs	
Adalimumab	Headache, CNS demyelinating disease
Balsalazide	Depression (uncommon), headache
Certolizumab pegol	Anxiety, CNS demyelinating disease, mood instability (rare)
Cyclosporine	Delirium, tremor, depression, mania, seizures, PML (rare)
Golimumab	CNS demyelinating disease
Infliximab	Fatigue, headache, CNS demyelinating disease, seizures (rare)
Mesalamine	Dizziness, headache
Natalizumab	Depression, headache, PML, herpes encephalitis (rare)
Olsalazine	Insomnia, irritability, mood swings, tremor (rare)
Vedolizumab	Headache, fatigue, PML
Proton pump inhibitors	
Esomeprazole, lansoprazole, omeprazole, and pantoprazole	Dizziness
Weight loss drugs	
Semaglutide injection	Headache, dizziness, fatigue, suicidal ideation and behavior, depression, mood changes

Note.   EPS = extrapyramidal side effects; PML = progressive multifocal leukoencephalopathy.

Table 4–6.   Gastrointestinal medication–psychotropic medication interactions

Medication	Interaction mechanism	Effects on psychotropic medications and management
Medications for gastric acidity, peptic ulcers, and GERD		
Antacids	Increased gastric pH and delayed gastric emptying Increased sodium excretion	May reduce drug absorption; take antacids 2–3 hours apart from other drugs. Sodium bicarbonate may increase renal excretion of lithium.
Cimetidine	Inhibits CYP1A2, CYP2C9/ 19, CYP2D6, and CYP3A4	Inhibits oxidative metabolism of most drugs. Reduce psychotropic dosage. Avoid cimetidine or use psychotropics eliminated by conjugation.
Esomeprazole	Induces CYP1A2	Increased elimination and reduced levels of clozapine and olanzapine.
Lansoprazole	Induces CYP1A2	Increased elimination and reduced levels of clozapine and olanzapine.
Omeprazole	Inhibits CYP2C19	Increased levels and toxicity of diazepam, flunitrazepam, phenytoin, and mephenytoin.
Sucralfate	Drug binding	May reduce drug absorption; take at least 2 hours before other drugs.
Antidiarrheal agents		
Kaolin/attapulgite	Drug binding	May bind drugs and reduce absorption; avoid within 2–3 hours of taking other medications.

Table 4–6. Gastrointestinal medication–psychotropic medication interactions (*continued*)

Medication	Interaction mechanism	Effects on psychotropic medications and management
Medications for irritable bowel syndrome		
Antispasmodics (clidinium-chlordiazepoxide, dicyclomine, glycopyrrolate, hyoscyamine, and methscopolamine)	Additive anticholinergic effects	Increased risk of cognitive impairment and delirium in combination with anticholinergic psychotropics (TCAs, antipsychotics, benztropine, tranylcypromine). Reduced therapeutic effect of cholinesterase inhibitors and memantine.
Tegaserod	Inhibits CYPA2 and CYP2D6	May reduce metabolism and increase levels of atomoxetine, clozapine, chlorpromazine, olanzapine, risperidone, TCAs, maprotiline, mirtazapine, trazodone, and venlafaxine.
Medications for inflammatory bowel disease		
Adalimumab, golimumab, and infliximab	Increased CYP enzymes by suppression of inflammation	May reduce levels of pimozide and iloperidone.
Cyclosporine	Inhibits CYP3A4	Increased risk of oversedation with alprazolam, midazolam, or triazolam.

Table 4–6.   Gastrointestinal medication–psychotropic medication interactions *(continued)*

Medication	Interaction mechanism	Effects on psychotropic medications and management
Antinauseants and antiemetic agents		
5-HT$_3$ antagonists (dolasetron, granisetron, ondansetron, palonosetron, and ramosetron)	QT prolongation	Increased risk of cardiac arrhythmias with other QT-prolonging agents, including TCAs, typical antipsychotics, pimozide, risperidone, paliperidone, iloperidone, quetiapine, ziprasidone, and lithium.
Amisulpride, domperidone, droperidol, and metoclopramide	Dopamine antagonist QT prolongation	Increased risk of EPS when combined with antipsychotics. Increased risk of cardiac arrhythmias with other QT-prolonging agents, including TCAs, typical antipsychotics, pimozide, risperidone, paliperidone, iloperidone, quetiapine, ziprasidone, and lithium.
Aprepitant and rolapitant	Inhibit CYP3A4, CYP2D6, CYP1A2	Increased risk of side effects with alprazolam, midazolam, triazolam, clozapine, vilazodone, donepezil, carbamazepine, aripiprazole, quetiapine, and pimozide (contraindicated).
Dimenhydrinate and diphenhydramine	Additive anticholinergic effects	Increased risk of cognitive impairment and delirium in combination with anticholinergic psychotropics (TCAs, antipsychotics, benztropine, tranylcypromine). Reduced therapeutic effect of cholinesterase inhibitors and memantine.
Domperidone and droperidol	Dopamine antagonist QT prolongation	Increased risk of EPS when combined with antipsychotics. Increased risk of cardiac arrhythmias with other QT-prolonging agents, including TCAs, typical antipsychotics, pimozide, risperidone, paliperidone, iloperidone, quetiapine, ziprasidone, and lithium.

Table 4–6. Gastrointestinal medication–psychotropic medication interactions *(continued)*

Medication	Interaction mechanism	Effects on psychotropic medications and management
Antinauseants and antiemetic agents *(continued)*		
Dronabinol and nabilone	Additive sympathomimetic effects	Additive hypertension, tachycardia, and possible cardiotoxicity with amphetamines, methylphenidate, and other sympathomimetics. Additive hypertension, tachycardia, and drowsiness with TCAs. Additive drowsiness and CNS depression with benzodiazepines, lithium, opioids, buspirone, and other CNS depressants.
Palonosetron–netupitant/ fosnetupitant combinations	Fosnetupitant is a prodrug of netupitant, which is a moderate inhibitor of CYP3A4 for at least 6 days	Monitor for increased side effects if used with psychotropics metabolized via CYP3A4, which include aripiprazole, haloperidol, lurasidone, quetiapine, alprazolam, diazepam, clonazepam, and triazolam. Avoid use with carbamazepine.
	Palonosetron is a 5-HT$_3$ receptor antagonist	Increased risk of serotonin syndrome with SSRI or SNRI.
Glucocorticoids	Induce CYP3A4	Increased metabolism and reduced levels of oxidatively metabolized benzodiazepines, buspirone, carbamazepine, quetiapine, ziprasidone, and pimozide. Adjust benzodiazepine dosage or consider oxazepam, lorazepam, or temazepam. Monitor carbamazepine levels. Adjust antipsychotic dosage or switch to another agent.
Metoclopramide	Dopamine antagonist	Increased risk of EPS when combined with antipsychotics.

Table 4–6. Gastrointestinal medication–psychotropic medication interactions *(continued)*

Medication	Interaction mechanism	Effects on psychotropic medications and management
Antinauseants and antiemetic agents *(continued)*		
Prochlorperazine, promethazine, and trimethobenzamide	Additive anticholinergic effects	Increased risk of cognitive impairment and delirium in combination with anticholinergic psychotropics (TCAs, antipsychotics, benztropine, tranylcypromine). Reduced therapeutic effect of cholinesterase inhibitors and memantine.
Direct-acting antiviral agents		
Dasabuvir	Unknown mechanism	Increased levels of buprenorphine and alprazolam.
Ritonavir	Inhibits CYP3A4, CYP2D6	Increased risk of side effects with alprazolam, aripiprazole, quetiapine, midazolam, diazepam, TCAs, lurasidone, trazodone, eszopiclone, zolpidem, clomipramine, and nefazodone.
Simeprevir	Inhibits CYP3A4	Increased risk of oversedation with alprazolam, midazolam, or triazolam.

Note. 5-HT$_3$=serotonin type 3; CYP=cytochrome P450; EPS=extrapyramidal side effects; GERD=gastroesophageal reflux disease; SNRI=serotonin-norepinephrine reuptake inhibitor; SSRI=selective serotonin reuptake inhibitor; TCAs=tricyclic antidepressants.
Source. Compiled from Cozza et al. 2003; Wynn et al. 2007; and product monographs.

Table 4–7. Psychotropic medication–gastrointestinal medication interactions

Medication	Interaction mechanism	Effects on gastrointestinal medications and management
Antidepressants		
Bupropion, duloxetine, moclobemide, and paroxetine	Inhibit CYP2D6	Increased levels and toxicity of tropisetron.
Fluoxetine	Inhibits CYP1A2, CYP2C19, CYP2D6, CYP3A4	Increased levels of antiemetics aprepitant, fosnetupitant, netupitant, rolapitant, granisetron, ondansetron, palonosetron, and tropisetron; μ opioid antagonists naldemedine and naloxegol; and corticosteroids, including budesonide.
Fluvoxamine	Inhibits CYP1A2, CYP2C9/19, CYP3A4	Increased levels and toxicity of alosetron such that coadministration is not advised. May increase levels and toxicity of antiemetics aprepitant, fosnetupitant, netupitant, rolapitant, granisetron, ondansetron, palonosetron, and tropisetron; μ opioid antagonists naldemedine and naloxegol; and corticosteroids, including budesonide. Increased cyclosporine levels and toxicity.
Nefazodone	Inhibits CYP3A4	Increased levels and toxicity of antiemetics aprepitant, fosnetupitant, netupitant, rolapitant, granisetron, ondansetron, palonosetron, and tropisetron; μ opioid antagonists naldemedine and naloxegol; and corticosteroids, including budesonide.
TCAs	QT prolongation	Increased risk of cardiac arrhythmias with other QT-prolonging agents, including domperidone, droperidol, dolasetron, granisetron, ondansetron, palonosetron, and ramosetron.

Table 4–7.   Psychotropic medication–gastrointestinal medication interactions *(continued)*

Medication	Interaction mechanism	Effects on gastrointestinal medications and management
Antipsychotics		
Typical and atypical antipsychotics (iloperidone, paliperidone, pimozide, quetiapine, risperidone, and ziprasidone)	QT prolongation	Increased risk of cardiac arrhythmias with other QT-prolonging agents, including domperidone, droperidol, amisulpride, dolasetron, granisetron, ondansetron, palonosetron, and ramosetron.
Mood stabilizers		
Carbamazepine, phenytoin, and oxcarbazepine	Induce CYP1A2, CYP2C9/19, CYP3A4	Increased metabolism and reduced therapeutic effects of aprepitant, fosnetupitant, netupitant, alosetron, rolapitant, granisetron, ondansetron, palonosetron, cyclosporine, and direct-acting antiviral agents for hepatitis C; μ opioid antagonists naldemedine and naloxegol; and corticosteroids, including budesonide.
Lithium	QT prolongation	Increased risk of cardiac arrhythmias with other QT-prolonging agents, including amisulpride, domperidone, droperidol, dolasetron, granisetron, ondansetron, palonosetron, and ramosetron; and μ opioid antagonists naldemedine and naloxegol.

Table 4–7. Psychotropic medication–gastrointestinal medication interactions *(continued)*

Medication	Interaction mechanism	Effects on gastrointestinal medications and management
Psychostimulants		
Armodafinil and modafinil	Induce CYP3A4	Increased metabolism and reduced therapeutic effects of aprepitant, fosnetupitant, netupitant, rolapitant, and granisetron; μ opioid antagonists naldemedine and naloxegol; direct-acting antiretroviral elbasvir/grazoprevir; and corticosteroids, including budesonide.
Atomoxetine	Inhibits CYP2D6	Increased levels and toxicity of tropisetron.

Note. CYP = cytochrome P450; TCAs = tricyclic antidepressants.
Source. Compiled from Cozza et al. 2003; Wynn et al. 2007; and product monographs.

Key Points

- Nearly all disorders of the gastrointestinal (GI) system are associated with significant distress and psychopathology.

- Psychopharmacological management of GI disorders requires careful consideration of absorption, distribution, and metabolism of psychotropic drugs; commonplace GI side effects of psychotropic drugs; and the potential interactions of psychotropic drugs with drugs used to treat GI disorders.

- GI disorders involving significant pain may respond to agents that modulate pain sensitivity and pain perception in patients with comorbid psychiatric illness. Trazodone, tricyclic antidepressants (TCAs), selective serotonin reuptake inhibitors (SSRIs), and serotonin-norepinephrine reuptake inhibitors have shown effectiveness for pain in many GI disorders.

- Disorders that involve significant nausea and vomiting may be particularly difficult to treat. Nausea and vomiting due to gastroparesis, pregnancy, or cancer treatment may respond to augmentation of standard antiemetics with olanzapine or mirtazapine.

- Gastric bypass and celiac disease may alter drug absorption, reducing therapeutic effect. Liquid or orally disintegrating tablets should be used instead of extended-release preparations, and therapeutic drug monitoring should be used when applicable.

- Available data suggest that SSRIs are preferable for constipation-predominant irritable bowel syndrome (IBS), and TCAs and mirtazapine are preferable for diarrhea-predominant IBS.

- In hepatic disease, psychotropic drug dosing may need to be reduced. The Child-Pugh score, a clinical measure that estimates the severity of cirrhosis, can help guide dosing.

- The risk of upper GI bleeding due to SSRIs appears to be low in healthy adults, but caution should be used in patient groups considered at higher risk for upper GI bleeding (e.g., those with a history of GI bleeding, those taking antiplatelet or anticoagulant medications, older adults). Proton pump inhibitors appear to lower risk.

- Transient aminotransferase elevation less than three times the upper limit of normal is associated with multiple psychotropic drugs and does not warrant discontinuation of psychotropic medication for an otherwise asymptomatic patient. Drug-induced hepatitis remains uncommon. Routine drug levels and aminotransferase monitoring are encouraged for patients prescribed valproate and clozapine.

- Patients taking clozapine are at risk for serious GI complications and death arising from constipation. Attention to bowel habits and drug dosage, the use of other anticholinergic agents, and coadministration of laxatives are advisable.

References

Abramowitz A, Miller ES, Wisner KL: Treatment options for hyperemesis gravidarum. Arch Womens Ment Health 20(3):363–372, 2017 28070660

Adamo D, Pecoraro G, Coppola N, et al: Vortioxetine versus other antidepressants in the treatment of burning mouth syndrome: an open-label randomized trial. Oral Dis 27(4):1022–1041, 2021 32790904

Adedoyin A, Branch RA: Pharmacokinetics, in Hepatology: A Textbook of Liver Disease, 3rd Edition. Edited by Zakim D, Boyer TD. Philadelphia, PA, WB Saunders, 1996, pp 307–322

Alam A, Raouf S, Recio FO: Lithium toxicity following vertical sleeve gastrectomy: a case report. Clin Psychopharmacol Neurosci 14(3):318–320, 2016 27489390

Alastal Y, Hasan S, Chowdhury MA, et al: Hypertriglyceridemia-induced pancreatitis in psychiatric patients: case report and review of literature. Am J Ther 23(3):e947–e949, 2016 24987947

Albers I, Hartmann H, Bircher J, et al: Superiority of the Child-Pugh classification to quantitative liver function tests for assessing prognosis of liver cirrhosis. Scand J Gastroenterol 24(3):269–276, 1989 2734585

Ali A, Anugwom GO, Naqvi W, et al: A case of carbamazepine-induced acute pancreatitis: a rare etiology. Cureus 13(5):e15199, 2021 34178519

American Association for the Study of Liver Diseases: Initial treatment of HCV infection. September 29, 2021. Available at: www.hcvguidelines.org/treatment-naive/gt1. Accessed March 9, 2022.

Anderson RJ, Gambertoglio JG, Schrier RW: Clinical Use of Drugs in Renal Failure. Springfield, IL, Charles C Thomas, 1976

Andrade C, Sharma E: Serotonin reuptake inhibitors and risk of abnormal bleeding. Psychiatr Clin North Am 39(3):413–426, 2016 27514297

Anglin R, Yuan Y, Moayyedi P, et al: Risk of upper gastrointestinal bleeding with selective serotonin reuptake inhibitors with or without concurrent nonsteroidal anti-inflammatory use: a systematic review and meta-analysis. Am J Gastroenterol 109(6):811–819, 2014 24777151

Arasteh A, Mostafavi S, Zununi Vahed S, et al: An association between incontinence and antipsychotic drugs: a systematic review. Biomed Pharmacother 142:112027, 2021 34392083

Arkfeld DV, Svingen LA, Sutton S, et al: Repeat ischemic colitis in a patient taking quetiapine. Prim Care Companion CNS Disord 20(6):17102250, 2018 30476377

Atluri DK, Chandar AK, Fass R, et al: Systematic review with meta-analysis: selective serotonin reuptake inhibitors for noncardiac chest pain. Aliment Pharmacol Ther 41(2):167–176, 2015 25412947

Austin K, Wilson K, Saha S: Hyperemesis gravidarum. Nutr Clin Pract 34(2):226–241, 2019 30334272

Aziz I, Palsson OS, Whitehead WE, et al: Epidemiology, clinical characteristics, and associations for Rome IV functional nausea and vomiting disorders in adults. Clin Gastroenterol Hepatol 17(5):878–886, 2019 29857155

Badar T, Cortes J, Borthakur G, et al: Phase II, open label, randomized comparative trial of ondansetron alone versus the combination of ondansetron and aprepitant for the prevention of nausea and vomiting in patients with hematologic malignancies receiving regimens containing high-dose cytarabine. Biomed Res Int 2015:497597, 2015 25654108

Bahin FF, Chu G, Rhodes G: Development of microscopic colitis secondary to duloxetine. J Clin Gastroenterol 47(1):89–90, 2013 23090036

Balon R, Starcevic V: Role of benzodiazepines in anxiety disorders. Adv Exp Med Biol 1191:367–388, 2020 32002938

Bashashati M, Hejazi RA, Andrews CN, et al: Gastroesophageal reflux symptoms not responding to proton pump inhibitor: GERD, NERD, NARD, esophageal hypersensitivity or dyspepsia? Can J Gastroenterol Hepatol 28(6):335–341, 2014 24719900

Bender SD: Burning mouth syndrome. Dent Clin North Am 62(4):585–596, 2018 30189984

Bhandari S, Jha P, Thakur A, et al: Cyclic vomiting syndrome: epidemiology, diagnosis, and treatment. Clin Auton Res 28(2):203–209, 2018 29442203

Bielefeldt K: Ischemic colitis as a complication of medication use: an analysis of the Federal Adverse Event Reporting System. Dig Dis Sci 61(9):2655–2665, 2016 27073073

Bixby AL, VandenBerg A, Bostwick JR: Clinical management of bleeding risk with antidepressants. Ann Pharmacother 53(2):186–194, 2019 30081645

Black CJ, Yuan Y, Selinger CP, et al: Efficacy of soluble fibre, antispasmodic drugs, and gut-brain neuromodulators in irritable bowel syndrome: a systematic review and network meta-analysis. Lancet Gastroenterol Hepatol 5(2):117–131, 2020 31859183

Blaschke TF: Protein binding and kinetics of drugs in liver diseases. Clin Pharmacokinet 2(1):32–44, 1977 322909

Boelig RC, Barton SJ, Saccone G, et al: Interventions for treating hyperemesis gravidarum: a Cochrane systematic review and meta-analysis. J Matern Fetal Neonatal Med 31(18):2492–2505, 2018 28614956

Bošnjak SM, Gralla RJ, Schwartzberg L: Prevention of chemotherapy-induced nausea: the role of neurokinin-1 (NK1) receptor antagonists. Support Care Cancer 25(5):1661–1671, 2017 28108820

Bowers RD, Valanejad SM, Holombo AA: Mirtazapine-induced pancreatitis: a case report. J Pharm Pract 32(5):586–588, 2019 29486665

Brietzke E, Lafer B: Long-acting injectable risperidone in a bipolar patient submitted to bariatric surgery and intolerant to conventional mood stabilizers (letter). Psychiatry Clin Neurosci 65(2):205, 2011 21414098

Burgstaller JM, Jenni BF, Steurer J, et al: Treatment efficacy for non-cardiovascular chest pain: a systematic review and meta-analysis. PLoS One 9(8):e104722, 2014 25111147

Burke KE, D'Amato M, Ng SC, et al: Microscopic colitis. Nat Rev Dis Primers 7(1):39, 2021 34112810

Camilleri M, Sanders KM: Gastroparesis. Gastroenterology 162(1):68–87, 2022 34717924

Camilleri M, Stanghellini V: Current management strategies and emerging treatments for functional dyspepsia. Nat Rev Gastroenterol Hepatol 10(3):187–194, 2013 23381190

Camilleri M, Chedid V, Ford AC, et al: Gastroparesis. Nat Rev Dis Primers 4(1):41, 2018 30385743

Canaparo R, Finnström N, Serpe L, et al: Expression of CYP3A isoforms and P-glycoprotein in human stomach, jejunum and ileum. Clin Exp Pharmacol Physiol 34(11):1138–1144, 2007 17880367

Cangemi DJ, Kuo B: Practical perspectives in the treatment of nausea and vomiting. J Clin Gastroenterol 53(3):170–178, 2019 30614944

Cao J, Ouyang Q, Wang S, et al: Mirtazapine, a dopamine receptor inhibitor, as a secondary prophylactic for delayed nausea and vomiting following highly emetogenic chemotherapy: an open label, randomized, multicenter phase III trial. Invest New Drugs 38(2):507–514, 2020 32036491

Cappetta K, Beyer C, Johnson JA, et al: Meta-analysis: risk of dry mouth with second generation antidepressants. Prog Neuropsychopharmacol Biol Psychiatry 84(Pt A):282–293, 2018 29274375

Celinski K, Konturek SJ, Konturek PC, et al: Melatonin or L-tryptophan accelerates healing of gastroduodenal ulcers in patients treated with omeprazole. J Pineal Res 50(4):389–394, 2011 21362032

Chen HK, Hsieh CJ: Risk of gastrointestinal hypomotility in schizophrenia and schizoaffective disorder treated with antipsychotics: a retrospective cohort study. Schizophr Res 195:237–244, 2018 29107449

Cheng YC, Chen CC, Ho AS, et al: Prolonged psychosis associated with interferon therapy in a patient with hepatitis C: case study and literature review. Psychosomatics 50(5):538–542, 2009 19855041

Chial HJ, Camilleri M, Burton D, et al: Selective effects of serotonergic psychoactive agents on gastrointestinal functions in health. Am J Physiol Gastrointest Liver Physiol 284(1):G130–G137, 2003 12488239

Cicala G, Barbieri MA, Spina E, et al: A comprehensive review of swallowing difficulties and dysphagia associated with antipsychotics in adults. Expert Rev Clin Pharmacol 12(3):219–234, 2019 30700161

Ciovica R, Riedl O, Neumayer C, et al: The use of medication after laparoscopic antireflux surgery. Surg Endosc 23(9):1938–1946, 2009 19169748

Clavé P, Shaker R: Dysphagia: current reality and scope of the problem. Nat Rev Gastroenterol Hepatol 12(5):259–270, 2015 25850008

Cockburn N, Pradhan A, Taing MW, et al: Oral health impacts of medications used to treat mental illness. J Affect Disord 223:184–193, 2017 28759866

Cohen D: Clozapine and gastrointestinal hypomotility. CNS Drugs 31(12):1083–1091, 2017 29230675

Coss-Adame E, Erdogan A, Rao SSC: Treatment of esophageal (noncardiac) chest pain: an expert review. Clin Gastroenterol Hepatol 12(8):1224–1245, 2014 23994670

Cozza KL, Armstrong S, Oesterheld J: Concise Guide to the Cytochrome P450 System: Drug Interaction Principles for Medical Practice. Washington, DC, American Psychiatric Publishing, 2003

Crone CC, Gabriel GM, DiMartini A: An overview of psychiatric issues in liver disease for the consultation-liaison psychiatrist. Psychosomatics 47(3):188–205, 2006 16684936

Cruz JE, Cocchio C, Lai PT, et al: Gluten content of medications. Am J Health Syst Pharm 72(1):54–60, 2015 25511839

Cui Y, Xu H, Chen FM, et al: Efficacy evaluation of clonazepam for symptom remission in burning mouth syndrome: a meta-analysis. Oral Dis 22(6):503–511, 2016 26680638

Daghaghzadeh H, Naji F, Afshar H, et al: Efficacy of duloxetine add on in treatment of inflammatory bowel disease patients: a double-blind controlled study. J Res Med Sci 20(6):595–601, 2015 26600836

Dall M, Schaffalitzky de Muckadell OB, Lassen AT, et al: There is an association between selective serotonin reuptake inhibitor use and uncomplicated peptic ulcers: a population-based case-control study. Aliment Pharmacol Ther 32(11–12):1383–1391, 2010 21050241

de Beaurepaire R, Trinh I, Guirao S, et al: Colitis possibly induced by quetiapine. BMJ Case Rep 2015:bcr2014207912, 2015 25721830

Dellon ES, Ringel Y: Treatment of functional diarrhea. Curr Treat Options Gastroenterol 9(4):331–342, 2006 16836952

den Hollander WJ, Kuipers EJ: Current pharmacotherapy options for gastritis. Expert Opin Pharmacother 13(18):2625–2636, 2012 23167300

DeSanty KP, Amabile CM: Antidepressant-induced liver injury. Ann Pharmacother 41(7):1201–1211, 2007 17609231 de Souza FTA, Teixeira AL, Amaral TMP, et al: Psychiatric disorders in burning mouth syndrome. J Psychosom Res 72(2):142–146, 2012 22281456

Dhir R, Brown DK, Olden KW: Drug-induced pancreatitis: a practical review. Drugs Today (Barc) 43(7):499–507, 2007 17728850

Dolovich C, Bernstein CN, Singh H, et al: Anxiety and depression leads to anti-tumor necrosis factor discontinuation in inflammatory bowel disease. Clin Gastroenterol Hepatol 19(6):1200.e1–1208.e1, 2021 32668341

Drossman DA, Tack J, Ford AC, et al: Neuromodulators for functional gastrointestinal disorders (disorders of gut-brain interaction): a Rome Foundation working team report. Gastroenterology 154(4):1140.e1–1171.e1, 2018 29274869

Economos G, Lovell N, Johnston A, et al: What is the evidence for mirtazapine in treating cancer-related symptomatology? A systematic review. Support Care Cancer 28(4):1597–1606, 2020 31858251

Eijsbouts C, Zheng T, Kennedy NA, et al: Genome-wide analysis of 53,400 people with irritable bowel syndrome highlights shared genetic pathways with mood and anxiety disorders. Nat Genet 53(11):1543–1552, 2021 34741163

Enweluzo C, Aziz F: Gastroparesis: a review of current and emerging treatment options. Clin Exp Gastroenterol 6:161–165, 2013 24039443

European Association for the Study of the Liver; Clinical Practice Guidelines Panel: Chair; EASL Governing Board representative, et al: EASL recommendations on treatment of hepatitis C: final update of the series. J Hepatol 73(5):1170–1218, 2020 32956768

Every-Palmer S, Ellis PM: Clozapine-induced gastrointestinal hypomotility: a 22-year bi-national pharmacovigilance study of serious or fatal "slow gut" reactions, and comparison with international drug safety advice. CNS Drugs 31(8):699–709, 2017 28623627

Every-Palmer S, Nowitz M, Stanley J, et al: Clozapine-treated patients have marked gastrointestinal hypomotility, the probable basis of life-threatening gastrointestinal complications: a cross sectional study. EBioMedicine 5:125–134, 2016 27077119

Every-Palmer S, Inns SJ, Ellis PM: Constipation screening in people taking clozapine: a diagnostic accuracy study. Schizophr Res 220:179–186, 2020 32245597

Faramarzi M, Kheirkhah F, Shokri-Shirvani J, et al: Psychological factors in patients with peptic ulcer and functional dyspepsia. Caspian J Intern Med 5(2):71–76, 2014 24778780

Feller L, Fourie J, Bouckaert M, et al: Burning mouth syndrome: aetiopathogenesis and principles of management. Pain Res Manag 2017:1926269, 2017 29180911

Fernandes SR, Alves R, Araújo Correia L, et al: Severe ischemic colitis following olanzapine use: a case report. Rev Esp Enferm Dig 108(9):595–598, 2016 26786111

Fonseca Mora MC, Milla Matute CA, Alemán R, et al: Medical and surgical management of gastroparesis: a systematic review. Surg Obes Relat Dis 17(4):799–814, 2021 33722476

Ford AC, Quigley EM, Lacy BE, et al: Effect of antidepressants and psychological therapies, including hypnotherapy, in irritable bowel syndrome: systematic review and meta-analysis. Am J Gastroenterol 109(9):1350–1365, quiz 1366, 2014 24935275

Ford AC, Lacy BE, Harris LA, et al: Effect of antidepressants and psychological therapies in irritable bowel syndrome: an updated systematic review and meta-analysis. Am J Gastroenterol 114(1):21–39, 2019 30177784

Ford AC, Mahadeva S, Carbone MF, et al: Functional dyspepsia. Lancet 396(10263):1689–1702, 2020 33049222

Fosnes GS, Lydersen S, Farup PG: Constipation and diarrhoea—common adverse drug reactions? A cross sectional study in the general population. BMC Clin Pharmacol 11:2, 2011 21332973

Franco JM, Vallabhajosyula S, Griffin T: Quetiapine-induced hypertriglyceridemia causing acute pancreatitis. BMJ Case Rep 2015:bcr201509571, 2015 25976202

Fu R, Zhang Y, Yu K, et al: Bariatric surgery alleviates depression in obese patients: a systematic review and meta-analysis. Obes Res Clin Pract 16(1):10–16, 2022 34802982

Gerstner T, Büsing D, Bell N, et al: Valproic acid-induced pancreatitis: 16 new cases and a review of the literature. J Gastroenterol 42(1):39–48, 2007 17322992

Goh T, Dhillon R, Bastiampillai T: Manic induction with interferon alpha therapy (letter). Aust N Z J Psychiatry 45(11):1004, 2011 21981775

Greenblatt DJ, Koch-Weser J: Clinical toxicity of chlordiazepoxide and diazepam in relation to serum albumin concentration: a report from the Boston Collaborative Drug Surveillance Program. Eur J Clin Pharmacol 7(4):259–262, 1974 4851053

Grover M, Farrugia G, Stanghellini V: Gastroparesis: a turning point in understanding and treatment. Gut 68(12):2238–2250, 2019 31563877

Guo CG, Cheung KS, Zhang F, et al: Risks of hospitalization for upper gastrointestinal bleeding in users of selective serotonin reuptake inhibitors after Helicobacter pylori eradication therapy: a propensity score matching analysis. Aliment Pharmacol Ther 50(9):1001–1008, 2019 31583734

Guo HL, Jing X, Sun JY, et al: Valproic acid and the liver injury in patients with epilepsy: an update. Curr Pharm Des 25(3):343–351, 2019 30931853

Han P, Suarez-Durall P, Mulligan R: Dry mouth: a critical topic for older adult patients. J Prosthodont Res 59(1):6–19, 2015 25498205

Hardy J, Davis MP: The management of nausea and vomiting not related to anticancer therapy in patients with cancer. Curr Treat Options Oncol 22(2):17, 2021 33443705

Herlihy JD, Reddy S, Shanker A, et al: Cyclic vomiting syndrome: an overview for clinicians. Expert Rev Gastroenterol Hepatol 13(12):1137–1143, 2019 31702939

Hershcovici T, Achem SR, Jha LK, et al: Systematic review: the treatment of noncardiac chest pain. Aliment Pharmacol Ther 35(1):5–14, 2012 22077344

Holtmann G, Shah A, Morrison M: Pathophysiology of functional gastrointestinal disorders: a holistic overview. Dig Dis 35(Suppl 1):5–13, 2017 29421808

Hou XJ, Xu JH, Wang J, et al: Can antidepressants prevent pegylated interferon-α/ribavirin-associated depression in patients with chronic hepatitis C: meta-analysis of randomized, double-blind, placebo-controlled trials? PLoS One 8(10):e76799, 2013 24204676

Houghton LA, Fell C, Whorwell PJ, et al: Effect of a second-generation alpha2delta ligand (pregabalin) on visceral sensation in hypersensitive patients with irritable bowel syndrome. Gut 56(9):1218–1225, 2007 17446306

Hussaini SH, Farrington EA: Idiosyncratic drug-induced liver injury: an update on the 2007 overview. Expert Opin Drug Saf 13(2):67–81, 2014 24073714

International Headache Society: International Classification of Orofacial Pain, 1st Edition (ICOP). Cephalalgia 40(2):129–221, 2020 32103673

Iwagami M, Tomlinson LA, Mansfield KE, et al: Gastrointestinal bleeding risk of selective serotonin reuptake inhibitors by level of kidney function: a population-based cohort study. Br J Clin Pharmacol 84(9):2142–2151, 2018 29864791

Jääskeläinen SK: Is burning mouth syndrome a neuropathic pain condition? Pain 159(3):610–613, 2018 29257770

Jacobson S: Psychopharmacology: prescribing for patients with hepatic or renal dysfunction. Psychiatric Times, November 2002, pp 65–70

Jamison SC, Aheron K: Lithium toxicity following bariatric surgery. SAGE Open Med Case Rep 8:2050313X20953000, 2020 32974026

Jiang HY, Chen HZ, Hu XJ, et al: Use of selective serotonin reuptake inhibitors and risk of upper gastrointestinal bleeding: a systematic review and meta-analysis. Clin Gastroenterol Hepatol 13(1):42.e3–50.e3, 2015 24993365

Jones MP: The role of psychosocial factors in peptic ulcer disease: beyond Helicobacter pylori and NSAIDs. J Psychosom Res 60(4):407–412, 2006 16581366

Jones MR, Hall OM, Kaye AM, et al: Drug-induced acute pancreatitis: a review. Ochsner J 15(1):45–51, 2015 25829880

Jordan K, Schaffrath J, Jahn F, et al: Neuropharmacology and management of chemotherapy-induced nausea and vomiting in patients with breast cancer. Breast Care (Basel) 9(4):246–253, 2014 25404883

Kast RE: Crohn's disease remission with phenelzine treatment. Gastroenterology 115(4):1034–1035, 1998 9786733

Kast RE, Altschuler EL: Remission of Crohn's disease on bupropion. Gastroenterology 121(5):1260–1261, 2001 11706830

Khalilian A, Ahmadimoghaddam D, Saki S, et al: A randomized, double-blind, placebo-controlled study to assess efficacy of mirtazapine for the treatment of diarrhea predominant irritable bowel syndrome. Biopsychosoc Med 15(1):3, 2021 33536043

Kingma JS, Burgers DMT, Monpellier VM, et al: Oral drug dosing following bariatric surgery: general concepts and specific dosing advice. Br J Clin Pharmacol 87(12):4560–4576, 2021 33990981

Kirkcaldy RD, Kim TJ, Carney CP: A somatoform variant of obsessive-compulsive disorder: a case report of OCD presenting with persistent vomiting. Prim Care Companion J Clin Psychiatry 6(5):195–198, 2004 15514688

Kisely S, Forbes M, Sawyer E, et al: A systematic review of randomized trials for the treatment of burning mouth syndrome. J Psychosom Res 86:39–46, 2016 27302545

Kjeldgaard HK, Eberhard-Gran M, Benth JS, et al: History of depression and risk of hyperemesis gravidarum: a population-based cohort study. Arch Womens Ment Health 20(3):397–404, 2017 28064341

Klein B, Thoppay JR, De Rossi SS, et al: Burning mouth syndrome. Dermatol Clin 38(4):477–483, 2020 32892856

Kovacic K, Li BUK: Cyclic vomiting syndrome: a narrative review and guide to management. Headache 61(2):231–243, 2021 33619730

Krieger CA, Cunningham JL, Reid JM, et al: Comparison of bioavailability of single-dose extended-release venlafaxine capsules in obese patients before and after gastric bypass surgery. Pharmacotherapy 37(11):1374–1382, 2017 28845898

Kristensen MS, Kjærulff TM, Ersbøll AK, et al: The influence of antidepressants on the disease course among patients with Crohn's disease and ulcerative colitis: a Danish nationwide register-based cohort study. Inflamm Bowel Dis 25(5):886–893, 2019 30551218

Kulkarni DP, Kamath VD, Stewart JT: Swallowing disorders in schizophrenia. Dysphagia 32(4):467–471, 2017 28447217

Kurokawa S, Kishimoto T, Mizuno S, et al: The effect of fecal microbiota transplantation on psychiatric symptoms among patients with irritable bowel syndrome, functional diarrhea and functional constipation: an open-label observational study. J Affect Disord 235:506–512, 2018 29684865

Lacy BE, Saito YA, Camilleri M, et al: Effects of antidepressants on gastric function in patients with functional dyspepsia. Am J Gastroenterol 113(2):216–224, 2018 29257140

Lacy BE, Tack J, Gyawali CP: AGA clinical practice update on management of medically refractory gastroparesis: expert review. Clin Gastroenterol Hepatol 20(3):491–500, 2022 34757197

Lally J, Al Kalbani H, Krivoy A, et al: Hepatitis, interstitial nephritis, and pancreatitis in association with clozapine treatment: a systematic review of case series and reports. J Clin Psychopharmacol 38(5):520–527, 2018 30059436

Laporte S, Chapelle C, Caillet P, et al: Bleeding risk under selective serotonin reuptake inhibitor (SSRI) antidepressants: a meta-analysis of observational studies. Pharmacol Res 118:19–32, 2017 27521835

Lebwohl B, Sanders DS, Green PHR: Coeliac disease. Lancet 391(10115):70–81, 2018 28760445

Lee MT, Park KY, Kim MS, et al: Concomitant use of NSAIDs or SSRIs with NOACs requires monitoring for bleeding. Yonsei Med J 61(9):741–749, 2020 32882758

Leipzig RM: Psychopharmacology in patients with hepatic and gastrointestinal disease. Int J Psychiatry Med 20(2):109–139, 1990 2203695

Levenstein S, Rosenstock S, Jacobsen RK, et al: Psychological stress increases risk for peptic ulcer, regardless of Helicobacter pylori infection or use of nonsteroidal anti-inflammatory drugs. Clin Gastroenterol Hepatol 13(3):498.e1–506.e1, 2015 25111233

Levenstein S, Jacobsen RK, Rosenstock S, et al: Mental vulnerability, Helicobacter pylori, and incidence of hospital-diagnosed peptic ulcer over 28 years in a population-based cohort. Scand J Gastroenterol 52(9):954–961, 2017 28503971

Levy RL, Olden KW, Naliboff BD, et al: Psychosocial aspects of the functional gastrointestinal disorders. Gastroenterology 130(5):1447–1458, 2006 16678558

Lewis C, Tesar GE, Dale R: Valproate-induced hyperammonemic encephalopathy in general hospital patients with one or more psychiatric disorders. Psychosomatics 58(4):415–420, 2017 28411969

Lichtwark IT, Newnham ED, Robinson SR, et al: Cognitive impairment in coeliac disease improves on a gluten-free diet and correlates with histological and serological indices of disease severity. Aliment Pharmacol Ther 40(2):160–170, 2014 24889390

Limketkai BN, LeBrett W, Lin L, et al: Nutritional approaches for gastroparesis. Lancet Gastroenterol Hepatol 5(11):1017–1026, 2020 33065041

Liu CL, Maruf AA, Bousman CA: Reporting of clozapine-induced gastrointestinal hypomotility and factors associated with fatal outcomes in Canada: a pharmacovigilance database study. Psychiatry Res 290:113048, 2020 32474068

London V, Grube S, Sherer DM, et al: Hyperemesis gravidarum: a review of recent literature. Pharmacology 100(3–4):161–171, 2017 28641304

Lu Y, Chen M, Huang Z, et al: Antidepressants in the treatment of functional dyspepsia: a systematic review and meta-analysis. PLoS One 11(6):e0157798, 2016 27310135

Lucendo AJ: Drug exposure and the risk of microscopic colitis: a critical update. Drugs R D 17(1):79–89, 2017 28101837

Luo L, Du L, Shen J, et al: Benefit of small dose antidepressants for functional dyspepsia: experience from a tertiary center in eastern China. Medicine (Baltimore) 98(41):e17501, 2019 31593119

Macer BJ, Prady SL, Mikocka-Walus A: Antidepressants in inflammatory bowel disease: a systematic review. Inflamm Bowel Dis 23(4):534–550, 2017 28267046

Mackay HP, Mitchell KG, Pickard WR, et al: The effect of trimipramine (Surmontil) on the gastric secretion of acid and pepsin in patients with duodenal ulceration. J Int Med Res 12(5):303–306, 1984 6437892

Malamood M, Roberts A, Kataria R, et al: Mirtazapine for symptom control in refractory gastroparesis. Drug Des Devel Ther 11:1035–1041, 2017 28408802

Maleki A, Ghadiyani M, Salamzadeh J, et al: Comparison of mirtazapine and olanzapine on nausea and vomiting following anthracycline-cyclophosphamide chemotherapy regimen in patients with breast cancer. Iran J Pharm Res 19(3):451–464, 2020 33680044

Martín-Merino E, Ruigómez A, García Rodríguez LA, et al: Depression and treatment with antidepressants are associated with the development of gastro-oesophageal reflux disease. Aliment Pharmacol Ther 31(10):1132–1140, 2010 20199498

Marwick KFM, Taylor M, Walker SW: Antipsychotics and abnormal liver function tests: systematic review. Clin Neuropharmacol 35(5):244–253, 2012 22986798

Mawardi G, Markman TM, Muslem R, et al: SSRI/SNRI therapy is associated with a high risk of gastrointestinal bleeding in LVAD patients. Heart Lung Circ 29(8):1241–1246, 2020 31635997

McCain KR, Sawyer TS, Spiller HA: Evaluation of centrally acting cholinesterase inhibitor exposures in adults. Ann Pharmacother 41(10):1632–1637, 2007 17848422

McConachie SM, Caputo RA, Wilhelm SM, et al: Efficacy of capsaicin for the treatment of cannabinoid hyperemesis syndrome: a systematic review. Ann Pharmacother 53(11):1145–1152, 2019 31104487

McLean AJ, Morgan DJ: Clinical pharmacokinetics in patients with liver disease. Clin Pharmacokinet 21(1):42–69, 1991 1914341

Miarons Font M, Rofes Salsench L: Antipsychotic medication and oropharyngeal dysphagia: systematic review. Eur J Gastroenterol Hepatol 29(12):1332–1339, 2017 29023321

Mikocka-Walus A, Ford AC, Drossman DA: Antidepressants in inflammatory bowel disease. Nat Rev Gastroenterol Hepatol 17(3):184–192, 2020 32071420

Monti JM, Pandi-Perumal SR: Eszopiclone: its use in the treatment of insomnia. Neuropsychiatr Dis Treat 3(4):441–453, 2007 19300573

Na KS, Jung HY, Cho SJ, Cho SE: Can we recommend mirtazapine and bupropion for patients at risk for bleeding? A systematic review and meta-analysis. J Affect Disord 225:221–226, 2018 28841484

Navari RM: Nausea and vomiting in advanced cancer. Curr Treat Options Oncol 21(2):14, 2020 32025954

Neuendorf R, Harding A, Stello N, et al: Depression and anxiety in patients with inflammatory bowel disease: a systematic review. J Psychosom Res 87:70–80, 2016 27411754

Nguyen TMT, Eslick GD: Systematic review: the treatment of noncardiac chest pain with antidepressants. Aliment Pharmacol Ther 35(5):493–500, 2012 22239853

Nielsen J, Meyer JM: Risk factors for ileus in patients with schizophrenia. Schizophr Bull 38(3):592–598, 2012 21112965

Nieves JE, Stack KM, Harrison ME, et al: Dysphagia: a rare form of dyskinesia? J Psychiatr Pract 13(3):199–201, 2007 17522565

Nitsche CJ, Jamieson N, Lerch MM, et al: Drug induced pancreatitis. Best Pract Res Clin Gastroenterol 24(2):143–155, 2010 20227028

Nochaiwong S, Ruengorn C, Awiphan R, et al: Use of serotonin reuptake inhibitor antidepressants and the risk of bleeding complications in patients on anticoagulant or antiplatelet agents: a systematic review and meta-analysis. Ann Med 54(1):80–97, 2022 34955074

Nwokediuko SC: Current trends in the management of gastroesophageal reflux disease: a review. ISRN Gastroenterol 2012:391631, 2012 22844607

Oka Y, Okamoto K, Kawashita N, et al: Meta-analysis of the risk of upper gastrointestinal hemorrhage with combination therapy of selective serotonin reuptake inhibitors and non-steroidal anti-inflammatory drugs. Biol Pharm Bull 37(6):947–953, 2014 24681541

Oustamanolakis P, Tack J: Dyspepsia: organic versus functional. J Clin Gastroenterol 46(3):175–190, 2012 22327302

Overland MK: Dyspepsia. Med Clin North Am 98(3):549–564, 2014 24758960

Owyang C: Treatment of chronic secretory diarrhea of unknown origin by lithium carbonate. Gastroenterology 87(3):714–718, 1984 6430744

Pacifici GM, Viani A, Franchi M, et al: Conjugation pathways in liver disease. Br J Clin Pharmacol 30(3):427–435, 1990 2223421

Padwal R, Brocks D, Sharma AM: A systematic review of drug absorption following bariatric surgery and its theoretical implications. Obes Rev 11(1):41–50, 2010 19493300

Pae CU, Lee SJ, Han C, et al: Atypical antipsychotics as a possible treatment option for irritable bowel syndrome. Expert Opin Investig Drugs 22(5):565–572, 2013 23506326

Paik KY, Seok HE, Chung JH: The analysis of risk for peptic ulcer disease using Korean national health and nutrition examination survey: a cross-sectional analysis of a national survey sample. Ann Transl Med 8(7):460, 2020 32395504

Palsson OS, Drossman DA: Psychiatric and psychological dysfunction in irritable bowel syndrome and the role of psychological treatments. Gastroenterol Clin North Am 34(2):281–303, 2005 15862936

Panebianco M, Marchese-Ragona R, Masiero S, et al: Dysphagia in neurological diseases: a literature review. Neurol Sci 41(11):3067–3073, 2020 32506360

Pardi DS: Microscopic colitis. Clin Geriatr Med 30(1):55–65, 2014 24267602

Park SJ, Gunn N, Harrison SA: Olanzapine and benztropine as a cause of ischemic colitis in a 27-year-old man. J Clin Gastroenterol 46(6):515–517, 2012 22011585

Parkman HP, Van Natta ML, Abell TL, et al: Effect of nortriptyline on symptoms of idiopathic gastroparesis: the NORIG randomized clinical trial. JAMA 310(24):2640–2649, 2013 24368464

Passmore MJ, Devarajan S, Ghatavi K, et al: Serotonin syndrome with prolonged dysphagia. Can J Psychiatry 49(1):79–80, 2004 14763689

Patten SB: Psychiatric side effects of interferon treatment. Curr Drug Saf 1(2):143–150, 2006 18690925

Peery AF, Crockett SD, Murphy CC, et al: Burden and cost of gastrointestinal, liver, and pancreatic disease in the United States: update 2018. Gastroenterology 156(1):254.e11–272.e11, 2019 30315778

Periseti A, Gajendran M, Dasari CS, et al: Cannabis hyperemesis syndrome: an update on the pathophysiology and management. Ann Gastroenterol 33(6):571–578, 2020 33162734

Piacentino D, Cantarini R, Alfonsi M, et al: Psychopathological features of irritable bowel syndrome patients with and without functional dyspepsia: a cross sectional study. BMC Gastroenterol 11:94, 2011 21871075

Puasripun S, Thinrungroj N, Pinyopornpanish K, et al: Efficacy and safety of clidinium/chlordiazepoxide as an add-on therapy in functional dyspepsia: a randomized, controlled trial. J Neurogastroenterol Motil 26(2):259–266, 2020 32235033

Quigley EMM, Lacy BE: Overlap of functional dyspepsia and GERD—diagnostic and treatment implications. Nat Rev Gastroenterol Hepatol 10(3):175–186, 2013 23296247

Rask SM, Luoto KE, Solismaa A, et al: Clozapine-related diarrhea and colitis: report of 4 cases. J Clin Psychopharmacol 40(3):293–296, 2020 32332465

Remes-Troche JM: The hypersensitive esophagus: pathophysiology, evaluation, and treatment options. Curr Gastroenterol Rep 12(5):417–426, 2010 20669058

Reyad AA, Mishriky R, Girgis E: Pharmacological and non-pharmacological management of burning mouth syndrome: a systematic review. Dent Med Probl 57(3):295–304, 2020 33113291

Richards JR: Cannabinoid hyperemesis syndrome: pathophysiology and treatment in the emergency department. J Emerg Med 54(3):354–363, 2018 29310960

Rifai MA, Gleason OC, Sabouni D: Psychiatric care of the patient with hepatitis C: a review of the literature. Prim Care Companion J Clin Psychiatry 12(6):PCC.09r00877, 2010 21494349

Ritchie A, Kramer JM: Recent advances in the etiology and treatment of burning mouth syndrome. J Dent Res 97(11):1193–1199, 2018 29913093

Roerig JL, Steffen KJ, Zimmerman C, et al: A comparison of duloxetine plasma levels in postbariatric surgery patients versus matched nonsurgical control subjects. J Clin Psychopharmacol 33(4):479–484, 2013 23771193

Roncero C, Villegas JL, Martínez-Rebollar M, et al: The pharmacological interactions between direct-acting antivirals for the treatment of chronic hepatitis C and psychotropic drugs. Expert Rev Clin Pharmacol 11(10):999–1030, 2018 30199279

Roquin G, Peres M, Lerolle N, et al: First report of lamotrigine-induced drug rash with eosinophilia and systemic symptoms syndrome with pancreatitis. Ann Pharmacother 44(12):1998–2000, 2010 21098750

Ruepert L, Quartero AO, de Wit NJ, et al: Bulking agents, antispasmodics and antidepressants for the treatment of irritable bowel syndrome. Cochrane Database Syst Rev (8):CD003460, 2011 21833945

Russo MW, Watkins PB: Are patients with elevated liver tests at increased risk of drug-induced liver injury? Gastroenterology 126(5):1477–1480, 2004 15131809

Saito YA, Almazar AE, Tilkes KE, et al: Randomised clinical trial: pregabalin vs placebo for irritable bowel syndrome. Aliment Pharmacol Ther 49(4):389–397, 2019 30663077

Salter TG, Williams MD: Antidepressant-associated microscopic colitis: a case report and literature review. Psychosomatics 58(3):307–312, 2017 28347506

Santoro GA, Eitan BZ, Pryde A, et al: Open study of low-dose amitriptyline in the treatment of patients with idiopathic fecal incontinence. Dis Colon Rectum 43(12):1676–1681, discussion 1681–1682, 2000 11156450

Scarpellini E, Arts J, Karamanolis G, et al: International consensus on the diagnosis and management of dumping syndrome. Nat Rev Endocrinol 16(8):448–466, 2020 32457534

Seaman JS, Bowers SP, Dixon P, et al: Dissolution of common psychiatric medications in a Roux-en-Y gastric bypass model. Psychosomatics 46(3):250–253, 2005 15883146

Shah AV, Serajuddin ATM, Mangione RA: Making all medications gluten free. J Pharm Sci 107(5):1263–1268, 2018 29287928

Shah V, Anderson J: Clozapine-induced ischaemic colitis. BMJ Case Rep 2013:bcr2012007933, 2013 23345490

Shamash J, Miall L, Williams F, et al: Dysphagia in the neuroleptic malignant syndrome. Br J Psychiatry 164(6):849–850, 1994 7953002

Shrivastava RK, Siegal H, Lawlor R, et al: Doxepin therapy for duodenal ulcer: a controlled trial in patients who failed to respond to cimetidine. Clin Ther 7(3):319–326, 1985 3888393

Siebenhüner AR, Rossel JB, Schreiner P, et al: Effects of anti-TNF therapy and immunomodulators on anxiety and depressive symptoms in patients with inflammatory bowel disease: a 5-year analysis. Therap Adv Gastroenterol 14:17562848211033763, 2021 34484421

Silva MA, Key S, Han E, et al: Acute pancreatitis associated with antipsychotic medication: evaluation of clinical features, treatment, and polypharmacy in a series of cases. J Clin Psychopharmacol 36(2):169–172, 2016 26859276

Simons-Linares CR, Elkhouly MA, Salazar MJ: Drug-induced acute pancreatitis in adults: an update. Pancreas 48(10):1263–1273, 2019 31688589

Ślebioda Z, Lukaszewska-Kuska M, Dorocka-Bobkowska B: Evaluation of the efficacy of treatment modalities in burning mouth syndrome: a systematic review. J Oral Rehabil 47(11):1435–1447, 2020 32979878

Sockalingam S, Tseng A, Giguere P, et al: Psychiatric treatment considerations with direct acting antivirals in hepatitis C. BMC Gastroenterol 13:86, 2013 23672254

Sockalingam S, Sheehan K, Feld JJ, et al: Psychiatric care during hepatitis C treatment: the changing role of psychiatrists in the era of direct-acting antivirals. Am J Psychiatry 172(6):512–516, 2015 26029803

Sorensen CJ, DeSanto K, Borgelt L, et al: Cannabinoid hyperemesis syndrome: diagnosis, pathophysiology, and treatment—a systematic review. J Med Toxicol 13(1):71–87, 2017 28000146

Sperber AD, Bangdiwala SI, Drossman DA, et al: Worldwide prevalence and burden of functional gastrointestinal disorders, results of Rome Foundation global study. Gastroenterology 160(1):99.e3–114.e3, 2021 32294476

Spiegel DR, Kolb R: Treatment of irritable bowel syndrome with comorbid anxiety symptoms with mirtazapine. Clin Neuropharmacol 34(1):36–38, 2011 21242743

Spieker MR: Evaluating dysphagia. Am Fam Physician 61(12):3639–3648, 2000 10892635

Spina E, Barbieri MA, Cicala G, et al: Clinically relevant drug interactions between newer antidepressants and oral anticoagulants. Expert Opin Drug Metab Toxicol 16(1):31–44, 2020 31795773

Sutherland A, Naessens K, Plugge E, et al: Olanzapine for the prevention and treatment of cancer-related nausea and vomiting in adults. Cochrane Database Syst Rev 9(9):CD012555, 2018 30246876

Tack J, Janssen P, Masaoka T, et al: Efficacy of buspirone, a fundus-relaxing drug, in patients with functional dyspepsia. Clin Gastroenterol Hepatol 10(11):1239–1245, 2012 22813445

Tan ECK, Lexomboon D, Sandborgh-Englund G, et al: Medications that cause dry mouth as an adverse effect in older people: a systematic review and metaanalysis. J Am Geriatr Soc 66(1):76–84, 2018 29071719

Tan PC, Vani S, Lim BK, et al: Anxiety and depression in hyperemesis gravidarum: prevalence, risk factors and correlation with clinical severity. Eur J Obstet Gynecol Reprod Biol 149(2):153–158, 2010 20097465

Tandra S, Chalasani N, Jones DR, et al: Pharmacokinetic and pharmacodynamic alterations in the Roux-en-Y gastric bypass recipients. Ann Surg 258(2):262–269, 2013 23222033

Telles-Correia D, Barbosa A, Cortez-Pinto H, et al: Psychotropic drugs and liver disease: a critical review of pharmacokinetics and liver toxicity. World J Gastrointest Pharmacol Ther 8(1):26–38, 2017 28217372

Törnblom H, Drossman DA: Psychopharmacologic therapies for irritable bowel syndrome. Gastroenterol Clin North Am 50(3):655–669, 2021 34304793

Tripp AC: Lithium toxicity after Roux-en-Y gastric bypass surgery. J Clin Psychopharmacol 31(2):261–262, 2011 21364348

Tuqan W, Lee S, Hanson J, et al: Carbamazepine-associated hypersensitivity colitis. Dig Dis Sci 63(2):334–337, 2018 29238897

Upala S, Wijarnpreecha K, Jaruvongvanich V, et al: Antipsychotics-induced ischemic colitis. Am J Emerg Med 33(11):1716.e5–1716.e6, 2015 25886897

Vaidyanathan S, Subramanian K, Bharadwaj B, et al: Acute necrotizing pancreatitis associated with orally disintegrating formulation of olanzapine: implications on clinical presentation and management. J Clin Psychopharmacol 39(5):519–521, 2019 31433336

Van Oudenhove L, Levy RL, Crowell M, et al: Biopsychosocial aspects of functional gastrointestinal disorders: how central and environmental processes contribute to the development and expression of functional gastrointestinal disorders. Gastroenterology 150(6):P1335–P1367, 2016 27144624

van Veggel M, Olofinjana O, Davies G, et al: Clozapine and gastro-oesophageal reflux disease (GORD): an investigation of temporal association. Acta Psychiatr Scand 127(1):69–77, 2013 22901096

Venkatesan T, Levinthal DJ, Li BUK, et al: Role of chronic cannabis use: cyclic vomiting syndrome vs cannabinoid hyperemesis syndrome. Neurogastroenterol Motil 31(Suppl 2):e13606, 2019a 31241817

Venkatesan T, Levinthal DJ, Tarbell SE, et al: Guidelines on management of cyclic vomiting syndrome in adults by the American Neurogastroenterology and Motility Society and Vomiting Syndrome Association. Neurogastroenterol Motil 31(Suppl 2):e13604, 2019b 31241819

Viazis N, Keyoglou A, Kanellopoulos AK, et al: Selective serotonin reuptake inhibitors for the treatment of hypersensitive esophagus: a randomized, double-blind, placebo-controlled study. Am J Gastroenterol 107(11):1662–1667, 2012 21625270

Videlock EJ, Chang L: Latest insights on the pathogenesis of irritable bowel syndrome. Gastroenterol Clin North Am 50(3):505–522, 2021 34304785

Villa A, Connell CL, Abati S: Diagnosis and management of xerostomia and hyposalivation. Ther Clin Risk Manag 11:45–51, 2014 25653532

Voican CS, Corruble E, Naveau S, et al: Antidepressant-induced liver injury: a review for clinicians. Am J Psychiatry 171(4):404–415, 2014 24362450

Wald A: Chronic constipation: advances in management. Neurogastroenterol Motil 19(1):4–10, 2007 17187583

Wang M, Zeraatkar D, Obeda M, et al: Drug-drug interactions with warfarin: a systematic review and meta-analysis. Br J Clin Pharmacol 87(11):4051–4100, 2021 33769581

Weijenborg PW, de Schepper HS, Smout AJ, et al: Effects of antidepressants in patients with functional esophageal disorders or gastroesophageal reflux disease: a systematic review. Clin Gastroenterol Hepatol 13(2):251.e1–259.e1, 2015 24997325

West S, Rowbotham D, Xiong G, et al: Clozapine induced gastrointestinal hypomotility: a potentially life threatening adverse event: a review of the literature. Gen Hosp Psychiatry 46:32–37, 2017 28622812

Whitehead WE, Wald A, Norton NJ: Treatment options for fecal incontinence. Dis Colon Rectum 44(1):131–142, discussion 142–144, 2001 11805574

Whitehead WE, Palsson OS, Levy RR, et al: Comorbidity in irritable bowel syndrome. Am J Gastroenterol 102(12):2767–2776, 2007 17900326

Whitehead WE, Borrud L, Goode PS, et al: Fecal incontinence in US adults: epidemiology and risk factors. Gastroenterology 137(2):512–517, 517.e1–517.e2, 2009 19410574

Whitehead WE, Rao SS, Lowry A, et al: Treatment of fecal incontinence: state of the science summary for the National Institute of Diabetes and Digestive and Kidney Diseases workshop. Am J Gastroenterol 110(1):138–146, quiz 147, 2015 25331348

Wolff A, Joshi RK, Ekström J, et al: A guide to medications inducing salivary gland dysfunction, xerostomia, and subjective sialorrhea: a systematic review sponsored by the World Workshop on Oral Medicine VI. Drugs R D 17(1):1–28, 2017 27853957

Wynn GH, Sandson NB, Cozza KL: Gastrointestinal medications. Psychosomatics 48(1):79–85, 2007 17209156

Xue F, Strombom I, Turnbull B, et al: Duloxetine for depression and the incidence of hepatic events in adults. J Clin Psychopharmacol 31(4):517–522, 2011 21694615

Zaccara G, Franciotta D, Perucca E: Idiosyncratic adverse reactions to antiepileptic drugs. Epilepsia 48(7):1223–1244, 2007 17386054

Zamani M, Alizadeh-Tabari S, Zamani V: Systematic review with meta-analysis: the prevalence of anxiety and depression in patients with irritable bowel syndrome. Aliment Pharmacol Ther 50(2):132–143, 2019 31157418

5

Renal and Urological Disorders

James L. Levenson, M.D.

Renal disease and the procedures and medications used to manage renal and urological disorders often cause psychiatric symptoms, including depression, anxiety, sleep disorders, and cognitive impairment. Surprisingly, the literature provides little specific guidance on the management of psychiatric symptoms in patients with renal disease, even though pharmacotherapy is confounded by disease-related alterations in pharmacokinetics (metabolism, excretion) for both hepatically and renally eliminated drugs, medication adverse effects, and drug interactions. Similar issues surround the safe and effective use of psychotropics for patients with urological disorders. In this chapter, I review psychiatric symptoms related to renal and urological disorders, psychopharmacotherapy in renal disease, and interactions between psychiatric drugs and renal and urological drugs.

Differential Diagnosis

Psychiatric Symptoms in Patients With Renal Disease

The diagnosis of psychiatric disorders in patients with end-stage renal disease (ESRD) is complicated because many somatic symptoms are extremely common as a result of renal insufficiency itself or comorbid medical disorders (especially diabetes). A systematic review of symptoms in ESRD found the following weighted mean prevalence rates: fatigue, 71%; pruritus, 55%; constipation, 53%; anorexia, 49%; pain, 47%; sleep disturbance, 44%; dyspnea, 35%; and nausea, 33% (Murtagh et al. 2007). It is not easy to determine the etiology of a particular symptom, which is often multifactorial in any case.

Depression is the most common psychiatric disorder in patients with ESRD (Kimmel et al. 2007). Prevalence estimates vary depending on definitions and methods, but the prevalence of major depression may be as high as 30% (Palmer et al. 2013), with minor depression in another 25% of patients. Metabolic, psychological, and social factors all contribute to increased risk for depression in ESRD. The diagnosis of depression in uremic patients is complicated because anorexia, anergia, insomnia, constipation, poor concentration, and diminished libido may all be caused by renal insufficiency. Depression in patients undergoing dialysis may be intermittent or chronic (Cukor et al. 2008b). Depression in patients with chronic kidney disease (CKD) has been shown to be associated with multiple poor outcomes, including increased mortality and hospitalization rates, as well as poorer treatment compliance and quality of life (Bautovich et al. 2014).

Significant anxiety is also frequent in almost half of patients with ESRD, intermittent in one-third, and persistent in 15% (Cukor et al. 2008a, 2008b). As with depression, metabolic, psychological, and social factors contribute to etiology. Fluid and electrolyte shifts that are too rapid may physiologically cause anxiety. Specific phobic anxiety may arise from a fear of needles or the sight of blood, as well as a reaction to removal of blood into a machine and its return to the patient's body. In one study, the prevalence of PTSD symptoms was 17%, with most related to the experience of hemodialysis (Tagay et al. 2007).

Acute renal failure with uremia often causes delirium with cognitive dysfunction and, at times, psychotic symptoms. Acute onset of renal failure accompanied by hallucinations should lead to consideration of a toxic exposure (e.g., poisonous mushrooms, herbal "remedies," insecticides). Psychotic symptoms in patients with ESRD may be due to a primary psychotic disorder (10% of patients at one urban dialysis center; Cukor et al. 2007), electrolyte disturbance, comorbid medical disorder (e.g., stroke, dementia), or toxicity of a renally excreted drug (e.g., acyclovir; Yang et al. 2007).

Subtle cognitive dysfunction is often present in patients with partial renal insufficiency (Elias et al. 2009). Cognitive disorders are common in patients with ESRD as a consequence of uremia, electrolyte disturbances, toxicity of renally excreted drugs, and comorbid medical disorders (e.g., cerebrovascular disease). The signs and symptoms of uremia vary in severity, depending on both the extent to which and the rate at which renal function is lost. Mild or chronic uremia may cause mild cognitive dysfunction, fatigue, and headache. Untreated uremia progresses to lethargy, hypoactive delirium, and coma. Up to 70% of patients older than 55 years undergoing hemodialysis have moderate to severe chronic cognitive impairment (Murray 2008). Cognitive impairment from CKD improves after renal transplantation (Drew et al. 2019). Vascular dementia is especially common because of the high prevalence of diabetes, hypertension, and atherosclerosis in patients with ESRD.

Sleep disorders, most commonly insomnia, affect 50%–80% of patients undergoing dialysis (Losso et al. 2015; Novak et al. 2006). Metabolic changes, lifestyle factors, depression, anxiety, and other underlying sleep disorders may all contribute to the development of chronic insomnia. Restless legs syndrome (RLS) is especially common, affecting 10%–30% of patients undergoing maintenance hemodialysis and up to 50% of those undergoing ambulatory peritoneal dialysis (Losso et al. 2015; Molnar et al. 2006; Murtagh et al. 2007) (see the subsection "Dopamine Agonists and Restless Legs Syndrome" later in this chapter). Antidepressants and antipsychotics are associated with increased risk for RLS in ESRD (Bliwise et al. 2014).

Renal Symptoms of Psychiatric Disorders: Psychogenic Polydipsia

Psychogenic polydipsia (PPD), also called primary polydipsia, occurs in 6%–20% of psychiatric patients, most commonly in patients with schizophrenia (Verghese et al. 1996), with higher risk during prolonged hospitalization and in smokers (de Leon et al. 2002). Excessive thirst, probably caused by abnormal hypothalamic thirst control, causes chronic and excessive fluid intake, often beyond the renal ability to excrete dilute urine. Hyponatremia, which is present in 10%–20% of compulsive drinkers, is often mild and asymptomatic unless accompanied by the syndrome of inappropriate antidiuretic hormone secretion (SIADH) or other impairment of water excretion. PPD can be distinguished from diabetes insipidus by water restriction. Although both PPD and diabetes insipidus have low urine osmolality before water restriction (<100 mOsm/L), after water restriction, urine becomes very concentrated with PPD (>600 mOsm/L) but remains dilute with diabetes insipidus (<600 mOsm/L) (Dundas et al. 2007). PPD can be managed by water restriction, although compliance is problematic, or by pharmacotherapy. No pharmacotherapy has been proven beneficial in a randomized clinical trial (Havens et al. 2021). Case reports suggest efficacy for atypical antipsychotics (clozapine, risperidone, olanzapine) and β-blockers. Acetazolamide was effective in a small case series (Takagi et al. 2011). In a small randomized controlled trial of clonidine or enalapril in chronically psychotic patients with PPD, both agents demonstrated improvement of measures reflecting fluid consumption in 60% of patients (Greendyke et al. 1998). Demeclocycline was reported to be effective in case reports but was ineffective in randomized controlled trials. Vasopressin V_2 antagonists (vaptans), including tolvaptan and conivaptan, were said to be effective for the treatment of hyponatremia resulting from PPD (Bhardwaj et al. 2013), but there have been no reports of their use since that report.

Pharmacotherapy in Renal Disease

Pharmacokinetics in Renal Disease

Although most psychotropic drugs, as the parent compounds, do not depend on the kidney for excretion, renal failure may alter the pharmacokinetics of practically all drugs through changes in distribution, protein binding, and metabolism (see Chapter 1, "Pharmacokinetics, Pharmacodynamics, and Principles of Drug-Drug Interactions"). Edema present in ESRD will increase the volume of distribution for hydrophilic drugs. Uremic products circulating in ESRD may displace highly bound drugs from plasma proteins, increasing the proportion of drug circulating free in plasma. This shift in ratio of free to bound drug may cause therapeutic drug monitoring methods that measure total drug to suggest lower, possibly subtherapeutic levels. For those highly bound drugs for which therapeutic drug monitoring guides dosing (e.g., phenytoin, valproate), clinicians should use drug monitoring methods that are selective for free drug (see Chapter 1); otherwise, seemingly lower levels might prompt a dosage increase, with possibly toxic results.

Renal disease can also significantly modify Phase I hepatic drug metabolism, although the effects vary markedly. In general, hepatic metabolism mediated by cytochrome P450 2C9 (CYP2C9), CYP2C19, CYP2D6, and CYP3A4 is reduced in chronic renal disease, possibly through reduced CYP gene expression. Phase II metabolic reactions, including acetylation, glucuronidation, sulfation, and methylation, are also impaired in chronic renal disease (Pichette and Leblond 2003). The metabolic effect of renal disease on renal metabolism is often overlooked. Renal metabolism, which ordinarily represents about 15% of hepatic metabolic capacity, is reduced in renal insufficiency (Anders 1980).

Despite the complexity of pharmacokinetic changes in renal failure, most psychotropics do not require drastic dosage adjustment. The exceptions include drugs for which the parent compound or active metabolites undergo significant renal elimination (e.g., lithium, gabapentin, pregabalin, topiramate, paliperidone, risperidone, paroxetine, desvenlafaxine, venlafaxine, and memantine) (Table 5–1). However, many problems associated with use of psychotropics in patients with ESRD are related to comorbid illnesses rather than to the renal failure per se. Specific dosing guidelines based on creatinine clearance are not available for most psychotropics, but many clinicians use the rule of two-thirds (Levy 1990); that is, for patients with renal insufficiency, use two-thirds of the dosage (except for drugs listed in Table 5–1) used for patients with normal renal function. Table 5–1 provides recommendations for dosing psychotropics in patients with renal disease.

Drug clearance also may be influenced by hemodialysis or peritoneal dialysis. Most psychotropics are not dialyzable because of their lipophilicity and large volumes of distribution. Dialyzable psychotropics are listed in Table 5–2. Significant fluid shifts occur during and several hours after each hemodialysis treatment, making these patients more prone to orthostasis. Therefore, drugs that often cause orthostatic hypotension should be avoided.

Pharmacodynamics in Renal Disease

Electrolyte disturbances associated with renal failure or diuretic therapy may increase the risk of cardiac arrhythmias. Significant QT prolongation is observed with tricyclic antidepressants (TCAs), lithium (van Noord et al. 2009),

Table 5–1. Psychotropic medications in renal insufficiency (RI)

Medication	Effect and management
Antidepressants	
SSRIs	
Most	Mild to moderate RI: no dosage adjustment needed.
	Severe RI: may need to reduce dosage or lengthen dosing interval.
Paroxetine	Mild RI: no dosage adjustment needed.
	Moderate RI: 50%–75% of usual dosage.
	Severe RI: initial dosage of 10 mg/day; increase as needed by 10 mg at weekly intervals to a maximum of 40 mg/day.
	Controlled-release formulation: initial dosage of 12.5 mg/day; increase as needed by 12.5 mg at weekly intervals to a maximum of 50 mg/day.
SNRIs and novel agents	
Bupropion	Water-soluble active metabolites may accumulate. Reduce initial dosage.
Desvenlafaxine	Approximately 45% of desvenlafaxine is excreted unchanged in urine.
	Mild RI: no dosage adjustment needed.
	The dosage should not exceed 50 mg/day in moderate RI or 50 mg every other day in severe RI according to manufacturer.
Duloxetine	Mild RI: population creatine kinase analyses suggest no significant effect on apparent clearance.
	No data regarding use in moderate to severe RI.
	Not recommended for patients with ESRD.
Levomilnacipran	Moderate RI: maximum dose 80 mg.
	Severe RI: clearance maximum dose 40 mg.

Table 5–1.   Psychotropic medications in renal
insufficiency (RI) *(continued)*

Medication	Effect and management
Antidepressants *(continued)*	
SNRIs and novel agents *(continued)*	
Mirtazapine	Moderate RI: clearance decreased by 30%.
	Severe RI: clearance decreased by 50%.
Nefazodone	No dosage adjustment needed.
Trazodone	Mild RI: use with caution.
	No data regarding use in moderate to severe RI.
Venlafaxine	Mild to moderate RI: 75% of usual dosage.
	Severe RI: 50% of usual dosage.
	Patients undergoing hemodialysis should have dosage reduced by 50% and receive the dose after dialysis session.
Vilazodone	No dosage adjustment needed.
Vortioxetine	No dosage adjustment needed.
MAOIs	May accumulate in RI.
Selegiline	Active metabolite (methamphetamine) renally eliminated. Use with caution in renal impairment. No dosing guidelines.
TCAs	Water-soluble active metabolites may accumulate. No recommended dosage adjustments.
Brexanolone	No dosage adjustment needed.
Esketamine	No dosage adjustment needed.

Table 5–1.   Psychotropic medications in renal insufficiency (RI) *(continued)*

Medication	Effect and management
Antipsychotics	
Atypical agents	
Aripiprazole, asenapine, cariprazine, clozapine, lumateperone, olanzapine, and quetiapine	No dosage adjustment needed.
Brexpiprazole	Mild RI: no dosage adjustment needed.
	Moderate to severe RI: reduce dosage.
Iloperidone	Dosage adjustment not needed in mild to moderate RI, according to manufacturer. No recommendations for dosing in severe RI.
Lurasidone	Moderate to severe impairment: reduce by 50%.
Paliperidone	Clearance decreased in RI.
	Mild impairment: start at 3 mg/day, increasing to a maximum of 6 mg/day.
	Moderate to severe impairment: start at 1.5 mg/day, increasing to 3 mg/day, as tolerated.
Pimavanserin	No dosage adjustment needed.
Risperidone	Clearance decreased in RI. Initiate therapy at 0.25–0.5 mg bid.
	Increases beyond 1.5 mg should be made at intervals of at least 7 days.
Ziprasidone	No recommendations made regarding dosage adjustment.
Typical agents	
Haloperidol	No dosage adjustment needed.

Table 5–1. Psychotropic medications in renal
insufficiency (RI) *(continued)*

Medication	Effect and management
Anxiolytics and sedative-hypnotics	
Benzodiazepines	
Most	No dosage adjustment needed.
Chlordiazepoxide	Severe RI: 50% of usual dosage.
Nonbenzodiazepines	
Buspirone	Severe RI: use not recommended.
Lemborexant	No dosage adjustment needed.
Ramelteon	No dosage adjustment needed.
Suvorexant	No dosage adjustment needed.
Tasimelteon	No dosage adjustment needed.
Zaleplon	Mild to moderate RI: no dosage adjustment needed.
	Severe RI: not adequately studied.
Zolpidem	Dosage adjustment may not be needed in RI.
Zopiclone and eszopiclone	No dosage adjustment needed.
Anticonvulsant and antimanic agents	
Carbamazepine	Severe RI: 75% of usual dosage.
Gabapentin	$Cl_{cr} > 60$ mL/min: 1,200 mg/day (400 mg tid).
	Cl_{cr} 30–60 mL/min: 600 mg/day (300 mg bid).
	Cl_{cr} 15–30 mL/min: 300 mg/day.
	$Cl_{cr} < 15$ mL/min: 150 mg/day (300 mg every other day).
	Hemodialysis: 300- to 400-mg loading dose to patients who have never received gabapentin, then 200–300 mg after each dialysis session.
Lamotrigine	Reduced dosage may be effective in significant RI.

Table 5–1.   Psychotropic medications in renal insufficiency (RI) *(continued)*

Medication	Effect and management
Anticonvulsant and antimanic agents *(continued)*	
Lithium	Moderate RI: 50%–75% of usual dosage.
	Hemodialysis: supplemental dose of 300 mg once after each dialysis session.
Oxcarbazepine	Initiate therapy at 300 mg/day (50% of usual starting dosage).
Pregabalin	Cl_{cr} 30–60 mL/min: 50% of usual dosage.
	Cl_{cr} 15–30 mL/min: 25% of usual dosage.
	Cl_{cr} <15 mL/min: 12.5% of usual dosage.
	Hemodialysis: supplemental dose may be needed after each 4-hour dialysis session. See manufacturer's recommendations.
Topiramate	Mild RI: 100% of usual dosage.
	Moderate RI: 50% of usual dosage.
	Severe RI: 25% of usual dosage.
	Supplemental dose may be needed after hemodialysis.
Valproate	No dosage adjustment needed in RI, but valproate level measurements are misleading.
Cholinesterase inhibitors and memantine	
Donepezil	Limited data suggest no dosage adjustment needed.
Galantamine	Moderate RI: maximum dosage 16 mg/day. Severe RI: use not recommended.
Memantine	Extensive renal elimination.
	Mild to moderate RI: no dosage reduction needed.
	Severe RI: reduce dosage to 5 mg bid.
Rivastigmine	Dosage adjustment not recommended.

Table 5–1. Psychotropic medications in renal insufficiency (RI) *(continued)*

Medication	Effect and management
Psychostimulants and drugs for narcolepsy	
Atomoxetine	No dosage adjustment needed.
Dextroamphetamine	No dosage adjustment needed.
Lisdexamfetamine	Mild RI: no dosage adjustment needed.
	Moderate RI: maximum dose 50 mg.
	Severe RI: maximum dose 30 mg.
Methylphenidate	No dosage adjustment needed.
Modafinil and armodafinil	No dosage adjustment needed.
Pitolisant	Mild RI: no dosage adjustment needed.
	Moderate RI: reduce dosage.
	Severe RI: use not recommended.
Solriamfetol	Mild to moderate RI: reduce dosage. Dialyzable (21%).
Viloxazine	Moderate to severe RI: reduce dosage.
Dopamine agonists	
Amantadine	Cl_{cr} 80 mL/min: 100 mg bid.
	Cl_{cr} 60 mL/min: 100 mg qd alternated with 100 mg bid every other day.
	Cl_{cr} 40 mL/min: 100 mg/day.
	Cl_{cr} 30 mL/min: 200 mg twice weekly.
	Cl_{cr} 20 mL/min: 100 mg three times weekly.
	Cl_{cr} 10 mL/min: 200 mg alternated with 100 mg every 7 days.

Table 5–1. Psychotropic medications in renal insufficiency (RI) *(continued)*

Medication	Effect and management
Dopamine agonists *(continued)*	
Pramipexole	90% renal elimination: clearance of pramipexole is 75% lower for severe renal impairment (Cl_{cr} 20 mL/min) and 60% lower for patients with moderate impairment (Cl_{cr} 40 mL/min) compared with healthy volunteers. The interval between titration steps should be increased to 14 days for patients with restless legs syndrome and severe or moderate renal impairment (Cl_{cr} 20–60 mL/min).
α_2 Agonists	
Clonidine	Excreted primarily renally unchanged (40%–60%). No dosage adjustment needed in mild RI. Otherwise, cautious low dosage.
Guanfacine	No specific recommendations. Titrate cautiously.
Lofexidine	Mild RI: no dosage adjustment needed.
	Moderate to severe RI: reduce dosage.
Prazosin	No specific recommendations. Titrate cautiously.
Drugs for tardive dyskinesia	
Deutetrabenazine	No dosage adjustment needed.
Valbenazine	No dosage adjustment needed.
Drugs for substance use disorder	
Methadone	May need lower starting dose. Caution in hemodialysis.
Buprenorphine/ naloxone	No dosage adjustment needed.
Naloxone	No dosage adjustment needed.
Naltrexone	May need lower dosage because of increased plasma levels in ESRD.
Disulfiram	No dosage adjustment needed.

Table 5–1. Psychotropic medications in renal insufficiency (RI) *(continued)*

Medication	Effect and management
Drugs for substance use disorder *(continued)*	
Acamprosate	Mild to moderate RI: reduce dosage.
	Severe RI, ESRD: contraindicated.
Varenicline	Mild to moderate RI: no dosage adjustment needed.
	Severe RI, ESRD: recommended dosage 0.5 mg/day.

Note. Mild RI is >50 mL/min; moderate RI is 10–50 mL/min; severe RI is <10 mL/min. Cl_{cr}=creatinine clearance; ESRD=end-stage renal disease; MAOIs=monoamine oxidase inhibitors; SNRIs=serotonin-norepinephrine reuptake inhibitors; SSRIs=selective serotonin reuptake inhibitors; TCAs=tricyclic antidepressants.
Source. Cohen et al. 2004; Crone et al. 2006; Jacobson 2002; Periclou et al. 2006; and manufacturers' product information.

Table 5–2. Dialyzable psychotropic drugs

Medication	Conventional hemodialysis	High-permeability hemodialysis	Peritoneal dialysis
Carbamazepine		Yes	
Gabapentin	Yes	Likely	
Lamotrigine		Clearance increased 20%	
Lithium	Yes	Yes	Yes
Pregabalin	Yes	Likely	
Topiramate	Yes	Likely	
Valproate	Yes	Likely	

Note. Likely=no data, but increased clearance likely on the basis of conventional hemodialysis observations; Yes=studies indicate clearance increased by ≥30%.
Source. Bassilios et al. 2001; Israni et al. 2006; Lacerda et al. 2006; MedlinePlus 2015; Ward et al. 1994.

and typical and atypical antipsychotics (for a list of QT-prolonging drugs, see Funk et al. 2018).

Psychotropic Drugs in Renal Disease

Antidepressants

Despite the high prevalence of depression, few studies have been done on the effectiveness of antidepressants in patients undergoing dialysis. A 2016 Cochrane review concluded that evidence for antidepressants in patients undergoing dialysis was sparse and generally inconclusive (Palmer et al. 2016). Sertraline was not effective in a randomized controlled trial of 201 patients with major depression and patients with CKD not undergoing dialysis (Hedayati et al. 2017). The largest randomized trial to date of antidepressants in patients undergoing dialysis illustrates the difficult challenge in conducting such studies (Friedli et al. 2017). After 709 patients were screened, 30 were randomly assigned to receive sertraline or placebo. Half of the patients taking sertraline dropped out, and there were no differences in outcomes. Part of the problem is that patients undergoing chronic hemodialysis with depression (and their nephrologists) are often not interested in modifying or initiating antidepressant treatment (Pena-Polanco et al. 2017).

Nearly all antidepressants may be used for patients with renal failure. Patients with ESRD tend to be more sensitive to the side effects of TCAs, including sedation, anticholinergic toxicity (urinary retention, dry mouth that encourages excessive drinking), orthostatic hypotension, and QT prolongation. Hydroxylated metabolites have been shown to be markedly elevated in patients with ESRD and may be responsible for some TCA side effects. Nortriptyline and desipramine are considered preferred TCAs for patients with renal failure because these drugs are less likely than other TCAs to cause anticholinergic effects or orthostatic hypotension (Gillman 2007). Limited data are available on the use of newer antidepressants for patients with renal failure. The half-life of venlafaxine is prolonged in renal insufficiency; its clearance is reduced by more than 50% in patients undergoing dialysis. Desvenlafaxine undergoes significant renal elimination, necessitating dosage reduction for patients with moderate or severe renal impairment. Paroxetine levels are two to four times higher in renal insufficiency. Because most antidepressants are metabolized by the liver and excreted by the kidney, the prudent action is to initially reduce the dosage of all antidepressants to minimize the potential accumulation of active metabolites. However, a large retrospective study found no increased adverse effects of higher versus lower dosages of paroxetine, mirtazapine, and venlafaxine (Dev et al. 2014), and a small case series detected effective antidepressant responses to fluoxetine up to 180 mg/week without serious adverse effects (Kauffman et al. 2021).

Antipsychotics

Little evidence is available to guide the use of antipsychotics for patients undergoing dialysis. A 2021 systematic review identified only 14 case reports and 1 case series (Sutar et al. 2021). All antipsychotics may be used for patients with renal failure. However, paliperidone clearance is significantly decreased in all degrees of renal impairment, necessitating a reduction in initial and target dosages. Difficulties with other antipsychotics can arise from the complications of renal failure and dialysis or from the chronic disease causing renal failure (e.g., diabetes). For example, patients with ESRD who also have diabetic autonomic neuropathy will be at higher risk for drug side effects, including postural hypotension and bladder, gastrointestinal, and sexual dysfunction. Antipsychotics associated with hyperglycemia (e.g., clozapine, olanzapine) should be avoided in patients with comorbid diabetes. For patients with electrolyte disturbances, the risk of cardiac arrhythmias can be minimized by using antipsychotics with the least QT-prolonging effect. Second-generation antipsychotics have been associated with a small increase in risk for acute kidney injury (Jiang et al. 2017) and CKD (Højlund et al. 2020; Wang et al. 2018), but the association may be attributable to confounding (Ryan et al. 2017).

Anxiolytics and Sedative-Hypnotics

We found no clinical trials of pharmacotherapy for anxiety in patients with ESRD. Benzodiazepine and zolpidem use by patients undergoing dialysis has been associated with an increase in mortality, but this appears to be partially explained by greater use of these medications by patients with comorbid chronic obstructive pulmonary disease (Winkelmayer et al. 2007). In Japan, benzodiazepines were associated with higher mortality (RR=1.27; 95% CI=1.01–1.59) in patients undergoing hemodialysis with symptoms of depression, most of whom had not received antidepressants, even after confounders were controlled for (Fukuhara et al. 2006). Fukuhara et al. (2006) suggested that these benzodiazepine-related deaths may have been caused by inappropriate use of benzodiazepines instead of antidepressants to treat depression and the medications' adverse cognitive and psychomotor effects. A 2020 retrospective cohort study found almost a doubling of mortality in patients undergoing hemodialysis who were co-prescribed short-acting benzodiazepines and opioids but no increase with longer-acting benzodiazepines (Muzaale et al. 2020).

Nearly all sedative-hypnotics except barbiturates can be used by patients with renal failure. Barbiturates should be avoided because they may increase osteomalacia and cause excessive sedation. Preferred benzodiazepines include those with inactive metabolites, such as lorazepam and oxazepam; however, there is a risk of propylene glycol toxicity with continuous infusion of lorazepam for patients with ESRD (Horinek et al. 2009). Other benzodiazepines with inactive metabolites include clonazepam and temazepam, but less is known about changes in their half-lives in ESRD.

Mood Stabilizers

Lithium is almost entirely excreted by the kidneys. It is contraindicated for patients with acute renal failure but not those with chronic renal failure. For patients with stable partial renal insufficiency, clinicians should dose conservatively and monitor renal function frequently. For patients undergoing dialysis, lithium is completely dialyzed and may be given as a single oral dose (300–600 mg) just on dialysis days after hemodialysis treatment. Lithium levels should not be checked until at least 2 hours after dialysis because reequilibration from tissue stores occurs in the immediate postdialysis period. For patients undergoing peritoneal dialysis, lithium can be given in the dialysate. Lithium prolongs the QT interval and may increase the risk of cardiac arrhythmias in patients with electrolyte disturbances. Dosage adjustment recommendations based on creatinine clearance are available for gabapentin, lithium, topiramate, and carbamazepine (Baghdady et al. 2009).

Cholinesterase Inhibitors and Memantine

From the limited data available, it appears that dosage adjustment of donepezil and rivastigmine is not necessary in renal disease. Galantamine should be used cautiously in patients with moderate renal insufficiency; according to the manufacturer, its use by patients with severe renal insufficiency is not recommended. Memantine undergoes extensive renal elimination, necessitating dosage reduction for patients with severe renal insufficiency.

Psychostimulants

Methylphenidate and atomoxetine do not require dosage adjustment. The maximum recommended dose of mixed amphetamine salts in severe renal impairment is 20 mg. Recommendations for other agents are shown in Table 5–1.

Dopamine Agonists and Restless Legs Syndrome

Dopaminergic therapy (levodopa or the dopamine receptor agonists pramipexole, ropinirole, and rotigotine) has been recommended as first-line treatment for RLS. Although dopamine agonists and gabapentin have been found to be effective in reducing RLS symptoms in the general population, data supporting their use by patients with ESRD come from small, mostly unblinded trials (Aurora et al. 2012; Giannaki et al. 2014). Side effects of dopamine agonists can be problematic, including altered mental status and fall risk (Ishida et al. 2018), but are less frequent with other dopamine agonists than with levodopa. Alternative treatment options for RLS include benzodiazepines (especially clonazepam), opioids, and other anticonvulsants, but only limited data are available on their effectiveness and side-effect profiles in patients with ESRD (Molnar et al. 2006). If iron deficiency is present, repletion of iron will improve RLS.

Psychiatric Adverse Effects of Renal and Urological Agents

Drugs used in the treatment of renal and urological disorders sometimes have psychiatric adverse effects (Table 5–3). In the following subsections, I describe these effects for a variety of drug classes. Psychiatric adverse effects of other medications frequently used to treat renal disease are covered elsewhere in this book: corticosteroids for autoimmune nephritis in Chapter 10, "Endocrine and Metabolic Disorders"; antihypertensives in Chapter 6, "Cardiovascular Disorders"; and immunosuppressants after renal transplantation in Chapter 16, "Organ Transplantation."

Antispasmodics

Anticholinergic medications commonly used to treat overactive bladder are associated with psychiatric adverse effects, including cognitive impairment,

Table 5–3.   Psychiatric adverse effects of renal and urological medications

Medication	Psychiatric adverse effects
Urinary antispasmodics	
Oxybutynin > tolterodine, solifenacin, darifenacin > fesoterodine > trospium chloride	Cognitive impairment, confusion, fatigue, psychosis
Thiazide and thiazide-like diuretics	
Bendroflumethiazide, chlorothiazide, chlorthalidone, hydrochlorothiazide, hydroflumethiazide, indapamide, metolazone, and trichlormethiazide	Hyponatremia-induced lethargy, stupor, confusion, psychosis, irritability, seizures
α_1 **Antagonists**	
Alfuzosin, silodosin, terazosin	Dizziness
Doxazosin	Anxiety, insomnia, impotence
Tamsulosin	Insomnia, impotence
5α-Reductase inhibitors	
Dutasteride and finasteride	Impotence, decreased libido
Vasopressin antagonists	
Conivaptan	Confusion, insomnia

confusion, fatigue, and psychosis (Table 5–3). Cumulative use of strong anticholinergics, including bladder antimuscarinics, is associated with an increase in incident dementia (Gray et al. 2015). Among the available agents, penetration of the blood-brain barrier appears to be highest for oxybutynin; lower for tolterodine, solifenacin, and darifenacin; and lowest for fesoterodine and trospium chloride (Kerdraon et al. 2014). A large longitudinal cohort study identified mild cognitive impairment in 80% of patients receiving anticholinergics for overactive bladder, compared with 35% of age-matched control subjects (Ancelin et al. 2006). Cognitive impairment is well documented, and cases of frank psychosis have been reported for first-generation anticholinergics, such as oxybutynin and tolterodine (Chancellor and Boone 2012). Oxybutynin appears to be most likely to cause cognitive impairment. Few CNS side effects have been reported in clinical trials of the newer agents. However, it should be remembered that older adults with dementia would have been excluded from the trials, and they would be most vulnerable to anticholinergic effects on cognition.

Diuretics

Thiazide diuretics are the most common cause of hyponatremia (Liamis et al. 2008). Psychiatric symptoms of hyponatremia include lethargy, stupor, confusion, psychosis, irritability, and seizures.

α_1-Adrenergic Antagonists

The α_1 antagonists, including alfuzosin, doxazosin, silodosin, tamsulosin, and terazosin, are used in the treatment of benign prostatic hyperplasia and prostatitis. All α-blockers can cause hypotension. Doxazosin and tamsulosin have also been associated with insomnia and impotence. Increased anxiety may occur with doxazosin.

5α-Reductase Inhibitors

Dutasteride and finasteride, indicated for benign prostatic hyperplasia, may cause impotence and decreased libido.

Vasopressin Antagonists

Conivaptan, a vasopressin V_2-selective receptor antagonist, is associated with confusion and insomnia in safety and efficacy trials (Cumberland Pharmaceuticals 2009). Tolvaptan appears to have a more benign psychiatric adverse-effect profile but often causes fatigue and dizziness (Gheorghiade et al. 2003).

Renal and Urological Adverse Effects of Psychotropics

Psychotropic drugs have a variety of renal and urological adverse effects (Table 5–4), including hyponatremia or hypernatremia, nephropathy, urinary retention or incontinence, and sexual dysfunction.

Table 5–4. Renal and urological adverse effects of psychiatric medications

Medication	Renal and urological adverse effects
Mood stabilizers	
Lithium	Nephrogenic diabetes insipidus, hypernatremia
Carbamazepine and oxcarbazepine	SIADH, psychogenic polydipsia, hyponatremia
Lamotrigine	Urinary frequency
Antidepressants	
SSRIs or SNRIs	Sexual dysfunction, SIADH, psychogenic polydipsia, hyponatremia
Duloxetine, milnacipran	Urinary retention
TCAs	Urinary hesitancy, urinary retention, SIADH, psychogenic polydipsia, hyponatremia
Esketamine	Urinary frequency
Antipsychotics	SIADH, psychogenic polydipsia, hyponatremia
Low-potency typical antipsychotics	Urinary hesitancy, urinary retention
Anxiolytics and sedative-hypnotics	
Tasimelteon	Frequent urinary tract infection
Anticholinergic agents for extrapyramidal side effects	
Trihexyphenidyl, benztropine	Urinary hesitancy, urinary retention
Drugs for tardive dyskinesia	
Deutetrabenazine	Frequent urinary tract infection

Note.   SIADH=syndrome of inappropriate antidiuretic hormone secretion; SNRIs=serotonin-norepinephrine reuptake inhibitors; SSRIs=selective serotonin reuptake inhibitors; TCAs=tricyclic antidepressants.

Renal Effects of Psychotropics

Hyponatremia, which can manifest as lethargy, stupor, confusion, psychosis, irritability, and seizures, has many different precipitants, including thiazide diuretics (see Table 5–3), but two have particular psychiatric relevance: 1) SIADH, which can be caused by many psychotropic drugs, especially oxcarbazepine and carbamazepine but also selective serotonin reuptake inhibitors (SSRIs), TCAs, and antipsychotics; and 2) PPD (discussed earlier in the subsection "Renal Symptoms of Psychiatric Disorders: Psychogenic Polydipsia"). In an acutely psychotic patient with hyponatremia, urinary concentration can help distinguish drug-induced SIADH from PPD: the concentration will be high in the former and low in the latter (Atsariyasing and Goldman 2014). A recent algorithm helps differentiate SIADH from other causes of hyponatremia (Pinkhasov et al. 2021). Hyponatremia is most common with oxcarbazepine and is more common in older adults. Among antidepressants, SSRIs and serotonin-norepinephrine reuptake inhibitors (SNRIs) are much more likely than TCAs to cause hyponatremia (De Picker et al. 2014). The risk increases considerably if the patient is also taking other drugs that cause hyponatremia, such as thiazide diuretics (Letmaier et al. 2012). Acute-onset symptomatic hyponatremia may necessitate emergent treatment with hypertonic (3%) saline. In chronic cases, correction should be gradual to minimize the risk of pontine myelinolysis, relying on fluid restriction and vasopressin receptor antagonists (Siegel 2008).

Hypernatremia can result in cognitive dysfunction, delirium, seizures, and lethargy, progressing to stupor and coma. Hypernatremia is usually caused by dehydration with significant total body water deficits. The only psychotropic drug that causes hypernatremia is lithium, via nephrogenic diabetes insipidus (NDI). Most patients receiving lithium have polydipsia and polyuria, reflecting mild benign NDI, as measured in reduction in concentrating ability (Doornebal et al. 2019). Lithium-induced NDI sometimes persists long after lithium discontinuation and varies from mild polyuria to hyperosmolar coma. NDI has been treated with nonsteroidal anti-inflammatory drugs, thiazides, and amiloride, as well as sodium restriction (Bockenhauer and Bichet 2015; Kavanagh and Uy 2019). Amiloride is considered the treatment of choice for lithium-induced NDI.

The effect of lithium on renal function remains under study, with variable results from more recent retrospective and cohort studies (Kessing et al. 2015; Nielsen et al. 2018; Rej et al. 2020; Schoot et al. 2020). Most recently, a historical cohort study reported that the risk of CKD in patients receiving long-term lithium was 27% (Pahwa et al. 2021), similar to the 25.5% calculated in a recent meta-analysis (Schoretsanitis et al. 2022). In a study of more than 1,000 patients treated with lithium from 2000 to 2015, the incidence of CKD was 0.012 cases per exposed patient-year. The incidence of CKD stage 4 was only 0.0004 per patient-year. No cases of ESRD occurred in that cohort (Van Alphen et al. 2021). Some of the apparent risk is attributable to surveillance bias and failure to control for other causes (Kessing et al. 2015; Nielsen et al. 2018). In general, more recent studies and more methodologically sound studies show lower risks (Nielsen et al. 2018; Rej et al. 2020). Some studies report that longer duration of lithium therapy is predictive of a decrease in esti-mated glomerular filtration ("creeping creatinine") (e.g., Łukawska et al. 2021; Van Alphen et al. 2021), whereas others do not. In patients who do develop CKD while taking lithium, continuation of treatment with lithium may not necessarily lead to an increase in the risk of end-stage kidney disease (Kessing et al. 2017). For those with CKD whose lithium was discontinued, most showed either an increase in glomerular filtration rate or a decrease in the rate of decline (Hoekstra et al. 2022). Chronic lithium use may result in altered kidney mor-phology, including interstitial fibrosis, tubular atrophy, urinary casts, and oc-casionally glomerular sclerosis, in some patients, but these changes are not always associated with impaired renal function. When lithium induced ne-phrotic syndrome with acute kidney injury, the underlying pathology was mainly minimal change disease, which quickly reversed after lithium was stopped (Łukawska et al. 2021). Although long-term lithium treatment is the only well-established factor associated with lithium-induced nephropathy, changes in renal function are often associated with other factors, including age, episodes of lithium toxicity, other medications (analgesics), substance abuse, and the presence of comorbid disorders (hypertension, diabetes). Higher lith-ium dosages appear to be associated with higher risk of kidney injury. Rej et al. (2020) found a small increase in risk of renal function decline in older adults with average lithium levels greater than 0.7 mEq/L compared with those re-ceiving valproate (hazard ratio=1.14) but no difference between lithium and valproate when lithium levels were less than 0.7 mEq/L. A Danish nationwide cohort study in patients with bipolar disorder found that lithium was associated with an increase in CKD but not ESRD. Patients with bipolar disorder receiv-ing valproate had an increase in both CKD and ESRD (Kessing et al. 2015).

In summary, the progression of lithium nephrotoxicity to ESRD is rare and requires lithium use for several decades. Lithium is so efficacious in bipolar disorder that the risk of renal dysfunction during chronic use is considered acceptable, with yearly monitoring of renal function, aiming for the lowest effective dosage. The presence of CKD does not preclude prescribing lithium (Kessing et al. 2017).

Urological Effects of Psychotropics

Many psychotropics cause disorders of micturition. Urinary retention is associated with drugs with significant anticholinergic activity, including TCAs, SNRIs, and antipsychotics, especially low-potency typical agents but also atypical agents (Trinchieri et al. 2021). Antipsychotics can also cause urinary incontinence and other lower urinary tract symptoms (frequency, urgency, or incomplete emptying) (Sinha et al. 2016; Trinchieri et al. 2021), and these effects may persist for the duration of treatment. Treatment of antipsychotic-induced urinary incontinence with sympathomimetics, anticholinergics, and desmopressin has not proved consistently useful.

SSRIs and SNRIs cause sexual side effects (delayed or absent orgasm or ejaculation or reduced libido) in 30%–70% of users. Bupropion and mirtazapine are not associated with sexual dysfunction. Antidepressant-induced sexual dysfunction can be managed by switching to a less problematic agent or by as-needed use of the phosphodiesterase type 5 (PDE5) inhibitor sildenafil, which has been shown to be effective in controlled trials in men and women (Nurnberg et al. 2003, 2008). Other agents have been recommended but lack evidence of efficacy (Luft et al. 2021). Rarely, sexual dysfunction may persist after discontinuation of serotonergic antidepressants (Rothmore 2020). Antipsychotics, TCAs, and irreversible monoamine oxidase inhibitors (MAOIs) also can impair sexual function (see the subsection "Hyperprolactinemia" in Chapter 10).

Drug-Drug Interactions

Several pharmacodynamic and pharmacokinetic drug interactions frequently occur between drugs prescribed for renal and urological disorders and psychotropic drugs (Tables 5–5 and 5–6). See Chapter 1 for a discussion of pharmacokinetics, pharmacodynamics, and principles of drug-drug interactions.

Table 5–5.   Renal and urological medication–psychotropic medication interactions

Medication	Interaction mechanism	Effects on psychotropic medications and management
Diuretics		
All	Additive hypotensive effect	Increased risk of hypotensive effects with antipsychotics, TCAs, and MAOIs.
Thiazide diuretics	Blocked sodium and lithium reabsorption	Reduced lithium clearance leads to increased lithium levels and risk of toxicity. Monitor lithium levels.
	Additive hyponatremia	Potential for additive hyponatremic effects when combined with oxcarbazepine, carbamazepine, and, to a lesser degree, SSRIs, TCAs, and antipsychotics. Monitor electrolytes.
	Electrolyte abnormalities, hypokalemia, hypomagnesemia	Increased risk of cardiac arrhythmias with other QT-prolonging agents, including TCAs, typical antipsychotics, pimozide, risperidone, paliperidone, iloperidone, quetiapine, ziprasidone, and lithium.
Indapamide	QT prolongation	Increased risk of cardiac arrhythmias with other QT-prolonging agents, including TCAs, typical antipsychotics, pimozide, risperidone, paliperidone, iloperidone, quetiapine, ziprasidone, and lithium.
Loop diuretics	Electrolyte abnormalities, hypokalemia, hypomagnesemia	Increased risk of cardiac arrhythmias with other QT-prolonging agents, including TCAs, typical antipsychotics, pimozide, risperidone, paliperidone, iloperidone, quetiapine, ziprasidone, and lithium.
	Urine acidification	Increased excretion and reduced effect of amphetamine, amitriptyline, imipramine, meperidine, methadone, memantine, and flecainide.

Table 5–5. Renal and urological medication–psychotropic medication interactions *(continued)*

Medication	Interaction mechanism	Effects on psychotropic medications and management
Diuretics *(continued)*		
Carbonic anhydrase inhibitors	Urine alkalinization	Reduced excretion and prolonged effect of amphetamine, amitriptyline, imipramine, meperidine, methadone, memantine, and flecainide.
Eplerenone, osmotic diuretics, and spironolactone	Increased lithium clearance	Reduced lithium levels and possible loss of therapeutic effect. Monitor lithium levels. Amiloride has little effect on lithium levels.
Phosphate binders		
Calcium acetate, calcium carbonate, and lanthanum carbonate	Urine alkalinization	Reduced excretion and prolonged effect of amphetamine, amitriptyline, imipramine, meperidine, methadone, memantine, and flecainide.
Anticholinergic urinary antispasmodics		
Darifenacin, oxybutynin, solifenacin, tolterodine, and trospium	Additive anticholinergic effects	Increased peripheral and central anticholinergic adverse effects of TCAs and antipsychotics. Reduced therapeutic effects of cognitive enhancers. Avoid combination if possible. Darifenacin has less central effect and is preferred.
Phosphodiesterase type 5 inhibitors		
Sildenafil and tadalafil	Additive hypotensive effect	Increased risk of hypotensive effects with antipsychotics, TCAs, and MAOIs.

Table 5–5. Renal and urological medication–psychotropic medication interactions (*continued*)

Medication	Interaction mechanism	Effects on psychotropic medications and management
Phosphodiesterase type 5 inhibitors (*continued*)		
Vardenafil	Additive hypotensive effect QT prolongation	Increased risk of hypotensive effects with antipsychotics, TCAs, and MAOIs. Increased risk of cardiac arrhythmias with other QT-prolonging agents, including TCAs, typical antipsychotics, pimozide, risperidone, paliperidone, iloperidone, quetiapine, ziprasidone, and lithium.
α₁ Antagonists for benign prostatic hyperplasia		
All	Additive hypotensive effect	Increased risk of hypotensive effects with antipsychotics, TCAs, and MAOIs.
Alfuzosin	QT prolongation	Increased risk of cardiac arrhythmias with other QT-prolonging agents, including TCAs, typical antipsychotics, pimozide, risperidone, paliperidone, iloperidone, quetiapine, ziprasidone, and lithium.
Vasopressin antagonists		
Conivaptan	Inhibits cytochrome P450 3A4	Reduced metabolism of oxidatively metabolized benzodiazepines, buspirone, tasimelteon, lemborexant, pitolisant, carbamazepine, lumateperone, quetiapine, ziprasidone, and pimozide. Midazolam area under the concentration-time curve is increased two- to threefold. Adjust benzodiazepine dosage or consider oxazepam, lorazepam, or temazepam. Avoid combination with buspirone or pimozide. Monitor carbamazepine levels. Adjust antipsychotic dosage or switch to another agent.

Note. MAOIs = monoamine oxidase inhibitors; SSRIs = selective serotonin reuptake inhibitors; TCAs = tricyclic antidepressants.

Table 5–6. Psychotropic medication–renal and urological medication interactions

Medication	Interaction mechanism	Effects on renal and urological medications and management
Antidepressants		
Fluoxetine	Inhibits CYP3A4	Increased levels of the following: • Vasopressin antagonists: conivaptan, tolvaptan • α_1 Antagonists for BPH: alfuzosin, doxazosin, tamsulosin • 5α-Reductase inhibitors: dutasteride, finasteride • PDE5 inhibitors: sildenafil, tadalafil, vardenafil • Anticholinergic urinary antispasmodics: darifenacin, oxybutynin, solifenacin • Potassium-sparing diuretics: eplerenone Avoid concurrent use of CYP3A4 inhibitors.
	Inhibits CYP2D6	Increased levels of tamsulosin, possibly increasing hypotensive adverse effect. Caution with strong CYP3A4 or CYP2D6 inhibitors.
Nefazodone	Inhibits CYP3A4	Increased levels of the following: • Vasopressin antagonists: conivaptan, tolvaptan • α_1 Antagonists for BPH: alfuzosin, doxazosin, tamsulosin • 5α-Reductase inhibitors: dutasteride, finasteride • PDE5 inhibitors: sildenafil, tadalafil, vardenafil • Anticholinergic urinary antispasmodics: darifenacin, oxybutynin, solifenacin • Potassium-sparing diuretics: eplerenone Avoid concurrent use of CYP3A4 inhibitors.

Table 5–6. Psychotropic medication–renal and urological medication interactions *(continued)*

Medication	Interaction mechanism	Effects on renal and urological medications and management
Antidepressants *(continued)*		
Bupropion, duloxetine, moclobemide, and paroxetine	Inhibit CYP2D6	Increased levels of tamsulosin, possibly increasing hypotensive adverse effect. Paroxetine increased area under the concentration-time curve 1.6-fold. Caution with strong CYP3A4 or CYP2D6 inhibitors.
Tricyclic antidepressants	Additive hypotensive effects	Increased risk of severe hypotension with the following: • PDE5 inhibitors: sildenafil, tadalafil, vardenafil • α_1 Antagonists for BPH: alfuzosin, doxazosin, tamsulosin, terazosin
	QT prolongation	Increased risk of cardiac arrhythmias with other QT-prolonging agents, including alfuzosin, indapamide, and vardenafil.
Monoamine oxidase inhibitors	Additive hypotensive effects	Increased risk of severe hypotension with the following: • PDE5 inhibitors: sildenafil, tadalafil, vardenafil • α_1 Antagonists for BPH: alfuzosin, doxazosin, tamsulosin, terazosin
St. John's wort	Induces CYP3A4	Decreased conivaptan and tolvaptan levels. Avoid use of CYP3A4 inducers.
Antipsychotics		
Typical and atypical: pimozide, risperidone, paliperidone, iloperidone, quetiapine, and ziprasidone	QT prolongation	Increased risk of cardiac arrhythmias with other QT-prolonging agents, including alfuzosin, indapamide, and vardenafil.

Table 5–6. Psychotropic medication–renal and urological
medication interactions *(continued)*

Medication	Interaction mechanism	Effects on renal and urological medications and management
Antipsychotics *(continued)*		
Typical and atypical	Additive hypotensive effects	Increased risk of severe hypotension with the following: • PDE5 inhibitors: sildenafil, tadalafil, vardenafil • α_1 Antagonists for BPH: alfuzosin, doxazosin, tamsulosin, terazosin
Mood stabilizers		
Carbamazepine, oxcarbazepine, and phenytoin	Induce CYP3A4	Decreased conivaptan and tolvaptan levels. Avoid use of CYP3A4 inducers.
Lithium	QT prolongation	Increased risk of cardiac arrhythmias with other QT-prolonging agents, including alfuzosin, indapamide, and vardenafil.
Psychostimulants		
Armodafinil and modafinil	Induce CYP3A4	Decreased conivaptan and tolvaptan levels. Avoid use of CYP3A4 inducers.
Atomoxetine	Inhibits CYP2D6	Increased levels of tamsulosin, possibly increasing hypotensive adverse effect. Caution with strong CYP3A4 or CYP2D6 inhibitors.

Note. BPH = benign prostatic hyperplasia; CYP = cytochrome P450; PDE5 = phosphodiesterase type 5.

Pharmacodynamic Interactions

Several urological agents have effects on cardiac conduction (see Table 5–5). Thiazides and loop diuretics may cause conduction abnormalities through electrolyte disturbances, including hypokalemia and hypomagnesemia. Alfuzosin, indapamide, and vardenafil prolong the QT interval. These agents should be used with caution in the presence of psychotropic drugs with QT-prolonging effects, such as TCAs, antipsychotics, and lithium (Funk et al. 2018). The anticholinergic properties of urinary antispasmodics can interact in an additive manner to increase the anticholinergic adverse effects of TCAs and antipsychotics (dry mouth, dry eyes, urinary retention, constipation, decreased sweating, and cognitive impairment). Anticholinergic antispasmodics may impair cognitive function and decrease the cognitive benefits of cholinesterase inhibitors and memantine. The hypotensive adverse effects of α_1 antagonists (e.g., doxazosin) for benign prostatic hyperplasia and PDE5 inhibitors (sildenafil, vardenafil, and tadalafil) may exacerbate the hypotensive effects of psychotropic agents, including TCAs, antipsychotics, and MAOIs. Hyponatremic effects may be enhanced when thiazide diuretics are used in combination with oxcarbazepine and carbamazepine and, to a lesser degree, with SSRIs, TCAs, and antipsychotics.

Pharmacokinetic Interactions

Diuretics alter lithium excretion but not in a consistent direction. Thiazide diuretics reduce lithium excretion, giving rise to clinically significant increases in lithium levels. Acute administration of loop diuretics (furosemide, ethacrynic acid, bumetanide) increases lithium excretion, causing a decrease in lithium levels; with chronic use of loop diuretics, compensatory changes leave lithium levels somewhat unpredictable but not greatly changed. Carbonic anhydrase inhibitors (acetazolamide, dichlorphenamide, methazolamide) and osmotic diuretics (e.g., mannitol) reduce lithium levels. Potassium-sparing diuretics, including both epithelial sodium channel blockers (amiloride, triamterene) and aldosterone antagonists (spironolactone, eplerenone), may increase lithium excretion (Finley 2016). Furosemide and amiloride are considered to have the least effect on lithium excretion.

Metabolic drug interactions can change the levels of drugs used to treat renal and urological disorders, thereby increasing the drugs' toxicity or reducing their therapeutic effect. Many renal and urological agents are CYP3A4 substrates (see Table 5–6); coadministration of a CYP3A4 inhibitor (fluoxetine, nefazodone) may increase renal and urological drug bioavailability and blood levels and increase toxicity. Inhibition of CYP3A4 (and probably P-glycoprotein) has the potential to greatly increase oxybutynin's bioavailability (normally only 6%) and increase anticholinergic toxicity. CYP3A4 inhibitors increase alfuzosin and vardenafil blood levels and increase cardiac conduction toxicity (QT prolongation). Severe hypotensive effects have been reported with sildenafil in the presence of potent CYP3A4 inhibitors; PDE5 inhibitors (sildenafil, tadalafil, vardenafil) should not be combined with potent CYP3A4 inhibitors. Tamsulosin, a substrate for CYP3A4 and CYP2D6, may have increased toxicity when combined with CYP3A4 or CYP2D6 inhibitors (e.g., paroxetine). Conversely, the therapeutic effect of these CYP3A4 substrates may be lower in patients also receiving CYP3A4 inducers (e.g., carbamazepine). Coadministration of conivaptan, a potent CYP3A4 inhibitor as well as a substrate, increases the systemic exposure (area under the curve) of midazolam up to threefold (Cumberland Pharmaceuticals 2009). Similar effects would be expected with other oxidatively metabolized benzodiazepines, buspirone, carbamazepine, quetiapine, ziprasidone, and pimozide.

Changes in urine pH can modify the elimination of those compounds whose ratio of ionized to un-ionized forms is dramatically altered across the physiological range of urine pH (4.6–8.2) (i.e., the compound has a pK_a within this pH range). Un-ionized forms of drugs undergo greater glomerular resorption, whereas ionized drug forms have less resorption and greater urinary excretion. Thiazide and loop diuretics decrease urine pH and promote the excretion of amphetamines and possibly other basic drugs (e.g., amitriptyline, imipramine, methadone, and memantine). Conversely, carbonic anhydrase inhibitors and phosphate binders (calcium carbonate, calcium acetate, and lanthanum carbonate) alkalinize urine, which may reduce clearance and prolong the effect of these drugs.

Key Points

- Unless specific information is available for dosing of psychotropic drugs in renal failure, clinicians should start patients with two-thirds the dosage recommended for patients with normal renal function.

- Renal failure alters not only renal elimination of drugs but also hepatic metabolism. Clinicians should use therapeutic drug monitoring (methods selective for free drug) when possible in patients with renal disease.

- Lithium levels should be regularly monitored for patients receiving diuretic therapy. Furosemide and amiloride are considered to have the least effect on lithium excretion.

- Disease- and medication-induced electrolyte disturbances increase the risk of cardiac arrhythmias. Psychotropics should be chosen for their lack of QT-prolonging effects.

- Many renal and urological drugs are metabolized by cytochrome P450 (CYP) 3A4. Inhibitors of CYP3A4 should be avoided. This is especially relevant for alfuzosin and vardenafil, which prolong the QT interval.

- Amiloride is considered the treatment of choice for lithium-induced diabetes insipidus.

- Lorazepam and oxazepam are preferred benzodiazepines for patients with end-stage renal disease because of the absence of active metabolites. Because the half-lives of lorazepam and oxazepam may increase up to fourfold, smaller than usual dosages are needed.

- Of the common anticholinergic urinary antispasmodics, oxybutynin has the most anticholinergic adverse effects on the CNS.

References

Ancelin ML, Artero S, Portet F, et al: Non-degenerative mild cognitive impairment in elderly people and use of anticholinergic drugs: longitudinal cohort study. BMJ 332(7539):455–459, 2006 16452102

Anders MW: Metabolism of drugs by the kidney. Kidney Int 18(5):636–647, 1980 7463957

Atsariyasing W, Goldman MB: A systematic review of the ability of urine concentration to distinguish antipsychotic- from psychosis-induced hyponatremia. Psychiatry Res 217(3):129–133, 2014 24726819

Aurora RN, Kristo DA, Bista SR, et al: The treatment of restless legs syndrome and periodic limb movement disorder in adults—an update for 2012: practice parameters with an evidence-based systematic review and meta-analyses: an American Academy of Sleep Medicine Clinical Practice Guideline. Sleep 35(8):1039–1062, 2012 22851801

Baghdady NT, Banik S, Swartz SA, et al: Psychotropic drugs and renal failure: translating the evidence for clinical practice. Adv Ther 26(4):404–424, 2009 19444657

Bassilios N, Launay-Vacher V, Khoury N, et al: Gabapentin neurotoxicity in a chronic haemodialysis patient. Nephrol Dial Transplant 16(10):2112–2113, 2001 11572915

Bautovich A, Katz I, Smith M, et al: Depression and chronic kidney disease: a review for clinicians. Aust N Z J Psychiatry 48(6):530–541, 2014 24658294

Bhardwaj SB, Motiwala FB, Morais M, et al: Vaptans for hyponatremia induced by psychogenic polydipsia. Prim Care Companion CNS Disord 15(1):PCC.12l01444, 2013 23724348

Bliwise DL, Zhang RH, Kutner NG: Medications associated with restless legs syndrome: a case-control study in the US Renal Data System (USRDS). Sleep Med 15(10):1241–1245, 2014 25156752

Bockenhauer D, Bichet DG: Pathophysiology, diagnosis and management of nephrogenic diabetes insipidus. Nat Rev Nephrol 11(10):576–588, 2015 26077742

Chancellor M, Boone T: Anticholinergics for overactive bladder therapy: central nervous system effects. CNS Neurosci Ther 18(2):167–174, 2012 22070184

Cohen LM, Tessier EG, Germain MJ, et al: Update on psychotropic medication use in renal disease. Psychosomatics 45(1):34–48, 2004 14709759

Crone CC, Gabriel GM, DiMartini A: An overview of psychiatric issues in liver disease for the consultation-liaison psychiatrist. Psychosomatics 47(3):188–205, 2006 16684936

Cukor D, Coplan J, Brown C, et al: Depression and anxiety in urban hemodialysis patients. Clin J Am Soc Nephrol 2(3):484–490, 2007 17699455

Cukor D, Coplan J, Brown C, et al: Anxiety disorders in adults treated by hemodialysis: a single-center study. Am J Kidney Dis 52(1):128–136, 2008a 18440682

Cukor D, Coplan J, Brown C, et al: Course of depression and anxiety diagnosis in patients treated with hemodialysis: a 16-month follow-up. Clin J Am Soc Nephrol 3(6):1752–1758, 2008b 18684897

Cumberland Pharmaceuticals: Vaprisol (conivaptan). Cumberland Pharmaceuticals, 2009. Available at: www.vaprisol.com. Accessed April 12, 2016.

de Leon J, Tracy J, McCann E, et al: Polydipsia and schizophrenia in a psychiatric hospital: a replication study. Schizophr Res 57(2–3):293–301, 2002 12223261

De Picker L, Van Den Eede F, Dumont G, et al: Antidepressants and the risk of hyponatremia: a class-by-class review of literature. Psychosomatics 55(6):536–547, 2014 25262043

Dev V, Dixon SN, Fleet JL, et al: Higher anti-depressant dose and major adverse outcomes in moderate chronic kidney disease: a retrospective population-based study. BMC Nephrol 15:79, 2014 24884589

Doornebal J, Diepenbroek A, van de Luijtgaarden MWM, et al: Renal concentrating ability and glomerular filtration rate in lithium-treated patients. Neth J Med 77(4):139–149, 2019 31502545

Drew DA, Weiner DE, Sarnak MJ: Cognitive impairment in CKD: pathophysiology, management, and prevention. Am J Kidney Dis 74(6):782–790, 2019 31378643

Dundas B, Harris M, Narasimhan M: Psychogenic polydipsia review: etiology, differential, and treatment. Curr Psychiatry Rep 9(3):236–241, 2007 17521521

Elias MF, Elias PK, Seliger SL, et al: Chronic kidney disease, creatinine and cognitive functioning. Nephrol Dial Transplant 24(8):2446–2452, 2009 19297357

Finley PR: Drug interactions with lithium: an update. Clin Pharmacokinet 55(8):925–941, 2016 26936045

Friedli K, Guirguis A, Almond M, et al: Sertraline versus placebo in patients with major depressive disorder undergoing hemodialysis: a randomized, controlled feasibility trial. Clin J Am Soc Nephrol 12(2):280–286, 2017 28126706

Fukuhara S, Green J, Albert J, et al: Symptoms of depression, prescription of benzodiazepines, and the risk of death in hemodialysis patients in Japan. Kidney Int 70(10):1866–1872, 2006 17021611

Funk MC, Beach SR, Bostwick JR, et al: APA Resource Document: Resource document on QTc prolongation and psychotropic medications. 2018. Available at: http://www.psychiatry.org/File%20Library/Psychiatrists/Directories/Library-and-Archive/resource_documents/Resource-Document-2018-QTc-Prolongation-and-Psychotropic-Med.pdf. Accessed September 19, 2022.

Gheorghiade M, Niazi I, Ouyang J, et al: Vasopressin V2-receptor blockade with tolvaptan in patients with chronic heart failure: results from a double-blind, randomized trial. Circulation 107(21):2690–2696, 2003 12742979

Giannaki CD, Hadjigeorgiou GM, Karatzaferi C, et al: Epidemiology, impact, and treatment options of restless legs syndrome in end-stage renal disease patients: an evidence-based review. Kidney Int 85(6):1275–1282, 2014 24107848

Gillman PK: Tricyclic antidepressant pharmacology and therapeutic drug interactions updated. Br J Pharmacol 151(6):737–748, 2007 17471183

Gray SL, Anderson ML, Dublin S, et al: Cumulative use of strong anticholinergics and incident dementia: a prospective cohort study. JAMA Intern Med 175(3):401–407, 2015 25621434

Greendyke RM, Bernhardt AJ, Tasbas HE, et al: Polydipsia in chronic psychiatric patients: therapeutic trials of clonidine and enalapril. Neuropsychopharmacology 18(4):272–281, 1998 9509495

Havens TH, Innamorato G, Nemec EC 2nd: Non-antipsychotic pharmacotherapy of psychogenic polydipsia: a systematic review. J Psychosom Res 152:110674, 2021 34856427

Hedayati SS, Gregg LP, Carmody T, et al: Effect of sertraline on depressive symptoms in patients with chronic kidney disease without dialysis dependence: the CAST randomized clinical trial. JAMA 318(19):1876–1890, 2017 29101402

Hoekstra R, Lekkerkerker MN, Kuijper TM, et al: Renal function after withdrawal of lithium. Bipolar Disord January 25, 2022 35075735 Epub ahead of print

Højlund M, Lund LC, Herping JLE, et al: Second-generation antipsychotics and the risk of chronic kidney disease: a population-based case-control study. BMJ Open 10(8):e038247, 2020 32784262

Horinek EL, Kiser TH, Fish DN, et al: Propylene glycol accumulation in critically ill patients receiving continuous intravenous lorazepam infusions. Ann Pharmacother 43(12):1964–1971, 2009 19920159

Ishida JH, McCulloch CE, Steinman MA, et al: Gabapentin and pregabalin use and association with adverse outcomes among hemodialysis patients. J Am Soc Nephrol 29(7):1970–1978, 2018 29871945

Israni RK, Kasbekar N, Haynes K, et al: Use of antiepileptic drugs in patients with kidney disease. Semin Dial 19(5):408–416, 2006 16970741

Jacobson S: Psychopharmacology: prescribing for patients with hepatic or renal dysfunction. Psychiatric Times, November 2002, pp 65–70

Jiang Y, McCombs JS, Park SH: A retrospective cohort study of acute kidney injury risk associated with antipsychotics. CNS Drugs 31(4):319–326, 2017 28290080

Kauffman KM, Dolata J, Figueroa M, et al: Higher dose weekly fluoxetine in hemodialysis patients: a case series report. Int J Psychiatry Med 56(1):3–13, 2021 32216496

Kavanagh C, Uy NS: Nephrogenic diabetes insipidus. Pediatr Clin North Am 66(1):227–234, 2019 30454745

Kerdraon J, Robain G, Jeandel C, et al: Impact on cognitive function of anticholinergic drugs used for the treatment of overactive bladder in the elderly [in French]. Prog Urol 24(11):672–681, 2014 25214448

Kessing LV, Gerds TA, Feldt-Rasmussen B, et al: Use of lithium and anticonvulsants and the rate of chronic kidney disease: a nationwide population-based study. JAMA Psychiatry 72(12):1182–1191, 2015 26535805

Kessing LV, Feldt-Rasmussen B, Andersen PK, et al: Continuation of lithium after a diagnosis of chronic kidney disease. Acta Psychiatr Scand 136(6):615–622, 2017 29049864

Kimmel PL, Cukor D, Cohen SD, et al: Depression in end-stage renal disease patients: a critical review. Adv Chronic Kidney Dis 14(4):328–334, 2007 17904499

Lacerda G, Krummel T, Sabourdy C, et al: Optimizing therapy of seizures in patients with renal or hepatic dysfunction. Neurology 67(12 Suppl 4):S28–S33, 2006 17190918

Letmaier M, Painold A, Holl AK, et al: Hyponatraemia during psychopharmacological treatment: results of a drug surveillance programme. Int J Neuropsychopharmacol 15(6):739–748, 2012 21777511

Levy NB: Psychopharmacology in patients with renal failure. Int J Psychiatry Med 20(4):325–334, 1990 2086520

Liamis G, Milionis H, Elisaf M: A review of drug-induced hyponatremia. Am J Kidney Dis 52(1):144–153, 2008 25214448

Losso RL, Minhoto GR, Riella MC: Sleep disorders in patients with end-stage renal disease undergoing dialysis: comparison between hemodialysis, continuous ambulatory peritoneal dialysis and automated peritoneal dialysis. Int Urol Nephrol 47(2):369–375, 2015 25358390

Luft MJ, Dobson ET, Levine A, et al: Pharmacologic interventions for antidepressant-induced sexual dysfunction: a systematic review and network meta-analysis of trials using the Arizona Sexual Experience Scale. CNS Spectr April 12, 2021 33843553 Epub ahead of print

Łukawska E, Frankiewicz D, Izak M, et al: Lithium toxicity and the kidney with special focus on nephrotic syndrome associated with the acute kidney injury: a case-based systematic analysis. J Appl Toxicol 41(12):1896–1909, 2021 33798272

MedlinePlus: Lamotrigine. 2015. U.S. National Library of Medicine. Available at: https://medlineplus.gov/druginfo/meds/a695007.html. Accessed July 6, 2016.

Molnar MZ, Novak M, Mucsi I: Management of restless legs syndrome in patients on dialysis. Drugs 66(5):607–624, 2006 16620140

Murray AM: Cognitive impairment in the aging dialysis and chronic kidney disease populations: an occult burden. Adv Chronic Kidney Dis 15(2):123–132, 2008 18334236

Murtagh FE, Addington-Hall J, Higginson IJ: The prevalence of symptoms in end-stage renal disease: a systematic review. Adv Chronic Kidney Dis 14(1):82–99, 2007 17200048

Muzaale AD, Daubresse M, Bae S, et al: Benzodiazepines, codispensed opioids, and mortality among patients initiating long-term in-center hemodialysis. Clin J Am Soc Nephrol 15(6):794–804, 2020 32457228

Nielsen RE, Kessing LV, Nolen WA, et al: Lithium and renal impairment: a review on a still hot topic. Pharmacopsychiatry 51(5):200–205, 2018 29346806

Novak M, Shapiro CM, Mendelssohn D, et al: Diagnosis and management of insomnia in dialysis patients. Semin Dial 19(1):25–31, 2006 16423179

Nurnberg HG, Hensley PL, Gelenberg AJ, et al: Treatment of antidepressant-associated sexual dysfunction with sildenafil: a randomized controlled trial. JAMA 289(1):56–64, 2003 12503977

Nurnberg HG, Hensley PL, Heiman JR, et al: Sildenafil treatment of women with antidepressant-associated sexual dysfunction: a randomized controlled trial. JAMA 300(4):395–404, 2008 18647982

Pahwa M, Joseph B, Nunez NA, et al: Long-term lithium therapy and risk of chronic kidney disease in bipolar disorder: a historical cohort study. Bipolar Disord 23(7):715–723, 2021 33548063

Palmer S, Vecchio M, Craig JC, et al: Prevalence of depression in chronic kidney disease: systematic review and meta-analysis of observational studies. Kidney Int 84(1):179–191, 2013 23486521

Palmer SC, Natale P, Ruospo M, et al: Antidepressants for treating depression in adults with end-stage kidney disease treated with dialysis. Cochrane Database Syst Rev (5):CD004541, 2016 27210414

Pena-Polanco JE, Mor MK, Tohme FA, et al: Acceptance of antidepressant treatment by patients on hemodialysis and their renal providers. Clin J Am Soc Nephrol 12(2):298–303, 2017 28126707

Periclou A, Ventura D, Rao N, et al: Pharmacokinetic study of memantine in healthy and renally impaired subjects. Clin Pharmacol Ther 79(1):134–143, 2006 16413248

Pichette V, Leblond FA: Drug metabolism in chronic renal failure. Curr Drug Metab 4(2):91–103, 2003 12678690

Pinkhasov A, Xiong G, Bourgeois JA, et al: Management of SIADH-related hyponatremia due to psychotropic medications: an expert consensus from the Association of Medicine and Psychiatry. J Psychosom Res 151:110654, 2021 34739943

Rej S, Herrmann N, Gruneir A, et al: Association of lithium use and a higher serum concentration of lithium with the risk of declining renal function in older adults: a population-based cohort study. J Clin Psychiatry 81(5):19m13045, 2020 32841553

Rothmore J: Antidepressant-induced sexual dysfunction. Med J Aust 212(7):329–334, 2020 32172535

Ryan PB, Schuemie MJ, Ramcharran D, et al: Atypical antipsychotics and the risks of acute kidney injury and related outcomes among older adults: a replication analysis and an evaluation of adapted confounding control strategies. Drugs Aging 34(3):211–219, 2017 28124262

Schoot TS, Molmans THJ, Grootens KP, et al: Systematic review and practical guideline for the prevention and management of the renal side effects of lithium therapy. Eur Neuropsychopharmacol 31:16–32, 2020 31837914

Schoretsanitis G, de Filippis R, Brady BM, et al: Prevalence of impaired kidney function in patients with long-term lithium treatment: a systematic review and meta-analysis. Bipolar Disord 24(3):264–274, 2022 34783413

Siegel AJ: Hyponatremia in psychiatric patients: update on evaluation and management. Harv Rev Psychiatry 16(1):13–24, 2008 18306096

Sinha P, Gupta A, Reddi VS, et al: An exploratory study for bladder dysfunction in atypical antipsychotic-emergent urinary incontinence. Indian J Psychiatry 58(4):438–442, 2016 28197002

Sutar R, Atlani MK, Chaudhary P: Antipsychotics and hemodialysis: a systematic review. Asian J Psychiatr 55:102484, 2021 33341539

Tagay S, Kribben A, Hohenstein A, et al: Posttraumatic stress disorder in hemodialysis patients. Am J Kidney Dis 50(4):594–601, 2007 17900459

Takagi S, Watanabe Y, Imaoka T, et al: Treatment of psychogenic polydipsia with acetazolamide: a report of 5 cases. Clin Neuropharmacol 34(1):5–7, 2011 21242740

Trinchieri M, Perletti G, Magri V, et al: Urinary side effects of psychotropic drugs: a systematic review and metanalysis. Neurourol Urodyn 40(6):1333–1348, 2021 34004020

Van Alphen AM, Bosch TM, Kupka RW, et al: Chronic kidney disease in lithium-treated patients, incidence and rate of decline. Int J Bipolar Disord 9(1):1, 2021 33392830

van Noord C, Straus SM, Sturkenboom MC, et al: Psychotropic drugs associated with corrected QT interval prolongation. J Clin Psychopharmacol 29(1):9–15, 2009 19142100

Verghese C, de Leon J, Josiassen RC: Problems and progress in the diagnosis and treatment of polydipsia and hyponatremia. Schizophr Bull 22(3):455–464, 1996 8873296

Wang HY, Huang CL, Feng IJ, et al: Second-generation antipsychotic medications and risk of chronic kidney disease in schizophrenia: population-based nested case-control study. BMJ Open 8(5):e019868, 2018 29794090

Ward ME, Musa MN, Bailey L: Clinical pharmacokinetics of lithium. J Clin Pharmacol 34(4):280–285, 1994 8006194

Winkelmayer WC, Mehta J, Wang PS: Benzodiazepine use and mortality of incident dialysis patients in the United States. Kidney Int 72(11):1388–1393, 2007 17851463

Yang HH, Hsiao YP, Shih HC, et al: Acyclovir-induced neuropsychosis successfully recovered after immediate hemodialysis in an end-stage renal disease patient. Int J Dermatol 46(8):883–884, 2007 17651180

6

Cardiovascular Disorders

Andrew Drysdale, M.D., Ph.D.

Alba Lara, M.D.

Peter A. Shapiro, M.D.

Comorbidity of psychiatric disorders and heart disease is extremely common. Psychopharmacological treatment for psychiatric disorders in patients with cardiovascular disease has been an important topic of active investigation from the beginning of the modern era of psychopharmacology, when psychoactive agents such as chlorpromazine, tricyclic antidepressants (TCAs), and lithium were noted to have significant cardiovascular effects. In addition, many psychiatric disorders are associated with higher cardiovascular morbidity and mortality in patients with existing heart disease, spurring even greater interest in the effects of psychopharmacological treatment in patients with cardiac disease.

Dr. Drysdale and Dr. Lara contributed equally to authorship of this chapter.

The most common psychiatric problems in patients with heart disease are depressive disorders and anxiety disorders. PTSD is increasingly recognized as both a risk factor for incident coronary disease and a complication of cardiac events that in turn increases the risk of recurrent events (De Hert et al. 2018). Patients who undergo long-term treatment with antipsychotic medications are at risk for heart disease due to metabolic side effects. Tobacco use disorder, substance use disorders, and sexual dysfunction also may be problems that warrant intervention.

Most clinical trials in psychopharmacology exclude patients with significant medical comorbidity, so contemporary psychopharmacotherapy practice for patients with cardiovascular disease is based on limited clinical trial data from this population, inferences from studies of patients without heart disease, and clinical lore. Additional specific evidence about treatment in patients with heart disease is needed. Nevertheless, some general guidelines apply.

Differential Diagnostic Considerations

In general, differential diagnosis of psychiatric problems in patients with cardiac disease begins with phenomenological characterization of the psychopathology. Next, one must evaluate whether the condition is secondary to a general medical condition or substance (including medications used to treat the medical condition) or is a primary psychiatric problem. Finally, comorbidity will help define treatment plans.

Some common errors involve misattribution of symptoms to a primary psychiatric diagnosis rather than to the cardiac problem. For example, patients with paroxysmal supraventricular tachycardia may appear to be anxious or to be having panic attacks. Patients with unrecognized congestive heart failure, pulmonary congestion, and nocturnal dyspnea may complain of insomnia and receive a diagnosis of depression or panic attacks. These patients will respond better to effective heart failure management than to psychotropics.

The workup of psychiatric symptoms in patients with cardiac disease should include a review of relevant organ systems and laboratory findings: assessment of cardiac rhythm; blood pressure; fluid and electrolyte status; glycemic control; blood gases; blood count; and hepatic, renal, and thyroid function. Hypotension and arrhythmias may reduce cerebral blood flow and perfusion of other vital organs, resulting in neurocognitive syndromes. Severe hyponatremia and anemia may lead to a variety of psychiatric symptoms. Hepatic and renal dysfunction often cause mood or cognitive disturbances. Hypothyroidism, which may occur as a complication of amiodarone therapy, causes mood and cognitive problems. The presence of infections and the role of medications and substance use or withdrawal symptoms should be considered. The history, examination, and neuroimaging studies may suggest the presence of CNS disease, including cerebrovascular disease and primary degenerative brain disorders (e.g., Alzheimer's disease, Parkinson's disease). The prevalence of small vessel ischemic cerebrovascular disease is high in patients with ischemic heart disease, even in patients without a known history of transient ischemic attack or stroke (Lazar et al. 2001). Electroencephalograms are often useful to distinguish encephalopathies (hypoactive delirium, dementia, recurring seizures, and interictal states) from depression with apathy, psychomotor retardation, or cognitive impairment.

Neuropsychiatric Side Effects of Cardiovascular Medications

Neuropsychiatric effects of cardiovascular medications should be considered in the differential diagnosis (Table 6–1). Noting the bidirectional relationship of heart disease with anxiety and mood disorders, evidence from animal models and clinical studies suggests that many cardiovascular medications have beneficial effects on anxiety and related symptoms (Repova et al. 2022), but one must also be aware of potential psychiatric adverse effects (Huffman and Stern 2007). α-Adrenergic-blocking agents may cause depression and sexual dysfunction. Fatigue and sexual dysfunction are uncommon dose-related adverse effects of β-blockers and may be mistaken for a depressive syndrome, but β-blocker treatment is not associated with an increased incidence of depressive illness (Ko et al. 2002; van Melle et al. 2006).

Digoxin may produce visual hallucinations, often of colored rings around objects (phosphenes). Some antiarrhythmic agents (especially lidocaine) cause confusion, hallucinations, or delirium. Angiotensin converting enzyme (ACE) inhibitors are occasionally associated with mood elevation or depression. Amiodarone treatment often leads to hypothyroidism, which may result in cognitive dulling or depression symptoms. Hypokalemia and hyponatremia from diuretic therapy may result in anorexia, weakness, and apathy; thiazide diuret-

Table 6–1.   Selected adverse neuropsychiatric effects of cardiovascular medications

Cardiovascular medication	Neuropsychiatric effects
α-Adrenergic blockers	Depression, sexual dysfunction
Amiodarone	Mood disorders secondary to thyroid effects
Angiotensin converting enzyme inhibitors	Mood elevation or depression (rare)
Antiarrhythmic agents	Hallucinations, confusion, delirium
β-Adrenergic blockers	Fatigue, sexual dysfunction
Digoxin	Visual hallucinations (phosphenes), delirium, depression
Diuretics	Anorexia, weakness, apathy secondary to electrolyte disturbances
Ivabradine	Phosphenes
Proprotein convertase subtilisin/kexin type 9 inhibitors	Confusion, depression, insomnia

ics sometimes cause erectile dysfunction. For more extensive discussion, see the reviews by Brown and Stoudemire (1998) and Keller and Frishman (2003).

Among newer agents for treatment of heart failure, sacubitril/valsartan and sodium/glucose transporter type 2 inhibitors such as empagliflozin have little neuropsychiatric effect, whereas ivabradine may cause phosphenes (Tomasoni et al. 2019). In a large uncontrolled observational study, beneficial psychiatric effects of adding sacubitril/valsartan to the heart failure regimen were found for patients with heart failure with reduced ejection fraction but not for patients with heart failure with preserved ejection fraction. In the reduced ejection fraction group, sacubitril/valsartan treatment was associated with subsequent reduction in mean Hamilton Depression Rating Scale and Hospital Anxiety and Depression Scale anxiety scores and in the proportion of patients with elevated depression and anxiety symptoms (Malik et al. 2021).

Many cardiac patients need lipid-lowering therapy. Statins (3-hydroxy-3-methylglutaryl–coenzyme A reductase inhibitors) are well tolerated, although several studies have suggested a possible risk of neuropsychiatric adverse effects, including depression and insomnia (Alghamdi et al. 2018). A new class of lipid-lowering agents, proprotein convertase subtilisin/kexin type 9 inhibitors, was approved by the U.S. FDA in 2015 for patients with clinical atherosclerotic cardiovascular disease on maximally tolerated statin therapy. Given recent safety data from the EudraVigilance database reporting increased rates of dizziness, depression, insomnia, and confusion with the use of proprotein convertase subtilisin/kexin type 9 inhibitors, more information is needed to make clinical recommendations regarding their neuropsychiatric adverse effects (di Mauro et al. 2021).

Pharmacokinetic Alterations in Heart Disease

For most patients, heart disease per se does not result in alterations in drug absorption, distribution, metabolism, and elimination, but there are some important exceptions (Table 6–2): severe right-sided heart failure with secondary hepatic congestion, ascites, or marked peripheral edema; severe left-sided heart failure with low cardiac output; and the effects of diuretics.

Right-sided congestive heart failure may result in elevated central venous pressure and impaired venous drainage from the hepatic venous system and the gut wall. Resulting gut wall edema may reduce drug absorption. Mild to moderate hepatic congestion has a limited effect on drug metabolism, but cirrhosis secondary to hepatic congestion leads to reduced serum albumin level, relatively increased α_1-acid glycoprotein level, and ascites, which may alter drug distribution and serum levels of free drug. Because the effects of diminished absorption and variable changes in drug distribution may be additive or offsetting, it is difficult to predict net effects. In general, as serum total protein and albumin levels decline with more advanced disease, the prudent action is to use smaller than usual dosages of psychotropic agents and increase dosages cautiously. When the ratio of protein-bound to free drug decreases, the plasma drug level is reduced, even though the amount of free drug, which is the amount that determines drug activity, remains the same. Therapeutic drug monitoring that measures only the total drug level would result in a lower level and may mislead the physician to increase drug dosage.

Left-sided heart failure results in reduced cardiac output and reduced blood flow through the hepatic and renal arteries. Decreased hepatic artery blood flow results in reduced drug metabolism, particularly Phase I pro-

Table 6–2.   Pharmacokinetic changes in heart disease

Condition	Physiological consequences	Pharmacokinetic effects	Significance
Drug absorption			
Right-sided heart failure	Hepatic congestion, gut wall edema	Decreased absorption	Uncertain
Drug distribution			
"Cardiac cirrhosis"	Reduced albumin, ascites, increased α_1-acid glycoprotein	Increased or decreased free drug levels	Uncertain
Drug metabolism			
Left-sided heart failure	Decreased hepatic artery blood flow, decreased Phase I hepatic metabolism	Reduced elimination of parent drug	Important for drugs with low therapeutic index and high hepatic extraction
Drug elimination			
Left-sided heart failure	Decreased renal artery blood flow, decreased glomerular filtration rate	Reduced elimination of water-soluble molecules	Increased blood levels of lithium, gabapentin, paliperidone. Increased risk of toxicity.

cesses—that is, oxidation (e.g., cytochrome P450 [CYP]) and reduction reactions. Conjugation reactions (Phase II metabolism) that make drug metabolites water soluble and subject to excretion through the kidneys are relatively spared. Because most psychotropic agents undergo hepatic Phase I metabolism, they tend to accumulate. Even agents that rely on Phase II metabolism (e.g., lorazepam, oxazepam, temazepam) tend to accumulate, but less than agents metabolized by Phase I processes (e.g., diazepam, amitriptyline). Again, as cardiac output falls, dosage reduction of most psychotropic agents may be necessary. Severe left-sided heart failure results in renal dysfunction due to hypotension and reduced renal artery blood flow. Thus, management of combined left- and right-sided heart failure, with combinations of β-blockers, ACE inhibitors, or angiotensin II receptor blockers and diuretics, is often limited by progressive renal dysfunction, necessitating inotropic support. Lithium is the most important psychotropic agent eliminated primarily by renal excretion—gabapentin, pregabalin, paliperidone, and memantine are others—and excretion of lithium and these other drugs declines along with creatinine clearance.

Lithium dosing should be closely monitored or withheld entirely for patients with congestive heart failure whose fluid and electrolyte status is unstable. Use of hepatically metabolized mood stabilizers (e.g., valproate) may be preferred for these patients.

Psychotropic Medication Use in Heart Disease

Mackin (2008) and Mladěnka et al. (2018) provide comprehensive discussions of cardiac side effects of psychotropic drugs. Some important effects are summarized in Table 6–3.

Anxiolytics and Sedative-Hypnotics

Relevant Treatment Literature

Although anxiety symptoms are common in patients with heart disease, studies are lacking of benzodiazepine and buspirone efficacy in the treatment of anxiety for patients with heart disease.

Prescribing Principles

Benzodiazepines, compared with buspirone, have the advantage of rapid onset of effect. Lorazepam, oxazepam, and temazepam may be the safest benzodiazepines to prescribe for patients with heart disease because these drugs do not undergo Phase I hepatic metabolism and are therefore relatively unaffected by altered metabolism in heart failure. Longer-acting agents and agents with active metabolites that extend their elimination half-life and duration of action—clonazepam, clorazepate, diazepam, chlordiazepoxide, flurazepam, halazepam, and quazepam—should be used cautiously and at low dosages because they may accumulate to a higher than expected steady-state level because of slowed elimination. Cognitive dysfunction or delirium can result

Table 6–3.   Cardiovascular adverse effects of psychotropic
medications

Medication	Cardiovascular effects
Antipsychotics	Hypotension, orthostatic hypotension, cardiac conduction disturbances, ventricular tachycardia or fibrillation, metabolic syndrome
Antidepressants	
Bupropion	Hypertension
Monoamine oxidase inhibitors	Orthostatic hypotension
Selective serotonin reuptake inhibitors	Reduced heart rate, occasional clinically significant sinus bradycardia or sinus arrest; QT prolongation, especially with citalopram
Serotonin-norepinephrine reuptake inhibitors	Hypertension, tachycardia
Tricyclic antidepressants	Hypotension, orthostatic hypotension, type 1A antiarrhythmic effects: slowed conduction through atrioventricular node and His bundle, heart block, QT prolongation, ventricular fibrillation
Trazodone	Orthostatic hypotension
Ketamine	Hypotension, hypertension, bradycardia, tachycardia, arrhythmias
Stimulants	Hypertension, tachycardia, tachyarrhythmias
Mood stabilizers	
Carbamazepine	Type 1A antiarrhythmic effects; atrioventricular block
Lithium	Sinus node dysfunction
Phosphodiesterase type 5 inhibitors	Hypotension, myocardial ischemia

when the CNS depressant effect of benzodiazepines is superimposed on a brain already compromised by microvascular disease, which may co-occur with atherosclerotic cardiovascular disease. After cardiac surgery, benzodiazepine or zolpidem use is associated with risk of developing delirium (Mangusan et al. 2015). Outpatients with heart failure have a higher risk of rehospitalization when taking benzodiazepines (vs. zolpidem, zopiclone, or zaleplon) for insomnia (Sato et al. 2020). Benzodiazepine use during acute coronary events may increase the risk of developing PTSD symptoms (von Känel et al. 2021).

Desirable Secondary Effects

Benzodiazepines have no significant effects of their own on heart rate and blood pressure, but reduction in acute anxiety can lead to reduction in anxiety-associated tachycardia, myocardial irritability, and myocardial work (Huffman and Stern 2003). Buspirone has no cardiovascular effects.

Antidepressants

Relevant Treatment Literature

Many studies have examined treatment of depression in patients with heart disease. Initial investigations of TCAs demonstrated their efficacy. However, TCAs also have a significant cardiovascular side-effect profile that is particularly pronounced in patients with heart disease: increased heart rate, orthostatic hypotension, and cardiac conduction disturbances. First-, second-, or third-degree heart block may develop, and a pacemaker may be necessary to avoid syncope, particularly for patients with an increased PR interval at baseline. TCAs have type 1A antiarrhythmic effects, similar to those of quinidine, and overdose may cause lethal ventricular arrhythmias. TCAs are associated with increased risk of myocardial infarction (MI) and mortality in patients with ischemic heart disease. Despite this risk profile, TCAs remain an option for patients who have not responded to other antidepressant trials. A series of studies on depressed patients with impaired left ventricular function suggested that nortriptyline, titrated to a blood level between 50 and 150 ng/mL, is well tolerated in patients with impaired left ventricular function (Roose and Glassman 1989).

Selective serotonin reuptake inhibitors (SSRIs) have limited cardiovascular side effects. SSRIs may reduce heart rate but generally by no more than 3 beats/min. Clinically significant sinus bradycardia and syncope occur rarely (Glassman et al. 1998). Citalopram and to a lesser degree escitalopram increase the QT interval more than other SSRIs. In a large retrospective cross-sectional study, citalopram resulted in significant dose-related QT prolongation, but other antidepressants did not (for bupropion, dosage was inversely associated with QT interval) (Castro et al. 2013). Analysis of the World Health Organization adverse drug event database, VigiBase, identified increased reporting of QT prolongation with citalopram and escitalopram but not with any other SSRIs (Ojero-Senard et al. 2017). However, epidemiological studies found no or very low extra risk of sudden cardiac death associated with citalopram use even at high dosages (Tampi et al. 2015; Zivin et al. 2013). In a cohort study of older adults starting an antidepressant, ventricular arrhythmias occurred in the first 90 days of treatment in 0.06% of patients taking citalopram compared with 0.04% of patients taking paroxetine or sertraline, yielding a number needed to harm of 5,000 (Qirjazi et al. 2016).

Randomized placebo-controlled trials of SSRIs for treatment of depression in patients with coronary heart disease, acute coronary syndrome (ACS), or heart failure have provided substantial evidence for safety and some evidence for efficacy of SSRI treatment. In the Canadian Cardiac Randomized Evaluation of Antidepressant and Psychotherapy Efficacy trial, citalopram, 20–40 mg/day, was more effective than placebo for treatment of depression in patients with stable coronary disease (Lespérance et al. 2007). In the Sertraline Antidepressant Heart Attack Randomized Trial (SADHART), sertraline treatment, 50–200 mg/day, for depression following an ACS was effective for patients with severe and prior or recurrent depression but not more effective than placebo for patients with first onset of depression following the cardiac event (Glassman et al. 2002, 2006; Shapiro et al. 1999). In the Escitalopram for Depression in Acute Coronary Syndrome (EsDEPACS) trial, escitalopram, 5–20 mg/day, was more effective than placebo with respect to both depression symptoms and several measures of functional status (Kim et al. 2015).

Prophylactic SSRI treatment after ACS was found to reduce incident depression over 12-month follow-up in one study (Hansen et al. 2012), but systematic review does not support prophylactic treatment (Christiansen et al. 2017).

Several studies have examined the effect of SSRI treatment of depression in patients with coronary disease on cardiovascular and all-cause morbidity and mortality, with inconclusive results. In SADHART, sertraline treatment was associated with a trend toward reduction of cardiovascular adverse events and mortality, but the number of subjects and the number of events were small, and the effect was not significant. In a post hoc exploration of non-randomized, open-label SSRI treatment adjunctive to psychotherapy for depression after MI, SSRI treatment was associated with a substantial reduction in recurrent cardiovascular events and deaths (Taylor et al. 2005). In the EsDEPACS study and the follow-up DEPACS study, Kim et al. (2021) found a significant beneficial effect of escitalopram treatment on long-term (mean 8.7-year follow-up) rates of recurrent cardiac events.

In summary, most available clinical trials support the benefit of SSRI treatment for depression in stable coronary artery disease and after ACS. However, in ACS the data are mixed on whether the benefits are limited to those with preexisting depression or include those who develop depression after their cardiac event. Finally, controlled clinical studies show little evidence of short-term benefit of SSRI treatment on cardiac outcomes but may support longer-term medical benefit in depressed patients.

Even fewer clinical trial data are available on the effects of SSRIs on anxiety in patients with coronary disease. In the Understanding the Benefits of Exercise and Escitalopram in Anxious Patients With Coronary Heart Disease trial, 128 patients with coronary disease and elevated anxiety or diagnosed anxiety disorders were randomly assigned to escitalopram only, exercise only, or pill placebo. Escitalopram was dosed at 5–20 mg/day (mean dosage = 14 mg/day). Exercise (three 35-minute sessions per week of supervised exercise) and escitalopram interventions were superior to placebo, and the effect of escitalopram was stronger than that of exercise (Blumenthal et al. 2021). In EsDEPACS, escitalopram significantly reduced anxiety, independent of effects on depression, in patients with ACS (Kang et al. 2017).

Bleeding risk is a concern when using SSRIs for patients who have undergone cardiac surgery or are taking concurrent anticoagulant or antiplatelet therapy, because SSRIs themselves inhibit platelet activation via multiple mechanisms (Lopez-Vilchez et al. 2017). Empirical findings in heart disease populations are mixed. Data from randomized clinical trials have not shown increased bleeding events in patients receiving SSRIs after ACS (e.g., Serebruany et al. 2003a) or anticoagulation for atrial fibrillation (Quinn et al. 2018), although the latter study found an insignificant trend toward more bleeding in patients receiving warfarin. However, larger analyses of observational data on large cohorts of patients have found significantly higher rates of severe bleeding, including gastrointestinal bleeding, in patients receiving SSRIs (Laporte et al. 2017). Bleeding rates seem to be selectively higher in patients receiving antiplatelet therapy, although this effect may be attenuated by concurrent proton pump inhibitor therapy (Jiang et al. 2015). Antidepressants with CYP2C19 activity are a notable exception and actually seem to decrease the effectiveness of clopidogrel, leading to higher risk of ischemic events (Bykov et al. 2017). Concomitant use of warfarin and SSRIs is also associated with increased bleeding risk (Wang et al. 2021), possibly more so than with other anticoagulants (Quinn et al. 2018). After cardiac surgery, most studies found no significant differences in bleeding, morbidity, or mortality with SSRI treatment, although the results of individual studies vary (Sepehripour et al. 2018). Few controlled studies of bleeding risk with non-SSRI agents are available. Although some studies have found lower risk of bleeding with serotonin-norepinephrine reuptake inhibitors (Cheng et al. 2015), the bulk of the evidence indicates that they confer a bleeding risk similar to that of SSRIs (Bixby et al. 2019). There is insufficient evidence to conclude whether other agents, such as mirtazapine or bupropion, are safer with regard to bleeding risk (Na et al. 2018).

In patients with heart failure, depression is common and is associated with lower quality of life, more rapid decline in functional status, and increased mortality. Antidepressants were linked to increased mortality and major cardiovascular events over 3-year follow-up in a prospective naturalistic follow-up study of 204 outpatients with heart failure. In a cohort of patients hospitalized for congestive heart failure, however, antidepressant use was not associated with increased mortality after adjustment for other relevant variables, including depression (O'Connor et al. 2008).

Several controlled trials have tested SSRIs for depression in patients with heart failure and found mixed results. In SADHART, randomization was stratified by ejection fraction. Sertraline effects were similar in subjects with left ventricular ejection fraction lower and higher than 35% (Glassman et al. 2002). A larger trial of sertraline limited to patients with heart failure did not find a beneficial effect of sertraline on depression or cardiovascular outcomes (O'Connor et al. 2010). In a very small ($n=28$) randomized placebo-controlled trial, depression response to treatment was 69% at 12 weeks for subjects who received paroxetine controlled release, 12.5–25 mg/day, versus only 23% for subjects given placebo (Gottlieb et al. 2007). A placebo-controlled trial of citalopram in elderly depressed patients with congestive heart failure was terminated prematurely after an interim analysis showed a very high placebo response rate and no separation of citalopram from placebo (Fraguas et al. 2009). The Effects of Selective Serotonin Re-Uptake Inhibition on Morbidity, Mortality, and Mood in

Depressed Heart Failure Patients trial randomly assigned 372 patients with New York Heart Association class II–IV heart failure and depression to escitalopram (10–20 mg/day) or placebo treatment; compared with placebo, escitalopram had no effect on depression, hospitalization, or mortality (Angermann et al. 2016).

The literature to guide use of other antidepressant classes in heart disease is limited. Mirtazapine was tested in a small randomized placebo-controlled trial involving 94 patients (Honig et al. 2007), nested within the larger Myocardial Infarction and Depression–Intervention Trial (van Melle et al. 2007). Mirtazapine dosing ranged from 30 to 45 mg/day. At week 8, the effect of mirtazapine on Hamilton Depression Rating Scale scores (the predefined primary outcome measure) was not significantly different from that of placebo, but mirtazapine was more efficacious as measured by the Depression scale of the Symptom Checklist–90 and by the Beck Depression Inventory. Patients with inadequate response at 8 weeks were offered alternative treatment, whereas the subset of patients with adequate response at 8 weeks continued with maintenance treatment to 24-week follow-up ($n=40$). In this small subset of patients, the efficacy of mirtazapine treatment was demonstrated on all measures at 24-week follow-up. Mirtazapine was well tolerated in this trial.

Hypertension sufficient to cause treatment discontinuation occurred in 2 of 40 patients in an open-label study of bupropion in patients with heart disease (Roose et al. 1991). A clinical trial of bupropion at a dosage of 300 mg/day for smoking cessation found no increase in major cardiac events (MI, stroke, cardiac death) over placebo, varenicline, or nicotine replacement (Benowitz et al. 2018). However, this study excluded any participants with MI, coronary artery bypass, stroke, or transient ischemic attack within the past 2 months. Hypertension is also a known adverse effect of venlafaxine. No studies have been reported of venlafaxine in patients with cardiac disease. One open-label study in patients older than 60 years found significant rates of hypertension and orthostatic hypotension and several instances of palpitations, dizziness, and QT prolongation (Johnson et al. 2006). Evidence is mixed on QT prolongation in particular. A secondary analysis of a broader clinical trial on depression in older adults (the Incomplete Response in Late-Life Depression: Getting to Remission study) found no evidence of QT or QTc interval prolongation with venlafaxine treatment (Behlke et al. 2020).

Duloxetine did not appear to be associated with significant cardiovascular risks in 42 placebo-controlled trials, 3 of which involved patients with diabetic neuropathy (Wernicke et al. 2007). A recent systematic review found that although some studies identified adverse cardiac events in duloxetine treatment groups, most often hypertension, meta-analysis indicated only small mean changes in heart rate (2.22 beats/min) and diastolic blood pressure (0.82 mm Hg) (Park et al. 2020). However, the medication has not been studied in patients with significant heart disease.

In a small placebo-controlled trial of patients with cardiac disease, trazodone had no significant adverse cardiac effects except postural hypotension (Bucknall et al. 1988). Numerous case reports (e.g., Service and Waring 2008) have described QT prolongation and ventricular arrhythmias after trazodone overdose, and a controlled study found a dose-dependent QT prolongation effect (Tellone et al. 2020).

Monoamine oxidase inhibitors have not been studied in patients with heart disease; their use is not appealing in view of their strong risk of orthostatic hypotension, the risk of interaction with pressors, and the risk of hypertensive reactions to dietary indiscretions.

Hierarchy of Drug Choice

On the basis of the available evidence, escitalopram, citalopram, and sertraline appear to be the first-line pharmacotherapy treatment options for depression in patients with coronary artery disease. In congestive heart failure, few data suggest efficacy for any antidepressant. The relative absence of CYP interactions associated with escitalopram and citalopram (and, to a lesser degree, with lower-dose sertraline) is an advantage for patients taking other medications. Citalopram use requires vigilance with respect to the QT interval and arrhythmia risk. Patients who cannot tolerate or have failed to respond to these agents might logically be offered second-line treatment with mirtazapine, bupropion, venlafaxine, or duloxetine, with special attention to blood pressure response during treatment. TCAs have a substantial side-effect burden and carry increased mortality risk. Nortriptyline might be a reasonable third-line option for patients who have not responded to adequate trials of other first- and second-line treatments and who are sufficiently impaired by depression that the additional adverse-effect risks are worth incurring.

Prescribing Principles

The agent of choice depends on the factors described previously, the patient's comorbid conditions, and the patient's other medications. Medication should be started at a low dosage—possibly below the lowest therapeutic dosage—and subjective tolerability and relevant electrocardiographic effects, vital signs, physical examination findings, and laboratory parameters should be reassessed before the dosage is increased. Dosage increases should be followed by reassessment for adverse effects. Appropriate clinical monitoring may include basic laboratory evaluation (e.g., of electrolytes, renal function), electrocardiogram (for QTc or conduction abnormalities), and therapeutic drug monitoring as indicated, although no specific guidelines exist. For patients in heart failure who also have hepatic or renal dysfunction, target dosages may need to be reduced to lower than normal levels because of slowed metabolism. However, if a patient is tolerating medication well but not responding adequately, it is worthwhile to consider a dose increase.

Desirable Secondary Effects

Antihistaminic agents (TCAs, trazodone, mirtazapine) may increase appetite and promote weight gain in patients with cardiac cachexia, and sedating effects may help patients with insomnia. Bupropion is one of the few psychotropic agents associated with weight loss and therefore may help patients who need to lose weight as part of their cardiac treatment program. Bupropion is also indicated as pharmacotherapy for smoking cessation (although the period of acute treatment of a depressive episode is probably an unfavorable time to attempt smoking cessation). Whether the antiplatelet effect of SSRIs is clinically valuable in patients with ischemic heart disease is unknown (Pollock et al. 2000; Serebruany et al. 2003b).

Antipsychotics

Relevant Treatment Literature

Agitation and psychotic symptoms occurring in delirium are often treated with antipsychotic medication, although such treatment is off label. Patients with heart disease and psychiatric disorders also may need antipsychotic drug therapy. No controlled studies of the risks and benefits of antipsychotic medications specifically in cardiac patients have been reported.

All antipsychotic agents may cause hypotension, especially orthostatic hypotension (Mackin 2008). The effect is particularly marked for low-potency agents such as chlorpromazine. Olanzapine, clozapine, and quetiapine may be associated with higher rates of orthostatic hypotension than other second-generation agents. Complaints of dizziness may occur even in the absence of hypotension or orthostatic hypotension. Increased heart rate is common in patients treated with clozapine, but bradycardia can also occur with clozapine and other second-generation antipsychotics. In a review of FDA data, syncope due to orthostatic hypotension occurred in up to 1% of patients taking quetiapine and up to 6% of patients taking clozapine. Most of the patients in these samples did not have heart disease. Tolerance to the blood pressure–lowering effects of antipsychotics may develop over time; initiating treatment at low dosages reduces the risk. Salt supplements, α-adrenergic agonists such as midodrine, and mineralocorticoids such as fludrocortisone can reduce the risk, but these agents may not be suitable for some cardiac patients; support stockings may be an acceptable alternative.

Metabolic syndrome—dyslipidemia, glucose intolerance, hypertension, and abdominal obesity—is an important side effect of second-generation antipsychotics, especially olanzapine and clozapine, and is a risk factor for coronary artery disease. Aripiprazole, ziprasidone, lurasidone, cariprazine, brexpiprazole, and lumateperone are less likely to lead to these effects than other second-generation antipsychotic medications (Kane et al. 2021; Pillinger et al. 2020). The novel antipsychotic pimavanserin apparently does not increase the risk of metabolic syndrome. Recommendations for prevention and treatment of metabolic side effects associated with second-generation antipsychotics emphasize antipsychotic choice, exercise, dietary modification, and concomitant treatment with agents such as metformin (Jiang et al. 2020) (see also Chapter 2, "Severe Drug Reactions").

All antipsychotic medications may prolong the QT interval, with the possible exception of aripiprazole, lurasidone, and lumateperone (Kane et al. 2021). Haloperidol, droperidol, thioridazine, sertindole, iloperidone, and ziprasidone tend to produce greater QT prolongation than do other agents (Beach et al. 2018; Funk et al. 2020). QT interval prolongation (QTc above 440 ms and especially above 500 ms) is associated with increased risk of polymorphic sustained ventricular tachycardia (torsades de pointes), which can degenerate into ventricular fibrillation. First-generation phenothiazine antipsychotics may also cause QT interval prolongation and torsades de pointes.

A comprehensive review concluded that at therapeutic dosages, antipsychotic medications alone, in the absence of other risk factors, are unlikely to cause torsades de pointes (Hasnain and Vieweg 2014). Women, patients with chronic heavy alcohol consumption, patients with familial long QT syndrome, and patients with anorexia nervosa are at higher risk for torsades de pointes. Other easily noted risk factors for torsades de pointes include severe heart disease, hypokalemia, hypomagnesemia, and concurrent treatment with one of the myriad other drugs that increase the QT interval (Table 6–4) (Beach et al. 2013; Brojmohun et al. 2013; Justo et al. 2005).

On the basis of Danish registry data, the risk of sudden death associated with antipsychotic medication is estimated to be only about 2–4 per 10,000 person-years of exposure in otherwise medically healthy subjects (Glassman and Bigger 2001). However, reviews of treatment studies addressing use of both first- and second-generation antipsychotic medications in behaviorally disturbed elderly patients have concluded that antipsychotic medications are associated with about a 1.9% absolute increase in short-term mortality in this patient population (4.5% vs. 2.6%, or about a 70% increase in adjusted RR), mostly due to cardiovascular events and infections. This finding resulted in an FDA-mandated warning about off-label treatment of agitation and psychotic symptoms in behaviorally disturbed elderly patients with dementia (Gill et al. 2007; Kuehn 2008; Liperoti et al. 2005; Rochon et al. 2008). A review of Tennessee Medicaid data found that nonusers of antipsychotic drugs had a sudden death rate of 0.0014 deaths per person-year, whereas antipsychotic drug users had a sudden death rate of 0.0028–0.0029 deaths per person-year. Thus, antipsychotic drugs were associated with an approximate doubling of risk for sudden death, but the absolute risk was only about 0.0015 deaths per person-year, yielding a number needed to treat to cause one additional sudden death in 1 year of 666 persons (Ray et al. 2009). The degree to which these findings apply in the treatment of delirium and acute psychotic symptoms in patients with cardiac disease is unknown. A large retrospective cohort study of hospitalized patients, controlling for ICU time, admission type, and comorbidities including delirium, found that typical antipsychotics were associated with an increase in the composite outcome of in-hospital mortality or cardiopulmonary arrest (hazard ratio = 1.6), whereas atypical antipsychotics were associated with risk only in adults age 65 and older (hazard ratio = 1.8) (Basciotta et al. 2020).

Clozapine is associated with a risk of myocarditis, which has been variously estimated to occur in 0.015%–8.5% of exposed patients. The mechanism of inflammation is uncertain, but an immune hypersensitivity reaction is suspected. The mortality rate of clozapine-induced myocarditis has been re-

Table 6–4.   Risk factors for torsades de pointes

Familial long QT syndrome

QT prolongation

Bradycardia

Female sex

Chronic heavy alcohol use

Anorexia nervosa

Low ejection fraction

Hypokalemia

Hypomagnesemia

Acute illness, including renal or hepatic dysfunction

Concurrent treatment with multiple drugs that prolong the QT interval or inhibit
   the metabolism of a QT-prolonging drug

ported to range from 21% to 64% and does not appear to be dose dependent; therefore, guidelines suggest that clozapine be titrated gradually in 25 mg/day increments over 4–6 weeks. The available literature reports the onset of symptoms at a median daily dose of 250 mg. Although the clinical presentation of the syndrome may be highly variable, the incidence is highest in the first 12 weeks of treatment, and the most common presenting signs and symptoms include shortness of breath, chest pain, flulike symptoms, malaise, fever, tachycardia, and hypotension. During clozapine initiation and up-titration, clinical monitoring and serial measurement of C-reactive protein and troponin are recommended (Bellissima et al. 2018).

Hierarchy of Drug Choice

Several new antipsychotic agents are relatively free from metabolic problems, although most carry at least mild or moderate risk of QTc interval prolongation. Antipsychotic choice should be individualized, weighing the likelihood of efficacy against baseline cardiac function. Given their favorable side-effect profiles, aripiprazole and lurasidone may be first-line antipsychotic agents for patients with heart disease or significant coronary risk factors. Olanzapine and aripiprazole are available as orally disintegrating tablets, which may be a convenient route of administration for patients who cannot swallow tablets, and many medications are available for intramuscular administration. Asenapine is absorbed through the buccal mucosa, which may obviate the need for intramuscular medication in patients unable to take oral medication. Intravenous haloperidol, in widely varying dosages, has been in use (off label) for decades. Ziprasidone and olanzapine can also be administered intravenously.

Prescribing Principles

Before antipsychotic drugs are prescribed, cardiology patients should be evaluated for risk factors for QTc interval prolongation and sudden cardiac death. Risk factors include history of syncope or cardiac arrest, family history of sudden death, familial long QT syndrome, long QT interval, low ejection fraction, treatment with other drugs that may prolong the QT interval either directly or through drug interactions, hypokalemia, and hypomagnesemia (Beach et al. 2018). Vital signs and electrocardiograms should be reviewed. Notably, there is a lack of consensus regarding the optimal formula to correct the QTc interval; however, Bazett's formula is the most commonly used in commercial electrocardiogram machines and is known to overestimate the QTc interval at heart rates greater than 60 beats/min and underestimate at rates less than 60 beats/min. Some authors suggest that the most accurate correction is obtained with Fridericia's formula, $QTc_{Fri} = QT/RR^{1/3}$ (Beach et al. 2018), which may allow greater liberty with the choice of antipsychotic agents. Patients taking known "offending" agents that prolong the QTc interval who develop cardiac symptoms such as syncope, dizziness, and palpitations, or who have a sudden increase in QTc interval more than 60 seconds from baseline, warrant a cardiology consultation (Funk et al. 2020).

For patients with congestive heart failure, lower than normal dosages may be adequate.

Mood Stabilizers

No studies have been reported of mood stabilizers as treatment for depression or bipolar disorder in cardiology patients. Lithium can cause sinus node dysfunction, manifesting in sinus bradycardia or sinus arrest. Lithium excretion is almost entirely through the kidney and is sensitive to the effects of left-sided heart failure, diuretics (see the section "Pharmacokinetic Alterations in Heart Disease" earlier in this chapter), ACE inhibitors, and angiotensin II receptor blockers. Long-term lithium use may cause impaired renal function, which may complicate heart failure management. Valproic acid has no cardiovascular effects; however, it may cause thrombocytopenia, which may be important for patients taking anticoagulants or those receiving antiplatelet therapy. It may increase plasma warfarin levels, but this effect has not been shown to be of clinical significance. An interaction with aspirin has been described that results in decreased protein binding, inhibited metabolism, and elevated free valproic acid level in blood. Lamotrigine at recommended dosages does not have significant cardiac effects; a case of complete heart block following lamotrigine overdose has been reported (French et al. 2011). Lamotrigine undergoes only Phase II hepatic metabolism, which may make it easier to dose in heart failure. Carbamazepine appears to be relatively free of cardiac effects in healthy patients (Kennebäck et al. 1995), but some electrocardiographic abnormalities have occurred in patients with heart disease (Kennebäck et al. 1991). Both carbamazepine and oxcarbazepine are associated with hyponatremia, especially in elderly women (see the section "Drug-Drug Interactions" later in this chapter). Gabapentin and pregabalin have no known cardiac effects.

Psychostimulants

Relevant Treatment Literature

Despite clinical lore supporting the value of stimulants to improve mood, increase energy, and improve subjective well-being in patients who are medically ill (Emptage and Semla 1996), including patients with heart disease (e.g., Kaufmann et al. 1984), no clinical trials have been reported of the risks and benefits of stimulants for depressed cardiac patients. A Cochrane review of a few small trials of psychostimulant treatment of depression, including several trials in patients who were medically ill, found no association between stimulant use and adverse cardiac effects but noted significant limitations in the quantity and quality of evidence available (Candy et al. 2008). Low dosages of stimulants (e.g., methylphenidate, 5–30 mg/day, dextroamphetamine, 5–20 mg/day) used as treatment for depression in medical patients have minimal effects on heart rate and blood pressure (Masand and Tesar 1996). A review of data from five clinical trials of stimulant and nonstimulant drugs for treatment of ADHD in adults concluded that amphetamine and methylphenidate both raise systolic and diastolic blood pressure by about 5 mm Hg; the dosages of stimulants were not described in this report (Wilens et al. 2005). Reviews of adverse events in young adults taking stimulants for ADHD reported very low rates of cardiac events (Cooper et al. 2011; Peyre et al. 2014). In older adults, stimulant prescription has been associated with increased risk of cardiovascular events within the first 30 days of a new prescription but not after 180 or 365 days (Tadrous et al. 2021).

Prescribing Principles

Contraindications to stimulant use as recorded in manufacturers' package inserts generally include broadly construed serious heart problems, structural cardiac abnormalities, serious cardiac rhythm abnormalities, cardiomyopathy, and coronary artery disease. Interpreting this language may require clinical judgment and consultation with a cardiologist. Stimulant treatment should not be started without a medical consultation for a patient with a history of heart disease or hypertension; symptoms of chest pain, palpitations, or shortness of breath; or physical examination findings of tachycardia, elevated blood pressure, or irregular heart rhythm. Stimulant treatment should be avoided in patients with acute ischemia, unstable angina, frequent ventricular premature contractions, or tachyarrhythmias. However, with concurrent medical supervision, in inpatient settings with cardiac monitoring, we have used stimulants in the treatment of numerous patients within days after coronary artery bypass graft surgery, MI, heart transplantation, and admission for decompensated heart failure and acute coronary events. Even ill patients can start with methylphenidate at dosages of 5 mg/day, with the dosage increased over a few days up to 30 mg/day. Vital signs and heart rhythm should be assessed with dosage changes. Benefit from stimulant medications for depressed cardiac patients should be observable within several days.

For alternative agents such as modafinil and atomoxetine, limited data are available. Both have hemodynamic effects, especially elevated systolic blood pressure and heart rate, which could be problematic for patients with heart failure or coronary artery disease (Liang et al. 2018; Taneja et al. 2005).

Cognitive Enhancers

Data on the use of cognitive enhancement medications specifically addressing patients with heart disease are limited. The cholinesterase inhibitors donepezil, rivastigmine, and galantamine have modest benefit for treatment of mild to moderate dementia and are increasingly used to treat patients with vascular dementia, many of whom also have atherosclerotic cardiac disease (Battle et al. 2021). Their procholinergic effects reduce heart rate and may occasionally result in sinus bradycardia, heart block, hypertension, and syncope. There have been several case reports of QTc interval prolongation leading to torsades de pointes with the use of donepezil (Beach et al. 2018). Although there was early concern about increased mortality and treatment discontinuation due to cardiovascular side effects in elderly patients with heart disease treated with cholinesterase inhibitors (Malone and Lindesay 2007), a meta-analysis found them to be associated with a 37% lower risk of cardiovascular events, including stroke, acute MI, and ACS (Isik et al. 2018). For the *N*-methyl-D-aspartate receptor antagonist memantine, which is indicated for the treatment of moderate dementia, the manufacturer reported hypertension as a rare event in premarketing trials.

Other Agents

Varenicline, a nicotinic receptor partial agonist, was introduced in 2006 as a medication to aid smoking cessation. Important side effects of varenicline are nausea and worsening of depression. Varenicline does not have significant cardiac effects. Varenicline should be titrated over 7 days from a starting dosage of 0.5 mg once daily to 1 mg twice daily.

Naltrexone hydrochloride, an opioid antagonist, is sometimes used to reduce craving and help prevent relapse in patients with a history of alcohol use disorder. This may be useful for patients with alcoholic cardiomyopathy, in concert with other measures to promote and maintain abstinence. Naltrexone has no cardiovascular effects. Intravenous naloxone, given as a competitive opioid receptor inhibitor to patients with opioid intoxication or overdose, may cause hypertension, hypotension, pulmonary edema, and cardiac arrest.

Methadone, frequently used for treatment of opioid use disorder, has a substantial dose-dependent effect on QTc interval prolongation and risk of torsades de pointes (Beach et al. 2018). There is no evidence that oral buprenorphine use is associated with torsades de pointes, but a recent study found that supratherapeutic dosing of transdermal buprenorphine was linked with dose-dependent QTc interval prolongation (Tran et al. 2020).

Acamprosate is indicated for maintenance of abstinence in patients with alcohol use disorder. Acamprosate has no cardiovascular effects.

Topiramate also has been reported to improve maintenance of abstinence from alcohol (Johnson et al. 2007). Topiramate has no cardiovascular side effects. Hydrochlorothiazide increases topiramate blood levels. Topiramate reduces digoxin blood levels slightly.

The phosphodiesterase type 5 (PDE5) inhibitors sildenafil, vardenafil, and tadalafil, used for the treatment of erectile dysfunction, cause vasodilation and increased blood flow into the penile corpus cavernosum. PDE5 inhibitors are also systemic and pulmonary arterial vasodilators and interact with numerous other agents that lower blood pressure. PDE5 inhibitors are also useful for the treatment of pulmonary hypertension (Wilkins et al. 2008). Concurrent use of nitrates is contraindicated because of severe hypotension, and extreme caution must be used when combining α-blocking agents with PDE5 inhibitors. PDE5 inhibitor use by patients with cardiovascular disease has resulted in syncope, chest pain, MI, tachycardia, and death, usually in conjunction with sexual activity.

Drug-Drug Interactions

The discussion of drug interactions in this section is based on several comprehensive reviews (Robinson and Owen 2005; Strain et al. 1999, 2002; Williams et al. 2007). Interactions between psychotropic and cardiac medications are due to pharmacodynamic properties of the drugs (i.e., they have overlapping and additive or offsetting effects) or pharmacokinetic effects (i.e., one drug affects metabolism, distribution, or elimination of the other), including effects on hepatic metabolism by the CYP system (Tables 6–5 and 6–6). For a complete review of drug-drug interactions, including cardiac medications, see Chapter 1, "Pharmacokinetics, Pharmacodynamics, and Principles of Drug-Drug Interactions."

Common pharmacodynamic interactions are additive effects on heart rate, blood pressure, and cardiac conduction. Many psychotropic drugs reduce blood pressure, and combining them with antihypertensive medications generally increases the hypotensive effect. SSRI antidepressants tend to reduce heart rate; combining them with β-blockers may exacerbate the bradycardic effect. In contrast, TCAs and mirtazapine suppress the centrally mediated antihypertensive effects of clonidine; the combination of TCA or mirtazapine with clonidine may result in severe hypertension. Drugs that slow cardiac conduction—TCAs, phenothiazines, and atypical antipsychotics—may interact with amiodarone, type 1A antiarrhythmic drugs, and ibutilide, resulting in

Table 6–5.　Clinically relevant cardiac medication–psychotropic medication interactions

Cardiac medication	Interaction mechanism	Clinical effects and management
Angiotensin converting enzyme inhibitors	Reduced lithium clearance	Elevated lithium levels. Monitor serum lithium levels.
Angiotensin II receptor blockers	Reduced lithium clearance	Elevated lithium levels. Monitor serum lithium levels.
Antianginals		
Isosorbide dinitrate	Anticholinergic activity	Impaired cognition. Reduced therapeutic effect of cholinesterase inhibitors and memantine.
Antiarrhythmics		
Amiodarone	Inhibition of CYP2C9, CYP2D6, and CYP3A4	Increased levels of phenytoin, TCAs, opiates, risperidone, aripiprazole, atomoxetine, benzodiazepines, buspirone, alfentanil, zopiclone, eszopiclone, modafinil. Impaired activation of codeine to morphine.
Disopyramide	Anticholinergic activity	Impaired cognition. Reduced therapeutic effect of cholinesterase inhibitors and memantine.
Mexiletine	CYP1A2 inhibition	Increased levels of olanzapine and clozapine.
Procainamide	Anticholinergic activity	Impaired cognition. Reduced therapeutic effect of cholinesterase inhibitors and memantine.
Propafenone	CYP1A2 inhibition	Increased levels of olanzapine and clozapine.
Quinidine	CYP2D6 inhibition	Increased levels of TCAs, opiates, risperidone, aripiprazole, atomoxetine. Impaired activation of codeine to morphine.

Table 6–5. Clinically relevant cardiac medication–psychotropic medication interactions *(continued)*

Cardiac medication	Interaction mechanism	Clinical effects and management
Antiarrhythmics *(continued)*		
	Anticholinergic activity	Impaired cognition. Reduced therapeutic effect of cholinesterase inhibitors and memantine.
Antihyperlipidemics		
Fluvastatin, gemfibrozil, lovastatin, and simvastatin	CYP2C9 inhibition	Increased levels of phenytoin. Monitor phenytoin levels.
Calcium channel blockers		
Diltiazem	CYP3A4 inhibition	Increased levels of benzodiazepines, buspirone, alfentanil, zopiclone, eszopiclone, modafinil.
Nifedipine and verapamil	Reduced lithium clearance	Elevated lithium levels. Monitor serum lithium levels.
Cardiac glycosides		
Digoxin	Anticholinergic activity	Impaired cognition. Reduced therapeutic effect of cholinesterase inhibitors and memantine.
Diuretics		
Acetazolamide and osmotic diuretics	Increased lithium clearance	Reduced lithium levels. Monitor serum lithium levels. Carbonic anhydrase inhibitors may decrease excretion of amphetamines.
Furosemide	Anticholinergic activity	Impaired cognition. Reduced therapeutic effect of cholinesterase inhibitors and memantine.
Thiazides	Reduced lithium clearance	Elevated lithium levels. Monitor serum lithium levels.

Note. CYP = cytochrome P450; TCAs = tricyclic antidepressants.

Table 6–6.   Clinically relevant psychotropic medication–cardiac medication interactions

Psychotropic medication	Interaction mechanism	Clinical effects and management
Antidepressants		
Bupropion	CYP2D6 inhibition	Increased β-blocker levels→decreased heart rate.
		Increased levels of many antiarrhythmics with possible conduction abnormalities.
Duloxetine	CYP2D6 inhibition	Increased β-blocker levels→decreased heart rate.
		Increased levels of many antiarrhythmics with possible conduction abnormalities.
Fluoxetine	CYP3A4 inhibition	Increased statin levels→myopathy, hepatic injury.
		Increased calcium channel blocker levels→hypotension.
Fluvoxamine	CYP2C9 inhibition	Increased warfarin levels, increased international normalized ratio→possible increased bleeding risk.
		Fluvoxamine contraindicated in patients receiving warfarin.
Mirtazapine	α_2-Receptor blockade	Possible severe hypertension with clonidine; avoid this combination.
Moclobemide	CYP2D6 inhibition	Increased β-blocker levels→decreased heart rate.
		Increased levels of many antiarrhythmics with possible conduction abnormalities.
Nefazodone	CYP3A4 inhibition	Increased statin levels→myopathy, hepatic injury.
		Increased calcium channel blocker levels→hypotension.

Table 6–6. Clinically relevant psychotropic medication–cardiac medication interactions *(continued)*

Psychotropic medication	Interaction mechanism	Clinical effects and management
Antidepressants (continued)		
Paroxetine	CYP2D6 inhibition	Increased β-blocker levels→decreased heart rate.
		Increased levels of many antiarrhythmics with possible conduction abnormalities.
Trazodone	Type 1A antiarrhythmic effects	QT prolongation, AV block with amiodarone, ibutilide, and type 1A antiarrhythmic agents. Monitor QT interval. Avoid trazodone in conjunction with antiarrhythmic therapy.
Monoamine oxidase inhibitors	Monoamine oxidase inhibition increases monoamine effect	Increased pressor effects of epinephrine and dopamine→hypertension.
SSRIs and SNRIs	Pharmacodynamic synergism: SIADH plus sodium wasting	SSRI/SNRI-induced SIADH and hyponatremia. Exacerbated with thiazide diuretic–induced sodium wasting. Monitor sodium levels. Consider nonthiazide diuretics.
TCAs	Type 1A antiarrhythmic effects	QT prolongation, AV block with amiodarone, ibutilide, and type 1A antiarrhythmic agents. Monitor QT interval. Avoid TCAs in conjunction with antiarrhythmic therapy.
	Unknown	Possible severe hypertension with clonidine; avoid this combination.

Table 6–6. Clinically relevant psychotropic medication–cardiac medication interactions *(continued)*

Psychotropic medication	Interaction mechanism	Clinical effects and management
Antipsychotics		
Atypical and typical	Type 1A antiarrhythmic effects	QT prolongation; AV block with amiodarone, ibutilide, and type 1A antiarrhythmic agents. Monitor QT interval. Use antipsychotics with minimal QT-prolonging effect (lurasidone, aripiprazole).
Mood stabilizers		
Carbamazepine	Pan-inducer of CYP metabolic enzymes	Increased metabolism and lower levels of most cardiac medications, including warfarin, β-blockers, antiarrhythmics, statins, calcium channel blockers. Avoid carbamazepine if possible. Monitor cardiovascular function. Increase cardiac agent dosage as necessary.
	Pharmacodynamic synergism: SIADH plus sodium wasting	SSRI/SNRI-induced SIADH and hyponatremia. Exacerbated with thiazide diuretic–induced sodium wasting. Monitor sodium levels. Consider nonthiazide diuretics.
Oxcarbazepine	Pharmacodynamic synergism: SIADH plus sodium wasting	SSRI/SNRI-induced SIADH and hyponatremia. Exacerbated with thiazide diuretic–induced sodium wasting. Monitor sodium levels. Consider nonthiazide diuretics.
Phenytoin	Pan-inducer of CYP metabolic enzymes	Increased metabolism and lower levels of most cardiac medications, including warfarin, β-blockers, antiarrhythmics, statins, calcium channel blockers. Avoid phenytoin if possible. Monitor cardiovascular function.

Table 6–6.   Clinically relevant psychotropic medication–cardiac medication interactions *(continued)*

Psychotropic medication	Interaction mechanism	Clinical effects and management
Cholinesterase inhibitors	Pharmacodynamic synergism: increased vagal tone	Increased β-blocker effect on heart rate. Monitor heart rate. Reduce β-blocker dosage as necessary.

Note.   AV = atrioventricular; CYP = cytochrome P450; SIADH = syndrome of inappropriate antidiuretic hormone secretion; SNRIs = serotonin-norepinephrine reuptake inhibitors; SSRIs = selective serotonin reuptake inhibitors; TCAs = tricyclic antidepressants.

atrioventricular block or prolonged QT interval. Several antibiotics, antifungal agents, methadone, tacrolimus, and cocaine also prolong the QT interval. Trazodone combined with amiodarone has resulted in QT prolongation and ventricular tachycardia.

Lithium clearance is an important example of a pharmacokinetic interaction that does not involve the hepatic CYP system. Thiazide diuretics block sodium reabsorption in the glomerular proximal convoluted tubule; as serum sodium is depleted, tubular reuptake of lithium from the glomerular filtrate is increased. Thus, thiazide diuretics increase serum lithium level and may increase the risk of lithium toxicity. Loop diuretics (furosemide, ethacrynic acid, bumetanide) have little effect on serum lithium levels. However, chronic use of any diuretic by patients with heart failure may reduce creatinine clearance, raising the serum lithium level and increasing the risk of lithium toxicity (Finley et al. 1995). Nifedipine, verapamil, lisinopril, ACE inhibitors, and angiotensin II receptor blockers all reduce lithium clearance and raise serum lithium levels. Acetazolamide and osmotic diuretics such as mannitol increase lithium clearance. Lithium toxicity may occur even when serum levels are not elevated in patients also taking diltiazem or verapamil.

Hyponatremia, a common side effect of SSRIs, oxcarbazepine, and carbamazepine, can be significantly exacerbated by interaction with the added hyponatremic effect of diuretics (Dong et al. 2005; Jacob and Spinler 2006; Ranta and Wooten 2004; Rosner 2004).

Many benzodiazepines, fluoxetine, paroxetine, and nefazodone can increase blood levels of digoxin, by an unknown mechanism.

Donepezil, rivastigmine, and galantamine have systemic and CNS procholinergic effects; these may be antagonized by medicines with anticholinergic activity, including disopyramide, procainamide, quinidine, isosorbide dinitrate, digoxin, and furosemide, resulting in cognitive worsening. Cholinesterase inhibitors plus β-blockers have additive bradycardic effects and may cause syncope.

Numerous pharmacokinetic interactions involve inhibition or induction of CYP isozymes involved in the metabolism of psychotropic and cardiac medications (see Chapter 1). The following discussion is limited to a few specific interactions of clinical importance.

Most β-blockers, including carvedilol, propranolol, and metoprolol, are metabolized mainly by CYP2D6, which is strongly inhibited by fluoxetine, paroxetine, and bupropion. Significant bradycardia could result. Most antiarrhythmic drugs are also metabolized by CYP2D6.

Warfarin is metabolized mainly by CYP2C9 and to a lesser extent through several other CYP isoenzymes. Fluvoxamine inhibition and carbamazepine induction of CYP2C9 may cause a clinically significant increase or decrease, respectively, in the international normalized ratio. Clopidogrel, argatroban, and heparin have not been reported to interact with psychotropic medications.

Most statins are metabolized by CYP3A4. Myopathy and hepatic injury as a result of statin toxicity may theoretically result from interaction with fluvoxamine, nefazodone, or other strong CYP3A4 inhibitors.

QT prolongation may occur when QTc-prolonging psychotropics are coprescribed with CYP inhibitors, and a thorough review of a patient's medication list is warranted. Cautious electrocardiographic monitoring is appropriate for patients with more than one risk factor for QTc interval prolongation (Beach et al. 2018). The combination of β-blockers and phenothiazines results in increased blood levels of both via mutual metabolic inhibition. Heart rate and blood pressure effects, as well as CNS effects, may be increased.

Key Points

- Differential diagnosis of psychiatric symptoms for patients with heart disease includes effects of the cardiac condition itself and of its treatment. Many cardiovascular medications have adverse neuropsychiatric effects.

- Many psychiatric medications have potential to cause adverse hemodynamic effects and cardiac rhythm abnormalities.

- Treatment requires attention to potential alterations in pharmacokinetics and to potential drug interactions, including effects mediated by the hepatic cytochrome P450 system.

- Despite these challenges, it is possible to use antipsychotic, antidepressant, mood stabilizer, and other medications to provide treatment for psychiatric disorders in patients with heart disease.

References

Alghamdi J, Matou-Nasri S, Alghamdi F, et al: Risk of neuropsychiatric adverse effects of lipid-lowering drugs: a Mendelian randomization study. Int J Neuropsychopharmacol 21(12):1067–1075, 2018 29986042

Angermann CE, Gelbrich G, Störk S, et al: Effect of escitalopram on all-cause mortality and hospitalization in patients with heart failure and depression: the MOOD-HF randomized clinical trial. JAMA 315(24):2683–2693, 2016 27367876

Basciotta M, Zhou W, Ngo L, et al: Antipsychotics and the risk of mortality or cardiopulmonary arrest in hospitalized adults. J Am Geriatr Soc 68(3):544–550, 2020 31743435

Battle CE, Abdul-Rahim AH, Shenkin SD, et al: Cholinesterase inhibitors for vascular dementia and other vascular cognitive impairments: a network meta-analysis. Cochrane Database Syst Rev 2(2):CD013306, 2021 33704781

Beach SR, Celano CM, Noseworthy PA, et al: QTc prolongation, torsades de pointes, and psychotropic medications. Psychosomatics 54(1):1–13, 2013 23295003

Beach SR, Celano CM, Sugrue AM, et al: QT prolongation, torsades de pointes, and psychotropic medications: a 5-year update. Psychosomatics 59(2):105–122, 2018 29275963

Behlke LM, Lenze EJ, Pham V, et al: The effect of venlafaxine on electrocardiogram intervals during treatment for depression in older adults. J Clin Psychopharmacol 40(6):553–559, 2020 33044352

Bellissima BL, Tingle MD, Cicović A, et al: A systematic review of clozapine-induced myocarditis. Int J Cardiol 259:122–129, 2018 29579587

Benowitz NL, Pipe A, West R, et al: Cardiovascular safety of varenicline, bupropion, and nicotine patch in smokers: a randomized clinical trial. JAMA Intern Med 178(5):622–631, 2018 29630702

Bixby AL, VandenBerg A, Bostwick JR: Clinical management of bleeding risk with antidepressants. Ann Pharmacother 53(2):186–194, 2019 30081645

Blumenthal JA, Smith PJ, Jiang W, et al: Effect of exercise, escitalopram, or placebo on anxiety in patients with coronary heart disease: the Understanding the Benefits of Exercise and Escitalopram in Anxious Patients With Coronary Heart Disease (UNWIND) randomized clinical trial. JAMA Psychiatry 78(11):1270–1278, 2021 34406354

Brojmohun A, Lou JY, Zardkoohi O, et al: Protected from torsades de pointes? What psychiatrists need to know about pacemakers and defibrillators. Psychosomatics 54(5):407–417, 2013 23756118

Brown TM, Stoudemire A: Cardiovascular agents, in Psychiatric Side Effects of Prescription and Over-the-Counter Medications. Washington, DC, American Psychiatric Press, 1998, pp 209–238

Bucknall C, Brooks D, Curry PV, et al: Mianserin and trazodone for cardiac patients with depression. Eur J Clin Pharmacol 33(6):565–569, 1988 3284752

Bykov K, Schneeweiss S, Donneyong MM, et al: Impact of an interaction between clopidogrel and selective serotonin reuptake inhibitors. Am J Cardiol 119(4):651–657, 2017 27939386

Candy M, Jones L, Williams R, et al: Psychostimulants for depression. Cochrane Database Syst Rev (2):CD006722, 2008 18425966

Castro VM, Clements CC, Murphy SN, et al: QT interval and antidepressant use: a cross sectional study of electronic health records. BMJ 346:f288, 2013 23360890

Cheng YL, Hu HY, Lin XH, et al: Use of SSRI, but not SNRI, increased upper and lower gastrointestinal bleeding: a nationwide population-based cohort study in Taiwan. Medicine (Baltimore) 94(46):e2022, 2015 26579809

Christiansen OG, Madsen MT, Simonsen E, et al: Prophylactic antidepressant treatment following acute coronary syndrome: a systematic review of randomized controlled trials. J Psychiatr Res 94:186–193, 2017 28746904

Cooper WO, Habel LA, Sox CM, et al: ADHD drugs and serious cardiovascular events in children and young adults. N Engl J Med 365(20):1896–1904, 2011 22043968

De Hert M, Detraux J, Vancampfort D: The intriguing relationship between coronary heart disease and mental disorders. Dialogues Clin Neurosci 20(1):31–40, 2018 29946209

di Mauro G, Zinzi A, Scavone C, et al: PCSK9 inhibitors and neurocognitive adverse drug reactions: analysis of individual case safety reports from the Eudravigilance database. Drug Saf 44(3):337–349, 2021 33351170

Dong X, Leppik IE, White J, et al: Hyponatremia from oxcarbazepine and carbamazepine. Neurology 65(12):1976–1978, 2005 16380624

Emptage RE, Semla TP: Depression in the medically ill elderly: a focus on methylphenidate. Ann Pharmacother 30(2):151–157, 1996 8835049

Finley PR, Warner MD, Peabody CA: Clinical relevance of drug interactions with lithium. Clin Pharmacokinet 29(3):172–191, 1995 8521679

Fraguas R, da Silva Telles RM, Alves TC, et al: A double-blind, placebo-controlled treatment trial of citalopram for major depressive disorder in older patients with heart failure: the relevance of the placebo effect and psychological symptoms. Contemp Clin Trials 30(3):205–211, 2009 19470312

French LK, McKeown NJ, Hendrickson RG: Complete heart block and death following lamotrigine overdose. Clin Toxicol (Phila) 49(4):330–333, 2011 21563910

Funk MC, Beach SR, Bostwick JR, et al: QTc prolongation and psychotropic medications. Am J Psychiatry 177(3):273–274, 2020 32114782

Gill SS, Bronskill SE, Normand SL, et al: Antipsychotic drug use and mortality in older adults with dementia. Ann Intern Med 146(11):775–786, 2007 17548409

Glassman AH, Bigger JT Jr: Antipsychotic drugs: prolonged QTc interval, torsade de pointes, and sudden death. Am J Psychiatry 158(11):1774–1782, 2001 11691681

Glassman AH, Rodriguez AI, Shapiro PA: The use of antidepressant drugs in patients with heart disease. J Clin Psychiatry 59(Suppl 10):16–21, 1998 9720478

Glassman AH, O'Connor CM, Califf RM, et al: Sertraline treatment of major depression in patients with acute MI or unstable angina. JAMA 288(6):701–709, 2002 12169073

Glassman AH, Bigger JT, Gaffney M, et al: Onset of major depression associated with acute coronary syndromes: relationship of onset, major depressive disorder history, and episode severity to sertraline benefit. Arch Gen Psychiatry 63(3):283–288, 2006 16520433

Gottlieb SS, Kop WJ, Thomas SA, et al: A double-blind placebo-controlled pilot study of controlled-release paroxetine on depression and quality of life in chronic heart failure. Am Heart J 153(5):868–873, 2007 17452166

Hansen BH, Hanash JA, Rasmussen A, et al: Effects of escitalopram in prevention of depression in patients with acute coronary syndrome (DECARD). J Psychosom Res 72(1):11–16, 2012 22200516

Hasnain M, Vieweg WV: QTc interval prolongation and torsade de pointes associated with second-generation antipsychotics and antidepressants: a comprehensive review. CNS Drugs 28(10):887–920, 2014 25168784

Honig A, Kuyper AMG, Schene AH, et al: Treatment of post-myocardial infarction depressive disorder: a randomized, placebo-controlled trial with mirtazapine. Psychosom Med 69(7):606–613, 2007 17846258

Huffman JC, Stern TA: The use of benzodiazepines in the treatment of chest pain: a review of the literature. J Emerg Med 25(4):427–437, 2003 14654185

Huffman JC, Stern TA: Neuropsychiatric consequences of cardiovascular medications. Dialogues Clin Neurosci 9(1):29–45, 2007 17506224

Isik AT, Soysal P, Stubbs B, et al: Cardiovascular outcomes of cholinesterase inhibitors in individuals with dementia: a meta-analysis and systematic review. J Am Geriatr Soc 66(9):1805–1811, 2018 29851022

Jacob S, Spinler SA: Hyponatremia associated with selective serotonin-reuptake inhibitors in older adults. Ann Pharmacother 40(9):1618–1622, 2006 16896026

Jiang HY, Chen HZ, Hu XJ, et al: Use of selective serotonin reuptake inhibitors and risk of upper gastrointestinal bleeding: a systematic review and meta-analysis. Clin Gastroenterol Hepatol 13(1):42.e3–50.e3, 2015 24993365

Jiang WL, Cai DB, Yin F, et al: Adjunctive metformin for antipsychotic-induced dyslipidemia: a meta-analysis of randomized, double-blind, placebo-controlled trials. Transl Psychiatry 10(1):117, 2020 32327628

Johnson BA, Rosenthal N, Capece JA, et al: Topiramate for treating alcohol dependence: a randomized controlled trial. JAMA 298(14):1641–1651, 2007 17925516

Johnson EM, Whyte E, Mulsant BH, et al: Cardiovascular changes associated with venlafaxine in the treatment of late-life depression. Am J Geriatr Psychiatry 14(9):796–802, 2006 16943176

Justo D, Prokhorov V, Heller K, et al: Torsade de pointes induced by psychotropic drugs and the prevalence of its risk factors. Acta Psychiatr Scand 111(3):171–176, 2005 15701100

Kane JM, Durgam S, Satlin A, et al: Safety and tolerability of lumateperone for the treatment of schizophrenia: a pooled analysis of late-phase placebo- and active-controlled clinical trials. Int Clin Psychopharmacol 36(5):244–250, 2021 34054112

Kang HJ, Bae KY, Kim SW, et al: Effects of escitalopram on anxiety in patients with acute coronary syndrome: a randomized controlled trial. Clin Psychopharmacol Neurosci 15(2):126–131, 2017 28449559

Kaufmann MW, Cassem N, Murray G, et al: The use of methylphenidate in depressed patients after cardiac surgery. J Clin Psychiatry 45(2):82–84, 1984 6693366

Keller S, Frishman WH: Neuropsychiatric effects of cardiovascular drug therapy. Cardiol Rev 11(2):73–93, 2003 12620132

Kennebäck G, Bergfeldt L, Vallin H, et al: Electrophysiologic effects and clinical hazards of carbamazepine treatment for neurologic disorders in patients with abnormalities of the cardiac conduction system. Am Heart J 121(5):1421–1429, 1991 2017974

Kennebäck G, Bergfeldt L, Tomson T: Electrophysiological evaluation of the sodium-channel blocker carbamazepine in healthy human subjects. Cardiovasc Drugs Ther 9(5):709–714, 1995 8573554

Kim JM, Bae KY, Stewart R, et al: Escitalopram treatment for depressive disorder following acute coronary syndrome: a 24-week double-blind, placebo-controlled trial. J Clin Psychiatry 76(1):62–68, 2015 25375836

Kim JM, Stewart R, Kang HJ, et al: Long-term cardiac outcomes of depression screening, diagnosis and treatment in patients with acute coronary syndrome: the DEPACS study. Psychol Med 51(6):964–974, 2021 31907104

Ko DT, Hebert PR, Coffey CS, et al: Beta-blocker therapy and symptoms of depression, fatigue, and sexual dysfunction. JAMA 288(3):351–357, 2002 12117400

Kuehn BM: FDA: antipsychotics risky for elderly. JAMA 300(4):379–380, 2008 18647971

Laporte S, Chapelle C, Caillet P, et al: Bleeding risk under selective serotonin reuptake inhibitor (SSRI) antidepressants: a meta-analysis of observational studies. Pharmacol Res 118:19–32, 2017 27521835

Lazar RM, Shapiro PA, Moskowitz A, et al: Randomized trial of on- vs off-pump CABG reveals baseline memory dysfunction. Paper presented at the annual meeting of the American Heart Association, Anaheim, CA, November 2001

Lespérance F, Frasure-Smith N, Koszycki D, et al: Effects of citalopram and interpersonal psychotherapy on depression in patients with coronary artery disease: the Canadian Cardiac Randomized Evaluation of Antidepressant and Psychotherapy Efficacy (CREATE) trial. JAMA 297(4):367–379, 2007 17244833

Liang EF, Lim SZ, Tam WW, et al: The effect of methylphenidate and atomoxetine on heart rate and systolic blood pressure in young people and adults with attention-deficit hyperactivity disorder (ADHD): systematic review, meta-analysis, and meta-regression. Int J Environ Res Public Health 15(8):E1789, 2018 30127314

Liperoti R, Gambassi G, Lapane KL, et al: Conventional and atypical antipsychotics and the risk of hospitalization for ventricular arrhythmias or cardiac arrest. Arch Intern Med 165(6):696–701, 2005 15795349

Lopez-Vilchez I, Jerez-Dolz D, Diaz-Ricart M, et al: Escitalopram impairs thrombin-induced platelet response, cytoskeletal assembly and activation of associated signalling pathways. Thromb Haemost 117(12):2312–2321, 2017 29212119

Mackin P: Cardiac side effects of psychiatric drugs. Hum Psychopharmacol 23(Suppl 1):3–14, 2008 18098218

Malik J, Shahid AW, Shah M, et al: Outcome of angiotensin receptor-neprilysin inhibitor on anxiety and depression in heart failure with reduced ejection fraction vs. heart failure with preserved ejection fraction. J Community Hosp Intern Med Perspect 11(5):629–634, 2021 34567453

Malone DM, Lindesay J: Cholinesterase inhibitors and cardiovascular disease: a survey of old age psychiatrists' practice. Age Ageing 36(3):331–333, 2007 17350975

Mangusan RF, Hooper V, Denslow SA, et al: Outcomes associated with postoperative delirium after cardiac surgery. Am J Crit Care 24(2):156–163, 2015 25727276

Masand PS, Tesar GE: Use of stimulants in the medically ill. Psychiatr Clin North Am 19(3):515–547, 1996 8856815

Mladěnka P, Applová L, Patočka J, et al: Comprehensive review of cardiovascular toxicity of drugs and related agents. Med Res Rev 38(4):1332–1403, 2018 29315692

Na KS, Jung HY, Cho SJ, et al: Can we recommend mirtazapine and bupropion for patients at risk for bleeding? A systematic review and meta-analysis. J Affect Disord 225:221–226, 2018 28841484

O'Connor CM, Jiang W, Kuchibhatla M, et al: Antidepressant use, depression, and survival in patients with heart failure. Arch Intern Med 168(20):2232–2237, 2008 19001200

O'Connor CM, Jiang W, Kuchibhatla M, et al: Safety and efficacy of sertraline for depression in patients with heart failure: results of the SADHART-CHF (Sertraline Against Depression and Heart Disease in Chronic Heart Failure) trial. J Am Coll Cardiol 56(9):692–699, 2010 20723799

Ojero-Senard A, Benevent J, Bondon-Guitton E, et al: A comparative study of QT prolongation with serotonin reuptake inhibitors. Psychopharmacology (Berl) 234(20):3075–3081, 2017 28770276

Park K, Kim S, Ko YJ, et al: Duloxetine and cardiovascular adverse events: a systematic review and meta-analysis. J Psychiatr Res 124:109–114, 2020 32135389

Peyre H, Hoertel N, Hatteea H, et al: Adulthood self-reported cardiovascular risk and ADHD medications: results from the 2004–2005 National Epidemiologic Survey on Alcohol and Related Conditions. J Clin Psychiatry 75(2):181–182, 2014 24602253

Pillinger T, McCutcheon RA, Vano L, et al: Comparative effects of 18 antipsychotics on metabolic function in patients with schizophrenia, predictors of metabolic dysregulation, and association with psychopathology: a systematic review and network meta-analysis. Lancet Psychiatry 7(1):64–77, 2020 31860457

Pollock BG, Laghrissi-Thode F, Wagner WR: Evaluation of platelet activation in depressed patients with ischemic heart disease after paroxetine or nortriptyline treatment. J Clin Psychopharmacol 20(2):137–140, 2000 10770450

Qirjazi E, McArthur E, Nash DM, et al: Risk of ventricular arrhythmia with citalopram and escitalopram: a population-based study. PLoS One 11(8):e0160768, 2016 27513855

Quinn GR, Hellkamp AS, Hankey GJ, et al: Selective serotonin reuptake inhibitors and bleeding risk in anticoagulated patients with atrial fibrillation: an analysis from the ROCKET AF trial. J Am Heart Assoc 7(15):e008755, 2018 30371223

Ranta A, Wooten GF: Hyponatremia due to an additive effect of carbamazepine and thiazide diuretics (letter). Epilepsia 45(7):879, 2004 15230718

Ray WA, Chung CP, Murray KT, et al: Atypical antipsychotic drugs and the risk of sudden cardiac death. N Engl J Med 360(3):225–235, 2009 19144938

Repova K, Aziriova S, Krajcirovicova K, et al: Cardiovascular therapeutics: a new potential for anxiety treatment? Med Res Rev 42(3):1202–1245, 2022 34993995

Robinson MJ, Owen JA: Psychopharmacology, in The American Psychiatric Publishing Textbook of Psychosomatic Medicine. Edited by Levenson JL. Washington, DC, American Psychiatric Publishing, 2005, pp 871–922

Rochon PA, Normand S-L, Gomes T, et al: Antipsychotic therapy and short-term serious events in older adults with dementia. Arch Intern Med 168(10):1090–1096, 2008 18504337

Roose SP, Glassman AH: Cardiovascular effects of tricyclic antidepressants in depressed patients with and without heart disease. J Clin Psychiatry 50(Suppl):S1–S18, 1989

Roose SP, Dalack GW, Glassman AH, et al: Cardiovascular effects of bupropion in depressed patients with heart disease. Am J Psychiatry 148(4):512–516, 1991 1900980

Rosner MH: Severe hyponatremia associated with the combined use of thiazide diuretics and selective serotonin reuptake inhibitors. Am J Med Sci 327(2):109–111, 2004 14770031

Sato Y, Yoshihisa A, Hotsuki Y, et al: Associations of benzodiazepine with adverse prognosis in heart failure patients with insomnia. J Am Heart Assoc 9(7):e013982, 2020 32200713

Sepehripour AH, Eckersley M, Jiskani A, et al: Selective serotonin reuptake inhibitor use and outcomes following cardiac surgery: a systematic review. J Thorac Dis 10(2):1112–1120, 2018 29607188

Serebruany VL, Glassman AH, Malinin AI, et al: Platelet/endothelial biomarkers in depressed patients treated with the selective serotonin reuptake inhibitor sertraline after acute coronary events: the Sertraline AntiDepressant Heart Attack Randomized Trial (SADHART) platelet substudy. Circulation 108(8):939–944, 2003a 12912814

Serebruany VL, Glassman AH, Malinin AI, et al: Selective serotonin reuptake inhibitors yield additional antiplatelet protection in patients with congestive heart failure treated with antecedent aspirin. Eur J Heart Fail 5(4):517–521, 2003b 12921813

Service JA, Waring WS: QT prolongation and delayed atrioventricular conduction caused by acute ingestion of trazodone. Clin Toxicol (Phila) 46(1):71–73, 2008 18167038

Shapiro PA, Lespérance F, Frasure-Smith N, et al: An open-label preliminary trial of sertraline for treatment of major depression after acute myocardial infarction (the SADHAT Trial). Sertraline Anti-Depressant Heart Attack Trial. Am Heart J 137(6):1100–1106, 1999 10347338

Strain JJ, Caliendo G, Alexis JD, et al: Cardiac drug and psychotropic drug interactions: significance and recommendations. Gen Hosp Psychiatry 21(6):408–429, 1999 10664901

Strain JJ, Karim A, Caliendo G, et al: Cardiac drug-psychotropic drug update. Gen Hosp Psychiatry 24(5):283–289, 2002 12220794

Tadrous M, Shakeri A, Chu C, et al: Assessment of stimulant use and cardiovascular event risks among older adults. JAMA Netw Open 4(10):e2130795, 2021 34694389

Tampi RR, Balderas M, Carter KV, et al: Citalopram, QTc prolongation, and torsades de pointes. Psychosomatics 56(1):36–43, 2015 25619672

Taneja I, Diedrich A, Black BK, et al: Modafinil elicits sympathomedullary activation. Hypertension 45(4):612–618, 2005 15753235

Taylor CB, Youngblood ME, Catellier D, et al: Effects of antidepressant medication on morbidity and mortality in depressed patients after myocardial infarction. Arch Gen Psychiatry 62(7):792–798, 2005 15997021

Tellone V, Rosignoli MT, Picollo R, et al: Effect of 3 single doses of trazodone on QTc interval in healthy subjects. J Clin Pharmacol 60(11):1483–1495, 2020 32488885

Tomasoni D, Adamo M, Lombardi CM, et al: Highlights in heart failure. ESC Heart Fail 6(6):1105–1127, 2019 31997538

Tran PN, Sheng J, Randolph AL, et al: Mechanisms of QT prolongation by buprenorphine cannot be explained by direct hERG channel block. PLoS One 15(11):e0241362, 2020 33157550

van Melle JP, Verbeek DEP, van den Berg MP, et al: Beta-blockers and depression after myocardial infarction: a multicenter prospective study. J Am Coll Cardiol 48(11):2209–2214, 2006 17161247

van Melle JP, de Jonge P, Honig A, et al: Effects of antidepressant treatment following myocardial infarction. Br J Psychiatry 190:460–466, 2007 17541103

von Känel R, Schmid JP, Meister-Langraf RE, et al: Pharmacotherapy in the management of anxiety and pain during acute coronary syndromes and the risk of developing symptoms of posttraumatic stress disorder. J Am Heart Assoc 10(2):e018762, 2021 33432839

Wang M, Zeraatkar D, Obeda M, et al: Drug-drug interactions with warfarin: a systematic review and meta-analysis. Br J Clin Pharmacol 87(11):4051–4100, 2021 33769581

Wernicke J, Lledó A, Raskin J, et al: An evaluation of the cardiovascular safety profile of duloxetine: findings from 42 placebo-controlled studies. Drug Saf 30(5):437–455, 2007 17472422

Wilens TE, Hammerness PG, Biederman J, et al: Blood pressure changes associated with medication treatment of adults with attention-deficit/hyperactivity disorder. J Clin Psychiatry 66(2):253–259, 2005 15705013

Wilkins MR, Wharton J, Grimminger F, et al: Phosphodiesterase inhibitors for the treatment of pulmonary hypertension. Eur Respir J 32(1):198–209, 2008 18591337

Williams S, Wynn G, Cozza K, et al: Cardiovascular medications. Psychosomatics 48(6):537–547, 2007 18071104

Zivin K, Pfeiffer PN, Bohnert ASB, et al: Evaluation of the FDA warning against prescribing citalopram at doses exceeding 40 mg. Am J Psychiatry 170(6):642–650, 2013 23640689

7

Respiratory Disorders

Yvette L. Smolin, M.D.
Catherine Daniels-Brady, M.D.

The modern era of treatment for depression was ushered in by the serendipitous discovery in 1952 that iproniazid, a potential antitubercular agent, caused an elevation of mood in patients with tuberculosis (TB; Lieberman 2003). Iproniazid was a poor antitubercular drug, but its secondary activity as a monoamine oxidase inhibitor opened the door to the use of drugs to treat depression.

In this chapter, we focus on asthma, chronic obstructive pulmonary disease (COPD), cystic fibrosis, TB, obstructive sleep apnea (OSA), and vocal cord dysfunction (VCD). In addition, we include aspects of coronavirus SARS-CoV-2 (COVID-19) that pertain to these patients. For both psychological and physiological reasons, patients with these disorders may present with symptoms that are a focus of psychopharmacological treatment (Table 7–1). Most conditions discussed (except cystic fibrosis) do not alter the metabolism of pulmonary or other drugs. The main concern is to avoid medica-

307

Table 7–1.   Psychiatric symptoms often associated with respiratory diseases

Respiratory disease	Symptoms
Asthma	Anxiety, depression, substance abuse (marijuana, crack cocaine), sleep disturbance
Chronic obstructive pulmonary disease	Anxiety, depression, chronic tobacco use, cognitive impairment, sleep disturbance, sexual dysfunction, fatigue
Cystic fibrosis	Depression, anxiety, eating disorder
Functional respiratory disorders	
Vocal cord dysfunction	Stress, anxiety, depression, conversion disorder
Hyperventilation syndrome	Anxiety, depression, pseudoseizures
Sleep apnea	Somnolence, sleep disturbance, irritability, depression, cognitive impairment
Tuberculosis	Psychosis, sleep disturbance, substance abuse, cognitive impairment, fatigue, lethargy, mania, delirium

tions that decrease respiratory drive or otherwise adversely affect ventilation. Psychiatric side effects of the medications used to treat pulmonary disease and drug-drug interactions are also reviewed.

Differential Diagnostic Considerations

All respiratory disorders discussed in this chapter are frequently associated with psychiatric symptoms that may warrant psychotropic medication. There is a complex interplay between psychiatric conditions and pulmonary diseases, with comorbidities often found to have a bidirectional association (Atlantis et al. 2013; Del Giacco et al. 2016). These comorbidities may occur because of the following factors: reaction to an illness and treatment, direct physiological consequence of an illness, complication of treatment, or psychiatric illness that may coincide with the respiratory illness without being etiologically related. Which diagnosis came first may be difficult to determine.

Anxiety

Patients with pulmonary disease often experience anxiety. These anxiety symptoms may be due to a comorbid anxiety disorder, an anxious response to a respiratory disease, an anxious response to the treatment of the disease, or the respiratory disease itself. Differentiation is important whenever possible; if the symptoms have a physiological basis (e.g., hypoxia), then this condition must be treated, either independently or in conjunction with treatment of the associated anxiety. Anxiety symptoms of air hunger, suffocation, chest tightness, or shortness of breath are similar in both panic disorder and respiratory illness, which can confound the diagnosis and treatment (Meuret et al. 2017). Anxiety disorders occur in 26% of patients with cystic fibrosis and almost one-third of asthmatic patients in outpatient settings (Ciprandi et al. 2015; Guta et al. 2021). There is a likelihood of bidirectional causality in that asthma precedes the onset of anxiety with similar frequency as anxiety precedes asthma (Del Giacco et al. 2016). Theophylline and many β agonists may induce or exacerbate anxiety (LiverTox 2020; Sher 2017). In addition, theophylline and psychosocial risk factors may contribute to an increase in suicidal ideation, independent of depressive disorders (Favreau et al. 2012). There is a higher risk of anxiety and panic disorder in patients with COPD, and recognition early in treatment can lead to an improvement in the patient's quality of life (Pothirat et al. 2015). There is an association between PTSD and asthma, but the mechanism of action remains unclear (Allgire et al. 2021; Hung et al. 2019).

Depression

The evaluation of depression in a patient with respiratory illness poses challenges in that it is sometimes difficult to determine whether the vegetative symptoms of depression (weight loss, fatigue, poor sleep, loss of interest in activities) are evidence of the psychiatric disorder, symptoms of the somatic disorder, or both (Pachi et al. 2013). Recognizing and treating depression in a timely manner may improve the patient's adherence with respiratory treatment. In patients with the pulmonary diseases discussed in this chapter, the prevalence of depression is higher than in the general population. The prevalence of depression has been reported as 27% in patients with COPD (Matte et al. 2016); 13% in patients with cystic fibrosis (Guta et al. 2021); 16% in those with asthma, with the additional caveat of increased risk of suicidal ideation regardless of severity (Vazquez et al. 2021); 41% in patients with TB (Shyamala et al. 2018); and 23% in patients with OSA (Jackson et al. 2019).

Sleep Disturbance

Sleep is an important activity needed to sustain mental and physical health. Disturbances may be caused by dyspnea or other respiratory symptoms, nicotine use or withdrawal, hypoxia-driven sympathetic activity, comorbid anxiety and depression, medication (i.e., β agonists), and sleep disorders such as sleep-disordered breathing, sleep apnea, snoring, and restless legs syndrome (Budhiraja et al. 2015). The association between anxiety, depression, and insomnia is probably bidirectional (Garbarino et al. 2020). OSA occurs in 10%–30% of people with COPD. This occurrence, called *overlap syndrome*, is found in 1% of the general population (McNicholas 2016). These patients have greater nocturnal desaturation, increased sleep time, and worse sleep quality, more so than if they had just one of the conditions (Shawon et al. 2017). In addition, overlap syndrome increases the risk of cardiovascular disease, thus increasing mortality (Singh et al. 2018). Anxiety and depression are more severe in patients with OSA and COPD than in patients with just COPD (Zhao et al. 2022). Similarly, there is a relationship between OSA and severe asthma whereby they share pathophysiological factors and bidirectional interactions. They both promote inflammatory responses by means of hypoxia, hypercapnia, and sleep fragmentation, resulting in an increase in C-reactive protein (Ragnoli et al. 2021).

Cognitive Deficits

Decreased pulmonary function contributes to decreased cognitive function (Emery et al. 2012). Up to 60% of people with COPD have signs of cognitive dysfunction (Dobric et al. 2022). These include impairments in executive function, memory, and attention, all of which affect older adults more (Tudorache et al. 2017). The most likely causes of cognitive dysfunction in COPD are hypoxia or hypercapnia, chronic inflammatory state, and oxidative stress (Dobric et al. 2022). OSA, a prevalent sleep-related breathing disorder, is associated with long-term health consequences such as hypertension, heart disease, diabetes, depression, metabolic disorders, and stroke. OSA can affect attention and vigilance, memory and learning, emotional regulation, and executive functioning. Continuous positive airway pressure (CPAP) appears to mitigate and slow the rate of cognitive decline (Morsy et al. 2019). Cognitive impairment is also observed in adults with asthma and is more prevalent in older people and those with longer duration of the disease and poorer lung function (Rhyou and Nam 2021).

COVID-19

COVID-19 causes pulmonary disease in humans ranging in severity from mild respiratory symptoms to severe pneumonia and respiratory failure necessitating ventilator support. There is a complex interplay between psychiatric symptoms and COVID-19. These symptoms can result from psychological reactions to the virus and its treatment, physiological consequences of COVID, complications of treatment, or psychiatric illness that is independent of the medical condition. Acutely, patients can experience anxiety, depression, and delirium (López-Atanes et al. 2021), as well as agitation, paranoia, and psychosis (Ferrando et al. 2020).

Although patients using ventilators experience the distress of being mechanically ventilated, patients with COVID also may not be able to see family and friends and sometimes are kept at a distance by staff so as not to spread the virus. Those with pulmonary disease at home can experience increased anxiety, depression, PTSD, and insomnia because of isolation and fear of the illness.

Neuropsychiatric Side Effects of Drugs Used to Treat Respiratory Diseases

Medications used to treat respiratory illnesses often cause neuropsychiatric side effects. These drugs and side effects are discussed in detail in this section and are summarized in Table 7–2.

Antibiotics

Antibiotics are used to treat infections associated with asthma, COPD, and cystic fibrosis. Although they usually have minimal side effects, case studies have reported psychosis, mania, delirium, and changes in behavior related to antibiotic treatment (Essali and Miller 2020; Meszaros et al. 2021; Palma-Alvarez et al. 2020). Psychiatric side effects of antibiotics are discussed in detail in Chapter 12, "Infectious Diseases."

Table 7–2. Neuropsychiatric side effects of medications used to treat respiratory diseases

Medication	Side effects
Antibiotics	Minimal side effects: rare cases of psychosis, mania, delirium, or mental status changes
Anticholinergics	
Atropine	Paranoia; tactile, visual, and auditory hallucinations; memory loss; delirium; agitation
Antituberculars	
Cycloserine and isoniazid	Depression, hallucinations, psychosis
Ethambutol	Confusion; auditory and visual hallucinations (rare)
Rifampin	May reduce effectiveness of other medications
Bronchodilators	
β Agonists	
Albuterol and levalbuterol	Anxiety, insomnia, paranoia, hallucinations, tremor, palpitations
Formoterol and arformoterol	Insomnia, anxiety, tremor, palpitations
Isoproterenol	Anxiety, insomnia, tremor
Metaproterenol	Anxiety, insomnia
Pirbuterol	Anxiety, tremor
Salmeterol	Anxiety, tremor, palpitations
Other bronchodilators	
Theophylline and aminophylline	Anxiety, insomnia, tremor, restlessness, withdrawal, hyperactivity, psychosis, delirium, mutism

Table 7–2.   Neuropsychiatric side effects of medications used to treat respiratory diseases *(continued)*

Medication	Side effects
Corticosteroids	
Inhaled	Uncommon
Oral (e.g., prednisone, prednisolone, dexamethasone)	Depression, mania, lability, anxiety, insomnia, psychosis, hallucinations, paranoia, personality changes
Leukotriene inhibitors	
Montelukast, zafirlukast, and zileuton	Fatigue, asthenia, suicidal ideation
Mixed α and β agonists	
Epinephrine	Anxiety, tremor, psychosis
Phenylephrine	Depression, hallucinations, paranoia
Phenylpropanolamine	Restlessness, anxiety, insomnia, psychosis, hallucinations, aggressiveness

Source.   American Thoracic Society et al. 2003; Breen et al. 2006; Flume et al. 2007; Pachi et al. 2013; Polosa 2008; Thompson and Sullivan 2006.

Anticholinergics

Atropine, an anticholinergic that is used rarely for the treatment of asthma, can cause paranoia; visual, tactile, and auditory hallucinations; memory loss; delirium; and agitation (Lakstygal et al. 2019). Inhaled tiotropium, also an anticholinergic, has a duration of action that is much longer than that of ipratropium bromide, which has not been reported to cause psychiatric side effects.

Antitubercular Drugs

Drugs such as isoniazid and cycloserine produce side effects such as depression, hallucinations, and psychosis (Chand et al. 2019; Sharma et al. 2014; Yadav and Rawal 2019). There is a single case report of a drug-induced violent suicide (Behara et al. 2014). Rifampin, another antitubercular drug, may reduce the effectiveness of other medications by increasing enzyme induction actions. Ethambutol can cause confusion, and there have been case reports of this drug causing auditory or visual hallucinations (Doherty et al. 2013; Testa et al. 2013) and depressive disorders (Yen et al. 2015).

Bronchodilators

The most common side effects of the β-adrenergic bronchodilators are nervousness and tremor. Albuterol can also cause insomnia. Mixed α and β agonists are often used in over-the-counter asthma medications. Epinephrine, ephedrine, phenylephrine, and phenylpropanolamine can cause anxiety, insomnia, tremor, and, in high dosages, psychosis.

Aminophylline and Theophylline

Aminophylline is a less potent and shorter-acting xanthine than theophylline. These drugs can produce dose-related side effects such as anxiety, insomnia, tremor, psychosis, delirium, and mutism. Theophylline has a narrow therapeutic window. Adverse effects can occur even at therapeutic serum levels. This is one of the reasons that the use of theophylline has decreased significantly. Toxicity is characterized by marked anxiety, severe nausea, and insomnia and may progress to psychosis and delirium. When there are signs of toxicity, theophylline should be stopped until the symptoms abate and the blood level returns to the therapeutic range. Theophylline may induce tremor or exacerbate essential tremor. There is an association with an increased risk of suicide attempts by asthmatic adults taking theophylline, which should be considered when this medication is being prescribed (Favreau et al. 2012). This can occur even in patients with no psychiatric history (Kapoor et al. 2015).

Corticosteroids

It is uncommon to have side effects from inhaled steroids. Steroids such as prednisone, prednisolone, and dexamethasone can produce neuropsychiatric symptoms that are probably dose related. The side effects can include euphoria, irritability, anxiety, mania, psychosis, delirium, and mixed states. Cognitive deficits can also occur (Dubovsky et al. 2012; Judd et al. 2014). Discontinuation of long-term glucocorticoid therapy is associated with increased risk of depression, delirium, and confusion (Fardet et al. 2013). There are case reports of persistent side effects long after corticosteroids were discontinued (Gable and Depry 2015; Roxanas 2018). Corticosteroid-induced psychiatric symptoms are reviewed in more detail in Chapter 10, "Endocrine and Metabolic Disorders."

Leukotriene Inhibitors

Montelukast, zafirlukast, and zileuton are leukotriene inhibitors, which can cause fatigue, dizziness, and suicidal ideation, as well as sleep disorders, behavioral disorders, and depression. The most recent evidence suggests that there is no association between modifying agents and suicide (Khalid et al. 2018; Law et al. 2018).

Drugs for COVID-19

Many different drugs have been used against COVID-19, some despite no evidence of efficacy. Psychiatric side effects of antibiotics, hydroxychloroquine/chloroquine, antivirals, ivermectin, and corticosteroids are covered elsewhere in this book.

There is no evidence of psychiatric side effects with remdesivir (Gulati and Kelly 2021) or baricitinib. Sotrovimab can cause an infusion reaction that includes altered mental status.

Alteration of Pharmacokinetics

For the most part, respiratory illnesses do not affect pharmacokinetics, with one major exception: cystic fibrosis. Cystic fibrosis–related abnormalities in cellular ion transport may alter drug pharmacokinetics because of abnormalities in the ion transport function of the cell membrane. The rate of drug absorption is slowed, but the extent of absorption is generally unchanged, and bioavailability and volume of distribution are unaffected (Akkerman-Nijland et al. 2021). Cystic fibrosis increases oxidative hepatic metabolism, but only for drug substrates of cytochrome P450 1A2 (CYP1A2) and CYP2C8; metabolism by other cytochromes is unchanged (Rey et al. 1998). There is little in the literature about the use of lithium by patients with cystic fibrosis, and what is there is contradictory. Brager et al. (1996) reported that renal clearance is reduced, resulting in higher lithium levels. However, in a case reported by Turkel and Cafaro (1992), no alteration in the lithium level occurred with standard dosages. It appears prudent for patients with cystic fibrosis to be started on a low dosage of lithium, with careful monitoring to avoid toxicity.

Smoking affects both the pharmacodynamics and the pharmacokinetics of many drugs. Smoking-induced bronchoconstriction is countertherapeutic, resulting in a poorer response to bronchodilators. In addition, the therapeutic response to corticosteroids is impaired in smokers with asthma compared with nonsmokers with asthma and in patients with COPD (Braganza et al. 2008). Smoking induces CYP1A2, which increases the metabolism of drug substrates of this hepatic enzyme, including clozapine, olanzapine, duloxetine, fluvoxamine, and theophylline (Moschny et al. 2021). Unless drug dosage is increased accordingly, lower, possibly subtherapeutic, drug levels will result. If the patient stops smoking, a week or more is needed before CYP1A2 activity declines to normal (Kroon 2007). In this case, a dosage reduction of substrate drugs may be necessary to prevent toxicity. Switching from tobacco to an electronic delivery system can increase the serum level of medications metabolized by the CYP1A2 system, such as clozapine. One patient experienced rebound psychosis, probably from switching back and forth between tobacco delivery systems (Montville et al. 2021).

Effects of Psychotropic Drugs on Pulmonary Function

Antidepressants

The safety of commonly used antidepressants in respiratory disease can be inferred from some recent studies of antidepressants used to treat chronic dyspnea of various etiologies. Although Currow et al. (2019) did not find a positive effect of sertraline in the treatment of chronic breathlessness, no adverse effects of sertraline were reported in this patient population, which included patients with various medical diagnoses. Mirtazapine may reduce breathlessness by specifically reducing activity in fear circuits in the brain (Lovell et al. 2019). One study has specifically looked at mirtazapine for use in chronic breathlessness, finding that there were few adverse events in patients who received mirtazapine (Higginson et al. 2020).

There have been individual case reports of eosinophilic pneumonia associated with various antidepressants, including sertraline, fluoxetine, duloxetine, venlafaxine, and amitriptyline, but this appears to be a very rare adverse event (Adhikari et al. 2020; Bartal et al. 2018; De Giacomi et al. 2018). Interstitial lung disease is a rare condition that is known to be triggered in some cases by drug exposure. Recent cases and case series show an association between interstitial lung disease and selective serotonin reuptake inhibitors (SSRIs), including fluoxetine and sertraline (Deidda et al. 2017; Izhakian et al. 2021). A case-control series showed significantly higher rates of SSRI and serotonin-norepinephrine reuptake inhibitor (SNRI) use in patients diagnosed with interstitial lung disease, although causality could not be inferred because of the retrospective design of this study (Rosenberg et al. 2017).

Esketamine has no known respiratory side effects, although it may cause sedation. The major concerns with monoamine oxidase inhibitors are drug-drug interactions, which are addressed later in the chapter in the section "Drug-Drug Interactions."

Anxiolytics and Sedative-Hypnotics

Respiratory depression resulting from sedative-hypnotics and opioids is the most common adverse respiratory effect associated with psychotropic medications. The respiratory depressant effects of benzodiazepines can significantly reduce the ventilatory response to hypoxia. This may precipitate respiratory failure in a patient with marginal respiratory reserve and contraindicates their use by patients with carbon dioxide retention.

Recent studies confirm the risk of combining opioids with sedative-hypnotic drugs (Cho et al. 2020). Combining opioids and benzodiazepines or nonbenzodiazepine benzodiazepine receptor agonists (z-drugs) is dangerous; combining trazodone with opioids has been shown to be safer (Ray et al. 2021). Reports are mixed regarding the safety of benzodiazepines in COPD, with studies raising significant concerns about the potential of benzodiazepines to decrease tidal volume, oxygen saturation, and minute ventilation. Benzodiazepines may also depress respiratory functions that maintain homeostasis of blood gases during sleep (Roth 2009). A prospective cohort study showed that in patients with COPD receiving long-term oxygen therapy, benzodiazepine use was associated with a 20% increase in mortality over patients who did not use benzodiazepines (Ekström et al. 2014). Benzodiazepines also may precipitate cough. Zolpidem did not impair respiratory drive or pulmonary function tests in patients with mild to moderate COPD (Girault et al. 1996). One small randomized controlled trial showed ramelteon to be free of respiratory effects in patients with moderate to severe COPD (Kryger et al. 2009). The oxrexin antagonists suvorexant and lemborexant do not appear to cause a drop in blood oxygenation or an increase in apnea-hypopnea index at usual or high dosages (Cheng et al. 2020; Uemura et al. 2015).

In the treatment of alcohol withdrawal, barbiturate use is not associated with more respiratory depression than benzodiazepine use (Mo et al. 2016); however, barbiturates, especially phenobarbital, should be avoided by patients with impaired respiratory drive, severe COPD, or OSA. Chronic treatment of epilepsy with phenobarbital may be an exception. Attention is required when combining sedating antidepressants and other sedating drugs such as anxiolytics and sedative-hypnotics in patients with severe COPD or OSA; the additive sedating effects may reduce respiratory drive.

In a small randomized controlled trial in patients with mild COPD, buspirone was shown to increase exercise tolerance and reduce the sensation of dyspnea (Argyropoulou et al. 1993). Buspirone was also reported to be well tolerated in combination with bronchodilators (Kiev and Domantay 1988). Buspirone reduced the occurrence of central apnea in patients with heart failure or spinal cord injury, by decreasing their sensitivity to carbon dioxide (Giannoni et al. 2021; Maresh et al. 2020). Buspirone was not found to be helpful for symptomatic dyspnea in patients with cancer (Peoples et al. 2016). No major safety concerns have emerged in studies of buspirone.

Antipsychotics

Patients using antipsychotics have been found to have a twofold higher risk of acute respiratory failure; this risk was dose dependent (Wang et al. 2020). In a Canadian study, patients using atypical antipsychotics were found to have a significantly greater risk of death or near death from asthma (Joseph et al. 1996). Patients who had recently discontinued antipsychotic use were at a particularly high risk. Patients with asthma and COPD are particularly susceptible to cardiac arrhythmias (De Bruin et al. 2003). If antipsychotic drugs are used, those most likely to cause QTc interval prolongation (ziprasidone, thioridazine) should be avoided, or the patients should be monitored. Abrupt discontinuation of antipsychotics with significant anticholinergic activity, such as clozapine, may cause cholinergic rebound, reducing the effectiveness of anticholinergic asthma medication (Szafrański and Gmurkowski 1999). Acute pulmonary edema[1] as been reported with phenothiazine overdose (Li and Gefter 1992).

In the last several decades, several studies have shown a correlation between antipsychotic use and pulmonary embolism and venous thromboembolism (VTE) (Barbui et al. 2014; Conti et al. 2015). A recent meta-analysis of 28 studies found a 50% increase in VTE and a greater than threefold increase in pulmonary embolism in patients receiving antipsychotics, but caution is warranted in interpreting the results because of high heterogeneity among studies (Liu et al. 2021). The results included that younger patients are at higher risk for VTE, that low-potency agents are more associated with VTE than are higher-potency agents, and that the risk is higher early in the course of treatment with antipsychotics (Di et al. 2021; Liu et al. 2021). During anticoagulation treatment after an episode of VTE, antipsychotic prescription was not associated with a recurrent episode of VTE (Ferraris et al. 2019).

Laryngeal dystonia, presenting as acute dyspnea, is a rare form of acute dystonic reaction. It is usually associated with high-potency typical antipsychotics but has also been reported with atypical antipsychotics (Erdoğan and İlhan 2022; Ganesh et al. 2015). It generally occurs, like other dystonic reactions, within 24–48 hours after antipsychotic therapy is initiated or, in a small number of cases, when dosage is increased. The reaction can be life-threatening but usually responds dramatically to intramuscular injection of anticholinergic agents. Tardive laryngeal dystonia has also been very rarely reported (Jiwanmall et al. 2021). Tardive dyskinesia affecting the respiratory musculature is rare, generally occurs with long-term typical antipsychotic use, and can severely impede breathing in patients with reduced respiratory capacity (Jann and Bitar 1982; Kruk et al. 1995). Several cases of respiratory muscle dyskinesia were reported to occur when the antipsychotic drug was discontinued (e.g., Mendhekar and Inamdar 2010).

Weight gain caused by antipsychotics may further impair respiratory capacity in patients with decreased respiratory function, especially in restrictive lung disease. An FDA black box warning for antipsychotic medications cautions against their use by older adults with dementia because of increased risk for death secondary to cardiovascular complications and infection, particularly pneumonia. The latter effect may be due to aspiration of secretions secondary to sedation and dysphagia.

Mood Stabilizers

Carbamazepine may cause cough, dyspnea, pulmonary infiltrates, and idiopathic pulmonary fibrosis. Valproate has been reported to cause pleural effusion (most often eosinophilic) (Tryfon et al. 2021).

Psychostimulants

Methylphenidate has been reported to cause dyspnea, asthma, pulmonary infiltrates, respiratory failure from idiopathic pulmonary fibrosis, and pulmonary vascular disease (Ben-Noun 2000).

Cognitive Enhancers

There is scant literature on the use of cognitive enhancers in patients with respiratory illnesses. Several pulmonary side effects have been reported with these drugs, frequently dyspnea and bronchitis and infrequently pneumonia, hyperventilation, pulmonary congestion, wheezing, hypoxia, pleurisy, pulmonary collapse, sleep apnea, and snoring.

Prescribing Psychotropic Medications in Respiratory Disease

Asthma

Antidepressants

The SSRIs citalopram and escitalopram have been studied for the treatment of depression in patients with asthma in randomized, double-blind trials. In these studies, remission rates for depression were numerically higher, but not statistically significantly higher, in the active medication groups. Both SSRIs were well tolerated. Patients treated with citalopram or escitalopram had a significant decrease in corticosteroid use, suggesting that treating depression in patients with asthma may improve the asthma outcomes as well as mood (Brown et al. 2005, 2012, 2018). Treating patients with optimal dosages of antidepressant medications may be key to improving asthma-related outcomes in this population (Shoair et al. 2020). Depressed asthmatic patients receiving open-label bupropion experienced improvement in depressive and asthmatic symptoms (Brown et al. 2007), as did depressed and nondepressed patients treated with sertraline (Smoller et al. 1998). There are no studies of other antidepressants for use by patients with asthma.

Sedative-Hypnotics

One study found that benzodiazepine or zopiclone use by asthmatic patients was significantly associated with the occurrence of asthma exacerbations and an increase in 2-year all-cause mortality (Nakafero et al. 2015). In the hospital setting, dexmedetomidine may be a safer sedative for use in patients with asthma (Motamed et al. 2021). There are no studies of orexin receptor antagonists for insomnia in patients with respiratory disorders. Respiratory adverse events have not been frequently reported in studies of melatonin (Besag et al. 2019), although there are theoretical concerns that melatonin could have a net pro-inflammatory effect, especially in patients with nocturnal asthma (Marseglia et al. 2014).

Antipsychotics

Inhaled loxapine is contraindicated in patients with asthma (Teva Pharmaceuticals 2016). In a study of inhaled loxapine in patients with asthma, 53% of subjects experienced symptomatic bronchospasm of mild or moderate severity. Eleven of 15 of these respiratory events responded to rescue bronchodilator (albuterol) (Gross et al. 2014). There are no other published clinical trials of antipsychotics in patients with asthma.

Chronic Obstructive Pulmonary Disease

Antidepressants

The tricyclic antidepressant (TCA) nortriptyline was found to be safe and effective for depression and improved functional outcomes in COPD (Borson et al. 1992). There have been multiple other studies of SSRIs and TCAs in COPD patients with depression and anxiety, but these studies have been limited in utility because of methodological problems, and there is little clarity about the effectiveness of antidepressants in patients with COPD (Pollok et al. 2018; Yohannes and Alexopoulos 2014). The studies have not consistently shown improvements in respiratory symptoms or physiological measures of respiratory function in patients taking antidepressants. A retrospective cohort study (Vozoris et al. 2018) demonstrated that SSRI and SNRI users had a small but significant increase in the rate of hospital contact for COPD or pneumonia and an increase in mortality. At the same time, outpatient respiratory exacerbations were lower in SSRI and SNRI users. Patients with COPD taking antidepressant drugs should be closely followed up.

Sedative-Hypnotics

Benzodiazepine use in patients with COPD requires caution. Although benzodiazepines are very often prescribed to patients with COPD (Vozoris et al. 2014), reports of their safety are mixed (Roth 2009). Adverse respiratory effects of benzodiazepines in COPD are more likely to occur in older adults and in patients with more severe disease (Ekström et al. 2014; Vozoris et al. 2014). Studies of benzodiazepine use by patients with COPD show higher rates of various negative outcomes—outpatient COPD exacerbations, emergency department visits and inpatient hospitalizations for COPD, and pneumonia (Vozoris et al. 2014). Benzodiazepine prescription has been associated with a modest increase in mortality in patients who have severe COPD (Ekström et al. 2014).

Several studies have compared benzodiazepine use with nonbenzodiazepine sedative use (z-drugs). Z-drug use was associated with fewer outpatient exacerbations of COPD but no difference in mortality, emergency department visits, or inpatient admissions, compared with benzodiazepine use (Liao et al. 2020). In patients with episodes of respiratory failure, benzodiazepine users had a higher risk of respiratory failure than did z-drug users; in fact, patients who used more than one type of benzodiazepine or a benzodiazepine plus a z-drug had a twofold higher risk of respiratory failure (Chen et al. 2015). A population-based study showed similar rates of adverse respiratory events in patients with COPD who used benzodiazepines and those who used z-drugs (Chung et al. 2015). Overall, there are concerns about respiratory outcomes with both benzodiazepines and z-drugs.

Despite these findings, benzodiazepines should not be rejected automatically for use in all patients with COPD. A few small studies found short-term use of low-dose benzodiazepines safe in patients with stable normocapnic COPD and no comorbid sleep apnea (Stege et al. 2010). Anxiety can reduce respiratory efficiency, and benzodiazepines may actually improve respiratory status in some patients, especially those with asthma or emphysema ("pink puffers") (Mitchell-Heggs et al. 1980). In patients with stable, mild to moderate, normocapnic COPD, benzodiazepines show safety and efficacy on polysomnographic measures of sleep (Lu et al. 2016). In patients with stable COPD, zopiclone moderately increased carbon dioxide pressure without reducing minimum oxygen saturation and improved sleep quality. In patients with combined features of COPD and OSA, zopiclone reduced apnea and hypopnea (Holmedahl et al. 2015).

Particular caution must be exercised in patients with COPD who use both opioids and benzodiazepines, especially when initiating combined therapy. In a study of Medicare beneficiaries with COPD, patients were at higher risk for respiratory events and death in the first 60 days of combined use. Longer-term users actually had a lower risk of these adverse events, suggesting relative safety once the patient is acclimated to both types of medication (Le et al. 2020).

In patients with COPD, ramelteon and melatonin have been found to improve length of sleep and sleep quality with no worsening of pulmonary function (Halvani et al. 2013; Kryger et al. 2007). Limited data demonstrate the safety of the orexin antagonists suvorexant and daridorexant for patients with mild to moderate COPD (Boof et al. 2021; Sun et al. 2015).

Mood Stabilizers

There is a theoretical concern that the inhibition of histone deacetylase by valproic acid could worsen pulmonary function in patients with COPD. However, a study did not show an increase in hospital admissions or emergency department visits for COPD exacerbation or a change in the initiation of oral corticosteroids in patients commencing treatment with valproic acid versus phenytoin (Antoniou et al. 2015).

Antipsychotics

Patients with COPD have been rarely reported to experience respiratory failure after initiation of antipsychotic medication; however, in the first 2 weeks of antipsychotic use, the risk of acute respiratory failure is 66% higher in antipsychotic users compared with nonusers (Wang et al. 2017). Inhaled loxapine is contraindicated in patients with COPD (Teva Pharmaceuticals 2016). In a study of inhaled loxapine in patients with COPD, symptomatic bronchospasm of mild to moderate severity occurred in 19% of patients with COPD (Gross et al. 2014).

Cognitive Enhancers

Because of their cholinomimetic effects, cholinesterase inhibitors increase acetylcholine levels and would be expected to cause bronchoconstriction. Also, they are likely to block the therapeutic effects of bronchodilators, especially anticholinergic agents such as ipratropium and tiotropium. Results of studies have been mixed, with some showing an increase in COPD-related adverse events in new users of cholinesterase inhibitors and some showing no increase in adverse events (Mahan and Blaszczyk 2016; Stephenson et al. 2012). Caution is still advised in using cholinesterase inhibitors for patients with COPD; however, memantine does not have respiratory side effects.

Sleep Apnea

Antidepressants

In theory, increasing serotonin might increase the tone of upper airway muscles, ameliorating symptoms of OSA. In clinical practice, however, the effect of antidepressants on OSA is complex. SSRIs and TCAs have not been found to improve sleep parameters in patients with OSA (Smith et al. 2006). Trazodone has been studied in patients with OSA and has been found to have variable effects on measures such as apnea-hypopnea index and respiratory arousal threshold; it has not been associated with worsening hypoxemia (Eckert et al. 2014; Smales et al. 2015). Trazodone may be particularly helpful for patients with OSA who have had acute ischemic strokes; a small study showed that trazodone improved OSA severity and was well tolerated in poststroke patients (Chen et al. 2021). Mirtazapine has been found to reduce the apnea-hypopnea index but did not reduce sleepiness or sleep efficiency. It was found to cause an unacceptable level of lethargy and to cause weight gain, which are treatment-limiting side effects (AbdelFattah et al. 2020). Mirtazapine may worsen central and mixed sleep apnea in stroke patients (Brunner 2008).

Sedative-Hypnotics

Benzodiazepines are considered potentially harmful in patients with OSA. Benzodiazepine-induced respiratory suppression occurs when patients with OSA are awake as well as asleep, potentially prolonging sleep apneic episodes, with dangerous consequences. Benzodiazepines have muscle relaxant properties, which can increase upper airway collapsibility in patients with OSA (Jullian-Desayes et al. 2017). Apneic episodes may become longer and more frequent when patients with OSA take benzodiazepines (Mason et al. 2015).

Z-drugs have been shown to be relatively safe and effective in patients with OSA. Zolpidem and zopiclone have been shown to promote sleep in patients with severe OSA without reducing the efficiency of CPAP therapy (Berry and Patel 2006; Rosenberg et al. 2007). Caution is advised, as zolpidem at a dose of 20 mg is associated with decreasing oxygen saturation (Mason et al. 2015). Zaleplon use during CPAP titration in patients with OSA improves sleep latency without adverse effects on apnea-hypopnea index or oxygenation (Park et al. 2013). In patients with central sleep apnea, zolpidem caused an overall improvement in apnea or hypopnea and sleep efficiency; however, some patients had an increase in obstructive apneas while having fewer central apneas, highlighting the need for caution when treating this population (Quadri et al. 2009).

In patients with sleep apnea, the melatonin agonist ramelteon improved length of sleep with no worsening of their pulmonary function (Kryger et al. 2007). An industry-sponsored study did not find respiratory adverse effects of lemborexant in patients with mild-severity OSA (Cheng et al. 2020). Buspirone may improve the respiratory status of patients with sleep apnea (Mendelson et al. 1991).

Antipsychotics

Weight gain with olanzapine, quetiapine, and other atypical antipsychotics is particularly problematic for patients with OSA; the additional weight will worsen the sleep apnea. Additionally, antipsychotic medication may worsen indexes of sleep apnea through other mechanisms, such as effects on muscle tone (Khazaie et al. 2018).

Stimulants

Chronic respiratory illnesses often lead to insomnia and daytime sleepiness. The few studies of stimulants have been in sleep apnea. Modafinil and armodafinil are beneficial for patients with OSA. They can increase daytime wakefulness when used as an adjunctive treatment for patients with OSA and daytime sleepiness despite CPAP treatment. Driving performance and subjective sleepiness may improve, even for patients not receiving CPAP (Chapman et al. 2014; Kay and Feldman 2013). These medications are well tolerated in the OSA population (Chapman et al. 2016; Kuan et al. 2016). Atomoxetine improved wakefulness in patients with mild to moderate OSA without worsening the respiratory distress index (Bart Sangal et al. 2008). Despite these encouraging findings, psychostimulants should be used with caution in this population given the limited breadth of this literature and the increased risk for cardiac arrhythmia in chronic respiratory disease.

Cognitive Enhancers

Two small randomized, double-blind, placebo-controlled studies found that donepezil reduced sleep apnea, increased rapid eye movement sleep, and improved cognition in patients with Alzheimer's disease (Moraes et al. 2006,

2008). Two later investigations found no effect of donepezil on sleep parameters in patients who had OSA without Alzheimer's disease (Hunchaisri and Chalermsuwiwattanakan 2016; Li et al. 2016).

Cystic Fibrosis

Scant literature exists regarding the use of psychotropic medications by patients with cystic fibrosis. In theory, the anticholinergic effects of TCAs could exacerbate the difficulty that patients with cystic fibrosis have with clearing their secretions. However, there is interest in the use of amitriptyline as a therapeutic agent for cystic fibrosis, because of its ability to reduce fatty acid derivatives (ceramide) in the respiratory tract. Amitriptyline is safe and well tolerated by patients with cystic fibrosis and has been associated with improvements in indexes of lung function with long-term use (Adams et al. 2016; Nährlich et al. 2013; Riethmüller et al. 2009). In a single case study of lithium treatment for bipolar mania in a patient with cystic fibrosis, mood improved with no apparent effect on pulmonary function (Turkel and Cafaro 1992).

Vocal Cord Dysfunction

Benzodiazepines can be used to terminate a severe episode of VCD (Hicks et al. 2008). If a benzodiazepine is prescribed, reduced dosages of a shorter-acting benzodiazepine (e.g., lorazepam) should be used so that adverse effects are mild and rapidly reversible with drug discontinuation. Some evidence indicates that low-dose amitriptyline can be helpful and well tolerated to reduce symptoms of VCD (Varney et al. 2009).

COVID-19

SSRIs, especially fluoxetine and fluvoxamine, may reduce the risk of mortality from COVID-19, through anti-inflammatory mechanisms. The association is strongest if the medication is taken during the hospitalization for COVID rather than during the 3 months before infection. From these studies, it appears that it is safe to use antidepressant agents in patients with COVID-19 (Hoertel et al. 2021; Oskotsky et al. 2021). Caution should be exercised when patients with COVID who have respiratory distress use antipsychotic and sedative agents. Antipsychotic and anxiolytic drug exposure is associated with mortality in patients with COVID-19 (Ostuzzi et al. 2020; Vai et al. 2021).

Dyspnea in Advanced and Terminal Disease

Several pharmacological agents, including opioids, have been tried for patients with advanced pulmonary disease whose dyspnea could not be managed by treating the underlying disease. A meta-analysis of 16 small studies in COPD patients showed a statistically significant positive effect of opioids on the sensation of dyspnea, with no reported serious adverse outcomes. Opioids are more effective when administered orally or parenterally rather than nebulized (Ekström et al. 2015). Opioids have been found to be effective for dyspnea in advanced disease across indications and do not cause a clinically relevant increase in respiratory adverse effects (Barnes et al. 2016; Verberkt et al. 2017). Benzodiazepines are considered second- or third-line interventions for relief of dyspnea in patients with advanced disease, with the advantage that they may cause less sedation than morphine (Simon et al. 2016). Looking specifically at advanced cancer, a recent meta-analysis did not find overall usefulness of opioids or benzodiazepines, and although opioids were not found to be seriously harmful, they were associated with side effects (Feliciano et al. 2021). Overall, opioids and benzodiazepines should be used cautiously, weighing the risks and benefits for the individual patient. Opioids (usually morphine) are also used in terminal weaning from ventilatory support (Campbell 2007).

Drug-Drug Interactions

Several pharmacokinetic and pharmacodynamic drug interactions may occur between drugs prescribed for chronic respiratory disease and psychotropic drugs (Table 7–3).

It is important to note that smoking, a cause of or contributor to multiple respiratory illnesses, can increase the metabolism of multiple psychotropic drugs via induction of CYP1A2, CYP2B6, and CYP2D6 (Kroon 2007). This includes benzodiazepines, zolpidem, antipsychotics (notable exceptions are aripiprazole, quetiapine, risperidone, and ziprasidone), and antidepressants, including fluvoxamine, duloxetine, TCAs, and mirtazapine. Reduction or cessation of smoking may necessitate reduction in dosage of psychotropic medications whose metabolism has been induced. This lifting of metabolism inhibition as a result of smoking cessation should be taken into consideration for patients who remain in the hospital for more than 2 days (Chui et al. 2019).

Table 7–3.   Respiratory medication–psychotropic medication interactions

Medication	Interaction mechanism	Clinical effect
Anticholinergics		
Atropine (systemic)	Additive anticholinergic effect	Additive anticholinergic effects with TCAs, antipsychotics, and other anticholinergic agents. Countertherapeutic effects with cholinesterase inhibitor cognitive enhancers.
β Agonists		
Albuterol	QT prolongation	Increased QT interval: avoid QT-prolonging drugs (TCAs, antipsychotics [pimozide, quetiapine, risperidone, ziprasidone]).
Bronchodilators		
Theophylline	Increased renal clearance	Increased clearance and lower levels of renally eliminated drugs (lithium, gabapentin, pregabalin, paliperidone, memantine, desvenlafaxine).
Leukotriene inhibitors		
Zafirlukast	Moderate inhibitor of CYP2C9, CYP2C8, CYP3A4	Possible increased levels of carbamazepine, phenytoin, benzodiazepines, pimozide, quetiapine, ziprasidone.

Note.   CYP=cytochrome P450; TCAs=tricyclic antidepressants.
Source.   Wynn et al. 2009.

Many anti-infective agents, including macrolide and fluoroquinolone antibacterials and conazole antifungals, are potent inhibitors of one or more CYP isozymes, whereas several rifamycins such as rifampin induce multiple CYP enzymes. Anti-infective drugs can cause significant psychotropic drug toxicities or loss of therapeutic effect unless the psychotropic drug dosage is suitably adjusted.

Isoniazid, a TB drug, possesses some monoamine oxidase inhibitor properties; although only a single case exists of serotonin syndrome being caused by isoniazid plus a serotonergic antidepressant, dietary tyramine restriction should be used when isoniazid is combined with an antidepressant (DiMartini 1995; O'Brien et al. 2020). Inhaled β agonists appear to be safe to use because little is absorbed systemically. SSRI and SNRI antidepressants are safe to use with the selective β_2 agonists (e.g., terbutaline, metaproterenol, albuterol, isoetarine).

Elexacaftor/tezacaftor/ivacaftor (Trikafta), a new agent for cystic fibrosis, may increase the serum concentration of risperidone, and patients taking this combination should be closely monitored (Vertex Pharmaceuticals 2021). Theophylline can lower alprazolam and possibly other benzodiazepine levels (Tuncok et al. 1994) and may counteract the therapeutic effects of benzodiazepines by exacerbating anxiety and insomnia. Theophylline may also increase lithium clearance (Holstad et al. 1988); lithium levels should be monitored when these drugs are coadministered.

Several psychotropic medications, including TCAs, low-potency typical antipsychotics, and anticholinergic agents for extrapyramidal symptoms, have anticholinergic effects that may increase the bronchodilator effects of atropine and inhaled anticholinergic bronchodilators such as ipratropium and tiotropium.

Respiratory disease drugs are also susceptible to pharmacokinetic interactions from psychotropic drugs. Fluvoxamine inhibits CYP1A2 and can significantly increase theophylline levels (Dawson et al. 1995). Carbamazepine and phenobarbital, both general metabolic inducers, significantly reduce blood levels of many drugs, including Trikafta, theophylline, and doxycycline. St. John's wort is also a CYP1A2 inducer and can lower theophylline levels to subtherapeutic values (Hu et al. 2005).

Key Points

- Most antidepressants have little or no effect on respiratory status; however, anticholinergic antidepressants may have functional and bronchodilating benefits.

- Generally, sedating agents should be avoided in carbon dioxide retainers. If necessary, short-acting benzodiazepines with no active metabolites, prescribed at a low dosage, are best tolerated.

- Polypharmacy contributes to unwanted drug-drug interactions and increases the risk of respiratory side effects.

- Drugs known to cause QTc interval prolongation should be avoided in patients with asthma and chronic obstructive pulmonary disease. If these drugs are used, cardiac status should be carefully monitored.

- Smoking induces cytochrome P450 (CYP) 1A2, CYP2B6, and CYP2D6, thereby lowering the levels of many psychotropic medications. When smoking is reduced or stopped, or the delivery system is changed (i.e., e-cigarettes), psychotropic side effects and blood levels should be monitored and dosages adjusted as necessary.

- Rifampin induces metabolism of some psychiatric medications. Higher dosages of these psychiatric medications may be needed for adequate response in patients treated for tuberculosis.

- Isoniazid is a weak irreversible monoamine oxidase inhibitor that may cause serotonin syndrome or hypertensive crisis when combined with selective serotonin reuptake inhibitors and sympathomimetic psychotropics and agents used to treat pulmonary diseases.

- Theophylline has multiple activating psychiatric side effects. Its levels can be reduced by CYP1A2 inducers such as carbamazepine and increased by CYP1A2 inhibitors such as fluvoxamine.

- The side effects of steroids can include euphoria, irritability, depression, mania, psychosis, and mixed states. It is important to remember that discontinuation after long-term therapy can be associated with increased risk of depression, delirium, and confusion.

References

AbdelFattah MR, Jung SW, Greenspan MA, et al: Efficacy of antidepressants in the treatment of obstructive sleep apnea compared to placebo: a systematic review with meta-analyses. Sleep Breath 24(2):443–453, 2020 31720982

Adams C, Icheva V, Deppisch C, et al: Long-term pulmonal therapy of cystic fibrosis patients with amitriptyline. Cell Physiol Biochem 39(2):565–572, 2016 27395380

Adhikari P, Alexander K, Ademiluyi AO, et al: Sertraline-induced acute eosinophilic pneumonia. Cureus 12(12):e12022, 2020 33457126

Akkerman-Nijland AM, Akkerman OW, Grasmeijer F, et al: The pharmacokinetics of antibiotics in cystic fibrosis. Expert Opin Drug Metab Toxicol 17(1):53–68, 2021 33213220

Allgire E, McAlees JW, Lewkowich IP, et al: Asthma and posttraumatic stress disorder (PTSD): emerging links, potential models and mechanisms. Brain Behav Immun 97:275–285, 2021 34107349

American Thoracic Society; CDC; Infectious Diseases Society of America: Treatment of tuberculosis. MMWR Recomm Rep 52:1–77, 2003

Antoniou T, Yao Z, Camacho X, et al: Safety of valproic acid in patients with chronic obstructive pulmonary disease: a population-based cohort study. Pharmacoepidemiol Drug Saf 24(3):256–261, 2015 25656984

Argyropoulou P, Patakas D, Koukou A, et al: Buspirone effect on breathlessness and exercise performance in patients with chronic obstructive pulmonary disease. Respiration 60(4):216–220, 1993 8265878

Atlantis E, Fahey P, Cochrane B, et al: Bidirectional associations between clinically relevant depression or anxiety and COPD: a systematic review and meta-analysis. Chest 144(3):766–777, 2013 23429910

Barbui C, Conti V, Cipriani A: Antipsychotic drug exposure and risk of venous thromboembolism: a systematic review and meta-analysis of observational studies. Drug Saf 37(2):79–90, 2014 24403009

Barnes H, McDonald J, Smallwood N, et al: Opioids for the palliation of refractory breathlessness in adults with advanced disease and terminal illness. Cochrane Database Syst Rev 3:CD011008, 2016 27030166

Bartal C, Sagy I, Barski L: Drug-induced eosinophilic pneumonia: a review of 196 case reports. Medicine (Baltimore) 97(4):e9688, 2018 29369189

Bart Sangal R, Sangal JM, Thorp K: Atomoxetine improves sleepiness and global severity of illness but not the respiratory disturbance index in mild to moderate obstructive sleep apnea with sleepiness. Sleep Med 9(5):506–510, 2008 17900980

Behara C, Krishna K, Singh H: Antitubercular drug-induced violent suicide of a hospitalized patient. BMJ 2014:bcr2013201469, 2014 24395874

Ben-Noun L: Drug-induced respiratory disorders: incidence, prevention and management. Drug Saf 23(2):143–164, 2000 10945376

Berry RB, Patel PB: Effect of zolpidem on the efficacy of continuous positive airway pressure as treatment for obstructive sleep apnea. Sleep 29(8):1052–1056, 2006 16944674

Besag FMC, Vasey MJ, Lao KSJ, et al: Adverse events associated with melatonin for the treatment of primary or secondary sleep disorders: a systematic review. CNS Drugs 33(12):1167–1186, 2019 31722088

Boof ML, Dingemanse J, Brunke M, et al: Effect of the novel dual orexin receptor antagonist daridorexant on night-time respiratory function and sleep in patients with moderate chronic obstructive pulmonary disease. J Sleep Res 30(4):e13248, 2021 33417730

Borson S, McDonald GJ, Gayle T, et al: Improvement in mood, physical symptoms, and function with nortriptyline for depression in patients with chronic obstructive pulmonary disease. Psychosomatics 33(2):190–201, 1992 1557484

Braganza G, Chaudhuri R, Thomson NC: Treating patients with respiratory disease who smoke. Ther Adv Respir Dis 2(2):95–107, 2008 19124362

Brager NP, Campbell NR, Reisch H, et al: Reduced renal fractional excretion of lithium in cystic fibrosis. Br J Clin Pharmacol 41(2):157–159, 1996 8838443

Breen RA, Miller RF, Gorsuch T, et al: Adverse events and treatment interruption in tuberculosis patients with and without HIV co-infection. Thorax 61(9):791–794, 2006 16844730

Brown ES, Vigil L, Khan DA, et al: A randomized trial of citalopram versus placebo in outpatients with asthma and major depressive disorder: a proof of concept study. Biol Psychiatry 58(11):865–870, 2005 15993860

Brown ES, Vornik LA, Khan DA, et al: Bupropion in the treatment of outpatients with asthma and major depressive disorder. Int J Psychiatry Med 37(1):23–28, 2007 17645195

Brown ES, Howard C, Khan DA, et al: Escitalopram for severe asthma and major depressive disorder: a randomized, double-blind, placebo-controlled proof-of-concept study. Psychosomatics 53(1):75–80, 2012 22221724

Brown ES, Sayed N, Van Enkevort E, et al: A randomized, double-blind, placebo-controlled trial of escitalopram in patients with asthma and major depressive disorder. J Allergy Clin Immunol Pract 6(5):1604–1612, 2018 29409976

Brunner H: Success and failure of mirtazapine as alternative treatment in elderly stroke patients with sleep apnea—a preliminary open trial. Sleep Breath 12(3):281–285, 2008 18369672

Budhiraja R, Siddiqi TA, Quan SF: Sleep disorders in chronic obstructive pulmonary disease: etiology, impact, and management. J Clin Sleep Med 11(3):259–270, 2015 25700872

Campbell ML: How to withdraw mechanical ventilation: a systematic review of the literature. AACN Adv Crit Care 18(4):397–403, quiz 344–345, 2007 17978613

Chand S, Bhandari R, Girish HN, et al: Isoniazid induced psychosis. Journal of Global Pharma Technology 11(3):11–14, 2019

Chapman JL, Kempler L, Chang CL, et al: Modafinil improves daytime sleepiness in patients with mild to moderate obstructive sleep apnoea not using standard treatments: a randomised placebo-controlled crossover trial. Thorax 69(3):274–279, 2014 24287166

Chapman JL, Vakulin A, Hedner J, et al: Modafinil/armodafinil in obstructive sleep apnoea: a systematic review and meta-analysis. Eur Respir J 47(5):1420–1428, 2016 26846828

Chen CY, Chen CL, Yu CC: Trazodone improves obstructive sleep apnea after ischemic stroke: a randomized, double-blind, placebo-controlled, crossover pilot study. J Neurol 268(8):2951–2960, 2021 33625584

Chen SJ, Yeh CM, Chao TF, et al: The use of benzodiazepine receptor agonists and risk of respiratory failure in patients with chronic obstructive pulmonary disease: a nationwide population-based case-control study. Sleep 38(7):1045–1050, 2015 25669186

Cheng JY, Filippov G, Moline M, et al: Respiratory safety of lemborexant in healthy adult and elderly subjects with mild obstructive sleep apnea: a randomized, double-blind, placebo-controlled, crossover study. J Sleep Res 29(4):e13021, 2020 32187781

Cho J, Spence MM, Niu F, et al: Risk of overdose with exposure to prescription opioids, benzodiazepines, and non-benzodiazepine sedative-hypnotics in adults: a retrospective cohort study. J Gen Intern Med 35(3):696–703, 2020 31919729

Chui CY, Taylor SE, Thomas D, et al: Prevalence and recognition of highly significant medication-smoking cessation interactions in a smoke-free hospital. Drug Alcohol Depend 200:78–81, 2019 31108404

Chung WS, Lai CY, Lin CL, et al: Adverse respiratory events associated with hypnotics use in patients of chronic obstructive pulmonary disease: a population-based case-control study. Medicine (Baltimore) 94(27):e1110, 2015 26166105

Ciprandi G, Schiavetti I, Rindone E, et al: The impact of anxiety and depression on outpatients with asthma. Ann Allergy Asthma Immunol 115(5):408–414, 2015 26392047

Conti V, Venegoni M, Cocci A, et al: Antipsychotic drug exposure and risk of pulmonary embolism: a population-based, nested case-control study. BMC Psychiatry 15:92, 2015 25924683

Currow DC, Ekström M, Louw S, et al: Sertraline in symptomatic chronic breathlessness: a double blind, randomised trial. Eur Respir J 53(1):1801270, 2019 30361250

Dawson JK, Earnshaw SM, Graham CS: Dangerous monoamine oxidase inhibitor interactions are still occurring in the 1990s. J Accid Emerg Med 12(1):49–51, 1995 7640830

De Bruin ML, Hoes AW, Leufkens HG: QTc-prolonging drugs and hospitalizations for cardiac arrhythmias. Am J Cardiol 91(1):59–62, 2003 12505572

De Giacomi F, Vassallo R, Yi ES, et al: Acute eosinophilic pneumonia: causes, diagnosis, and management. Am J Respir Crit Care Med 197(6):728–736, 2018 29206477

Deidda A, Pisanu C, Micheletto L, et al: Interstitial lung disease induced by fluoxetine: systematic review of literature and analysis of VigiAccess, EudraVigilance and a national pharmacovigilance database. Pharmacol Res 120:294–301, 2017 28411001

Del Giacco SR, Cappai A, Gambula L, et al: The asthma-anxiety connection. Respir Med 120:44–53, 2016 27817815

Di X, Chen M, Shen S, et al: Antipsychotic use and risk of venous thromboembolism: a meta-analysis. Psychiatry Res 296:113691, 2021 33421839

DiMartini A: Isoniazid, tricyclics and the "cheese reaction." Int Clin Psychopharmacol 10(3):197–198, 1995 8675973

Dobric A, DeLuca SN, Spencer SJ, et al: Novel pharmacological strategies to treat cognitive dysfunction in chronic obstructive pulmonary disease. Pharmacol Ther 233:108017, 2022 34626675

Doherty AM, Kelly J, McDonald C, et al: A review of the interplay between tuberculosis and mental health. Gen Hosp Psychiatry 35(4):398–406, 2013 23660587

Dubovsky AN, Arvikar S, Stern TA, et al: The neuropsychiatric complications of glucocorticoid use: steroid psychosis revisited. Psychosomatics 53(2):103–115, 2012 22424158

Eckert DJ, Malhotra A, Wellman A, et al: Trazodone increases the respiratory arousal threshold in patients with obstructive sleep apnea and a low arousal threshold. Sleep 37(4):811–819, 2014 24899767

Ekström MP, Bornefalk-Hermansson A, Abernethy AP, et al: Safety of benzodiazepines and opioids in very severe respiratory disease: national prospective study. BMJ 348:g445, 2014 24482539

Ekström M, Nilsson F, Abernethy AA, et al: Effects of opioids on breathlessness and exercise capacity in chronic obstructive pulmonary disease: a systematic review. Ann Am Thorac Soc 12(7):1079–1092, 2015 25803110

Emery CF, Finkel D, Pedersen NL: Pulmonary function as a cause of cognitive aging. Psychol Sci 23(9):1024–1032, 2012 22864997

Erdoğan A, İlhan F: Risperidone-associated acute laryngeal dystonia: a case report. J Clin Psychopharmacol 42(1):98–99, 2022 34508055

Essali N, Miller BJ: Psychosis as an adverse effect of antibiotics. Brain Behav Immun Health 19;9:100148, 2020 34589893

Fardet L, Nazareth I, Whitaker HJ, et al: Severe neuropsychiatric outcomes following discontinuation of long-term glucocorticoid therapy: a cohort study. J Clin Psychiatry 74(4):e281–e286, 2013 23656853

Favreau H, Bacon SL, Joseph M, et al: Association between asthma medications and suicidal ideation in adult asthmatics. Respir Med 106(7):933–941, 2012 22495109

Feliciano JL, Waldfogel JM, Sharma R, et al: Pharmacologic interventions for breathlessness in patients with advanced cancer: a systematic review and meta-analysis. JAMA Netw Open 4(2):e2037632, 2021 33630086

Ferrando SJ, Klepacz L, Lynch S, et al: COVID-19 psychosis: a potential new neuropsychiatric condition triggered by novel coronavirus infection and the inflammatory response? Psychosomatics 61(5):551–555, 2020 32593479

Ferraris A, Szmulewicz AG, Posadas-Martínez ML, et al: The effect of antipsychotic treatment on recurrent venous thromboembolic disease: a cohort study. J Clin Psychiatry 80(5):18m12656, 2019 31509358

Flume PA, O'Sullivan BP, Robinson KA, et al: Cystic fibrosis pulmonary guidelines: chronic medications for maintenance of lung health. Am J Respir Crit Care Med 176(10):957–969, 2007 17761616

Gable M, Depry D: Sustained corticosteroid-induced mania and psychosis despite cessation: a case study and brief literature review. Int J Psychiatry Med 50(4):398–404, 2015 26644319

Ganesh M, Jabbar U, Iskander FH: Acute laryngeal dystonia with novel antipsychotics: a case report and review of literature. J Clin Psychopharmacol 35(5):613–615, 2015 26252439

Garbarino S, Bardwell WA, Guglielmi O, et al: Association of anxiety and depression in obstructive sleep apnea patients: a systematic review and meta-analysis. Behav Sleep Med 18(1):35–57, 2020 30453780

Giannoni A, Borrelli C, Mirizzi G, et al: Benefit of buspirone on chemoreflex and central apnoeas in heart failure: a randomized controlled crossover trial. Eur J Heart Fail 23(2):312–320, 2021 32441857

Girault C, Muir JF, Mihaltan F, et al: Effects of repeated administration of zolpidem on sleep, diurnal and nocturnal respiratory function, vigilance, and physical performance in patients with COPD. Chest 110(5):1203–1211, 1996 8915222

Gross N, Greos LS, Meltzer EO, et al: Safety and tolerability of inhaled loxapine in subjects with asthma and chronic obstructive pulmonary disease: two randomized controlled trials. J Aerosol Med Pulm Drug Deliv 27(6):478–487, 2014 24745666

Gulati G, Kelly BD: Does remdesivir have any neuropsychiatric adverse effects? Ir J Psychol Med 38(4):313–314, 2021 32641172.

Guta MT, Tekalign T, Awoke N, et al: Global burden of anxiety and depression among cystic fibrosis patient: systematic review and meta-analysis. Int J Chronic Dis 2021:6708865, 2021 34307644

Halvani A, Mohsenpour F, Nasiriani K: Evaluation of exogenous melatonin administration in improvement of sleep quality in patients with chronic obstructive pulmonary disease. Tanaffos 12(2):9–15, 2013 25191456

Hicks M, Brugman SM, Katial R: Vocal cord dysfunction/paradoxical vocal fold motion. Prim Care 35(1):81–103, vii, 2008 18206719

Higginson IJ, Wilcock A, Johnson MJ, et al: Randomised, double-blind, multicentre, mixed-methods, dose-escalation feasibility trial of mirtazapine for better treatment of severe breathlessness in advanced lung disease (BETTER-B feasibility). Thorax 75(2):176–179, 2020 31915308

Hoertel N, Sánchez-Rico M, Vernet R, et al: Association between antidepressant use and reduced risk of intubation or death in hospitalized patients with COVID-19: results from an observational study. Mol Psychiatry 26(9):5199–5212, 2021 33536545

Holmedahl NH, Øverland B, Fondenes O, et al: Zopiclone effects on breathing at sleep in stable chronic obstructive pulmonary disease. Sleep Breath 19(3):921–930, 2015 25501294

Holstad SG, Perry PJ, Kathol RG, et al: The effects of intravenous theophylline infusion versus intravenous sodium bicarbonate infusion on lithium clearance in normal subjects. Psychiatry Res 25(2):203–211, 1988 2845461

Hu Z, Yang X, Ho PC, et al: Herb-drug interactions: a literature review. Drugs 65(9):1239–1282, 2005 15916450

Hunchaisri N, Chalermsuwiwattanakan W: Efficacy of donepezil in the treatment of obstructive sleep apnea: a placebo-controlled trial. J Med Assoc Thai 99(Suppl 8):S31–S35, 2016 29901379

Hung Y-H, Cheng CM, Lin WC, et al: Post-traumatic stress disorder and asthma risk: a nationwide longitudinal study. Psychiatry Res 276:25–30, 2019 30991276

Izhakian S, Rosengarten D, Pertzov B, et al: Sertraline-associated interstitial lung disease: a case series and literature review. Sarcoidosis Vasc Diffuse Lung Dis 38(3):e2021027, 2021 34744423

Jackson ML, Tolson J, Bartlett D, et al: Clinical depression in untreated obstructive sleep apnea: examining predictors and a meta-analysis of prevalence rates. Sleep Med 62:22–28, 2019 31525678

Jann MW, Bitar AH: Respiratory dyskinesia. Psychosomatics 23(7):764–765, 1982 6126912

Jiwanmall SA, Gopalakrishnan R, Kuruvilla A: Tardive laryngeal dystonia with risperidone: a case report. Indian J Psychiatry 63(3):306–307, 2021 34211231

Joseph KS, Blais L, Ernst P, et al: Increased morbidity and mortality related to asthma among asthmatic patients who use major tranquillisers. BMJ 312(7023):79–82, 1996 8555932

Judd LL, Schettler PJ, Brown ES, et al: Adverse consequences of glucocorticoid medication: psychological, cognitive and behavioral effects. Am J Psychiatry 171(10):1045–1051, 2014 25272344

Jullian-Desayes I, Revol B, Chareyre E, et al: Impact of concomitant medications on obstructive sleep apnoea. Br J Clin Pharmacol 83(4):688–708, 2017 27735059

Kapoor S, Thakkar J, Aggarwal V: Theophylline toxicity leading to suicidal ideation in a patient with no prior psychiatric illness. SAGE Open Med Case Rep 3:2050313X15583208, 2015 27489687

Kay GG, Feldman N: Effects of armodafinil on simulated driving and self-report measures in obstructive sleep apnea patients prior to treatment with continuous positive airway pressure. J Clin Sleep Med 9(5):445–454, 2013 23674935

Khalid F, Aftab A, Khatri S: The association between leukotriene-modifying agents and suicidality: a review of literature. Psychosomatics 59(1):19–27, 2018 28919375

Khazaie H, Sharafkhaneh A, Khazaie S, et al: A weight-independent association between atypical antipsychotic medications and obstructive sleep apnea. Sleep Breath 22(1):109–114, 2018 28707161

Kiev A, Domantay AG: A study of buspirone coprescribed with bronchodilators in 82 anxious ambulatory patients. J Asthma 25(5):281–284, 1988 3053607

Kroon LA: Drug interactions with smoking. Am J Health Syst Pharm 64(18):1917–1921, 2007 17823102

Kruk J, Sachdev P, Singh S: Neuroleptic-induced respiratory dyskinesia. J Neuropsychiatry Clin Neurosci 7(2):223–229, 1995 7626967

Kryger M, Wang-Weigand S, Roth T: Safety of ramelteon in individuals with mild to moderate obstructive sleep apnea. Sleep Breath 11(3):159–164, 2007 17294232

Kryger M, Roth T, Wang-Weigand S, et al: The effects of ramelteon on respiration during sleep in subjects with moderate to severe chronic obstructive pulmonary disease. Sleep Breath 13(1):79–84, 2009 18584227

Kuan YC, Wu D, Huang KW, et al: Effects of modafinil and armodafinil in patients with obstructive sleep apnea: a meta-analysis of randomized controlled trials. Clin Ther 38(4):874–888, 2016 26923035

Lakstygal AM, Kolesnikova TO, Khatsko SL, et al: DARK classics in chemical neuroscience: atropine, scopolamine, and other anticholinergic deliriant hallucinogens. ACS Chem Neurosci 10(5):2144–2159, 2019 30566832

Law SWY, Wong AYS, Anand S, et al: Neuropsychiatric events associated with leukotriene-modifying agents: a systematic review. Drug Saf 41(3):253–265, 2018 29076063

Le TT, Park S, Choi M, et al: Respiratory events associated with concomitant opioid and sedative use among Medicare beneficiaries with chronic obstructive pulmonary disease. BMJ Open Respir Res 7(1):e000483, 2020 32213535

Li C, Gefter WB: Acute pulmonary edema induced by overdosage of phenothiazines. Chest 101(1):102–104, 1992 1729053

Li Y, Owens RL, Sands S, et al: The effect of donepezil on arousal threshold and apnea-hypopnea index: a randomized, double-blind, cross-over study. Ann Am Thorac Soc 13(11):2012–2018, 2016 27442715

Liao YH, Chen LY, Liao KM, et al: Drug safety of benzodiazepines in Asian patients with chronic obstructive pulmonary disease. Front Pharmacol 11:592910, 2020 33424603

Lieberman JA III: History of the use of antidepressants in primary care. Prim Care Companion J Clin Psychiatry 5(Suppl 7):6–10, 2003

Liu Y, Xu J, Fang K, et al: Current antipsychotic agent use and risk of venous thromboembolism and pulmonary embolism: a systematic review and meta-analysis of observational studies. Ther Adv Psychopharmacol 11:2045125320982720, 2021 33505665

LiverTox: Clinical and research information on drug-induced liver injury. Bethesda, MD, National Institute of Diabetes and Digestive and Kidney Diseases, 2012-. Xanthine Derivatives. Updated July 18, 2020. Available at: https://www.ncbi.nlm.nih.gov/books/NBK548950. Accessed March 26, 2023.

López-Atanes M, González-Briceño JP, Abeal-Adham A, et al: Liaison psychiatry during the peak of the coronavirus pandemic: a description of referrals and interventions. Front Psychiatry 12:555080, 2021 34955903

Lovell N, Wilcock A, Bajwah S, et al: Mirtazapine for chronic breathlessness? A review of mechanistic insights and therapeutic potential. Expert Rev Respir Med 13(2):173–180, 2019 30596298

Lu XM, Zhu JP, Zhou XM: The effect of benzodiazepines on insomnia in patients with chronic obstructive pulmonary disease: a meta-analysis of treatment efficacy and safety. Int J Chron Obstruct Pulmon Dis 11:675–685, 2016 27110106

Mahan RJ, Blaszczyk AT: COPD exacerbation and cholinesterase therapy in dementia patients. Consult Pharm 31(4):221–225, 2016 27056359

Maresh S, Prowting J, Vaughan S, et al: Buspirone decreases susceptibility to hypocapnic central sleep apnea in chronic SCI patients. J Appl Physiol (1985) 129(4):675–682, 2020 32816639

Marseglia L, D'Angelo G, Manti S, et al: Melatonin and atopy: role in atopic dermatitis and asthma. Int J Mol Sci 15(8):13482–13493, 2014 25093714

Mason M, Cates CJ, Smith I: Effects of opioid, hypnotic and sedating medications on sleep-disordered breathing in adults with obstructive sleep apnoea. Cochrane Database Syst Rev (7):CD011090, 2015 26171909

Matte DL, Pizzichini MM, Hoepers AT, et al: Prevalence of depression in COPD: a systematic review and meta-analysis of controlled studies. Respir Med 117:154–161, 2016 27492526

McNicholas WT: Chronic obstructive pulmonary disease and obstructive sleep apnea: the overlap syndrome. J Thorac Dis 8(2):236–242, 2016 ,

Mendelson WB, Maczaj M, Holt J: Buspirone administration to sleep apnea patients. J Clin Psychopharmacol 11(1):71–72, 1991 2040719

Mendhekar DN, Inamdar A: Withdrawal-emergent respiratory dyskinesia with risperidone treated with clozapine. J Neuropsychiatry Clin Neurosci 22(2):E24, 2010 20463136

Meszaros EP, Stancu C, Costanza A, et al: Antibiomania: a case report of clarithromycin and amoxicillin-clavulanic acid induced mania episodes separately. BMC Psychiatry 21(1):399, 2021 34380446

Meuret AE, Kroll J, Ritz T: Panic disorder comorbidity with medical conditions and treatment implications. Annu Rev Clin Psychol 13:209–240, 2017 28375724

Mitchell-Heggs P, Murphy K, Minty K, et al: Diazepam in the treatment of dyspnoea in the "pink puffer" syndrome. Q J Med 49(193):9–20, 1980 6776586

Mo Y, Thomas MC, Karras GE Jr: Barbiturates for the treatment of alcohol withdrawal syndrome: a systematic review of clinical trials. J Crit Care 32:101–107, 2016 26795441

Montville DJ, Lindsey JM, Leung JG: Fluctuation between cigarette smoking and use of electronic nicotine delivery systems: impact on clozapine concentrations and clinical effect. Ment Health Clin 11(6):365–368, 2021 34824961

Moraes W, Poyares DR, Guilleminault C, et al: The effect of donepezil on sleep and REM sleep EEG in patients with Alzheimer disease: a double-blind placebo-controlled study. Sleep 29(2):199–205, 2006 16494088

Moraes W, Poyares D, Sukys-Claudino L, et al: Donepezil improves obstructive sleep apnea in Alzheimer disease: a double-blind, placebo-controlled study. Chest 133(3):677–683, 2008 18198262

Morsy NE, Farrag NS, Zaki NFW, et al: Obstructive sleep apnea: personal, societal, public health, and legal implications. Rev Environ Health 34(2):153–169, 2019 31085749

Moschny N, Hefner G, Grohmann R, et al: Therapeutic drug monitoring of second- and third-generation anti-psychotic drugs: influence of smoking behavior and inflammation on pharmacokinetics. Pharmaceuticals (Basel) 14(6):1–32, 2021 34071813

Motamed H, Forouzan A, Moezzi M, et al: Dexmedetomidine as an adjunctive treatment for acute asthma. Clin Exp Emerg Med 8(2):89–93, 2021 34237813

Nährlich L, Mainz JG, Adams C, et al: Therapy of CF-patients with amitriptyline and placebo—a randomised, double-blind, placebo-controlled phase IIb multicenter, cohort-study. Cell Physiol Biochem 31(4–5):505–512, 2013 23572075

Nakafero G, Sanders RD, Nguyen-Van-Tam JS, et al: Association between benzodiazepine use and exacerbations and mortality in patients with asthma: a matched case-control and survival analysis using the United Kingdom Clinical Practice Research Datalink. Pharmacoepidemiol Drug Saf 24(8):793–802, 2015 26013409

O'Brien ME, Gandhi RG, Kotton CN, et al: Risk of serotonin syndrome with isoniazid (letter). Antimicrob Agents Chemother 65(1):e01455-20, 2020 33077663

Oskotsky T, Maric I, Tang A, et al: Mortality risk among patients with COVID-19 prescribed selective serotonin reuptake inhibitor antidepressants. JAMA Netw Open 4(11):e2133090, 2021 34779847

Ostuzzi G, Papola D, Gastaldon C, et al: Safety of psychotropic medications in people with COVID-19: evidence review and practical recommendations. BMC Med 18(1):215, 2020 32664944

Pachi A, Bratis D, Moussas G, et al: Psychiatric morbidity and other factors affecting treatment adherence in pulmonary tuberculosis patients. Tuberc Res Treat 2013:489865, 2013 23691305

Palma-Alvarez RF, Duque-Yemail J, Ros-Cucurull E, et al: Quinolone-induced psychosis: an updated review. Actas Esp Psiquiatr 48(3):126–137, 2020 32905605

Park JG, Olson EJ, Morgenthaler TI: Impact of zaleplon on continuous positive airway pressure therapy compliance. J Clin Sleep Med 9(5):439–444, 2013 23674934

Peoples AR, Bushunow PW, Garland SN, et al: Buspirone for management of dyspnea in cancer patients receiving chemotherapy: a randomized placebo-controlled URCC CCOP study. Support Care Cancer 24(3):1339–1347, 2016 26329396

Pollok J, van Agteren JE, Carson-Chahhoud KV: Pharmacological interventions for the treatment of depression in chronic obstructive pulmonary disease. Cochrane Database Syst Rev 12:CD012346, 2018 30566235

Polosa R: An overview of chronic severe asthma. Intern Med J 38(3):190–198, 2008 18028366

Pothirat C, Chaiwong W, Phetsuk N, et al: Major affective disorders in chronic obstructive pulmonary disease compared with other chronic respiratory diseases. Int J Chron Obstruct Pulmon Dis 10:1583–1590, 2015 26300637

Quadri S, Drake C, Hudgel DW: Improvement of idiopathic central sleep apnea with zolpidem. J Clin Sleep Med 5(2):122–129, 2009 19968044

Ragnoli B, Pochetti P, Raie A, et al: Interrelationship between obstructive sleep apnea syndrome and severe asthma: from endo-phenotype to clinical aspects. Front Med (Lausanne) 8:640636, 2021 34277650

Ray WA, Chung CP, Murray KT, et al: Mortality and concurrent use of opioids and hypnotics in older patients: a retrospective cohort study. PLoS Med 18(7):e1003709, 2021 34264928

Rey E, Tréluyer JM, Pons G: Drug disposition in cystic fibrosis. Clin Pharmacokinet 35(4):313–329, 1998 9812180

Rhyou HII, Nam Y-H: Association between cognitive function and asthma in adults. Ann Allergy Asthma Immunol 126(1):69–74, 2021 32858237

Riethmüller J, Anthonysamy J, Serra E, et al: Therapeutic efficacy and safety of amitriptyline in patients with cystic fibrosis. Cell Physiol Biochem 24(1–2):65–72, 2009 19590194

Rosenberg R, Roach JM, Scharf M, et al: A pilot study evaluating acute use of eszopiclone in patients with mild to moderate obstructive sleep apnea syndrome. Sleep Med 8(5):464–470, 2007 17512799

Rosenberg T, Lattimer R, Montgomery P, et al: The relationship of SSRI and SNRI usage with interstitial lung disease and bronchiectasis in an elderly population: a case-control study. Clin Interv Aging 12:1977–1984, 2017 29200837

Roth T: Hypnotic use for insomnia management in chronic obstructive pulmonary disease. Sleep Med 10(1):19–25, 2009 18693067

Roxanas MG: Persistent mania following cessation of corticosteroids. Australas Psychiatry 26(5):520–523, 2018 29446641

Sharma B, Handa R, Nagpal K, et al: Cycloserine-induced psychosis in a young female with drug-resistant tuberculosis. Gen Hosp Psychiatry 36(4):451.e3–451.e4, 2014 24766906

Shawon MS, Perret JL, Senaratna CV, et al: Current evidence on prevalence and clinical outcomes of co-morbid obstructive sleep apnea and chronic obstructive pulmonary disease: a systematic review. Sleep Med Rev 32:58–68, 2017 28169105

Sher Y: Psychiatric aspects of lung disease in critical care. Crit Care Clin 33(3):601–617, 2017 28601136

Shoair OA, Cook EA, Shipman D, et al: Antidepressant target dose optimization and control of severe asthma exacerbations in uninsured and underinsured patients with anxiety and/or depression. Pharmacotherapy 40(4):320–330, 2020 32060937

Shyamala KK, Naveen RS, Khatri B: Depression: a neglected comorbidity in patients with tuberculosis. J Assoc Physicians India 66(12):18–21, 2018 31313544

Simon ST, Higginson IJ, Booth S, et al: Benzodiazepines for the relief of breathlessness in advanced malignant and non-malignant diseases in adults. Cochrane Database Syst Rev 10:CD007354, 2016 27764523

Singh S, Kaur H, Singh S, et al: The overlap syndrome. Cureus 10(10):e3453, 2018 30564532

Smales ET, Edwards BA, Deyoung PN, et al: Trazodone effects on obstructive sleep apnea and non-REM arousal threshold. Ann Am Thorac Soc 12(5):758–764, 2015 25719754

Smith I, Lasserson TJ, Wright J: Drug therapy for obstructive sleep apnoea in adults. Cochrane Database Syst Rev (2):CD003002, 2006 16625567

Smoller JW, Pollack MH, Systrom D, et al: Sertraline effects on dyspnea in patients with obstructive airways disease. Psychosomatics 39(1):24–29, 1998 9538672

Stege G, Heijdra YF, van den Elshout FJ, et al: Temazepam 10mg does not affect breathing and gas exchange in patients with severe normocapnic COPD. Respir Med 104(4):518–524, 2010 19910177

Stephenson A, Seitz DP, Fischer HD, et al: Cholinesterase inhibitors and adverse pulmonary events in older people with chronic obstructive pulmonary disease and concomitant dementia: a population-based, cohort study. Drugs Aging 29(3):213–223, 2012 22332932

Sun H, Palcza J, Rosenberg R, et al: Effects of suvorexant, an orexin receptor antagonist, on breathing during sleep in patients with chronic obstructive pulmonary disease. Respir Med 109(3):416–426, 2015 25661282

Szafrański T, Gmurkowski K: Clozapine withdrawal: a review [in Polish]. Psychiatr Pol 33(1):51–67, 1999 10786215

Testa A, Giannuzzi R, Sollazzo F, et al: Psychiatric emergencies (part II): psychiatric disorders coexisting with organic diseases. Eur Rev Med Pharmacol Sci 17(Suppl 1):65–85, 2013 23436669

Teva Pharmaceuticals: Adasuve package insert. September 2016. Available at: http://www.accessdata.fda.gov/drugsatfda_docs/label/2016/022549s005lbl.pdf. Accessed September 20, 2022.

Thompson WL, Sullivan SP: Pulmonary disease, in Psychosomatic Medicine. Edited by Blumenfield M, Strain JJ. Philadelphia, PA, Lippincott Williams & Wilkins, 2006, pp 193–212

Tryfon S, Papadopoulou E, Saroglou M, et al: Clinical and pathophysiological characteristics of valproate-induced pleural effusion. Clin Toxicol (Phila) 59(10):869–876, 2021 34259092

Tudorache E, Fildan AP, Frandes M, et al: Aging and extrapulmonary effects of chronic obstructive pulmonary disease. Clin Interv Aging 12(12):1281–1287, 2017 28860729

Tuncok Y, Akpinar O, Guven H, et al: The effects of theophylline on serum alprazolam levels. Int J Clin Pharmacol Ther 32(12):642–645, 1994 7881701

Turkel SB, Cafaro DR: Lithium treatment of a bipolar patient with cystic fibrosis (letter). Am J Psychiatry 149(4):574, 1992 1554052

Uemura N, McCrea J, Sun H, et al: Effects of the orexin receptor antagonist suvorexant on respiration during sleep in healthy subjects. J Clin Pharmacol 55(10):1093–1100, 2015 25903940

Vai B, Mazza MG, Delli Colli C, et al: Mental disorders and risk of COVID-19-related mortality, hospitalisation, and intensive care unit admission: a systematic review and meta-analysis. Lancet Psychiatry 8(9):797–812, 2021 34274033

Varney V, Parnell H, Evans J, et al: The successful treatment of vocal cord dysfunction with low-dose amitriptyline—including literature review. J Asthma Allergy 2:105–110, 2009 21437148

Vazquez VS, de Lima VB, de Mello LM, et al: Depression, suicidal motivation and suicidal ideation among individuals with asthma: a cross-sectional study. J Thorac Dis 13(10):6082–6094, 2021 34795954

Verberkt CA, van den Beuken-van Everdingen MHJ, Schols JMGA, et al: Respiratory adverse effects of opioids for breathlessness: a systematic review and meta-analysis. Eur Respir J 50(5):1701153, 2017 29167300

Vertex Pharmaceuticals: Trikafta package insert. October 2021. Available at: http://www.accessdata.fda.gov/drugsatfda_docs/label/2021/212273s008lbl.pdf. Accessed September 20, 2022.

Vozoris NT, Fischer HD, Wang X, et al: Benzodiazepine drug use and adverse respiratory outcomes among older adults with COPD. Eur Respir J 44(2):332–340, 2014 24743966

Vozoris NT, Wang X, Austin PC, et al: Serotonergic antidepressant use and morbidity and mortality among older adults with COPD. Eur Respir J 52(1):1800475, 2018 29946006

Wang MT, Tsai CL, Lin CW, et al: Association between antipsychotic agents and risk of acute respiratory failure in patients with chronic obstructive pulmonary disease. JAMA Psychiatry 74(3):252–260, 2017 28055066

Wang MT, Lin CW, Tsai CL, et al: Use of antipsychotics and the risk of acute respiratory failure among adults: a disease risk score-matched nested case-control study. Br J Clin Pharmacol 86(11):2204–2216, 2020 32337738

Wynn G, Oesterheld JR, Cozza KL, et al: Clinical Manual of Drug Interaction: Principles for Medical Practice. Washington, DC, American Psychiatric Publishing, 2009

Yadav S, Rawal G: Adverse drug reactions due to cycloserine on the central nervous system in the multi-drug resistant tuberculosis cases: a case series. Pan Afr Med J 1(25):1–5, 2019

Yen Y-F, Chung M-S, Hu HY, et al: Association of pulmonary tuberculosis and ethambutol with incident depressive disorder: a nationwide, population-based cohort study. J Clin Psychiatry 76(4):e505–e511, 2015 25919843

Yohannes AM, Alexopoulos GS: Pharmacological treatment of depression in older patients with chronic obstructive pulmonary disease: impact on the course of the disease and health outcomes. Drugs Aging 31(7):483–492, 2014 24902934

Zhao Z, Zhang D, Sun H, et al: Anxiety and depression in patients with chronic obstructive pulmonary disease and obstructive sleep apnea: the overlap syndrome. Sleep Breath 26(4):1603–1611, 2022 34783978

Oncology

Philip A. Bialer, M.D.

Syed Rashdi Ahmed, M.D.

Stephen J. Ferrando, M.D.

Shirley Qiong Yan, Pharm.D., BCOP

P sychiatric symptoms are common in many patients with cancer, especially those with advanced cancer. Several factors, including the emotional stress of the cancer diagnosis, the effects of CNS tumors, neurotoxicity from immune reactions to non-CNS tumors, and the adverse effects of cancer chemotherapy or radiotherapy, may contribute to psychiatric comorbidity. In most situations, psychiatric symptoms can be safely managed with psychotropics; however, psychotropic agents must be carefully selected to avoid adverse interactions with chemotherapeutic agents, including interactions that potentially limit the therapeutic efficacy of chemotherapy. In this chapter, we review psychiatric symptoms related to cancer and cancer treatment, psychopharmacological treatment of psychiatric comorbidity, and interactions between psychiatric and oncological drugs.

Differential Diagnosis of Psychiatric Manifestations of Cancers

Cancer-Related Depression and Fatigue

Emotional distress accompanies the diagnosis of cancer and adversely affects the patient's quality of life. Surveys suggest that about 50% of patients with advanced cancer have symptoms that meet criteria for a psychiatric disorder, most commonly adjustment disorder (11%–35%), major depression (5%–26%), and anxiety disorders (6%–10%) (Traeger et al. 2012). Pancreatic, oropharyngeal, and breast cancers are often associated with symptoms of depression (Carvalho et al. 2014; Chen et al. 2013). Risk factors for depression include younger age, advanced disease, inadequate social support, and insecure attachment style. The diagnosis of cancer may also exacerbate preexisting psychiatric disorders. Depression and fatigue are common adverse effects of cancer chemotherapy and radiation therapy (discussed in the section "Neuropsychiatric Adverse Effects of Oncology Treatments" later in this chapter).

Differentiating transient adjustment-related depression and anxiety warranting at most short-term pharmacotherapy (e.g., benzodiazepines) from major depression or generalized anxiety disorder necessitating ongoing pharmacotherapy can be challenging. Furthermore, differentiating neurovegetative symptoms of depression and anxiety such as anorexia or fatigue from those produced by cancer or its treatment is often difficult. Addressing potential underlying causes of fatigue such as anemia and close monitoring of these symptoms during pharmacotherapy are warranted. These symptoms may be ameliorated with standard pharmacotherapy; however, if residual neurovegetative symptoms persist, adjunctive treatment should be initiated. In general, psychopharmacology in cancer is symptom focused, making use of both primary and secondary pharmacodynamic benefits of medications.

Psychiatric Symptoms of Brain Tumors

Brain tumors typically cause generalized or focal neurological symptoms and signs. However, some tumors, especially in neurologically silent areas, may give rise to only psychiatric symptoms such as depression, anxiety disorders, mania, psychosis, personality changes, anorexia, or cognitive dysfunction. Although there have been attempts to categorize psychiatric symptoms according to tumor location or histological type, a review indicated a lack of specific association (Madhusoodanan et al. 2015). Brain imaging should be considered for patients presenting with atypical psychiatric symptoms, onset of psychiatric symptoms after age 40, or a change in the clinical presentation of existing psychiatric symptoms (Cosci et al. 2015; Forbes et al. 2019; Masdeu 2011; Mugge et al. 2020) (see also Chapter 9, "Central Nervous System Disorders").

Paraneoplastic Limbic Encephalitis

Paraneoplastic limbic encephalitis (PLE) is a consequence of CNS damage from antineuronal antibodies expressed as an immune response to a non–nervous system cancer. Symptoms include rapidly progressive confusion and short-term memory deficits, depression, visual and auditory hallucinations, delusions, paranoia, and seizures (Voltz 2007). PLE occurs in 40% of small-cell lung cancers (Gozzard et al. 2015) and 20% of seminomas (Gultekin et al. 2000). PLE also occurs in lymphoma and tumors of the breast and thymus (Kelley et al. 2017). In most cases of PLE, neuropsychiatric symptoms precede cancer diagnosis, often by several years. PLE is identified by characteristic findings of bilateral temporal lobe hyperintensities on MRI, with supporting evidence from electroencephalographic and cerebrospinal fluid antibody studies (Shen et al. 2018). Symptoms have limited response to psychopharmacotherapy (Foster and Caplan 2009). Although antipsychotics and anticonvulsants have been tried, treatment is focused on eradication of the tumor and on immunosuppressant therapy.

Psychopharmacological Treatment of Psychiatric Disorders in Patients With Cancer

The research literature on psychopharmacological treatment of psychiatric disorders in cancer is sparse and is focused primarily on depression and somatic symptoms, including pain, nausea, and fatigue (for general clinical reviews of major psychotropic drug classes in cancer, see Caruso et al. 2013;

Reich and Bondenet 2018). Psychopharmacological treatment of pain and nausea is covered in Chapter 17, "Pain Management," and Chapter 4, "Gastrointestinal Disorders," respectively. Psychopharmacological treatment of depression, anxiety, cancer-related fatigue (CRF), and cognitive impairment is covered in the following subsections.

Depression

Depression has a prevalence ranging from 10.8% to 24% in patients with cancer (Ng et al. 2011) and a prevalence of 13.7% among cancer survivors (Zhao et al. 2014). Multiple case series and case reports suggest the effectiveness of tricyclic antidepressants (TCAs) and selective serotonin reuptake inhibitors (SSRIs) in a range of cancers; however, only a small number of randomized controlled trials (RCTs) have been conducted. Generally, RCTs have included predominantly women with breast and gynecological malignancies, many have been brief in duration (5–6 weeks), and several studies have been underpowered to detect drug-drug or drug-placebo differences. Of note, a large multicenter study that randomly assigned patients with cancer and depression either to a manualized program of collaborative depression care or to usual care by their oncologists found a significantly (and substantially) higher response rate in the depression care group (Sharpe et al. 2014; Walker et al. 2014).

Cyclic Antidepressants

Mianserin (a tetracyclic antidepressant not approved in the United States) up to 60 mg/day in depressed women with breast cancer has been reported by two groups to be superior to placebo in improving both depression and quality of life (Costa et al. 1985; Ostuzzi et al. 2015; van Heeringen and Zivkov 1996). Mianserin was well tolerated, and dropout rates were higher among placebo-treated patients because of lack of response. In a clinical sample, patients with gynecological malignancies and depression who were adherent to imipramine treatment (minimum 150 mg/day for 4 weeks) had significantly fewer depressive symptoms compared with patients who did not adhere to the treatment (Evans et al. 1988).

Selective Serotonin Reuptake Inhibitors

A 5-week RCT of fluoxetine ($n=45$) versus placebo ($n=46$) for depression in patients with cancer did not find a difference in the primary depression end point on the Montgomery-Åsberg Depression Rating Scale; however, fluoxe-tine yielded greater reduction in general distress as measured by the Symptom Checklist–90 (Razavi et al. 1996). In a 6-week multisite RCT comparing flu-oxetine (20–40 mg/day; $n=21$) and desipramine (25–100 mg/day; $n=17$) for depressed women with breast, colorectal, and gynecological malignancies, both treatments yielded significant improvements in depression, anxiety, and quality-of-life end points (Holland et al. 1998). However, 29% of patients treated with fluoxetine and 41% of patients treated with desipramine with-drew because of adverse events. The results of both of these studies were ham-pered by their brief duration. In two large RCTs of treatment for depressive or fatigue symptoms in women with breast cancer who were actively undergoing chemotherapy, paroxetine, 20 mg/day, initiated just after the start of chemo-therapy and discontinued a week after the end of chemotherapy was more effective than placebo in reducing depressive symptoms but not fatigue (Mor-row et al. 2003; Roscoe et al. 2005). A small multicenter RCT comparing par-oxetine ($n=13$) with desipramine ($n=11$) and placebo ($n=11$) showed no group differences, probably a result of high placebo response and lack of statistical power (Musselman et al. 2006). Additionally, paroxetine is not recommended for first-line treatment of patients with cancer because of its significant drug interactions and potentially detrimental side effects (Li et al. 2017).

Fluoxetine was superior to placebo in an oncologist-driven RCT for the treatment of nonmajor depression and diminished quality of life in patients with advanced cancer (3–24 months estimated survival) (Fisch et al. 2003; Perusinghe et al. 2021); however, this effect was accounted for by improve-ment in the patients with the most severe depression at baseline. Nausea and vomiting were also more common in the fluoxetine group. In another on-cologist-driven RCT comparing sertraline, 50 mg/day, with placebo for the amelioration of mild depression, anxiety, and other quality-of-life symptoms, sertraline showed no benefit over placebo and was associated with higher dropout rates (Stockler et al. 2007). This study was stopped because of higher mortality in the sertraline group at the first interim analysis on a subset of the patients; however, survival did not differ between the treatment groups when all enrolled patients were analyzed with a longer duration of follow-up. Cau-tion is recommended for prescribing medications with cytochrome P450 (CYP) interactions, specifically fluoxetine, fluvoxamine, paroxetine, and ser-traline (Yi and Syrjala 2017).

Other Antidepressants

A recent systematic review found that mirtazapine, a noradrenergic and specific serotonergic antidepressant, is effective in treating depression in patients with cancer (Economos et al. 2020). In a 6-week unblinded randomized trial in patients with advanced cancer and multiple somatic and psychiatric symptoms, mirtazapine (7.5–30 mg/day), but not imipramine (5–100 mg/day) or a no-medication control, was found to reduce depression and anxiety, as measured by the Hospital Anxiety and Depression Scale, and insomnia (Cankurtaran et al. 2008). Similarly, in a group of depressed patients with lung, breast, and gastrointestinal cancers experiencing nausea or vomiting and sleep disturbance, open-label treatment with mirtazapine (orally dissolving, 15–45 mg/day) was associated with improvement in depressive and somatic symptoms and quality of life within 7 days (Kim et al. 2008). Excessive sleepiness occurred in 36% of patients early in treatment but generally abated within 2 weeks (Kim et al. 2008).

Cao et al. (2018) aimed to assess the effectiveness of mirtazapine in addition to usual antiemetic therapies in the treatment of chemotherapy-induced emesis. The intervention group received mirtazapine in addition to aprepitant, a serotonin type 3 receptor antagonist, and dexamethasone (7.5 mg). The control group received the same medications except mirtazapine. In the first and third cycles of the study, overall complete response rates (no emesis and no rescue treatments) were significantly higher with mirtazapine (Economos et al. 2020). Mirtazapine also has been found to be useful for the treatment of cancer-related cachexia and anorexia (Riechelmann et al. 2010). Furthermore, mirtazapine significantly improves gastric emptying for patients with prostate and breast cancer experiencing cancer-associated anorexia (Kumar et al. 2017). A randomized prospective study showed mirtazapine's effectiveness in treating delayed emesis among patients with breast cancer receiving highly emetogenic chemotherapy (Cao et al. 2020).

Bupropion is a noradrenergic and dopaminergic antidepressant that has been shown to improve fatigue and focus in patients with cancer (Grassi et al. 2018). Bupropion sustained release (100–300 mg/day) was effective in an open-label trial for depressive symptoms in patients with cancer in which fatigue was the primary end point (Moss et al. 2006). A more recent randomized placebo-controlled clinical trial found that use of bupropion (150 mg/day) to treat CRF also improved depression and performance scores at the end of a 6-week trial of bupropion (Salehifar et al. 2020).

Psychostimulants

Methylphenidate and dextroamphetamine have also been found to be effective for depression in case series and small open-label trials in patients with advanced cancer, with onset of action generally within 2–5 days (Centeno et al. 2012; Huffman and Stern 2004; Sood et al. 2006). A double-blind, placebo-controlled study also reported the efficacy of methylphenidate as an add-on to mirtazapine therapy in terminally ill patients with cancer (Ng et al. 2014). Methylphenidate and modafinil have been found to reduce depression in RCTs in which CRF was the primary end point (Conley et al. 2016; Kerr et al. 2012; Lundorff et al. 2009).

Cholinesterase Inhibitors

In a small clinical trial in patients with irradiated brain tumors, donepezil led to limited improvements in acute fatigue, depression, and cognitive impairment (Shaw et al. 2006).

Melatonin

One RCT showed that melatonin may reduce the risk of developing depression in patients with breast cancer (Hansen et al. 2014).

Conclusion

The limited clinical trial literature generally supports the use of standard antidepressants for the treatment of moderate to severe depression in patients with cancer. Other symptoms such as fatigue, nausea, and anorexia may respond as well. Nonetheless, it should be kept in mind that those who are currently receiving chemotherapy or have widespread disease are likely to be sensitive to adverse effects. In patients with advanced malignancies and limited life expectancies, a psychostimulant should be considered because of the rapid onset of response and benefit for accompanying symptoms such as fatigue and cognitive impairment.

Anxiety

Anxiety is also prevalent in patients with cancer and is often comorbid with depression, in which case antidepressant treatment is effective in alleviating anxiety symptoms (see previous subsection, "Depression"). SSRI and serotonin-norepinephrine reuptake inhibitor (SNRI) antidepressants are the long-term treatments of choice for anxiety disorders such as generalized anxiety disorder and panic disorder. There are no studies of antidepressants among patients with cancer in which anxiety was the primary end point. Atypical antipsychotics such as olanzapine and quetiapine have also been used to treat anxiety symptoms in the clinical setting but have not been systematically studied.

Benzodiazepines are often used clinically to treat acute anxiety-related symptoms and nausea. Alprazolam (0.5–3.4 mg/day) and placebo were found to decrease anxiety symptoms within 1 week in 36 patients with mixed cancers enrolled in an RCT (Wald et al. 1993). Similarly, in a 10-day multicenter RCT that included 147 inpatients and outpatients with mixed cancers, alprazolam (0.5 mg three times daily) and progressive muscle relaxation were found to reduce anxiety symptoms (Holland et al. 1998). Alprazolam produced greater and more rapid symptom relief on some but not all outcome measures. In both studies, the structure and attention received by the patients were thought to be instrumental in alleviating symptoms. A more recent study examining the use of alprazolam in patients with bladder cancer undergoing cystoscopy found a reduction in anxiety and pain after treatment with alprazolam (Ozkan et al. 2017).

In clinical practice, clinicians often use lorazepam for patients with cancer because of its favorable pharmacokinetics, multiple routes of administration, and putative efficacy for treating nausea and other distressing symptoms (James et al. 2017). Clonazepam is also used because of its longer half-life. When patients with cancer are taking benzodiazepines, excessive sedation, cognitive impairment, rebound or withdrawal, and other adverse effects should be monitored closely (Costantini et al. 2011; Howard et al. 2014).

When benzodiazepines are used to treat anxiety, patients with a history of substance or alcohol misuse must be monitored carefully. Caution is also advised for patients receiving multiple sedating medications, particularly patients taking narcotics to treat pain. An alternative approach may be the use of gabapentin, which was shown to be effective in addressing anxiety in a cohort of breast cancer survivors (Lavigne et al. 2012). Both gabapentin and pregabalin are used off label for the treatment of various anxiety disorders (Greenblatt and Greenblatt 2018).

Cancer-Related Fatigue

CRF affects a majority of patients with cancer at some point during the course of illness. The most common disease-related correlates are active chemotherapy and anemia. Fatigue is often comorbid with anxiety and depression; however, it also occurs alone and can be a residual symptom even if the anxiety and depression are treated effectively. Anemia-related fatigue is ameliorated by treatment with erythropoietin or darbepoietin (see Mücke et al. 2015 for a review).

Psychostimulants and modafinil are the most commonly prescribed psychotropic agents for CRF. Methylphenidate, 10–50 mg daily in divided doses, has been studied in RCTs in patients with advanced cancer (Escalante et al. 2014; Moraska et al. 2010), patients receiving palliative care (Bruera et al. 2013), and patients with prostate cancer (Roth et al. 2010). In patients receiving palliative care, fatigue improved after 1 week in both methylphenidate and placebo groups; the latter was attributed to the powerful effects of research nurse support. Although one meta-analysis showed that placebo was inferior to other treatments, there was still a 29% response rate, and this effect must be considered when studying the treatment of CRF (Junior et al. 2020). A significant decrease in fatigue was seen in the prostate study. The benefits of methylphenidate in the other studies were mixed, although improvement in cognition and more severe fatigue was noted. A systematic review of systematic reviews of pharmacological interventions to improve CRF did show a statistically significant benefit for methylphenidate (Belloni et al. 2021). Modafinil has been studied in four open-label trials on CRF, including patients with breast cancer, cerebral tumor, and lung cancer, and in one RCT involving patients with mixed cancers receiving chemotherapy (Cooper et al. 2009; Spathis et al. 2014). In the controlled trial with 642 patients receiving concurrent chemotherapy, modafinil, 200 mg/day, was more efficacious than placebo in treating fatigue and excessive daytime sleepiness but not depressive symptoms (Spathis et al. 2014). Patients with the highest levels of fatigue at the beginning of their second cycle of chemotherapy benefited most. Adverse effects reported in these trials included headache, nausea, and activation symptoms such as insomnia and anxiety (Cooper et al. 2009; Spathis et al. 2014).

Armodafinil was studied in two RCTs and did not produce any significant improvement in fatigue compared with placebo (Berenson et al. 2015; Page et al. 2015). Although the patients with more baseline fatigue in the study by Page et al. did experience improved quality of life and reduced fatigue, the results of the study by Berenson et al. suggested a strong placebo effect.

Although potential etiological factors for CRF (e.g., anemia, depression) should be addressed whenever possible, methylphenidate and modafinil appear to be effective pharmacological treatments for CRF. Nonpharmacological treatments also should be considered. One meta-analysis indicated that exercise, psychological treatment, and exercise plus psychological treatment may all be more beneficial than medication (Mustian et al. 2017). Because many patients have residual symptoms of fatigue, which diminishes their quality of life, adjunctive treatment should not be unduly delayed. Excessive activation and anorexia are not a major clinical concern at usual therapeutic dosages, but these potential adverse effects should be monitored.

Cognitive Impairment

Chemotherapy-related cognitive impairment, or "chemo brain," has a reported incidence of 17%–70%. The pathogenesis is unclear and may be related to direct neurotoxic effects, inflammatory cytokines, oxidative stress, genetic polymorphism, or hormone levels (Lv et al. 2020).

A review of pharmacological management of chemotherapy-related cognitive impairment found no studies that identified medications that were protective. In terms of treatment, Karschnia et al. (2019) found that although stimulants such as methylphenidate could be helpful in the pediatric population, studies in adults were inconclusive. Donepezil has been found to be effective in several studies for treating chemotherapy-related cognitive impairment in patients with CNS cancer and in those given brain-directed cancer therapies. Donepezil was also found to be beneficial for patients with non-CNS cancer, particularly those with memory impairment and those with more severe deficits (Karschnia et al. 2019).

Adverse Oncological Effects of Psychotropics

Antipsychotics

Antipsychotics have been associated with cancer risk. Evaluation of this association is confounded by the fact that patients with schizophrenia, the primary population for which these agents are prescribed, have multiple risk factors for cancer, including alcohol use disorders, obesity, smoking, and poor self-care. Antipsychotic-induced hyperprolactinemia is also considered a risk factor for pituitary, breast, and endometrial cancers (see also Chapter 10, "Endocrine and Metabolic Disorders").

Several epidemiological studies have documented both increased and decreased rates of cancer in patients taking (mostly typical) antipsychotics (Dalton et al. 2006; Hippisley-Cox et al. 2007; Mortensen 1987, 1992; Wang et al. 2002), and it is difficult to design and implement a study that would conclusively prove or disprove an association. Risperidone (and possibly its major metabolite, paliperidone), in particular, may be associated with pituitary tumors. A retrospective pharmacovigilance study used the FDA Adverse Event Reporting System database through March 2005 to assess the association of pituitary tumors with atypical antipsychotics. Risperidone was associated with pituitary tumors at 18.7 times the expected rate (Szarfman et al. 2006). A survey of the World Health Organization's adverse drug reaction database supports this relationship between risperidone and pituitary neoplasms (Doraiswamy et al. 2007). However, a more recent retrospective review of more than 400,000 records found no greater risk for pituitary tumors with mass effect among patients taking risperidone compared with other atypical antipsychotics (McCarren et al. 2012).

One review and meta-analysis indicated that there may be a relationship between antipsychotic-induced hyperprolactinemia and breast cancer risk, but the risk is much lower than for other factors such as nulliparity, obesity, diabetes mellitus, and unhealthy lifestyle factors (De Hert et al. 2016). A large case-control study indicated that long-term use of prolactin-increasing, but not prolactin-sparing, antipsychotics was associated with increased risk of breast cancer (Taipale et al. 2021).

Reluctance to prescribe antipsychotics because of fear of increasing cancer risk is not supported by available studies, with the possible exception of increased risk for pituitary tumors with risperidone. Animal studies suggest a relationship between pituitary tumor growth and hyperprolactinemia secondary to dopamine D_2 receptor antagonism (Szarfman et al. 2006). Thus, it seems prudent to avoid antipsychotics associated with a high incidence of hyperprolactinemia (risperidone, paliperidone, ziprasidone, haloperidol, and aripiprazole) in patients with current or past history of pituitary endocrine tumors and possibly family history of breast cancer. Evidence that antipsychotics may reduce cancer risk is inconclusive.

Anxiolytics

Studies support the lack of cancer risk with benzodiazepine use for several cancers, including non-Hodgkin's lymphoma, Hodgkin's disease, malignant melanoma, and breast, large bowel, lung, endometrial, ovarian, testicular, thyroid, and liver cancer (Halapy et al. 2006; Pottegård et al. 2013; Rosenberg et al. 1995; Zhang et al. 2017). Although a more recent population-based retrospective cohort study suggested an overall increased risk of developing cancer among patients using benzodiazepines (Iqbal et al. 2017; Kao et al. 2012), the results may be misleading because of a lack of theoretical rationale and the presence of many confounding factors (Kao et al. 2012; Selaman et al. 2012).

Mood Stabilizers

Lithium salts often cause leukocytosis (Young 2009), which raised a concern that lithium may act as an inducer or reinducer of acute and chronic monocytic leukemia (Swierenga et al. 1987; Volf and Crismon 1991). However, no association of lithium and leukemia was observed in two retrospective studies of patients with leukemia (Lyskowski and Nasrallah 1981; Resek and Olivieri 1983). A third retrospective study observed a significant inverse trend for nonepithelial cancers with lithium dosage (Cohen et al. 1998). This report suggested that psychiatric patients have lower cancer prevalence than the general population and that lithium may have a protective effect. Another retrospective study also observed a lower incidence of overall cancer risk in patients with bipolar disorder taking lithium (Huang et al. 2016). Retrospective studies of the risk of long-term lithium use on the development of thyroid, renal cell, and other upper urinary tract tumors have produced mixed findings, with one study showing an increased risk and others showing no significant association (Ambrosiani et al. 2018; Pottegård et al. 2016; Zaidan et al. 2014). Other RCTs have shown that lithium may be protective or may actually enhance the chemotherapeutic treatment of non-small-cell lung cancer, hormone-independent prostate cancer, and pancreatic ductal adenocarcinoma (Hossein et al. 2012; Lan et al. 2013; Peng et al. 2013). Valproate, similar to other short-chain fatty acids, has been known to have anticancer effects on a variety of malignant cells in vitro. Several clinical trials have confirmed the efficacy of valproate in acute myeloid leukemia and myelodysplastic syndromes (Kuendgen et al. 2011; Voso et al. 2009). No human studies of carbamazepine carcinogenicity have been done.

Antidepressants

A relationship between antidepressant use and increased cancer risk has been suggested, but early epidemiological studies yielded inconsistent results. Serotonin-enhancing antidepressants elevate prolactin levels, and hyperprolactinemia has been associated with an increased risk of postmenopausal breast cancer. Large population-based case-control surveys and a meta-analysis reported no association between the risk of breast cancer and the use of antidepressants overall, by antidepressant class, or by individual agent (Chen et al. 2016). Similar methods have been used to examine the risk of ovarian, prostate, lung, and colorectal cancer with SSRIs and TCAs. No evidence of increased risk of ovarian cancer was observed with antidepressants in general or with SSRIs (Huo et al. 2018; Moorman et al. 2005). SSRI use did not increase the risk of prostate cancer (Lin et al. 2018; Tamim et al. 2008) and was associated with a decreased risk of lung cancer (Toh et al. 2007). Although one study found a decreased risk of colorectal cancer among SSRI users, more recent case-control studies disputed this finding (Coogan et al. 2009; Cronin-Fenton et al. 2011; Xu et al. 2006). A marginally elevated risk of lung and prostate cancer, possibly due to experimental bias, was observed among TCA users.

Conclusion

Based on conflicting findings in the literature and disparities in patient populations and potentially confounding factors, it is impossible at this time to substantiate any relationship, positive or negative, between psychotropics and cancer risk. In weighing the risks and benefits, it is not justifiable to withhold psychiatric medications on the basis of fear of increasing cancer risk, particularly when considering the morbidity (and even mortality) associated with untreated psychiatric disorder.

Neuropsychiatric Adverse Effects of Oncology Treatments

Radiotherapy

Fatigue is the most common neuropsychological acute reaction to brain radiation, often occurring within several weeks of the beginning of therapy and generally lasting 1–3 months. Delayed reactions, including decreased energy, depression, and cognitive dysfunction, occur months or years after radiotherapy and are generally irreversible.

Methylphenidate use in patients with brain tumors undergoing radiation therapy did not produce any improvement in fatigue or cognition (Butler et al. 2007). However, modafinil (Kaleita et al. 2006), donepezil (Shaw et al. 2006), and memantine (Day et al. 2014) have produced limited improvements in acute fatigue, depression, and cognitive impairment in small clinical trials involving patients with irradiated brain tumors.

Chemotherapy

Delirium

Delirium is common in cancer, with many possible causes, including adverse effects of chemotherapy, infection, brain metastases, and terminal delirium (delirium is covered comprehensively in Chapter 15, "Critical Care and Surgery"). Delirium occurs frequently with chemotherapeutic agents associated with CNS toxicity and those able to cross the blood-brain barrier, including 5-fluorouracil, ifosfamide, asparaginase, chlorambucil, cytarabine, methotrexate, interferons, interleukins, vincristine, and vinblastine (Caraceni 2013; Das et al. 2020). Corticosteroids (see also Chapter 10 for full discussion), antihistamines, and opioids are a few supportive medications that also potentially contribute to an acute confusional state (Agar and Lawlor 2008). Medication-related delirium often responds to dosage reduction or a change of drug. The incidence of delirium and other psychiatric symptoms may be exacerbated by the interaction of tumor-related factors and treatment-induced neurotoxicity. There are no RCTs of psychotropic drugs for cancer-related delirium (Breitbart 2011) (see Breitbart 2014 for a summary of RCTs in medically ill patients).

Cognitive Impairment

Chemotherapy-induced cognitive dysfunction, sometimes called "chemo brain," has been identified in patients with breast, colorectal, and testicular cancers (Joly et al. 2015; Matsos et al. 2017; Mounier et al. 2020). Inflammatory cytokines have been implicated in the pathogenesis of the cognitive dysfunction, and the demarcation between the cancer and the therapies is not always clear.

Chemotherapeutic Agents

Psychiatric adverse effects of oncology drugs are summarized in Table 8–1 and discussed in the following subsections.

Table 8–1. Psychiatric adverse effects of oncology medications

Medication	Psychiatric adverse effects
Alkylating agents	
Nitrogen mustards	
Ifosfamide	Seizures, drowsiness, confusion, hallucinations
Nonclassic alkylators	
Altretamine	Fatigue, anxiety, depression
Procarbazine	Psychosis, hallucinations, anxiety, depression, confusion, nightmares (Sigma-Tau Pharmaceuticals 2014)
Antimetabolites	
Pyrimidine analogs	
Cytarabine (cytosine arabinoside)	Confusion, somnolence, personality changes (high dose) (Baker et al. 1991; Pfizer 2020)
Purine analogs	
Nelarabine	Somnolence, headache, peripheral neuropathy, seizures, fatigue, hypoesthesia (Novartis 2005)
Interferons and interleukins	
Interferon-α-2a	Apathy, fatigue, depression, suicidal behaviors, agitation, mania, psychoses
Interferon-α-2b	Apathy, fatigue, depression, suicidal behaviors, confusion, mania
Interleukin-2 (aldesleukin)	Apathy, fatigue, confusion, sedation, anxiety, psychosis
Retinoic acid compounds	
Tretinoin (all-trans retinoic acid)	Anxiety, insomnia, depression, confusion, agitation, hallucinations
Enzymes	
Pegaspargase, *Erwinia* (recombinant)	Somnolence, fatigue, coma, seizures, confusion, agitation, hallucinations (Jazz Pharmaceuticals 2021; Servier 2021)

Table 8–1.   Psychiatric adverse effects of oncology
medications *(continued)*

Medication	Psychiatric adverse effects
Monoclonal antibodies	
Bortezomib	35% incidence of psychiatric disorders: agitation, confusion, mental status change, psychotic disorder, suicidal ideation (Takeda Pharmaceuticals 2021)
Bevacizumab, moxetumomab, ramucirumab, tagraxofusp-erzs	RPLS, a rare brain capillary leak syndrome (Jain and Litzow 2020)
Brentuximab, obinutuzumab, ofatumumab, polatuzumab	Progressive multifocal leukoencephalopathy (rare), peripheral neuropathy, headache, dizziness (Cortese et al. 2021)
Blinatumomab	Encephalopathy, convulsions, speech disorders, disturbances in consciousness, confusion, disorientation, fatigue, headache, tremor, dizziness, insomnia (Amgen 2018; Jain and Litzow 2020)
ICIs	
Ipilimumab, nivolumab, pembrolizumab	Serious neurological adverse events affect 1% of patients receiving ICIs: mild fatigue, headache, Guillain-Barré syndrome (rare), and meningitis (<1%) were seen more with ipilimumab (Guidon et al. 2021; Johnson et al. 2019).
Anti-GD2	
Dinutuximab, naxitamab	RPLS, hypotension, severe peripheral neuropathy, pain, anxiety, fatigue, headache, and irritability (United Therapeutics 2015; Y-mAbs Therapeutics 2020)

Note.   ICI=immune checkpoint inhibitor; RPLS=reversible posterior leukoencephalopathy syndrome.

Ifosfamide.   Ifosfamide encephalopathy, characterized by seizures, drowsiness, confusion, and hallucinations, occurs in 15%–30% of patients and is often dose limiting. Predisposing factors for ifosfamide-induced encephalopathy include previous cisplatin exposure, concomitant use of opioids and CYP2B6 inhibitors, low serum albumin, elevated serum creatinine, and elevated hemoglobin (Szabatura et al. 2015). Case reports suggest a lack of efficacy of psychoactive agents for ifosfamide-induced neurotoxicity and delirium. Symptoms usually resolve after drug withdrawal and treatment with oral or intravenous methylene blue (Dufour et al. 2006). Although methylene blue is widely used to treat ifosfamide delirium, its efficacy has not been confirmed in controlled clinical trials, and many patients experience positive outcomes without methylene blue (Alici-Evcimen and Breitbart 2007).

Nonclassic alkylating agents. Neuropsychiatric adverse events have been reported with procarbazine and altretamine. Case reports have identified psychosis as a side effect of procarbazine chemotherapy (e.g., van Eys et al. 1987). Other psychiatric adverse effects, including hallucinations, anxiety, depression, confusion, and nightmares, are also associated with procarbazine use (Leadiant Biosciences 2018). Altretamine was associated with fatigue (63%) and anxiety or depression (29%) of mild to moderate severity during a 6-month Phase II trial (Rothenberg et al. 2001).

Biological response modifiers. The immunomodulatory agents interferon-α (IFN-α) and interleukin-2 (IL-2) are often associated with psychiatric adverse effects, including apathy, fatigue, cognitive impairment, depression with suicidal ideation, and psychosis. Preexisting psychiatric illness increases vulnerability to psychiatric adverse effects (see Chapter 4 for a more thorough discussion of psychiatric symptoms associated with IFN-α).

IL-2 has been found to be elevated in patients with major depressive disorder (Nobis et al. 2020), and therapy with this agent has been reported to cause severe depressive symptoms in more than 20% of patients with cancer (Capuron et al. 2000). Neuropsychiatric symptoms may lead to treatment discontinuation. Recent studies suggest that measurement of IL-2 may be used as a valid laboratory diagnostic tool for depression in breast cancer (Ho et al. 2021).

IFN-α-induced depression in patients with cancer has been responsive to antidepressant treatment in controlled trials with paroxetine (Capuron et al. 2002; Pinto and Andrade 2016), but symptoms of fatigue and anorexia are less responsive to SSRI treatment (Capuron et al. 2002; Pinto and Andrade 2016). Use of an adjunctive antidepressant was associated with better adherence to IFN-α therapy (Musselman et al. 2001). Other neurobehavioral side effects of IFN-α, such as anxiety and cognitive dysfunction, have also been found to respond to treatment with paroxetine (McNutt et al. 2012; Udina et al. 2014).

Retinoic acid compounds.   Retinoic acid compounds, commonly used to treat acne (isotretinoin), are also used systemically for acute promyelocytic leukemia (tretinoin, all-trans retinoic acid) and brain and pancreatic cancer (isotretinoin). Tretinoin often causes psychiatric symptoms, including anxiety (17%), insomnia (14%), depression (14%), confusion (11%), agitation (9%), and hallucinations (6%). Several studies also suggest an association between isotretinoin use and depression, suicide, and psychosis. See Chapter 13, "Dermatological Disorders," for additional discussion of isotretinoin and depression and suicide.

Hormone therapy.   Tamoxifen has been reported to impair verbal memory in several clinical trials (Bakoyiannis et al. 2016; Jenkins et al. 2004; Schilder et al. 2009). However, a recent prospective longitudinal study of breast cancer survivors who had received endocrine therapy showed no effect on neuropsychological performance or impairment (Van Dyk et al. 2019). Despite early concerns about a link between tamoxifen and the development of depression, a large placebo-controlled cohort study of women with breast cancer concluded that tamoxifen administration does not increase risk (Lee et al. 2007). These results support the conclusion of an earlier multicenter placebo-controlled chemoprevention trial that tamoxifen does not increase risk for or exacerbate existing depression in women (Day et al. 2001). The effect of the aromatase inhibitor anastrozole on memory is unclear, with studies showing either greater impairment than with tamoxifen (Bender et al. 2015) or little or no impairment (Jenkins et al. 2008). On the other hand, a multinational trial showed less neurocognitive impairment with the aromatase inhibitor exemestane than with tamoxifen (Schilder et al. 2010).

Vinca alkaloids.   Posterior reversible encephalopathy syndrome has been reported in patients receiving vinflunine (Helissey et al. 2012) and vinorelbine (Chen and Huang 2012).

Monoclonal antibodies.   Novel immunotherapies have changed the landscape of how we treat cancers. Chimeric antigen receptor T cells and immune checkpoint inhibitors are two classes of treatment currently being used. Despite their clinical success, the use of chimeric antigen receptor T cells can result in significant toxicities that are associated with the induction of immune effector responses. The two primary toxicities following chimeric antigen receptor T-cell administration are cytokine release syndrome and immune-related neurotoxicity syndrome, which we have observed with bevacizumab, tagraxofusp-erzs, brentuximab, blinatumomab, ipilimumab, and dinutuximab (Morris et al. 2022). Symptoms of each of these syndromes may overlap and include headache, confusion, cognitive impairment, dizziness, seizures, hallucinations, decreased coordination, dysphagia, disarticulation, tremor, movement disorder, anxiety, and depression.

Drug-Drug Interactions

Drug-drug interactions are common in cancer therapy because of multiple medications, including cytotoxic chemotherapeutic agents, hormonal agents, and adjunctive medications for supportive care, as well as patients' preexisting medical problems. Because most patients with cancer are elderly (Yancik 2005), the drug burden from other medical conditions can be considerable.

Several complex pharmacokinetic and pharmacodynamic interactions can occur between chemotherapy and psychotropic medications. Pharmacokinetic interactions due to chemotherapy occur at several levels: inhibition of metabolic enzymes (CYP enzymes, monoamine oxidase), reduction of metabolism and excretion due to cytotoxic effects on hepatic and renal function, and altered distribution (hypoalbuminemia) and absorption (increased P-glycoprotein [P-gp] activity) (Tables 8–2 and 8–3). Many cancer agents are prodrugs (i.e., compounds that require metabolic activation for clinical effect), and many of them use CYP enzymes for their activation (Table 8–4). Drug-drug interactions from adjunctive medications, including psychotropic medications, can increase or reduce the metabolic activation of these prodrugs and affect their therapeutic benefit and adverse effects. Although clinicians should be vigilant about screening for any potential drug interactions, many of these interactions are theoretical in nature, and because oncological drug interactions are rarely reported, their clinical effect is uncertain (see Chapter 1, "Pharmacokinetics, Pharmacodynamics, and Principles of Drug-Drug Interactions").

Table 8–2.   Oncology medication–psychotropic medication interactions

Medication	Interaction mechanism	Effects on psychotropic medications and management
Alemtuzumab, arsenic trioxide, ceritinib, cetuximab, crizotinib, daunorubicin, denileukin, encorafenib, entrectinib, eribulin, etoposide, gemtuzumab, gilteritinib, glasdegib, homoharringtonine, idarubicin, inotuzumab, ivosidenib, lapatinib, lenvatinib, midostaurin, mitoxantrone, nilotinib, osimertinib, panobinostat, ribociclib, rituximab, selpercatinib, tamoxifen, tretinoin (systemic), vandetanib, vemurafenib	QT prolongation	Increased QT prolongation in combination with other QT-prolonging drugs such as TCAs, citalopram, typical antipsychotics, pimozide, risperidone, paliperidone, iloperidone, quetiapine, ziprasidone, and lithium
Asparaginase	Hypoalbuminemia	Therapeutic drug monitoring of total (free+bound) drug may give misleading results. Use methods selective for free drug levels (see Chapter 2, "Severe Drug Reactions").

Table 8–2. Oncology medication–psychotropic medication
interactions *(continued)*

Medication	Interaction mechanism	Effects on psychotropic medications and management
Cisplatin	Nephrotoxicity	Reduced elimination of renally eliminated drugs (e.g., lithium, paliperidone, desvenlafaxine, gabapentin, pregabalin, memantine); monitor lithium levels
	Unknown	Decreased levels of carbamazepine, phenytoin, valproate
Carboplatin, ifosfamide, methotrexate	Nephrotoxicity; acute and chronic reduction in GFR	Reduced elimination of renally eliminated drugs (e.g., lithium, paliperidone, desvenlafaxine, gabapentin, pregabalin, memantine); monitor lithium levels
Ceritinib, crizotinib, idelalisib, imatinib, larotrectinib	Inhibition of CYP3A4	Increased levels and toxicities for pimozide, quetiapine, ziprasidone, iloperidone, desvenlafaxine, oxidatively metabolized benzodiazepines, fentanyl, methadone, meperidine, tramadol
Mitotane, siltuximab, sotorasib, trametinib	Induction of CYP3A4	Increased metabolism and reduced exposure and therapeutic effect for pimozide, quetiapine, ziprasidone, iloperidone, desvenlafaxine, oxidatively metabolized benzodiazepines, fentanyl, methadone, meperidine, tramadol
5-Fluorouracil, alpelisib capecitabine	Reduced synthesis of CYP2C9	Reduced phenytoin metabolism with increased toxicity

Table 8–2. Oncology medication–psychotropic medication interactions *(continued)*

Medication	Interaction mechanism	Effects on psychotropic medications and management
Umbralisib	Inhibition of CYP2C9, CYP2C19, CYP3A4, P-gp	Increased levels and toxicities for phenytoin, pimozide, quetiapine, risperidone, ziprasidone, iloperidone, TCAs, bupropion, venlafaxine, fentanyl, meperidine, tramadol, atomoxetine, and benzodiazepines except oxazepam, lorazepam, and temazepam (see Chapter 2 for expanded list)
Interleukin-2 (aldesleukin)	QT prolongation	Increased QT prolongation in combination with other QT-prolonging drugs such as TCAs, citalopram, typical antipsychotics, pimozide, risperidone, paliperidone, iloperidone, quetiapine, ziprasidone, and lithium
	Nephrotoxicity and reduced renal function	Reduced elimination of renally eliminated drugs (e.g., lithium, paliperidone, desvenlafaxine, gabapentin, pregabalin, memantine); monitor lithium levels
	Reduced hepatic and renal function	Reduced hepatic metabolism and renal elimination of most drugs
Interferon-α	General inhibition of CYP450	Increased levels and adverse effects for oxidatively metabolized drugs, especially those metabolized by CYP1A2, CYP2C19, and CYP2D6

Table 8–2. Oncology medication–psychotropic medication interactions *(continued)*

Medication	Interaction mechanism	Effects on psychotropic medications and management
Interferon-α *(continued)*	QT prolongation	Increased QT prolongation in combination with other QT-prolonging drugs such as TCAs, citalopram, typical antipsychotics, pimozide, risperidone, paliperidone, iloperidone, quetiapine, ziprasidone, and lithium
Crizotinib, enasidenib, sotorasib	P-gp inhibition	Possible increased oral bioavailability of P-gp substrates (e.g., carbamazepine, phenytoin, lamotrigine, olanzapine, risperidone, quetiapine)
Procarbazine	MAO inhibition	Serotonin syndrome with selective serotonin reuptake inhibitors and serotonin-norepinephrine reuptake inhibitors, TCAs, MAO inhibitors, lithium, opiates (fentanyl, meperidine, methadone, tramadol, dextromethorphan, and propoxyphene) Hypertensive reaction with TCAs, sympathomimetics, and psychostimulants
Ceritinib, enasidenib, sorafenib, tamoxifen	Inhibition of CYP2C9	Reduced phenytoin metabolism with increased toxicity

Note. CYP = cytochrome P450; GFR = glomerular filtration rate; MAO = monoamine oxidase; P-gp = P-glycoprotein; TCAs = tricyclic antidepressants.

Interactions Affecting Drug Distribution

Asparaginase reduces serum albumin level by approximately 25% (Petros et al. 1992; Yang et al. 2008). Reductions in serum albumin level can have variable clinical effects on serum levels and clearance of highly protein-bound drugs,

Table 8–3.   Psychotropic medication–oncology medication interactions

Medication	Pharmacokinetic effect	Effects on oncology medications and management
Carbamazepine, phenytoin, and oxcarbazepine; armodafinil and modafinil; St. John's wort	Induction of CYP3A4 and other CYP enzymes	Increased metabolism and reduced exposure and therapeutic effect of CYP3A4 substrates, including abemaciclib, acalabrutinib, asciminib, avapritinib, axitinib, bexarotene, bosutinib, brentuximab, brigatinib, cabozantinib, capmatinib, ceritinib, cobimetinib, copanlisib, crizotinib, dabrafenib, dasatinib, docetaxel, doxorubicin, duvelisib, enfortumab, entrectinib, etoposide, everolimus, fedratinib, gefitinib, gilteritinib, glasdegib, ibrutinib, idelalisib, imatinib, infigratinib, ivosidenib, ixabepilone, ixazomib, lapatinib, larotrectinib, methotrexate, neratinib, olaparib, paclitaxel, palbociclib, panobinostat, pazopanib, pemigatinib, pomalidomide, ponatinib, pralsetinib, regorafenib, ribociclib, ruxolitinib, selpercatinib, sorafenib, sotorasib, sunitinib, tazemetostat, teniposide, tisotumab, tivozanib, topotecan, toremifene, tucatinib, umbralisib, vandetanib, vemurafenib, vinblastine, vincristine, and vinorelbine. Increased metabolism of cyclophosphamide and thiotepa and increased exposure to the toxic active metabolites. Reduce dosage to avoid excessive toxicity. Increased metabolic activation of prodrugs ifosfamide and procarbazine increases toxicity and shortens duration of effect. Increased metabolic inactivation of prodrug irinotecan reduces therapeutic effect.

Table 8–3.   Psychotropic medication–oncology medication interactions *(continued)*

Medication	Pharmacokinetic effect	Effects on oncology medications and management
Fluoxetine	Inhibition of CYP3A4	Reduced metabolism and increased exposure and toxicities of CYP3A4 substrates, including abemaciclib, acalabrutinib, asciminib, avapritinib, axitinib, bexarotene, bosutinib, brentuximab, brigatinib, cabozantinib, capmatinib, ceritinib, cobimetinib, copanlisib, crizotinib, dabrafenib, dasatinib, docetaxel, doxorubicin, enfortumab, etoposide, gefitinib, gilteritinib, glasdegib, ibrutinib, idelalisib, imatinib, infigratinib, ivosidenib, ixabepilone, ixazomib, lapatinib, larotrectinib, methotrexate, neratinib, olaparib, paclitaxel, palbociclib, panobinostat, pazopanib, pemigatinib, pomalidomide, ponatinib, pralsetinib, regorafenib, ribociclib, ruxolitinib, selpercatinib, sorafenib, sotorasib, sunitinib, tazemetostat, teniposide, tisotumab, tivozanib, topotecan, toremifene, tucatinib, umbralisib, vandetanib, vemurafenib, vinblastine, vincristine, and vinorelbine. Reduced metabolism of cyclophosphamide and thiotepa and reduced exposure to toxic active metabolites. Reduced metabolic activation of prodrugs ifosfamide, irinotecan, and procarbazine.
Fluvoxamine	Inhibition of CYP1A2	Reduced metabolism and increased exposure and toxicities of CYP1A2 substrates, including bendamustine, erlotinib, pomalidomide, and umbralisib.

Table 8–3. Psychotropic medication–oncology medication interactions *(continued)*

Medication	Pharmacokinetic effect	Effects on oncology medications and management
Fluvoxamine *(continued)*	Anticoagulant or antiplatelet	Increased anticoagulant or antiplatelet effects in combination with other antiplatelet drugs such as dasatinib and ibrutinib.
Atomoxetine, bupropion, duloxetine, fluoxetine, moclobemide, and paroxetine	Inhibition of CYP2D6	Reduced bioactivation of prodrug tamoxifen. Decreased therapeutic effect. Reduced metabolism and increased serum concentration and toxicities of gefitinib.
Carbamazepine	Downregulation of folate carrier	Reduced methotrexate cancer treatment efficacy.
Valproate	Inhibition of UGT1A1	Reduced metabolism of irinotecan active metabolite (SN-38) and increased toxicity. Possible reduced metabolism of sorafenib.
Carbamazepine, fosphenytoin, phenobarbital, and phenytoin	Induction of UGT1A1	Decreased metabolism of the active metabolite of sacituzumab (SN-38). Decreased SN-38 exposure may lead to a decreased response to treatment.
	Induction of P-gp	Increased metabolism and reduced exposure and therapeutic effect of P-gp substrates, including brigatinib, carfilzomib, ceritinib, crizotinib, enasidenib, gilteritinib, infigratinib, lapatinib, lenalidomide, lenvatinib, niraparib, and talazoparib.

Note. CYP=cytochrome P450; P-gp=P-glycoprotein; UGT=uridine 5′-diphosphate glucuronosyltransferase.

Table 8–4. Oncology prodrugs activated by cytochrome P450 (CYP) metabolism

Prodrug	Activating enzymes
Cyclophosphamide	CYP2B6
Dacarbazine	CYP1A2
Ifosfamide	CYP3A4
Procarbazine	Unidentified CYPs
Tamoxifen	CYP2D6, CYP3A4

Note. Refer to Chapter 1, "Pharmacokinetics, Pharmacodynamics, and Principles of Drug-Drug Interactions," for a list of relevant CYP metabolic inhibitors and inducers.

including carbamazepine, phenytoin, and valproate (see Chapter 1). When psychotropic drugs are coadministered with asparaginase, levels of the psychotropics should be monitored by methods selective for free drug; otherwise, lower total (free + bound) drug levels may prompt an inappropriate dosage increase.

Inhibition of Drug Metabolism by Chemotherapy Agents

The protein kinase inhibitors imatinib, nilotinib, and dasatinib and the anti-androgen nilutamide inhibit several CYP isozymes. Imatinib inhibits CYP2D6, CYP3A4, and CYP2C9 (Miguel and Albuquerque 2011; Novartis 2008), and the second-generation compound nilotinib has greater scope, inhibiting CYP2C8, CYP2C9, CYP2D6, CYP3A4, and P-gp (Deremer et al. 2008). Nilutamide may inhibit several isoenzymes, including CYP1A2 and CYP3A4, but this has not been firmly established (Sanofi-Aventis 2019). In the presence of one of these anticancer agents, many drugs, including many psychotropics, may experience increased bioavailability and reduced metabolism because of their metabolism pathways through CYP isozymes. Similarly, dasatinib is also a CYP3A4 inhibitor (Bristol-Myers Squibb 2021; Miguel and Albuquerque 2011), which may increase the bioavailability and plasma levels of several psychotropics, including pimozide, quetiapine, ziprasidone, iloperidone, desvenlafaxine, oxidatively metabolized benzodiazepines, fentanyl, and methadone, leading to unwanted toxicities and side effects.

Interferons and interleukins can give rise to drug interactions through inhibition of one or more CYP isozymes or the P-gp efflux transporter. Some small studies have shown that interferons significantly inhibit CYP1A2 and CYP2D6 immediately after the first interferon dose (Islam et al. 2002; Williams et al. 1987), followed by inhibition of CYP1A2, CYP2C19, and CYP2D6 over the course of treatment. However, other investigators have not found any consistent changes in CYP1A2 and CYP3A4 (Pageaux et al. 1998) or CYP2D6 and CYP3A4 (Becquemont et al. 2002). The reason for this variable effect is unclear. Given the wide scope of interferon's potential effects on CYP metabolism, the introduction of INF-α may require dosage reduction of narrow therapeutic range drugs metabolized by CYP isozymes.

Reduction in CYP isozyme activity has also been observed with IL-2 administration. Research suggests that high-dose ($\geq 9 \times 10^6$ U/m^2) IL-2 therapy may reduce metabolism of drugs metabolized by CYP1A2 (olanzapine and clozapine) and CYP3A4 (e.g., benzodiazepines, pimozide, quetiapine, ziprasidone, iloperidone, modafinil) (Elkahwaji et al. 1999; Vanda 2017).

Procarbazine inhibits monoamine oxidase and could trigger serotonin syndrome in combination with TCAs, SSRIs, SNRIs, monoamine oxidase inhibitors (MAOIs), or opiates with serotonin reuptake–inhibiting activity (meperidine, fentanyl, tramadol, methadone, dextromethorphan, and propoxyphene). Therefore, psychostimulants and other sympathomimetics should be avoided, and patients should be instructed to follow a tyramine-restricted diet.

Inhibition of Renal Elimination by Chemotherapy Agents

Several cancer agents are nephrotoxic, including the platinating agents cisplatin, carboplatin, and oxaliplatin; methotrexate; ifosfamide; and aldesleukin (Kintzel 2001) (see Table 8–2). A 20%–40% reduction in glomerular filtration rate after cisplatin therapy is common. Surprisingly, little evidence suggests that these drugs (with the exception of aldesleukin) alter renal drug elimination. In three case reports of patients receiving lithium, the introduction of cisplatin led to a transient decrease—not the expected increase—in lithium levels in two cases (Beijnen et al. 1992, 1994) and no change in a third (Pietruszka et al. 1985). In a survey of 123 children and adolescents, ifosfamide was shown to cause an average reduction in glomerular filtration rate of about 30% (Skinner et al. 2000). Caution is advised when administering a nephrotoxic agent with a drug that is primarily renally eliminated, including lithium, paliperidone, venlafaxine, desvenlafaxine, gabapentin, pregabalin, and memantine (Nagler et al. 2012).

Intentional Pharmacokinetic Interactions

Although drug-drug interactions are generally avoided in clinical practice because of unwanted side effects, some interactions or combinations of drugs are purposely used to increase therapeutic efficacy. For example, the oral bioavailability of the anticancer agent paclitaxel can be increased 10-fold by coadministration with cyclosporine, a CYP3A4 and P-gp inhibitor (Helgason et al. 2006). For other medications, including psychotropics, the pharmacokinetic effect of coadministering drugs for their interacting properties must be considered.

Interactions of Psychotropic Drugs With Chemotherapy Agents

Drug interactions that influence oncology drug levels may increase toxicity or reduce therapeutic effect, compromising overall survival rate. Many chemotherapy agents are CYP3A4 substrates. Coadministration of a CYP3A4 inhibitor (e.g., fluoxetine, fluvoxamine) may increase chemotherapy drug bioavailability and blood levels, increasing toxicity (see Table 8–3), which can decrease patients' medication adherence to these lifesaving chemotherapy agents.

Psychotropic Induction of Chemotherapeutic Metabolism

Concurrent use of the general CYP enzyme–inducing anticonvulsants carbamazepine, phenytoin, and phenobarbital with antileukemic chemotherapy has been shown to compromise the efficacy of the chemotherapy (Relling et al. 2000). Patients receiving long-term anticonvulsant therapy had significantly lower event-free survival (OR=2.67) than the anticonvulsant-free group. Systemic clearance of teniposide and methotrexate was shown to be faster in the anticonvulsant group. Other studies confirm increased clearance of imatinib (Pursche et al. 2008), irinotecan (Mathijssen et al. 2002a, 2002b), gefitinib (Swaisland et al. 2005), dasatinib (Johnson et al. 2010), nilotinib (Tanaka et al. 2011), and erlotinib (Hamilton et al. 2014; Pillai et al. 2013) in the presence of CYP enzyme inducers.

Psychotropic Inhibition of Chemotherapy Prodrug Bioactivation

Many chemotherapy agents are administered as prodrugs. Cyclophosphamide, dacarbazine, ifosfamide, procarbazine, tamoxifen, and trofosfamide undergo bioactivation via the CYP pathway (see Table 8–4). Drug interactions that inhibit the bioactivation of oncology prodrugs may reduce therapeutic effect and survival rate.

Tamoxifen is metabolized to the active metabolite endoxifen in a two-step process involving both CYP2D6 and CYP3A4 (Briest and Stearns 2009). For women with breast cancer taking tamoxifen, plasma levels of endoxifen were reduced with the strong CYP2D6 inhibitor paroxetine (>70%) or the mild CYP2D6 inhibitor sertraline (>40%). Conversion of tamoxifen was also reduced with even mild CYP3A4 inhibition (Jin et al. 2005). For women with breast cancer who were receiving tamoxifen therapy, concurrent use of a CYP2D6 inhibitor increased the recurrence of breast cancer 1.9-fold (Aubert et al. 2009). A large population-based cohort study of women taking tamoxifen found that concurrent use of paroxetine was associated with increased breast cancer mortality (Kelly et al. 2010). Paroxetine, fluoxetine, sertraline (CYP2D6 inhibition at >200 mg/day), duloxetine, bupropion, moclobemide, atomoxetine, and other CYP2D6 inhibitors should be avoided during tamoxifen therapy (Goetz et al. 2007). Citalopram, escitalopram, venlafaxine, and mirtazapine are preferred because of their lack of effect on CYP metabolism (Breitbart 2011; Miguel and Albuquerque 2011). Despite this concern, paroxetine and other antidepressants that inhibit CYP2D6 continue to be prescribed frequently to women who are taking tamoxifen (Binkhorst et al. 2013; Dieudonné et al. 2014; Dusetzina et al. 2013).

Irinotecan, a topoisomerase I inhibitor, has complex metabolism. It is metabolized to the active cytotoxic compound SN-38 by carboxylesterases but is inactivated by CYP3A4 isozymes. Drugs that induce CYP3A4, including carbamazepine, phenytoin, phenobarbital (Kuhn 2002), and St. John's wort (Mathijssen et al. 2002b), produce significant reductions in SN-38 levels, as does valproate (de Jong et al. 2007). Dosage adjustment may be needed in the presence of these and other psychotropic drugs that induce (armodafinil, modafinil) or inhibit (fluoxetine, fluvoxamine, nefazodone) CYP3A4.

Cyclophosphamide is converted by CYP2B6 metabolism to the active anticancer metabolite 4-hydroxycoumarin. Two case reports suggested that CYP enzyme induction by phenytoin (de Jonge et al. 2005) or carbamazepine (Ekhart et al. 2009) increases conversion to 4-hydroxycoumarin and may increase toxicities. Conversely, CYP2B6 inhibitors would be expected to reduce 4-hydroxycoumarin levels and decrease therapeutic effect. Common psychotropic drugs, including paroxetine, fluoxetine, and fluvoxamine, are also CYP2B6 inhibitors, and concurrent administration should be avoided.

Ifosfamide and trofosfamide (an ifosfamide prodrug), in contrast to cyclo-phosphamide, are activated by CYP3A4 and inactivated by CYP2B6 and CYP3A4. One study suggests that CYP3A4 inhibitors and inducers should be avoided when ifosfamide is administered and possibly during trofosfamide therapy (Kerbusch et al. 2001).

Pharmacodynamic Interactions

A wide variety of chemotherapy agents prolong the QT interval (see Table 8–2) (Arbel et al. 2007; Coppola et al. 2018; Duan et al. 2018; Ghatalia et al. 2015; Slovacek et al. 2008; Yeh 2006; see also https://crediblemeds.org). These agents should be used with caution in the presence of other QT-prolonging drugs such as TCAs, citalopram, typical antipsychotics, pimozide, risperidone, paliperidone, iloperidone, quetiapine, ziprasidone, and lithium (Beach et al. 2013; Kane et al. 2008; van Noord et al. 2009).

Hypotension is commonly associated with dinutuximab, etoposide, deni-leukin, naxitamab, systemic tretinoin, alemtuzumab, cetuximab, rituximab, INF-α, and IL-2 (aldesleukin). These agents may increase the hypotensive effects of psychotropic agents, including TCAs, antipsychotics, and MAOIs.

Antiemetics are often used to manage chemotherapy-induced nausea and vomiting during intense chemotherapy treatment. Antiemetic drug interactions are discussed in Chapter 4.

Drug Interaction Summary

Clinically significant drug-drug interactions are rarely reported in the literature, and many are speculative; however, several interactions deserve attention. The use of multiple QT-prolonging drugs should be avoided. Several chemotherapy agents inhibit metabolism of psychotropic drugs and may increase psychotropic toxicities. In this event, psychotropic clinical response and therapeutic drug–level monitoring should guide dosage adjustments. SSRIs, SNRIs, TCAs, MAOIs, and other agents known to precipitate serotonin syndrome should be avoided with procarbazine. Many oncological drugs are metabolized primarily through CYP3A4 isozymes; therefore, inducers and inhibitors of CYP3A4 should be avoided. Reduced therapeutic efficacy of oncological prodrugs may occur in the presence of drugs that inhibit their metabolic activation. Prodrug interactions that reduce therapeutic efficacy are becoming increasingly recognized. Conversely, the adverse effects of oncological prodrugs may be exacerbated by metabolic inducers, especially pan-inducers such as carbamazepine, phenytoin, and phenobarbital.

Key Points

- Psychiatric comorbidities of cancer or cancer therapy are often undertreated. Anxiety, depression, and fatigue can be treated effectively with psychotropics.

- Neuropsychiatric symptoms of chemotherapy—especially depression with interferon and interleukin—may lead to treatment discontinuation. Use of an adjunctive antidepressant increases adherence to chemotherapy.

- Studies to date do not support withholding any psychiatric medications on the basis of fear of increasing cancer risk, with the possible exception of antipsychotics with a high incidence of hyperprolactinemia in patients with current or past history of pituitary endocrine tumors.

- Many chemotherapeutic agents prolong the QT interval. Coadministration of other QT-prolonging drugs, including many psychotropics, should be avoided.

- Many chemotherapy agents are metabolized by cytochrome P450 (CYP) 3A4. Coadministration of a CYP3A4 inhibitor may increase chemotherapy toxicity and should be avoided.

- Use of psychotropics that do not inhibit metabolism is preferred in combination with oncology prodrugs such as tamoxifen.

References

Agar M, Lawlor P: Delirium in cancer patients: a focus on treatment-induced psychopathology. Curr Opin Oncol 20(4):360–366, 2008 18525328

Alici-Evcimen Y, Breitbart WS: Ifosfamide neuropsychiatric toxicity in patients with cancer. Psychooncology 16(10):956–960, 2007 17278152

Ambrosiani L, Pisanu C, Deidda A, et al: Thyroid and renal tumors in patients treated with long-term lithium: case series from a lithium clinic, review of the literature and international pharmacovigilance reports. Int J Bipolar Disord 6(1):17, 2018 30079440

Amgen: Blincyto (blinatumomab) injection package insert. March 2018. Available at: http://www.accessdata.fda.gov/drugsatfda_docs/label/2018/125557s013lbl.pdf. Accessed March 8, 2022.

Arbel Y, Swartzon M, Justo D: QT prolongation and torsades de pointes in patients previously treated with anthracyclines. Anticancer Drugs 18(4):493–498, 2007 17351403

Aubert RE, Stanek EJ, Yao J, et al: Risk of breast cancer recurrence in women initiating tamoxifen with CYP2D6 inhibitors (meeting abstracts). J Clin Oncol 27(18S):CRA508, 2009

Baker WJ, Royer GL Jr, Weiss RB: Cytarabine and neurologic toxicity. J Clin Oncol 9(4):679–693, 1991 1648599

Bakoyiannis I, Tsigka EA, Perrea D, et al: The impact of endocrine therapy on cognitive functions of breast cancer patients: a systematic review. Clin Drug Investig 36(2):109–118, 2016 26619839

Beach SR, Celano CM, Noseworthy PA, et al: QTc prolongation, torsades de pointes, and psychotropic medications. Psychosomatics 54(1):1–13, 2013 23295003

Becquemont L, Chazouilleres O, Serfaty L, et al: Effect of interferon alpha-ribavirin bitherapy on cytochrome P450 1A2 and 2D6 and N-acetyltransferase-2 activities in patients with chronic active hepatitis C. Clin Pharmacol Ther 71(6):488–495, 2002 12087352

Beijnen JH, Vlasveld LT, Wanders J, et al: Effect of cisplatin-containing chemotherapy on lithium serum concentrations. Ann Pharmacother 26(4):488–490, 1992 1576384

Beijnen JH, Bais EM, ten Bokkel Huinink WW: Lithium pharmacokinetics during cisplatin-based chemotherapy: a case report. Cancer Chemother Pharmacol 33(6):523–526, 1994 7511066

Belloni S, Arrigoni C, de Sanctis R, et al: A systematic review of systematic reviews and pooled meta-analysis on pharmacological interventions to improve cancer-related fatigue. Crit Rev Oncol Hematol 166:103373, 2021 34051301

Bender CM, Merriman JD, Gentry AL, et al: Patterns of change in cognitive function with anastrozole therapy. Cancer 121(15):2627–2636, 2015 25906766

Berenson JR, Yellin O, Shamasunder HK, et al: A phase 3 trial of armodafinil for the treatment of cancer-related fatigue for patients with multiple myeloma. Support Care Cancer 23(6):1503–1512, 2015 25370889

Binkhorst L, Mathijssen RH, van Herk-Sukel MP, et al: Unjustified prescribing of CYP2D6 inhibiting SSRIs in women treated with tamoxifen. Breast Cancer Res Treat 139(3):923–929, 2013 23760858

Breitbart W: Do antidepressants reduce the effectiveness of tamoxifen? Psychooncology 20(1):1–4, 2011 21182159

Breitbart WA: Treatment of delirium and confusional states in oncology and palliative care settings, in Psychopharmacology in Oncology and Palliative Care: A Practical Manual. Edited by Grassi L, Riba M. Heidelberg, Germany, Springer, 2014, pp 203–228

Briest S, Stearns V: Tamoxifen metabolism and its effect on endocrine treatment of breast cancer. Clin Adv Hematol Oncol 7(3):185–192, 2009 19398943

Bristol-Myers Squibb: Sprycel (dasatinib) package insert. June 2021. Available at: http://www.accessdata.fda.gov/drugsatfda_docs/label/2010/021986s7s8lbl.pdf. Accessed December 12, 2021.

Bruera E, Yennurajalingam S, Palmer JL, et al: Methylphenidate and/or a nursing telephone intervention for fatigue in patients with advanced cancer: a randomized, placebo-controlled, phase II trial. J Clin Oncol 31(19):2421–2427, 2013 23690414

Butler JM Jr, Case LD, Atkins J, et al: A phase III, double-blind, placebo-controlled prospective randomized clinical trial of d-threo-methylphenidate HCl in brain tumor patients receiving radiation therapy. Int J Radiat Oncol Biol Phys 69(5):1496–1501, 2007 17869448

Cankurtaran ES, Ozalp E, Soygur H, et al: Mirtazapine improves sleep and lowers anxiety and depression in cancer patients: superiority over imipramine. Support Care Cancer 16(11):1291–1298, 2008 18299900

Cao J, Wang B, Wang Z, et al: Efficacy of mirtazapine in preventing delayed nausea and vomiting induced by highly emetogenic chemotherapy: an open label, randomized, multicenter phase III trial. J Clin Oncol 36(15 Suppl):1078, 2018

Cao J, Ouyang QC, Wang BSS, et al: Mirtazapine, a dopamine receptor inhibitor, as a secondary prophylactic for delayed nausea and vomiting following highly emetogenic chemotherapy: an open label, randomized, multicenter phase III trial. Invest New Drugs 38(2):507–514, 2020 32036491

Capuron L, Ravaud A, Dantzer R: Early depressive symptoms in cancer patients receiving interleukin 2 and/or interferon alfa-2b therapy. J Clin Oncol 18(10):2143–2151, 2000 10811680

Capuron L, Gumnick JF, Musselman DL, et al: Neurobehavioral effects of interferon-alpha in cancer patients: phenomenology and paroxetine responsiveness of symptom dimensions. Neuropsychopharmacology 26(5):643–652, 2002 11927189

Caraceni A: Drug-associated delirium in cancer patients. EJC Suppl 11(2):233–240, 2013 26217132

Caruso R, Grassi L, Nanni MG, et al: Psychopharmacology in psycho-oncology. Curr Psychiatry Rep 15(9):393, 2013 23949568

Carvalho AF, Hyphantis T, Sales PM, et al: Major depressive disorder in breast cancer: a critical systematic review of pharmacological and psychotherapeutic clinical trials. Cancer Treat Rev 40(3):349–355, 2014 24084477

Centeno C, Sanz A, Cuervo MA, et al: Multicentre, double-blind, randomised placebo-controlled clinical trial on the efficacy of methylphenidate on depressive symptoms in advanced cancer patients. BMJ Support Palliat Care 2(4):328–333, 2012 24654216

Chen AM, Daly ME, Vazquez E, et al: Depression among long-term survivors of head and neck cancer treated with radiation therapy. JAMA Otolaryngol Head Neck Surg 139(9):885–889, 2013 23949013

Chen VCH, Liao YT, Yeh DC, et al: Relationship between antidepressant prescription and breast cancer: a population based study in Taiwan. Psychooncology 25(7):803–807, 2016 26274350

Chen YH, Huang CH: Reversible posterior leukoencephalopathy syndrome induced by vinorelbine. Clin Breast Cancer 12(3):222–225, 2012 22424944

Cohen Y, Chetrit A, Cohen Y, et al: Cancer morbidity in psychiatric patients: influence of lithium carbonate treatment. Med Oncol 15(1):32–36, 1998 9643528

Conley CC, Kamen CS, Heckler CE, et al: Modafinil moderates the relationship between cancer-related fatigue and depression in 541 patients receiving chemotherapy. J Clin Psychopharmacol 36(1):82–85, 2016 26658264

Coogan PF, Strom BL, Rosenberg L: Antidepressant use and colorectal cancer risk. Pharmacoepidemiol Drug Saf 18(11):1111–1114, 2009 19623565

Cooper MR, Bird HM, Steinberg M: Efficacy and safety of modafinil in the treatment of cancer-related fatigue. Ann Pharmacother 43(4):721–725, 2009 19318599

Coppola C, Rienzo A, Piscopo G, et al: Management of QT prolongation induced by anti-cancer drugs: target therapy and old agents. Different algorithms for different drugs. Cancer Treat Rev 63:135–143, 2018 29304463

Cortese I, Reich DS, Nath A: Progressive multifocal leukoencephalopathy and the spectrum of JC virus-related disease. Nat Rev Neurol 17(1):37–51, 2021 33219338

Cosci F, Fava GA, Sonino N: Mood and anxiety disorders as early manifestations of medical illness: a systematic review. Psychother Psychosom 84(1):22–29, 2015 25547421

Costa D, Mogos I, Toma T: Efficacy and safety of mianserin in the treatment of depression of women with cancer. Acta Psychiatr Scand Suppl 320:85–92, 1985 3901675

Costantini C, Ale-Ali A, Helsten T: Sleep aid prescribing practices during neoadjuvant or adjuvant chemotherapy for breast cancer. J Palliat Med 14(5):563–566, 2011 21388255

Cronin-Fenton DP, Riis AH, Lash TL, et al: Antidepressant use and colorectal cancer risk: a Danish population-based case-control study. Br J Cancer 104(1):188–192, 2011 20877356

Dalton SO, Johansen C, Poulsen AH, et al: Cancer risk among users of neuroleptic medication: a population-based cohort study. Br J Cancer 95(7):934–939, 2006 16926836

Das A, Ranadive N, Kinra M, et al: An overview on chemotherapy-induced cognitive impairment and potential role of antidepressants. Curr Neuropharmacol 18(9):838–851, 2020 32091339

Day J, Zienius K, Gehring K, et al: Interventions for preventing and ameliorating cognitive deficits in adults treated with cranial irradiation. Cochrane Database Syst Rev (12):CD011335, 2014 25519950

Day R, Ganz PA, Costantino JP: Tamoxifen and depression: more evidence from the National Surgical Adjuvant Breast and Bowel Project's Breast Cancer Prevention (P-1) Randomized Study. J Natl Cancer Inst 93(21):1615–1623, 2001 11698565

De Hert M, Peuskens J, Sabbe T, et al: Relationship between prolactin, breast cancer risk, and antipsychotics in patients with schizophrenia: a critical review. Acta Psychiatr Scand 133(1):5–22, 2016 26114737

de Jong FA, van der Bol JM, Mathijssen RH, et al: Irinotecan chemotherapy during valproic acid treatment: pharmacokinetic interaction and hepatotoxicity. Cancer Biol Ther 6(9):1368–1374, 2007 17873515

de Jonge ME, Huitema AD, van Dam SM, et al: Significant induction of cyclophosphamide and thiotepa metabolism by phenytoin. Cancer Chemother Pharmacol 55(5):507–510, 2005 15685452

Deremer DL, Ustun C, Natarajan K: Nilotinib: a second-generation tyrosine kinase inhibitor for the treatment of chronic myelogenous leukemia. Clin Ther 30(11):1956–1975, 2008 19108785

Dieudonné AS, De Nys K, Casteels M, et al: How often did Belgian physicians co-prescribe tamoxifen with strong CYP2D6 inhibitors over the last 6 years? Acta Clin Belg 69(1):47–52, 2014 24635399

Doraiswamy PM, Schott G, Star K, et al: Atypical antipsychotics and pituitary neoplasms in the WHO database. Psychopharmacol Bull 40(1):74–76, 2007 17285098

Duan J, Tao J, Zhai M, et al: Anticancer drugs-related QTc prolongation, torsade de pointes and sudden death: current evidence and future research perspectives. Oncotarget 9(39):25738–25749, 2018 29876021

Dufour C, Grill J, Sabouraud P, et al: Ifosfamide induced encephalopathy: 15 observations [in French]. Arch Pediatr 13(2):140–145, 2006 16364615

Dusetzina SB, Alexander GC, Freedman RA, et al: Trends in co-prescribing of antidepressants and tamoxifen among women with breast cancer, 2004–2010. Breast Cancer Res Treat 137(1):285–296, 2013 23149465

Economos G, Lovell N, Johnston A, et al: What is the evidence for mirtazapine in treating cancer-related symptomatology? A systematic review. Support Care Cancer 28(4):1597–1606, 2020 31858251

Ekhart C, Rodenhuis S, Beijnen JH, et al: Carbamazepine induces bioactivation of cyclophosphamide and thiotepa. Cancer Chemother Pharmacol 63(3):543–547, 2009 18437385

Elkahwaji J, Robin MA, Berson A, et al: Decrease in hepatic cytochrome P450 after interleukin-2 immunotherapy. Biochem Pharmacol 57(8):951–954, 1999 10086330

Escalante CP, Meyers C, Reuben JM, et al: A randomized, double-blind, 2-period, placebo-controlled crossover trial of a sustained-release methylphenidate in the treatment of fatigue in cancer patients. Cancer J 20(1):8–14, 2014 24445757

Evans DL, McCartney CF, Haggerty JJ Jr, et al: Treatment of depression in cancer patients is associated with better life adaptation: a pilot study. Psychosom Med 50(1):73–76, 1988 3344305

Fisch MJ, Loehrer PJ, Kristeller J, et al: Fluoxetine versus placebo in advanced cancer outpatients: a double-blinded trial of the Hoosier Oncology Group. J Clin Oncol 21(10):1937–1943, 2003 12743146

Forbes M, Stefler D, Velakoulis D, et al: The clinical utility of structural neuroimaging in first-episode psychosis: a systematic review. Aust N Z J Psychiatry 53(11):1093–1104, 2019 31113237

Foster AR, Caplan JP: Paraneoplastic limbic encephalitis. Psychosomatics 50(2):108–113, 2009 19377018

Ghatalia P, Je Y, Kaymakcalan MD, et al: QTc interval prolongation with vascular endothelial growth factor receptor tyrosine kinase inhibitors. Br J Cancer 112(2):296–305, 2015 25349964

Goetz MP, Knox SK, Suman VJ, et al: The impact of cytochrome P450 2D6 metabolism in women receiving adjuvant tamoxifen. Breast Cancer Res Treat 101(1):113–121, 2007 17115111

Gozzard P, Woodhall M, Chapman C, et al: Paraneoplastic neurologic disorders in small cell lung carcinoma: a prospective study. Neurology 85(3):235–239, 2015 26109714

Grassi L, Nanni MG, Rodin G, et al: The use of antidepressants in oncology: a review and practical tips for oncologists. Ann Oncol 29(1):101–111, 2018 29272358

Greenblatt HK, Greenblatt DJ: Gabapentin and pregabalin for the treatment of anxiety disorders. Clin Pharmacol Drug Dev 7(3):228–232, 2018 29579375

Guidon AC, Burton LB, Chwalisz BK, et al: Consensus disease definitions for neurologic immune-related adverse events of immune checkpoint inhibitors. J Immunother Cancer 9(7):e002890, 2021 34281989

Gultekin SH, Rosenfeld MR, Voltz R, et al: Paraneoplastic limbic encephalitis: neurological symptoms, immunological findings and tumour association in 50 patients. Brain 123(Pt 7):1481–1494, 2000 10869059

Halapy E, Kreiger N, Cotterchio M, et al: Benzodiazepines and risk for breast cancer. Ann Epidemiol 16(8):632–636, 2006 16406246

Hamilton M, Wolf JL, Drolet DW, et al: The effect of rifampicin, a prototypical CYP3A4 inducer, on erlotinib pharmacokinetics in healthy subjects. Cancer Chemother Pharmacol 73(3):613–621, 2014 24474302

Hansen MV, Andersen LT, Madsen MT, et al: Effect of melatonin on depressive symptoms and anxiety in patients undergoing breast cancer surgery: a randomized, double-blind, placebo-controlled trial. Breast Cancer Res Treat 145(3):683–695, 2014 24756186

Helgason HH, Kruijtzer CM, Huitema AD, et al: Phase II and pharmacological study of oral paclitaxel (Paxoral) plus ciclosporin in anthracycline-pretreated metastatic breast cancer. Br J Cancer 95(7):794–800, 2006 16969354

Helissey C, Chargari C, Lahutte M, et al: First case of posterior reversible encephalopathy syndrome associated with vinflunine. Invest New Drugs 30(5):2032–2034, 2012 21728021

Hippisley-Cox J, Vinogradova Y, Coupland C, et al: Risk of malignancy in patients with schizophrenia or bipolar disorder: nested case-control study. Arch Gen Psychiatry 64(12):1368–1376, 2007 18056544

Ho HY, Chin-Hung Chen V, Tzang BS, et al: Circulating cytokines as predictors of depression in patients with breast cancer. J Psychiatr Res 136:306–311, 2021 33636686

Holland JC, Romano SJ, Heiligenstein JH, et al: A controlled trial of fluoxetine and desipramine in depressed women with advanced cancer. Psychooncology 7(4):291–300, 1998 9741068

Hossein G, Zavareh VA, Fard PS: Combined treatment of androgen-independent prostate cancer cell line DU145 with chemotherapeutic agents and lithium chloride: effect on growth arrest and/or apoptosis. Avicenna J Med Biotechnol 4(2):75–87, 2012 23408470

Howard P, Twycross R, Shuster J, et al: Benzodiazepines. J Pain Symptom Manage 47(5):955–964, 2014 24681184

Huang RY, Hsieh KP, Huang WW, et al: Use of lithium and cancer risk in patients with bipolar disorder: population-based cohort study. Br J Psychiatry 209(5):393–399, 2016 27388574

Huffman JC, Stern TA: Using psychostimulants to treat depression in the medically ill. Prim Care Companion J Clin Psychiatry 6(1):44–46, 2004 15486600

Huo YL, Qiao JM, Gao S: Association between antidepressant medication use and epithelial ovarian cancer risk: a systematic review and meta-analysis of observational studies. Br J Clin Pharmacol 84(4):649–658, 2018 29292523

Iqbal U, Chang TH, Nguyen PA, et al: Benzodiazepines use and breast cancer risk: a population-based study and gene expression profiling evidence. J Biomed Inform 74:85–91, 2017 28851658

Islam M, Frye RF, Richards TJ, et al: Differential effect of IFNalpha-2b on the cytochrome P450 enzyme system: a potential basis of IFN toxicity and its modulation by other drugs. Clin Cancer Res 8(8):2480–2487, 2002 12171873

Jain T, Litzow MR: Management of toxicities associated with novel immunotherapy agents in acute lymphoblastic leukemia. Ther Adv Hematol 11:2040620719899897, 2020 32010436

James A, Nair MM, Abraham DS, et al: Effect of lorazepam in reducing psychological distress and anticipatory nausea and vomiting in patients undergoing chemotherapy. J Pharmacol Pharmacother 8(3):112–115, 2017 29081618

Jazz Pharmaceuticals: Rylaze (asparaginase erwinia chrysanthemi [recombinant]-rywn) product monograph. June 2021. Available at: http://www.accessdata.fda.gov/drugsatfda_docs/label/2021/761179s000lbl.pdf. Accessed March 8, 2022.

Jenkins V, Shilling V, Fallowfield L, et al: Does hormone therapy for the treatment of breast cancer have a detrimental effect on memory and cognition? A pilot study. Psychooncology 13(1):61–66, 2004 14745746

Jenkins VA, Ambroisine LM, Atkins L, et al: Effects of anastrozole on cognitive performance in postmenopausal women: a randomised, double-blind chemoprevention trial (IBIS II). Lancet Oncol 9(10):953–961, 2008 18768369

Jin Y, Desta Z, Stearns V, et al: CYP2D6 genotype, antidepressant use, and tamoxifen metabolism during adjuvant breast cancer treatment. J Natl Cancer Inst 97(1):30–39, 2005 15632378

Johnson DB, Manouchehri A, Haugh AM, et al: Neurologic toxicity associated with immune checkpoint inhibitors: a pharmacovigilance study. J Immunother Cancer 7(1):134, 2019 31118078

Johnson FM, Agrawal S, Burris H, et al: Phase 1 pharmacokinetic and drug-interaction study of dasatinib in patients with advanced solid tumors. Cancer 116(6):1582–1591, 2010 20108303

Joly F, Giffard B, Rigal O, et al: Impact of cancer and its treatments on cognitive function: advances in research from the Paris International Cognition and Cancer Task Force Symposium and update since 2012. J Pain Symptom Manage 50(6):830–841, 2015 26344551

Junior PNA, Barreto CMN, Cubero DIG, et al: The efficacy of placebo for the treatment of cancer-related fatigue: a systematic review and meta-analysis. Support Care Cancer 28(4):1755–1764, 2020 31302766

Kaleita T, Wellisch D, Graham C, et al: Pilot study of modafinil for treatment of neurobehavioral dysfunction and fatigue in adult patients with brain tumors. J Clin Oncol 24(18S):1503, 2006

Kane JM, Lauriello J, Laska E, et al: Long-term efficacy and safety of iloperidone: results from 3 clinical trials for the treatment of schizophrenia. J Clin Psychopharmacol 28(2 Suppl 1):S29–S35, 2008 18334910

Kao CH, Sun LM, Su KP, et al: Benzodiazepine use possibly increases cancer risk: a population-based retrospective cohort study in Taiwan. J Clin Psychiatry 73(4):e555–e560, 2012 22579162

Karschnia P, Parsons MW, Dietrich J: Pharmacologic management of cognitive impairment induced by cancer therapy. Lancet Oncol 20(2):e92–e102, 2019 30723041

Kelley BP, Patel SC, Marin HL, et al: Autoimmune encephalitis: pathophysiology and imaging review of an overlooked diagnosis. AJNR Am J Neuroradiol 38(6):1070–1078, 2017 28183838

Kelly CM, Juurlink DN, Gomes T, et al: Selective serotonin reuptake inhibitors and breast cancer mortality in women receiving tamoxifen: a population based cohort study. BMJ 340:c693, 2010 20142325

Kerbusch T, Jansen RL, Mathôt RA, et al: Modulation of the cytochrome P450-mediated metabolism of ifosfamide by ketoconazole and rifampin. Clin Pharmacol Ther 70(2):132–141, 2001 11503007

Kerr CW, Drake J, Milch RA, et al: Effects of methylphenidate on fatigue and depression: a randomized, double-blind, placebo-controlled trial. J Pain Symptom Manage 43(1):68–77, 2012 22208450

Kim SW, Shin IS, Kim JM, et al: Effectiveness of mirtazapine for nausea and insomnia in cancer patients with depression. Psychiatry Clin Neurosci 62(1):75–83, 2008 18289144

Kintzel PE: Anticancer drug-induced kidney disorders. Drug Saf 24(1):19–38, 2001 11219485

Kuendgen A, Bug G, Ottmann OG, et al: Treatment of poor-risk myelodysplastic syndromes and acute myeloid leukemia with a combination of 5-azacytidine and valproic acid. Clin Epigenetics 2(2):389–399, 2011 22704349

Kuhn JG: Influence of anticonvulsants on the metabolism and elimination of irinotecan: a North American Brain Tumor Consortium preliminary report. Oncology (Williston Park) 16(8 Suppl 7):33–40, 2002 12199631

Kumar N, Barai S, Gambhir S, et al: Effect of mirtazapine on gastric emptying in patients with cancer-associated anorexia. Indian J Palliat Care 23(3):335–337, 2017 28827942

Lan Y, Liu X, Zhang R, et al: Lithium enhances TRAIL-induced apoptosis in human lung carcinoma A549 cells. Biometals 26(2):241–254, 2013 23378009

Lavigne JE, Heckler C, Mathews JL, et al: A randomized, controlled, double-blinded clinical trial of gabapentin 300 versus 900 mg versus placebo for anxiety symptoms in breast cancer survivors. Breast Cancer Res Treat 136(2):479–486, 2012 23053645

Leadiant Biosciences: Matulane (procarbazine) package insert. August 2018. Available at: https://dailymed.nlm.nih.gov/dailymed/getFile.cfm?setid=1aa75a3a-18c9-49e1-91a6-293d0b7da756&type=pdf. Accessed December 12, 2021.

Lee KC, Ray GT, Hunkeler EM, et al: Tamoxifen treatment and new-onset depression in breast cancer patients. Psychosomatics 48(3):205–210, 2007 17478588

Li M, Kennedy EB, Byrne N, et al: Systematic review and meta-analysis of collaborative care interventions for depression in patients with cancer. Psychooncology 26(5):573–587, 2017 27643388

Lin WY, Chen VCH, Chiu WC, et al: Prostate cancer and antidepressants: a nationwide population-based nested case-control study. J Affect Disord 227:834–839, 2018 29689697

Lundorff LE, Jønsson BH, Sjøgren P: Modafinil for attentional and psychomotor dysfunction in advanced cancer: a double-blind, randomised, cross-over trial. Palliat Med 23(8):731–738, 2009 19648224

Lv L, Mao S, Dong H, et al: Pathogenesis, assessments, and management of chemotherapy-related cognitive impairment (CRCI): an updated literature review. J Oncol 2020:3942439, 2020 32684930

Lyskowski J, Nasrallah HA: Lithium therapy and the risk for leukemia (letter). Br J Psychiatry 139:256, 1981 7317712

Madhusoodanan S, Ting MB, Farah T, et al: Psychiatric aspects of brain tumors: a review. World J Psychiatry 5(3):273–285, 2015 26425442

Masdeu JC: Neuroimaging in psychiatric disorders. Neurotherapeutics 8(1):93–102, 2011 21274689

Mathijssen RH, Sparreboom A, Dumez H, et al: Altered irinotecan metabolism in a patient receiving phenytoin. Anticancer Drugs 13(2):139–140, 2002a 11901305

Mathijssen RH, Verweij J, de Bruijn P, et al: Effects of St. John's wort on irinotecan metabolism. J Natl Cancer Inst 94(16):1247–1249, 2002b 12189228

Matsos A, Loomes M, Zhou I, et al: Chemotherapy-induced cognitive impairments: white matter pathologies. Cancer Treat Rev 61:6–14, 2017 29073552

McCarren M, Qiu H, Ziyadeh N, et al: Follow-up study of a pharmacovigilance signal: no evidence of increased risk with risperidone of pituitary tumor with mass effect. J Clin Psychopharmacol 32(6):743–749, 2012 23131882

McNutt MD, Liu S, Manatunga A, et al: Neurobehavioral effects of interferon-a in patients with hepatitis-C: symptom dimensions and responsiveness to paroxetine. Neuropsychopharmacology 37(6):1444–1454, 2012 22353759

Miguel C, Albuquerque E: Drug interaction in psycho-oncology: antidepressants and antineoplastics. Pharmacology 88(5–6):333–339, 2011 22123153

Moorman PG, Berchuck A, Calingaert B, et al: Antidepressant medication use [corrected] and risk of ovarian cancer. Obstet Gynecol 105(4):725–730, 2005 15802397

Moraska AR, Sood A, Dakhil SR, et al: Phase III, randomized, double-blind, placebo-controlled study of long-acting methylphenidate for cancer-related fatigue: North Central Cancer Treatment Group NCCTG-N05C7 trial. J Clin Oncol 28(23):3673–3679, 2010 20625123

Morris EC, Neelapu SS, Giavridis T, et al: Cytokine release syndrome and associated neurotoxicity in cancer immunotherapy. Nat Rev Immunol 22(2):85–96, 2022 34002066

Morrow GR, Hickok JT, Roscoe JA, et al: Differential effects of paroxetine on fatigue and depression: a randomized, double-blind trial from the University of Rochester Cancer Center Community Clinical Oncology Program. J Clin Oncol 21(24):4635–4641, 2003 14673053

Mortensen PB: Neuroleptic treatment and other factors modifying cancer risk in schizophrenic patients. Acta Psychiatr Scand 75(6):585–590, 1987 2887088

Mortensen PB: Neuroleptic medication and reduced risk of prostate cancer in schizophrenic patients. Acta Psychiatr Scand 85(5):390–393, 1992 1351334

Moss EL, Simpson JS, Pelletier G, et al: An open-label study of the effects of bupropion SR on fatigue, depression and quality of life of mixed-site cancer patients and their partners. Psychooncology 15(3):259–267, 2006 16041840

Mounier NM, Abdel-Maged AES, Wahdan SA, et al: Chemotherapy-induced cognitive impairment (CICI): an overview of etiology and pathogenesis. Life Sci 258:118071, 2020 32673664

Mücke M, Cuhls H, Peuckmann-Post V, et al: Pharmacological treatments for fatigue associated with palliative care. Cochrane Database Syst Rev (5):CD006788, 2015 26026155

Mugge L, Mansour TR, Crippen M, et al: Depression and glioblastoma, complicated concomitant diseases: a systemic review of published literature. Neurosurg Rev 43(2):497–511, 2020 30094499

Musselman DL, Lawson DH, Gumnick JF, et al: Paroxetine for the prevention of depression induced by high-dose interferon alfa. N Engl J Med 344(13):961–966, 2001 11274622

Musselman DL, Somerset WI, Guo Y, et al: A double-blind, multicenter, parallel-group study of paroxetine, desipramine, or placebo in breast cancer patients (stages I, II, III, and IV) with major depression. J Clin Psychiatry 67(2):288–296, 2006 16566626

Mustian KM, Alfano CM, Heckler C, et al: Comparison of pharmaceutical, psychological, and exercise treatments for cancer-related fatigue: a meta-analysis. JAMA Oncol 3(7):961–968, 2017 28253393

Nagler EV, Webster AC, Vanholder R, et al: Antidepressants for depression in stage 3–5 chronic kidney disease: a systematic review of pharmacokinetics, efficacy and safety with recommendations by European Renal Best Practice (ERBP). Nephrol Dial Transplant 27(10):3736–3745, 2012 22859791

Ng CG, Boks MP, Zainal NZ, et al: The prevalence and pharmacotherapy of depression in cancer patients. J Affect Disord 131(1–3):1–7, 2011 20732716

Ng CG, Boks MP, Roes KCB, et al: Rapid response to methylphenidate as an add-on therapy to mirtazapine in the treatment of major depressive disorder in terminally ill cancer patients: a four-week, randomized, double-blinded, placebo-controlled study. Eur Neuropsychopharmacol 24(4):491–498, 2014 24503279

Nobis A, Zalewski D, Waszkiewicz N: Peripheral markers of depression. J Clin Med 9(12):3793, 2020 33255237

Novartis: Arranon (nelarabine) package insert. October 2005. Available at: https://www.accessdata.fda.gov/drugsatfda_docs/label/2005/021877lbl.pdf. Accessed September 20, 2022.

Novartis: Gleevec (imatinib) package insert. 2008. Available at: https://www.accessdata.fda.gov/drugsatfda_docs/label/2008/021588s024lbl.pdf. Accessed September 20, 2022.

Ostuzzi G, Benda L, Costa E, et al: Efficacy and acceptability of antidepressants on the continuum of depressive experiences in patients with cancer: systematic review and meta-analysis. Cancer Treat Rev 41(8):714–724, 2015 26118318

Ozkan TA, Koprulu S, Karakose A, et al: Does using alprazolam during outpatient flexible cystoscopy decrease anxiety and pain? Arch Esp Urol 70(9):800–805, 2017 29099383

Page BR, Shaw EG, Lu L, et al: Phase II double-blind placebo-controlled randomized study of armodafinil for brain radiation-induced fatigue. Neuro Oncol 17(10):1393–1401, 2015 25972454

Pageaux GP, le Bricquir Y, Berthou F, et al: Effects of interferon-alpha on cytochrome P-450 isoforms 1A2 and 3A activities in patients with chronic hepatitis C. Eur J Gastroenterol Hepatol 10(6):491–495, 1998 9855065

Peng Z, Ji Z, Mei F, et al: Lithium inhibits tumorigenic potential of PDA cells through targeting hedgehog-GLI signaling pathway. PLoS One 8(4):e61457, 2013 23626687

Perusinghe M, Chen KY, McDermott B: Evidence-based management of depression in palliative care: a systematic review. J Palliat Med 24(5):767–781, 2021 33720758

Petros WP, Rodman JH, Relling MV, et al: Variability in teniposide plasma protein binding is correlated with serum albumin concentrations. Pharmacotherapy 12(4):273–277, 1992 1518726

Pfizer: Cytosar (cytarabine) product monograph. Hospira, 2020. Available at: https://www.pfizer.com/products/product-detail/cytarabine-0. Accessed December 12, 2021.

Pietruszka LJ, Biermann WA, Vlasses PH: Evaluation of cisplatin-lithium interaction. Drug Intell Clin Pharm 19(1):31–32, 1985 4038480

Pillai VC, Venkataramanan R, Parise RA, et al: Ritonavir and efavirenz significantly alter the metabolism of erlotinib: an observation in primary cultures of human hepatocytes that is relevant to HIV patients with cancer. Drug Metab Dispos 41(10):1843–1851, 2013 23913028

Pinto EF, Andrade C: Interferon-related depression: a primer on mechanisms, treatment, and prevention of a common clinical problem. Curr Neuropharmacol 14(7):743–748, 2016 26733280

Pottegård A, Friis S, Andersen M, et al: Use of benzodiazepines or benzodiazepine related drugs and the risk of cancer: a population-based case-control study. Br J Clin Pharmacol 75(5):1356–1364, 2013 23043261

Pottegård A, Hallas J, Jensen BL, et al: Long-term lithium use and risk of renal and upper urinary tract cancers. J Am Soc Nephrol 27(1):249–255, 2016 25941353

Pursche S, Schleyer E, von Bonin M, et al: Influence of enzyme-inducing antiepileptic drugs on trough level of imatinib in glioblastoma patients. Curr Clin Pharmacol 3(3):198–203, 2008 18781906

Razavi D, Allilaire JF, Smith M, et al: The effect of fluoxetine on anxiety and depression symptoms in cancer patients. Acta Psychiatr Scand 94(3):205–210, 1996 8891089

Reich M, Bondenet X: Place of psychotropic drugs in oncology [in French]. Psycho-Oncologie 12(2):114–130, 2018

Relling MV, Pui CH, Sandlund JT, et al: Adverse effect of anticonvulsants on efficacy of chemotherapy for acute lymphoblastic leukaemia. Lancet 356(9226):285–290, 2000 11071183

Resek G, Olivieri S: No association between lithium therapy and leukemia (letter). Lancet 1(8330):940, 1983 6132264

Riechelmann RP, Burman D, Tannock IF, et al: Phase II trial of mirtazapine for cancer-related cachexia and anorexia. Am J Hosp Palliat Care 27(2):106–110, 2010 19776373

Roscoe JA, Morrow GR, Hickok JT, et al: Effect of paroxetine hydrochloride (Paxil) on fatigue and depression in breast cancer patients receiving chemotherapy. Breast Cancer Res Treat 89(3):243–249, 2005

Rosenberg L, Palmer JR, Zauber AG, et al: Relation of benzodiazepine use to the risk of selected cancers: breast, large bowel, malignant melanoma, lung, endometrium, ovary, non-Hodgkin's lymphoma, testis, Hodgkin's disease, thyroid, and liver. Am J Epidemiol 141(12):1153–1160, 1995 7771453

Roth AJ, Nelson C, Rosenfeld B, et al: Methylphenidate for fatigue in ambulatory men with prostate cancer. Cancer 116(21):5102–5110, 2010 20665492

Rothenberg ML, Liu PY, Wilczynski S, et al: Phase II trial of oral altretamine for consolidation of clinical complete remission in women with stage III epithelial ovarian cancer: a Southwest Oncology Group trial (SWOG-9326). Gynecol Oncol 82(2):317–322, 2001 11531286

Salehifar E, Azimi S, Janbabai G, et al: Efficacy and safety of bupropion in cancer-related fatigue, a randomized double blind placebo controlled clinical trial. BMC Cancer 20(1):158, 2020 32106832

Sanofi-Aventis: Nilandron (nilutamide) product monograph. 2019. Available at: https://products.sanofi.us/nilandron/nilandron.html. Accessed December 12, 2021.

Schilder CM, Eggens PC, Seynaeve C, et al: Neuropsychological functioning in postmenopausal breast cancer patients treated with tamoxifen or exemestane after AC-chemotherapy: cross-sectional findings from the neuropsychological TEAM-side study. Acta Oncol 48(1):76–85, 2009 18777410

Schilder CM, Seynaeve C, Beex LV, et al: Effects of tamoxifen and exemestane on cognitive functioning of postmenopausal patients with breast cancer: results from the neuropsychological side study of the Tamoxifen and Exemestane Adjuvant Multinational trial. J Clin Oncol 28(8):1294–1300, 2010 20142601

Selaman Z, Bolton JM, Oswald T, et al: Association of benzodiazepine use with increased cancer risk is misleading due to lack of theoretical rationale and presence of many confounding factors. J Clin Psychiatry 73(9):1264, author reply 1264–1265, 2012 23059153

Servier: Oncaspar (pegaspargase) product monograph. 2021. Available at: chrome-extension://efaidnbmnnnibpcajpcglclefindmkaj/https://pdf.hres.ca/dpd_pm/00063640.PDF. Accessed December 12, 2021.

Sharpe M, Walker J, Holm Hansen C, et al: Integrated collaborative care for comorbid major depression in patients with cancer (SMaRT Oncology-2): a multicentre randomised controlled effectiveness trial. Lancet 384(9948):1099–1108, 2014 25175478

Shaw EG, Rosdhal R, D'Agostino RB Jr, et al: Phase II study of donepezil in irradiated brain tumor patients: effect on cognitive function, mood, and quality of life. J Clin Oncol 24(9):1415–1420, 2006 16549835

Shen K, Xu Y, Guan H, et al: Paraneoplastic limbic encephalitis associated with lung cancer. Sci Rep 8(1):6792, 2018 29717222

Sigma-Tau Pharmaceuticals: Matulane (procarbazine). 2014. Available at: http://www.matulane.com. Accessed April 14, 2016.

Skinner R, Cotterill SJ, Stevens MC, et al: Risk factors for nephrotoxicity after ifosfamide treatment in children: a UKCCSG Late Effects Group study. Br J Cancer 82(10):1636–1645, 2000 10817497

Slovacek L, Ansorgova V, Macingova Z, et al: Tamoxifen-induced QT interval prolongation. J Clin Pharm Ther 33(4):453–455, 2008 18613864

Sood A, Barton DL, Loprinzi CL: Use of methylphenidate in patients with cancer. Am J Hosp Palliat Care 23(1):35–40, 2006 16450661

Spathis A, Fife K, Blackhall F, et al: Modafinil for the treatment of fatigue in lung cancer: results of a placebo-controlled, double-blind, randomized trial. J Clin Oncol 32(18):1882–1888, 2014 24778393

Stockler MR, O'Connell R, Nowak AK, et al: Effect of sertraline on symptoms and survival in patients with advanced cancer, but without major depression: a placebo-controlled double-blind randomised trial. Lancet Oncol 8(7):603–612, 2007 17548243

Swaisland HC, Ranson M, Smith RP, et al: Pharmacokinetic drug interactions of gefitinib with rifampicin, itraconazole and metoprolol. Clin Pharmacokinet 44(10):1067–1081, 2005 16176119

Swierenga SH, Gilman JP, McLean JR: Cancer risk from inorganics. Cancer Metastasis Rev 6(2):113–154, 1987 2439222

Szabatura AH, Cirrone F, Harris C, et al: An assessment of risk factors associated with ifosfamide-induced encephalopathy in a large academic cancer center. J Oncol Pharm Pract 21(3):188–193, 2015 24664476

Szarfman A, Tonning JM, Levine JG, et al: Atypical antipsychotics and pituitary tumors: a pharmacovigilance study. Pharmacotherapy 26(6):748–758, 2006 16716128

Taipale H, Solmi M, Lähteenvuo M, et al: Antipsychotic use and risk of breast cancer in women with schizophrenia: a nationwide nested case-control study in Finland. Lancet Psychiatry 8(10):883–891, 2021 34474013

Takeda Pharmaceuticals: Velcade (bortezomib). 2021. Available at: https://www.velcade.com. Accessed December 12, 2021.

Tamim HM, Mahmud S, Hanley JA, et al: Antidepressants and risk of prostate cancer: a nested case-control study. Prostate Cancer Prostatic Dis 11(1):53–60, 2008

Tanaka C, Yin OQ, Smith T, et al: Effects of rifampin and ketoconazole on the pharmacokinetics of nilotinib in healthy participants. J Clin Pharmacol 51(1):75–83, 2011 20702754

Toh S, Rodríguez LA, Hernández-Díaz S: Use of antidepressants and risk of lung cancer. Cancer Causes Control 18(10):1055–1064, 2007 17682831

Traeger L, Greer JA, Fernandez-Robles C, et al: Evidence-based treatment of anxiety in patients with cancer. J Clin Oncol 30(11):1197–1205, 2012 22412135

Udina M, Moreno-España J, Capuron L, et al: Cytokine-induced depression: current status and novel targets for depression therapy. CNS Neurol Disord Drug Targets 13(6):1066–1074, 2014 24923336

United Therapeutics: Unituxin (dinutuximab) prescribing information. March 2015. Available at: https://www.accessdata.fda.gov/drugsatfda_docs/label/2015/125516s000lbl.pdf. Accessed March 8, 2022.

Vanda: Fanapt (iloperidone). 2017. Available at: https://www.fanapt.com. Accessed December 12, 2021.

Van Dyk K, Crespi CM, Bower JE, et al: The cognitive effects of endocrine therapy in survivors of breast cancer: a prospective longitudinal study up to 6 years after treatment. Cancer 125(5):681–689, 2019 30485399

van Eys J, Cangir A, Pack R, et al: Phase I trial of procarbazine as a 5-day continuous infusion in children with central nervous system tumors. Cancer Treat Rep 71(10):973–974, 1987 3308081

van Heeringen K, Zivkov M: Pharmacological treatment of depression in cancer patients: a placebo-controlled study of mianserin. Br J Psychiatry 169(4):440–443, 1996 8894194

van Noord C, Straus SM, Sturkenboom MC, et al: Psychotropic drugs associated with corrected QT interval prolongation. J Clin Psychopharmacol 29(1):9–15, 2009 19142100

Volf N, Crismon ML: Leukemia in bipolar mood disorder: is lithium contraindicated? DICP 25(9):948–951, 1991 1949974

Voltz R: Neuropsychological symptoms in paraneoplastic disorders. J Neurol 254(Suppl 2):II84–II86, 2007 17503138

Voso MT, Santini V, Finelli C, et al: Valproic acid at therapeutic plasma levels may increase 5-azacytidine efficacy in higher risk myelodysplastic syndromes. Clin Cancer Res 15(15):5002–5007, 2009 19638460

Wald TG, Kathol RG, Noyes R Jr, et al: Rapid relief of anxiety in cancer patients with both alprazolam and placebo. Psychosomatics 34(4):324–332, 1993 8351307

Walker J, Hansen CH, Martin P, et al: Integrated collaborative care for major depression comorbid with a poor prognosis cancer (SMaRT Oncology-3): a multicentre randomised controlled trial in patients with lung cancer. Lancet Oncol 15(10):1168–1176, 2014 25175097

Wang PS, Walker AM, Tsuang MT, et al: Dopamine antagonists and the development of breast cancer. Arch Gen Psychiatry 59(12):1147–1154, 2002 12470131

Williams SJ, Baird-Lambert JA, Farrell GC: Inhibition of theophylline metabolism by interferon. Lancet 2(8565):939–941, 1987 2444839

Xu W, Tamim H, Shapiro S, et al: Use of antidepressants and risk of colorectal cancer: a nested case-control study. Lancet Oncol 7(4):301–308, 2006 16574545

Yancik R: Population aging and cancer: a cross-national concern. Cancer J 11(6):437–441, 2005 16393477

Yang L, Panetta JC, Cai X, et al: Asparaginase may influence dexamethasone pharmacokinetics in acute lymphoblastic leukemia. J Clin Oncol 26(12):1932–1939, 2008 18421047

Yeh ET: Cardiotoxicity induced by chemotherapy and antibody therapy. Annu Rev Med 57:485–498, 2006 16409162

Yi JC, Syrjala KL: Anxiety and depression in cancer survivors. Med Clin North Am 101(6):1099–1113, 2017 28992857

Y-mAbs Therapeutics: Danyelza (naxitamab-gqgk) package insert. November 2020. Available at: https://www.accessdata.fda.gov/drugsatfda_docs/label/2020/761171lbl.pdf. Accessed March 8, 2022.

Young W: Review of lithium effects on brain and blood. Cell Transplant 18(9):951–975, 2009 19523343

Zaidan M, Stucker F, Stengel B, et al: Increased risk of solid renal tumors in lithium-treated patients. Kidney Int 86(1):184–190, 2014 24451323

Zhang T, Yang X, Zhou J, et al: Benzodiazepine drug use and cancer risk: a dose-response meta analysis of prospective cohort studies. Oncotarget 8(60):102381–102391, 2017 29254253

Zhao G, Okoro CA, Li J, et al: Current depression among adult cancer survivors: findings from the 2010 Behavioral Risk Factor Surveillance System. Cancer Epidemiol 38(6):757–764, 2014 25455653

9

Central Nervous System Disorders

Curtis A. McKnight, M.D.
Jason P. Caplan, M.D.

The delicate neuronal meshwork of the human brain mediates both neurological and psychiatric function. Diseases that affect the CNS are therefore apt to cause both neurological and psychiatric symptoms, and their management requires care so as not to exacerbate symptoms in either domain. In this chapter, we discuss the treatment of neuropsychiatric manifestations of cognitive dysfunction, depression, anxiety, psychosis, and emotional and behavioral dysregulation that are common in CNS diseases.

The pharmacological management of psychiatric symptoms in neurological illness is almost exclusively "off label" because remarkably few agents have been specifically approved for use in this regard. When addressing these symptoms, it is advisable to leverage as many beneficial effects from a single agent as possible. For example, if a patient with a traumatic brain injury experiences both seizures and mood lability as a result, it may be beneficial to first try an antiepileptic drug that also has a mood-stabilizing effect (e.g., valproic acid) in an attempt to address both symptoms rather than using two drugs to target the two symptoms separately (e.g., levetiracetam and olanzapine). As is often the case when addressing multiple co-occurring illnesses, starting at a relatively low dose and titrating to efficacy is typically the preferred approach. It is important to stay up-to-date on emerging therapies for CNS disorders to maintain an awareness of the potential (useful and adverse) psychiatric effects of these treatments.

Dementia

Dementia is a clinical syndrome characterized by cognitive decline, emotional and behavioral dysregulation, and impairments in activities of daily living (ADLs). Anything that can result in neuronal death may be considered a cause of dementia. Alzheimer's disease (AD) is the most common type of dementia, accounting for almost 70% of all patients with dementia age 65 and older. Other types of dementia include Lewy body dementia, the frontotemporal dementias (FTDs), vascular dementia, dementia due to Parkinson's disease (PD), and dementias due to immune diseases, infectious diseases, or brain injury.

The target of treatment has historically been cognition, but over time more focus has come to rest on behavioral and psychological symptoms of dementia. We provide an outline of the salient features of these guidelines related to pharmacotherapy.

Alzheimer's Disease

Cognitive Deficits

An important but controversial development in the treatment of AD is monoclonal antibody therapy targeting amyloid beta plaques in the brain. Amyloid beta plaques are a defining pathophysiological feature of AD. Aducanumab is a human immunoglobulin γ1 monoclonal antibody directed against aggregated soluble and insoluble forms of amyloid beta, developed by Biogen. Aducanumab received accelerated approval in June 2021 from the U.S. FDA, the first drug approved for AD since 2003. The drug was approved for mild cognitive impairment and the mild dementia stage of AD. To date, Biogen has conducted two identically designed 18-month randomized double-blind, placebo-controlled, parallel-group studies. The primary and secondary end points involved cognitive and ADL function, and tertiary end points involved neuropsychiatric and safety outcomes. Both studies were terminated early for futility. High-dose aducanumab in one trial showed modest benefit for cognitive, ADL, and neuropsychiatric symptoms. At time of approval, the FDA acknowledged uncertainty about the expectation of clinical benefit (Cavazzoni 2021; Tampi et al. 2021). Because of this uncertainty, many expressed concern, saying that clinicians must explain to patients that the treatment risks may outweigh the benefits (Chiong et al. 2021). Aducanumab must be administered intravenously via a 60-minute infusion every 4 weeks. The most common adverse reaction is amyloid-related neuroimaging abnormalities, which can take the form of hemorrhagic edema or superficial siderosis hemosiderin deposition. These reactions appear to be dose related, can range from mild to severe, and may result in symptoms ranging from mild headache to confusion, coma, and death, so intensive monitoring is necessary. Overall, the benefit of aducanumab is not clearly established at this time, particularly in light of limited and conflicting evidence, administration and monitoring burden, and high cost.

Acetylcholinesterase Combination Therapy

Three acetylcholinesterase inhibitors (AchEIs)—donepezil, rivastigmine, and galantamine—are available to treat mild to moderate AD. The benefit of therapy with AchEIs is generally considered to be a slowing of AD progression by 6 months. The clinically relevant benefit is uncertain. These three AchEIs are similar in efficacy (Arvanitakis et al. 2019). Side effects include nausea, vomiting, and diarrhea. Rivastigmine is available as a transdermal patch that appears to have fewer side effects while retaining efficacy (Birks et al. 2015). If AD is identified in a mild stage, then initiation of a cholinesterase inhibitor alone is the recommended first step.

The *N*-methyl-D-aspartate receptor antagonist memantine is FDA approved for use in moderate to severe AD and has a low side-effect profile with isolated reports of delirium. Comparisons of the efficacy of AchEIs and memantine showed that AchEI had an advantage over memantine in mild to moderate AD, whereas memantine was more effective than donepezil in severe AD. If AD is moderate to advanced, memantine should be added to a cholinesterase inhibitor or used alone if the AchEI is not tolerated. A 2020 network meta-analysis found the combination of memantine and donepezil superior for outcomes of cognition, global assessment, ADLs, and neuropsychiatric symptoms than either drug individually (Guo et al. 2020), so earlier combination therapy can also be considered.

Behavioral and Psychological Symptoms of Dementia

Terminology surrounding the noncognitive, psychiatric, neurological, neuropsychiatric, behavioral, and neuropsychological aspects of dementia has been coalescing toward the term *behavioral and psychological symptoms of dementia*. This group of symptoms includes agitation, psychosis, depression, and apathy. It affects nearly all patients with AD over the course of the disease (Forester and Vahia 2019). Psychopharmacological treatment is aimed at mitigating symptoms as well as deterioration of family relationships, caregiver burden, and institutionalization.

Agitation, Aggression, and Psychosis

Agitation, aggression, and psychosis are common in patients with moderate to severe dementia, and it is critical to consider the safety of patients and their caregivers when choosing pharmacological interventions. Atypical antipsychotics used by elderly patients with dementia-related psychosis have an FDA black box warning. Since the Clinical Antipsychotic Trials of Intervention Effectiveness–Alzheimer's Disease authors concluded in 2006 that the adverse effects of the atypical antipsychotics outweigh the benefits when they are used for these indications (Schneider et al. 2006), this has remained a controversial area of psychopharmacology.

More recent reviews continue to draw mixed conclusions. It is generally agreed that atypical antipsychotics reduce agitation, probably through sedation. This effect may be of significant benefit to the patient, albeit indirectly, if it allows less disruption in caregiving. This is important because the behaviors of a person with dementia-related agitation or psychosis may profoundly affect their primary caregivers and level of function. Thus, caregiver burden should be considered as part of the overall treatment plan and risk-benefit discussion. Including the potential adverse effects as part of an informed consent discussion (often with a surrogate decision-maker) is important (Mühlbauer et al. 2021; Seibert et al. 2021).

Many other classes of medications, including benzodiazepines, mood stabilizers, dextromethorphan/quinidine, prazosin, cannabinoids (dronabinol, purified Δ-9-tetrahydrocannabinol, and nabilone), and antidepressants, have been used to treat behavior problems in patients with AD.

Available data, although limited, do not support the routine use of benzodiazepines (Tampi and Tampi 2014). The most current review of mood stabilizers was by Yeh and Ouyang (2012), which found that carbamazepine can be effective for management of agitation; however, valproate, oxcarbazepine, and lithium showed little or no evidence of efficacy.

The randomized controlled trial (RCT) of the combination dextromethorphan/quinidine in 194 patients showed improvement in the Neuropsychiatric Inventory Agitation/Aggression domain score compared with placebo (Cummings et al. 2015). Dextromethorphan/quinidine is discussed further in the subsection "Pseudobulbar Affect" later in this chapter.

At present, the effects (both positive and negative) of cannabinoids in dementia are unclear. If there are benefits of cannabinoids for people with dementia, the effects may be too small to be clinically meaningful (Bosnjak Kuharic et al. 2021).

There is modest evidence for the use of selective serotonin reuptake inhibitors (SSRIs) in AD-associated agitation. A 2011 Cochrane review reported significant reduction in agitation with the use of sertraline and citalopram (Seitz et al. 2011). A 2014 RCT further supported the use of citalopram for agitation in patients with AD, although the authors noted that the daily dose should be limited to 30 mg to minimize adverse cardiac effects (Porsteinsson et al. 2014). Patient selection may be refined by considering that those with moderate agitation and with less cognitive impairment are more likely to benefit from citalopram (Schneider et al. 2016).

Depressive Phenomena and Apathy

Depressed mood is the most common comorbid condition in dementia and can worsen cognitive deficits, resulting in a poorer quality of life, increased risk of hospitalization, and increased caregiver burnout. Apathy is related and often difficult to distinguish.

In a case of major depressive disorder (nine-question Patient Health Questionnaire score >9) and dementia, treatment algorithms may not differ from those for patients with major depressive disorder without dementia. Research literature on the antidepressant treatment of depression in AD is limited in scope, with significant methodological differences between RCTs; careful meta-analyses indicate no clear antidepressant benefits in the short or long term (Dudas et al. 2018; Orgeta et al. 2017).

In the case of depressive symptoms that are subsyndromal, nondrug interventions were found to be more efficacious than drug interventions for reducing symptoms of depression in people with dementia without a major depressive disorder (Watt et al. 2021).

Apathy is defined as a lack of initiative, reduced interest, reduced action, and reduced goal-directed behaviors. Apathy can range in severity from mild to severe. In very severe forms, there can be akinetic mutism or the appearance of catatonic symptoms. Apathy is associated with diminished quality of life and increased caregiving needs. A 2018 Cochrane review including 21 studies concluded that only methylphenidate may have benefit (Ruthirakuhan et al. 2018), and a randomized placebo-controlled trial of bupropion as treatment for apathy found that it was not superior to placebo (Maier et al. 2020). In a review of 33 studies, methylphenidate, olanzapine, cholinesterase inhibitors, choline alfoscerate, citalopram, memantine, and mibampator showed benefits for AD-related apathy to limited degrees (Azhar et al. 2022).

Anxiety

Anxiety is a common symptom of dementia, both as a comorbid condition and as a result of depression. SSRIs are generally considered to be the first-line agents. Benzodiazepines can occasionally have a role in treating patients with prominent anxiety or on an as-needed basis for patients with infrequent episodes of agitation. However, adverse effects of benzodiazepines in this population include sedation, worsening cognition, delirium, increased risk of falls, and worsening of respiratory disorders. Lorazepam and oxazepam, which have no active metabolites, are typically preferable to agents with a longer half-life, such as diazepam or clonazepam. Atypical antipsychotics should be used only for the short-term management of severe anxiety until SSRIs take effect because of the black box warning about atypical antipsychotic use in older adults, explained in the subsection "Agitation, Aggression, and Psychosis" earlier in this chapter.

Sleep Disturbances

Sleep disturbances, including decreased nocturnal sleep, sleep fragmentation, nocturnal wandering, and daytime sleepiness, are common among patients with AD and reduce the quality of life for both patients and their caregivers.

Melatonin is preferred as the initial option (Sumsuzzman et al. 2021). There-after, low-dose trazodone and orexin antagonists (lemborexant and suvorexant) can be used, according to small studies showing beneficial effects and no evidence of harm (McCleery and Sharpley 2020).

Lewy Body Dementia

Cognitive Deficits

Dementia with Lewy bodies (DLB) is a result of a disease process leading to the deposition of α-synuclein. Lewy body deposits have been found not only in patients with DLB but also in patients with AD and PD. This overlap in pathology is reflected in the overlap of treatment for these diseases.

Trials of AchEIs have shown the most robust positive effects on cognitive symptoms for both high-dose and low-dose donepezil (Chu et al. 2021; Matsunaga et al. 2015; Mori et al. 2015).

Psychosis and the Behavioral and Psychological Symptoms of Dementia

Hallucinations occur in as many as 80% of patients with DLB and tend to occur early in the progression of the disease, compared with the end stage of AD (Mehraram et al. 2022). The AchEIs have been shown to improve DLB-associated hallucinations, delusions, and paranoia. Furthermore, stopping medications that worsen neuropsychiatric symptoms, such as anticholinergic medications, amantadine, dopamine agonists, monoamine oxidase inhibitors (MAOIs), catechol O-methyltransferase inhibitors, and levodopa, is recommended (Wood et al. 2010). A slow discontinuation of dopaminergic agents is recommended to minimize the risk of neuroleptic malignant syndrome.

The use of antipsychotics in DLB is controversial because patients with DLB are exquisitely sensitive to extrapyramidal side effects in addition to having increased risk according to the FDA black box warning. However, short-term use of antipsychotics can still be beneficial, specifically if there is a high risk of harm to the patient because of psychosis (Wood et al. 2010). Of the antipsychotic options for patients with DLB, most evidence supports the use of quetiapine, clozapine, and pimavanserin. Clozapine is the second-line choice because of concern about agranulocytosis (Kyle and Bronstein 2020).

Similar to those of the treatment options for AD, the adverse effects of atypical antipsychotics should be carefully considered in the context of the patient's overall disease burden, and agents such as olanzapine, clozapine, and quetiapine should be avoided in patients at risk for hyperlipidemia or diabetes, and olanzapine and risperidone should be avoided in patients with elevated cerebrovascular risk. Pimavanserin, which is approved for psychosis in PD (and is discussed in detail later in this chapter), functions as a selective serotonin type 2A (5-HT$_{2A}$) inverse agonist (Cummings et al. 2014) and may have some off-label utility for treatment of psychosis in DLB.

Frontotemporal Dementia

Cognitive Deficits

FTD is a heterogeneous disorder with distinct clinical phenotypes associated with multiple neuropathological entities. To date, no medications have been shown to improve cognitive dysfunction in patients with FTD, and the FDA-approved treatments for AD have not shown benefit in FTD. Evidence indicates that AchEIs actually make symptoms worse (Olney et al. 2017). An RCT of memantine in this population found no improvement in symptoms, with a greater incidence of adverse cognitive effects than with placebo; thus, memantine is also not recommended for FTD (Boxer et al. 2013).

Behavioral Disruption and Behavioral and Psychological Symptoms of Dementia

The involvement of the frontal lobe in FTD can result in behaviors such as compulsions, gambling, stealing, sexual disinhibition, apathy, and carbohydrate craving, which can place the patient at risk and increase caregiver burden. SSRIs have shown some efficacy in addressing these behaviors in case reports and small observational studies (Olney et al. 2017). Trazodone, an atypical serotonergic antidepressant, has demonstrated improvement of the neuropsychiatric symptoms of FTD in randomized double-blind studies (Olney et al. 2017). Atypical antipsychotic use in this patient population carries the same risk-to-benefit considerations as discussed for AD and DLB, because patients with FTD also have greater extrapyramidal side-effect sensitivity.

AchEIs, antiepileptic medications, and MAOIs all have limited evidence for use in FTD. The available literature includes reports of both improvement and worsening of neuropsychiatric symptoms. Benzodiazepine use in this patient population is not recommended because of risks of delirium, cognitive worsening, and paradoxical agitation.

Vascular Dementia

Given the nature of pathology in vascular dementia, the most important intervention is prevention of further vasculopathy and stroke, including smoking cessation and control of hypertension, hyperlipidemia, and diabetes. In a meta-analysis of controlled trials of patients with vascular dementia, donepezil, galantamine, memantine, and rivastigmine were shown to improve cognitive function as measured by the Alzheimer's Disease Assessment Scale (Kavirajan and Schneider 2007). A more recent Cochrane review of AchEIs for vascular dementia concluded that donepezil and galantamine have beneficial effects on cognition (Battle et al. 2021).

Stroke

People who have had a stroke are at significant risk for a variety of neuropsychiatric disturbances, the presentation of which is heavily dependent on the location and extent of the stroke. These disturbances include dementia, depression, mania, anxiety, psychosis, disinhibition, apathy, and fatigue.

Cognitive Deficits

The pathophysiology of poststroke cognitive disorders is similar to that of vascular dementia, with evidence supporting use of the AchEIs as described previously in the subsection "Vascular Dementia."

Depression

Depression can be one of the most devastating neuropsychiatric symptoms after stroke. It has a prevalence of almost 30% at any time after a stroke (Ayerbe et al. 2013) and is associated with increased morbidity and mortality. Tricyclic antidepressants (TCAs), SSRIs, and mirtazapine have all shown some benefit in clinical trials for treatment of poststroke depression. SSRIs are considered first-line therapy (Mortensen and Andersen 2021).

The prevention of poststroke depression has been studied, with evidence that mirtazapine given prophylactically and acutely after stroke may prevent depression (Niedermaier et al. 2004). A meta-analysis of six studies found that early SSRI therapy was associated with a significant reduction in poststroke depression occurrence compared with placebo (Richter et al. 2021). However, there is a challenge in balancing the prophylactic benefits of SSRIs with increased bleeding risk, particularly for people who have had a hemorrhagic stroke. Post–hemorrhagic stroke SSRI use was found to be associated with unfavorable 3-month neurological outcomes (Liu et al. 2020), and SSRI exposure was associated with higher major hemorrhage risk in patients taking warfarin, which is common after stroke (Quinn et al. 2014).

Mania

Mania is a rare consequence of stroke, and no clear guidelines for treatment of poststroke mania have been published. A systematic review indicated that patients most at risk for poststroke mania are men with right-sided cerebral infarct who have no personal or family history of psychiatric illness (Santos et al. 2011). The treatment of poststroke mania is similar to that of bipolar mania, with evidence supporting the use of valproic acid, carbamazepine, and lithium (Bernardo et al. 2008). The use of antipsychotics for poststroke mania, especially by older adults, is recommended only for the short term in acute episodes to reduce the risk of imminent harm to the patient.

Anxiety

Like depression, anxiety is a common comorbid condition after stroke, affecting 29% of patients (Hoffmann et al. 2015), who may respond to antidepressant therapy. Duloxetine has shown greater efficacy than either sertraline or citalopram in the management of poststroke anxiety, and all three agents were equally efficacious in addressing poststroke depression, although there was no placebo control (Karaiskos et al. 2012). As in vascular dementia, the use of benzodiazepines should be avoided because of cognitive impairment and risk of delirium, falls, or further ischemic events due to hypotension.

Aggression and Irritability

The degree of aggression and irritability after stroke depends on many factors, including prestroke psychiatric illness and extent of cerebral involvement. Small studies on the prevalence and treatment of poststroke aggression and irritability have indicated that the prevalence may be as high as 35% (Choi-Kwon and Kim 2022). Data for the treatment of poststroke aggression and irritability are limited to antidepressants; for example, fluoxetine has been found to be effective in treating poststroke aggression and irritability (Choi-Kwon et al. 2006).

Traumatic Brain Injury

Traumatic brain injury (TBI) has become a major focus in the practice of neurological and psychiatric health care, with attention being drawn to the long-term effects of TBI on members of the military and professional athletes. Neuropsychiatric symptoms of TBI include impaired cognition, depression, mania, psychosis, mood lability, irritability, and anxiety.

This is a very active area of medication development. There are at least a dozen ongoing and recently completed Phase II and III trials of pharmacotherapies for TBI, many with disappointing results. Medications being studied currently include cyclosporine for its neuroprotective properties (Kelsen et al. 2019), calpain inhibitors (calcium-dependent cysteine proteases), dexanabinol (synthetic cannabinoid), deltibant (bradykinin antagonist), and etanercept (tumor necrosis factor inhibitor) (Diaz-Arrastia et al. 2014).

If acute TBI is complicated by elevated intracranial pressure, the treatment options of hypertonic saline, mannitol, or mannitol in combination with glycerol have been shown to have similar efficacy for reducing mortality in long-term management (Chen et al. 2020).

Cognitive Deficits

The cognitive deficits seen as a result of TBI span multiple domains, including arousal, attention, concentration, memory, language, sleep, and executive functioning. An increasing body of data suggests that stimulants (including dextroamphetamine, methylphenidate, modafinil, armodafinil, and lisdexamfetamine) have utility in the treatment of post-TBI cognitive deficits (Johansson et al. 2015; Menn et al. 2014; Tramontana et al. 2014). An RCT demonstrated significant dose-dependent improvement of long-lasting mental fatigue and processing speed with methylphenidate (Johansson et al. 2015). Dopamine agonists (including amantadine, levodopa or carbidopa, and bromocriptine) also have been shown to reduce the cognitive deficits associated with TBI (Khellaf et al. 2019). Animal models have shown that AchEIs confer some benefit for improved recovery after TBI, although this has yet to be confirmed in humans (Zhao et al. 2018). Preliminary investigations of the use of lithium and valproic acid for patients who have experienced a TBI have yielded promising data supporting a neuroprotective effect, which may lead to long-term improvement of neuropsychiatric sequelae of TBI, although clinical trials have yet to be completed (Chen et al. 2014; Leeds et al. 2014).

Anxiety and PTSD

The physical trauma resulting in brain injury and the circumstances surrounding it can result in post-TBI anxiety syndromes or PTSD. There have not been enough RCTs to provide a solid scientific consensus on treatment. SSRIs may not be as effective in this post-TBI population as in patients with PTSD without TBI (Hicks et al. 2019). Short-term benzodiazepine use may be necessary, and these drugs are often used as initial therapy while the patient awaits expected benefit from SSRI or serotonin-norepinephrine reuptake inhibitor (SNRI) therapy (Fann et al. 2022).

Depression and Apathy

It is important but also difficult to separate post-TBI apathy syndrome and diminished motivation from depression. Because post-TBI depression is caused by both traumatically damaged brain circuits and psychosocial sequelae, it is not surprising that the treatments are often less effective than for a primary depressive disorder. A 2016 meta-analysis showed that pharmacotherapy after TBI may be associated with a reduction in depressive symptoms (Salter et al. 2016), but a more recent analysis of antidepressants did not find benefit over placebo (Kreitzer et al. 2019). For major depressive disorder after TBI, SSRIs are considered first-line agents (Fann et al. 2022), with SNRIs a next step in treatment of post-TBI depression. If the SSRI or SNRI classes prove ineffective, psychostimulants or dopamine agents can be used for augmentation. Caution is advised with the use of bupropion because of its potential to reduce the seizure threshold at higher doses. Solriamfetol (a dopamine and norepinephrine reuptake inhibitor already FDA approved for daytime sleepiness associated with narcolepsy or obstructive sleep apnea) is being studied as a treatment option.

Mania

Mania due to a TBI is uncommon, but TBI can involve functional and structural damage to multiple neuroanatomical networks and neurotransmitter systems, leading to mania or mania-like behavioral disinhibition that manifests as activation, disinhibition, and impulsivity. Treatment selection should be similar to that for mania not due to TBI, with consideration of individual patient characteristics that may, for example, favor an antiepileptic drug in a patient with comorbid posttraumatic epilepsy.

Psychosis

Similar to mania, psychosis due to TBI is rare. In general, atypical antipsychotics are preferred over typical agents because of lower rates of extrapyramidal side effects. Case reports make up the majority of current data, describing positive results with olanzapine and risperidone (Guerreiro et al. 2009; Schreiber et al. 1998). Clozapine should be used with caution in patients with neurological insult because of the increased risk of seizures. It is important to keep in mind that unusual or treatment-resistant symptoms of psychosis in the setting of a neurological injury may be due to subclinical seizure activity, specifically complex partial seizures.

Aggression and Irritability

Aggression and irritability are common after TBI and may be transient, may resolve with neurological improvement, or may be persistent. Management of aggression and irritability in this population is similar to management of aggression and irritability after stroke, with judicious use of antipsychotics to avoid exacerbating neurological fragility. Unlike in patients with possible ischemia, such as those with risk factors for stroke or vascular dementia, β-blockers can be safely used for agitation by patients with TBI (Fleminger et al. 2006). Anticonvulsants, including lithium, valproate, and carbamazepine, have shown modest effect in decreasing mood lability (Chiu et al. 2013). Amantadine administered in the morning and at noon has been shown to decrease the intensity and frequency of post-TBI irritability and aggression (Hammond et al. 2014).

Antipsychotics remain controversial because their adverse effects on cognitive recovery may outweigh the benefits of reduction in irritability (Mehta et al. 2018).

Benzodiazepines can be useful in short-term abortive therapy for aggression. However, a conservative risk-benefit calculus should be used because long-term benzodiazepine use can perpetuate cognitive dulling, delirium, or a cycle of dose escalation.

Multiple Sclerosis

Multiple sclerosis (MS) can result in motor, cognitive, and psychiatric disturbances. The neuropsychiatric disturbances of MS (which include cognitive deficits, depression, mania, psychosis, and fatigue) may occur only during acute exacerbations or as a chronic feature of the disease.

Cognitive Deficits

Cognitive impairments, including deficits of attention and memory, executive dysfunction, and reduced information processing speed, may be present in almost 70% of patients with MS, and they may be present as early as at the time of initial diagnosis (Zhang et al. 2021). Disease-modifying agents such as β-interferon, glatiramer acetate, natalizumab, dimethyl fumarate, and fingolimod can prevent or reduce the progression of cognitive deficits in patients with MS, but no evidence supports treatment escalation on the basis of cognitive impairment (Landmeyer et al. 2020). A systematic review performed by Motavalli et al. (2020) concluded that no current convincing evidence supports the efficacy of pharmacological symptomatic treatment (including cholinesterase inhibitors and stimulants) of MS-associated cognitive impairment.

Depression and Fatigue

The prevalence of depression in patients with MS is about 30% (Boeschoten et al. 2017), and these patients have an increased risk for suicide (Smyrke et al. 2022). However, few RCTs have examined the use of antidepressants for patients with MS, resulting in a paucity of evidence to support their use (Patten et al. 2017). The SSRIs escitalopram, citalopram, and sertraline are typically considered first-line agents because of their lower drug interaction profiles (Kaplin 2007), although the potential of citalopram and escitalopram to prolong the QTc interval may limit their use in conjunction with the disease-modifying treatment fingolimod (Patten et al. 2017). The few RCTs that have examined the treatment of depression in patients with MS have shown that desipramine, sertraline, and paroxetine are effective pharmacological treatments, but they also indicated that there is a broadly heterogeneous response to both antidepressants and psychotherapeutic interventions (Fiest et al. 2016). The management of depression in patients with MS can be tailored to treat concurrent somatic conditions. For example, TCAs can be used for depression co-occurring with incontinence, whereas SNRIs may be used in depression co-occurring with neuropathic pain.

Previous reports have raised concerns about the risks of psychiatric adverse effects, including anxiety and depression, with disease-modifying treatments directed against MS. One systematic review found no increased risk of either depression or anxiety and reported that patients who received the disease-modifying treatment fingolimod actually had an improvement in symptoms of depression (Gasim et al. 2018). The authors stated that it remains unclear whether this improvement was a direct effect of the drug or an indirect effect stemming from an improvement in physical condition. Fatigue is common among patients with MS, an effect of the disease process or a neurovegetative symptom of an associated depression. For the management of concurrent depression and fatigue, bupropion may be a prudent choice, given the increased susceptibility to sexual dysfunction experienced by patients with MS taking SSRIs who have impairment of spinal cord function (Nathoo and Mackie 2017). Several RCTs and subsequent meta-analyses have produced mixed results for the efficacy of either modafinil or amantadine in the management of fatigue associated with MS, and one RCT indicated that paroxetine produced more benefit in this regard compared with placebo (Zielińska-Nowak et al. 2020). One recent crossover RCT found no superiority for amantadine, modafinil, or methylphenidate for alleviation of fatigue in MS compared with placebo (Nourbakhsh et al. 2021).

Mania

Lifetime prevalence of mania in patients with MS is 8.4%, more than twice that of the general population (Joseph et al. 2021). However, there have been no clinical trials on the treatment of MS-associated mania. For management of mania, pharmacological approaches typically mirror those used for patients without a diagnosis of MS, although close attention should be paid to adverse effects to which those with MS may be particularly susceptible (e.g., increased fall risk and fatigue) (Murphy et al. 2017).

Corticosteroids are a common treatment for MS flares and can precipitate mania. A 1979 chart review found that none of the 27 patients who were pretreated with lithium before corticosteroid administration developed mania, compared with 6 of 44 patients who did not receive prophylactic lithium (Falk et al. 1979). If a patient develops mania during steroid therapy, lithium or olanzapine may be used to manage the mania in lieu of discontinuing the steroids (Murphy et al. 2017).

Psychosis

Psychosis is rare in patients with MS, occurring in 2%–4% of patients, although these rates are still significantly higher than in the general population.

There are no published trials of the treatment of psychosis in MS. Atypical antipsychotics are usually preferred in this patient population because of the lower risk of extrapyramidal side effects (Murphy et al. 2017).

Parkinson's Disease

PD is characterized by motoric symptoms, including bradykinesia, resting tremor, rigidity, and postural and gait instability. The neuropsychiatric symptoms of PD are a significant cause of impairment in quality of life and increased caregiver burden. The pharmacological management of psychiatric disturbances in patients with PD is a delicate balance of neurotransmitter action and requires close longitudinal monitoring.

Cognitive Deficits

Cognitive symptoms, including psychomotor slowing, impaired verbal and working memory, executive dysfunction, and ultimately dementia, are common in patients with PD. PD-associated dementia has many of the clinical features of DLB. Some have suggested that these two diagnoses are variant presentations of the same illness, which may indicate similar efficacies of treatment approaches to cognitive dysfunction. Rivastigmine has the most evidence to support benefit for dementia-related cognitive deficits in PD, and evidence is not sufficient to recommend donepezil in this regard (Seppi et al. 2019). For patients with executive dysfunction or inattention associated with PD, modafinil and atomoxetine can be beneficial (Bassett 2005). Rasagiline has led to marked improvement in cognitive domains of attention, executive functioning, and verbal fluency (Hanagasi et al. 2011).

The effect of dopamine agonists on cognition is not completely established, with some studies indicating that certain ergot-derived dopamine agonists such as pergolide had no effect on cognition (Brusa et al. 2005), whereas some non-ergot-derived dopamine agonists (i.e., pramipexole) have caused impairment in verbal memory, executive functions, and attention (Brusa et al. 2003). The differences in receptor profile for dopamine agonists may explain the dichotomous outcomes. Newer studies continue to provide evidence that certain dopamine agonists can be used with little or no effect on cognition (Brusa et al. 2013).

Depression

Depression in patients with PD can exacerbate deficits of cognitive and motor function and is associated with a decreased quality of life. Although clinical trials for treatment of depression in patients with PD are limited, a 2019 review by the International Parkinson and Movement Disorder Society found venlafaxine to have the most evidence for efficacy and clinical utility in the treatment of depression in PD on the basis of a single high-quality RCT (Seppi et al. 2019). The same trial indicated efficacy for paroxetine, but because of conflicting evidence from other studies, this drug was classified as having "insufficient evidence" to support efficacy. Reports of motor impairment with SSRIs in patients with PD have resulted in cautious use of these medications, although there is also evidence that fluoxetine can be used with no effect on motor movement (Kostić et al. 2012). Although use of the TCAs, specifically nortriptyline and desipramine, has evidence for greater efficacy than use of the SSRIs (Laux 2022), SSRIs have a lower side-effect profile, although TCAs may help ease motoric symptoms of PD as a result of their anticholinergic activity and may have additional neuroprotective activity in PD (Kandil et al. 2016). Dopamine agonists, especially pramipexole, have evidence for effective treatment of depression (Laux 2022), but precipitation of psychosis may be a concern.

Psychosis

Approximately 60% of patients with PD experience psychosis at some point in their illness, with the common symptoms being visual hallucinations and persecutory delusions, most often occurring in patients also experiencing symptoms of dementia (Segal et al. 2021). Treatment of psychosis in PD has historically been complicated by the potential of dopamine antagonist antipsychotics to worsen motor symptoms. The serotonin receptors 5-HT_{2A} and 5-HT_{2C} are thought to contribute to the evolution of PD psychosis, with the basal unbound activity of upregulated 5-HT_{2A} receptors producing increased stimulation of downstream dopaminergic and glutamatergic pathways. Pimavanserin, a 5-HT_{2A} inverse agonist without dopaminergic, muscarinic, adrenergic, or histaminergic affinity, is indicated specifically for the management of PD psychosis. Clinical trials of pimavanserin have shown efficacy in the reduction of both hallucinations and delusions associated with PD psychosis without effect on motor function (Cummings et al. 2014).

If off-label management of PD psychosis is needed, clozapine remains the antipsychotic of choice, whereas quetiapine has mixed evidence for efficacy in controlling the symptoms of psychosis and for its effect on motor symptoms. The International Parkinson and Movement Disorder Society review classified both pimavanserin and clozapine as being efficacious and clinically useful in the management of PD psychosis while having acceptable levels of risk from a safety perspective (with additional notation underscoring the need for specialized monitoring for agranulocytosis with the use of clozapine) (Seppi et al. 2019). Quetiapine was found to have insufficient evidence to support efficacy but was noted as "possibly useful" in clinical practice. Olanzapine was classified as having insufficient evidence, no clinical utility, and unacceptable risk. Aripiprazole and risperidone have similarly been found to be ineffective and to worsen motor function in patients with PD, and they are not recommended (Divac et al. 2016).

One case report noted improvement of psychosis with the addition of mirtazapine (Godschalx-Dekker and Siegers 2014). Rivastigmine is the only AchEI with data indicating significant improvement of hallucinations in a large RCT (Burn et al. 2006). Donepezil has repeatedly failed to show efficacy, and galantamine has few data to support its use.

Fatigue

Modafinil has been shown to improve excessive daytime sleepiness in PD in multiple RCTs (Rodrigues et al. 2016). One RCT has shown benefit of methylphenidate in alleviating fatigue in PD (Mendonça et al. 2007), and rasagiline was shown to slow the progression of fatigue in PD in another RCT (Stocchi and ADAGIO investigators 2014). Typical stimulants should be used with caution in PD because of the theoretical risk of exacerbating psychosis.

Huntington's Disease

Huntington's disease (HD) is an autosomal dominant genetic disorder characterized by choreiform movements, dementia, and psychiatric symptoms, including depression, mania, obsessions and compulsions, and psychosis. Few controlled trials exist specifically for management of psychiatric symptoms in patients with HD, and the approach typically mirrors that for other basal ganglia disorders. A recent review by the International Parkinson and Movement

Disorder Society found no evidence to support any particular pharmacological approach to psychiatric conditions in HD, and thus treatment is guided largely by routine practice for the management of a specific psychiatric diagnosis or by more anecdotal reports (Ferreira et al. 2022). Pharmacological treatment of HD requires care because these patients are particularly susceptible to sedation, falls, cognitive impairment, and extrapyramidal symptoms (Rosenblatt 2007).

Depression

To date, there have been no RCTs for management of depression in patients with HD. A meta-analysis of available data from controlled trials, uncontrolled trials, observational studies, and case series found inadequate evidence to recommend any specific treatment (Moulton et al. 2014). SSRIs are commonly used as first-line agents because they also reduce the irritability and anxiety commonly reported by patients, and SNRIs and mirtazapine are also recommended (Bachoud-Lévi et al. 2019). Given the autosomal dominant transmission of HD, depression may precede the onset of symptoms if the person is aware of the likelihood of developing the illness via either knowledge of a parental diagnosis or confirmatory genetic testing.

Mania

Approximately 5%–10% of patients with HD become manic, exhibiting grandiosity and elevated or irritable mood (Rosenblatt 2007). Patients with HD may respond more positively to valproate or carbamazepine, with the available data indicating a less robust response to and more side effects with lithium (Rosenblatt 2007). Antipsychotics may be used as adjunctive treatment, but a specific agent should be selected with care, as described in the following subsection.

Psychosis

Delusions are the most prominent symptom of psychosis in patients with HD, followed by hallucinations. The choice of antipsychotic for patients with HD and psychosis (or those who need adjunctive medication for severe mania) should be determined by the severity of the choreiform movements. Atypical antipsychotics are recommended as first-line agents for the management of psychosis in HD, with clozapine specifically recommended in akinetic presentations of HD with severe parkinsonian symptoms (Bachoud-Lévi et al. 2019).

Epilepsy

Psychiatric disturbances in epilepsy include cognitive dysfunction, mood disorders, impulsive behavior, and psychosis, with these symptoms occurring as preictal, interictal, and postictal phenomena.

Cognitive Deficits

Cognitive disorders associated with epilepsy are common, and the most effective management depends on aggressive seizure control. Antiepileptic drugs with fewer cognitive side effects, specifically lamotrigine and levetiracetam, are generally preferred. Untreated depression can manifest as cognitive impairment (Feldman et al. 2018). One RCT of methylphenidate found a statistically significant improvement in cognitive performance in patients with epilepsy without increase in seizure frequency (Adams et al. 2017). AchEIs have not been found to be effective for cognitive deficits in epilepsy (Hamberger et al. 2007). Memantine has not shown any cognitive benefit in patients with epilepsy, and there is concern regarding increased seizure risk (Leeman-Markowski et al. 2018).

Depression

Depression is very common in patients with epilepsy, with a prevalence up to 10 times that of the general population and a risk of suicide more than three times that of the general population (Hesdorffer et al. 2012). Furthermore, antiepileptic drugs have been reported to increase suicidal behavior and completed suicides, although the risk is small and causal relationships are unclear, with the risk of completed suicide probably influenced by patients having access to drugs more likely to be lethal in overdose (Dreier et al. 2019). One meta-analysis found no increase in suicidality in those treated with antiepileptic drugs approved since 2008 compared with placebo (Klein et al. 2021). Despite the high prevalence of depression in epilepsy, a 2021 systematic review by the International League Against Epilepsy found only six controlled studies addressing medication use for depression in epilepsy (four involving antidepressants, two examining antiepileptic drugs) (Mula et al. 2022). In general, depressive symptoms that are acutely temporally related to seizure activity (either ictal or peri-ictal) are best managed with improved seizure control. Interictal depressive symptoms can be managed with SSRIs as first-line agents because they have little effect on the seizure threshold (Mula et al. 2022), with similar recommendations available for SNRIs (Tolchin et al. 2020). Conversely, bupropion and clomipramine are not recommended because of the risk of lowering the seizure threshold.

Mania

Mania is rare in patients with epilepsy, with the exception of patients who have undergone disease-modifying surgeries, specifically lobectomies. The use of mood-stabilizing antiepileptic medications such as lamotrigine, valproate, and carbamazepine is considered first line, with cautious use of lithium as a second-line agent because of possible epileptogenic activity (Prueter and Norra 2005).

Anxiety

Anxiety can be present as an ictal or peri-ictal symptom or may evolve as a chronic symptom as a result of anticipatory anxiety about a recurrence of seizure activity. No RCTs are available addressing medication selection for the treatment of anxiety in patients with epilepsy. As with depression, SSRIs are considered first-line agents because of minimal effect on seizure threshold. Benzodiazepines can be useful given their anxiolytic and anticonvulsant properties, but adverse motor and cognitive effects and the potential for dependence or abuse must be considered.

Psychosis

Patients with epilepsy have a risk of psychosis eight times as high as in the general population (Clancy et al. 2014). Psychosis in epilepsy may be classified as either ictal or postictal psychosis (psychoses closely linked to seizures), alternative psychosis (psychosis linked to seizure remission, also called *forced normalization*), interictal psychosis (intermittent episodes of psychosis not associated with seizures), or iatrogenic psychosis (psychosis related to anticonvulsant drugs, most notoriously levetiracetam). Anticonvulsants are the primary treatment for ictal and postictal psychosis. The treatment of interictal psychosis includes both anticonvulsants and antipsychotics. Antipsychotics with a high risk of lowering the seizure threshold, such as clozapine (and to a lesser degree quetiapine and olanzapine) and low-potency typical agents, should be avoided, whereas risperidone, aripiprazole, and haloperidol carry less risk of triggering seizures (Tolchin et al. 2020). If concerns are raised about the potential for an antipsychotic to exacerbate epilepsy, a careful risk-benefit analysis should be undertaken, weighing the potential contribution of the medication to the seizures against the risks of destabilizing or exacerbating psychosis.

Symptoms and Syndromes Common Across Neurological Disorders

Apathy

A Cochrane review of RCTs evaluating interventions for apathy in patients with TBI found no medication trials (Lane-Brown and Tate 2009). Methylphenidate has demonstrated safety and efficacy in treating apathy in patients with AD across several RCTs (Mintzer et al. 2021; Padala et al. 2018; Rosenberg et al. 2013). A study comparing sertraline, escitalopram, and nicergoline in patients with AD reported improved apathy scores in the sertraline cohort (Takemoto et al. 2020). Other RCTs have found no effect on apathy for modafinil (Frakey et al. 2012) or bupropion (Maier et al. 2020) in this population. Escitalopram has been shown to be effective in preventing apathy immediately after a stroke (within 3 months) (Mikami et al. 2013). Apathy is a common feature of PD, but RCTs have failed to demonstrate efficacy from a variety of pharmacological interventions (including SSRIs, SNRIs, and dopamine receptor agonists) for this symptom (Hauser et al. 2016; Takahashi et al. 2019).

Pseudobulbar Affect

A broad spectrum of neurological conditions have been associated with paroxysmal episodes of affective outbursts that are either exaggerated or grossly incongruent with the patient's internal mood state. This pathological separation of mood and affect has been referred to by several descriptors (including *affective lability, emotional incontinence, pathological laughing and crying,* and *involuntary emotional expression disorder*) but has most consistently been described by the term *pseudobulbar affect*. One study of patients with diagnoses of stroke, dementia, TBI, MS, PD, or amyotrophic lateral sclerosis found that more than one-third of these patients screened positive for symptoms of pseudobulbar affect (Brooks et al. 2013). Pseudobulbar affect may be misdiagnosed as a primary mood disorder.

The sole current FDA-approved treatment for pseudobulbar affect is the combination of low-dose dextromethorphan and quinidine, based on data from a large double-blind, placebo-controlled trial (Pioro et al. 2010). This formulation leverages inhibition of cytochrome P450 2D6 (CYP2D6) by quinidine to prevent metabolism of dextromethorphan to its active metabolite dextrorphan, increasing concentrations of the parent drug 30-fold. Dextromethorphan is postulated to have antiglutamatergic activity in the CNS via activity at the N-methyl-D-aspartate and σ_1 receptors (Pioro et al. 2010). Patients should be monitored for adverse effects, including diarrhea and dizziness. QTc interval monitoring may be indicated for patients with additional risk factors for arrhythmia. Patients receiving other medications that are metabolized by CYP2D6 should be observed for drug-drug interactions. SSRIs (which probably exert their effect in pseudobulbar affect by secondary modulation of glutamate by serotonin) and TCAs may be considered as second- and third-line approaches, with published studies limited by very small sample sizes (Chen 2017).

Sexual Disinhibition

Sexual disinhibition is common in patients with disturbances of frontal lobe function, particularly men. A 2021 systematic literature review identified no RCTs examining management of sexual disinhibition in dementia and no studies comparing efficacies of different agents (Sarangi et al. 2021). Small trials or case reports using SSRIs, gabapentin, pindolol, clomipramine, carbamazepine, cimetidine, or antipsychotics have found some clinical benefit (Sarangi et al. 2021). Estrogen therapy was effective in a double-blind study (Kyomen et al. 1999), and Ozkan and colleagues (2008) reported effectiveness with leuprolide and cyproterone. Medroxyprogesterone acetate was reported as effective and well tolerated in a case series of five geriatric patients with sexual disinhibition (Bardell et al. 2011). Dopamine agonists, discussed later in this chapter, also have been known to cause impulse-control problems, including the development of paraphilias.

Adverse Neurological Effects of Psychotropic Medications

Psychotropic medications have been associated with the potential to produce a number of adverse neurological effects, most notably extrapyramidal symptoms, including tardive dyskinesia (TD); lowering of the seizure threshold; cognitive impairment; delirium; and behavioral disinhibition (Table 9–1). Neuroleptic malignant syndrome, which may develop in patients taking antipsychotic medications, and serotonin syndrome, which may develop in patients taking any serotonergic agent, are covered in Chapter 2, "Severe Drug Reactions."

Extrapyramidal Symptoms

Psychotropic-induced extrapyramidal symptoms include acute dyskinesias, tremor, dystonia, and akathisia. Patients with PD, DLB, vascular dementia, or MS are at greatest risk for developing these symptoms. Antipsychotics are the most common cause of extrapyramidal symptoms, with risk increasing as dopamine D_2 receptor blockade increases. High-potency first-generation antipsychotics such as haloperidol present the greatest risk, followed by phenothiazines and atypical antipsychotics. Among the atypical antipsychotics, the hierarchy of extrapyramidal symptom risk was evaluated on the basis of average extrapyramidal symptom presentation in patients with schizophrenia or bipolar disorder. Based on data reported in the prescribing information for each drug (with some notable variability based on dosage and speed of titration), the hierarchy (greater to lesser) is as follows: ziprasidone > risperidone > cariprazine > paliperidone > olanzapine > asenapine > lurasidone > lumateperone > brexpiprazole > aripiprazole > iloperidone > quetiapine > clozapine > pimavanserin. Extrapyramidal symptoms have also been reported with antidepressants, including SSRIs, SNRIs, mirtazapine, vortioxetine, and bupropion. The symptoms are not dose related, and they can develop with short- or long-term use (Revet et al. 2020).

TD, characterized by repetitive, involuntary, purposeless movements, can be associated with chronic use or abrupt discontinuation of antipsychotic medications. It has also been reported with metoclopramide and phenothiazine antiemetics and very rarely with SSRIs. Medical complications may include pain and impairment of gait, swallowing, and respiration. Neurologically ill and elderly patients are thought to be at increased risk. Tardive dystonia and tardive akathisia also may result from prolonged antipsychotic

Table 9–1. Neurological adverse effects of psychotropic medications

Medication	Neurological adverse effects
Antidepressants	
Selective serotonin reuptake inhibitors and serotonin-norepinephrine reuptake inhibitors	Tremor, parkinsonism, sedation, apathy
Tricyclic antidepressants	Cognitive impairment (tertiary > secondary amines), seizure (particularly clomipramine), sedation (tertiary > secondary amines)
Amoxapine and maprotiline	Lower seizure threshold at therapeutic dosages
Monoamine oxidase inhibitors	Sedation
Bupropion	Seizure (increased risk with dosages exceeding 400 mg/day; however, overall risk is low) (Ruffmann et al. 2006)
Antipsychotics	
Atypical and typical agents	Extrapyramidal symptoms and tardive dyskinesia, seizure (particularly clozapine, chlorpromazine, and loxapine), cognitive impairment (particularly low-potency typical agents), orthostatic hypotension, neuroleptic malignant syndrome
Mood stabilizers	
Carbamazepine	Dizziness, drowsiness, incoordination, blurred vision, nystagmus, ataxia
Lithium	Seizure, ataxia, delirium, slurred speech, dystonia, tics, tremor; deficits can be acute and chronic and are generally dose and serum concentration dependent
Valproate	Somnolence, dizziness, tremor, insomnia
Anticholinergics	
Benztropine and trihexyphenidyl	Delirium, visual hallucinations, cognitive impairment

Table 9–1. Neurological adverse effects of psychotropic medications *(continued)*

Medication	Neurological adverse effects
Anxiolytics	
Benzodiazepines	Withdrawal seizures, delirium, disinhibition, cognitive impairment, sedation, dysarthria
Buspirone	Sedation, dizziness

exposure. First-line treatment of TD features use of an inhibitor of the vesicular monoamine transporter 2. Although tetrabenazine is a vesicular monoamine transporter 2 inhibitor that was previously used for management of TD, its use has been curtailed by significant risk of depression and suicide. Two newer vesicular monoamine transporter 2 inhibitors—valbenazine and deutetrabenazine—are indicated specifically for the management of TD, without concern for increasing depression or suicide risk (Solmi et al. 2018). There are no head-to-head trials to allow direct comparison, so drug choice is based largely on tolerability and adherence. Use of anticholinergic antiparkinsonian drugs (i.e., benztropine) has been found to have no therapeutic benefit and may worsen TD (Ward et al. 2018).

Seizures

Use of psychotropics for patients with epilepsy is generally approached with caution. However, in a retrospective study assessing the effect of psychotropics on seizure frequency, Gross and colleagues (2000) found that seizure frequency decreased in 33% of patients, was unchanged in 44%, and increased in 23%. No significant difference in average seizure frequency was found between pretreatment and treatment periods. The authors concluded that psychotropic medications can be used safely by patients with epilepsy and psychopathology if introduced slowly in low to moderate doses. However, certain psychotropics, such as chlorpromazine, clozapine, maprotiline, bupropion, and clomipramine, have been associated with increased seizure frequency, and the calculus of relative risk and benefit should be carefully considered and documented if these drugs are prescribed for patients with epilepsy (i.e., a relative increase in the risk of seizure may be preferred to decompensation of co-occurring psychiatric illness). Haloperidol and atypical antipsychotics other than clozapine have a lower risk of causing seizures than do phenothiazine antipsychotics (Guarnieri et al. 2004). The rate of seizures with bupropion is dose related, with the greatest risk (about 0.4%) in patients without a co-occurring neurological diagnosis noted at dosages of 450 mg/day. Psychostimulants, including dextroamphetamine and methylphenidate, do not appear to increase seizure risk in patients with ADHD who have epilepsy and good seizure control (Kanner 2008). However, patients whose seizures are not well controlled may be at further risk with the addition of a stimulant medication (Gonzalez-Heydrich et al. 2007).

Cognitive Impairment and Delirium

The psychotropic medications most likely to cause or exacerbate cognitive impairment and delirium are benzodiazepines, medications with anticholinergic properties (e.g., benztropine, phenothiazines, tertiary-amine TCAs), lithium (especially at supratherapeutic levels), and topiramate. Behavioral disinhibition is often caused by benzodiazepines, particularly in patients with neurological illness and in children and older adults. Behavioral disinhibition often co-occurs with cognitive impairment and delirium. In general, benzodiazepines and lithium should be used with caution and monitored closely in patients with neurological conditions because each medication has a relatively low therapeutic index.

Adverse Psychiatric Effects of Neurological Medications

Dopamine Agonists

Dopamine agonists (Table 9–2), including levodopa, amantadine, pramipexole, and ropinirole, have been associated with hallucinations, delusions, and complex behavior problems in patients with PD. Patients at greatest risk include those with advanced disease, prolonged treatment, cognitive impairment, and dyskinesias.

Complex behavior problems associated with dopamine receptor stimulation in patients with PD include pathological gambling, hypersexuality, punding (intense fascination with repetitive handling, examining, sorting, and arranging of objects), compulsive shopping, and compulsive medication

Table 9–2. Psychiatric adverse effects of neurological medications

Medication	Psychiatric adverse effects
Dopamine agonists	
Amantadine, levodopa/carbidopa	Psychosis, agitation, insomnia, confusion
Pramipexole and ropinirole	Hallucinations, delusions, psychosis, agitation, somnolence, confusion, impulse-control disorders, paraphilias
Anticonvulsants	
Gabapentin	Sedation
Lamotrigine	Euphoria
Levetiracetam	Mood disorder, psychosis, aggressive behavior
Topiramate	Cognitive impairment, decreased appetite, mood disorder, psychosis, aggressive behavior
Valproate	Cognitive impairment, increased appetite
Interferons	
Interferon-β-1a/1b	Depression, affective lability, irritability
Monoamine oxidase B inhibitors	
Selegiline	Dizziness, vivid dreams, agitation, insomnia; risk for hypertensive crisis and serotonin syndrome at dosages exceeding 10 mg/day
Rasagiline	Dizziness, vivid dreams, anxiety
Catechol O-methyltransferase inhibitors	
Entacapone and tolcapone	Dyskinesia, sleep disorders, hallucinations, agitation
α_2-Adrenoceptor agonists	
Clonidine and guanfacine	Depression, anxiety, vivid dreams, restlessness, fatigue

Table 9–2. Psychiatric adverse effects of neurological
medications *(continued)*

Medication	Psychiatric adverse effects
Cholinesterase inhibitors	
Donepezil, rivastigmine, and galantamine	Insomnia, fatigue, anorexia, vivid dreams
Aducanumab-avwa	Headache, falls, amyloid-related imaging abnormalities (microhemorrhage or edema)

use (Weintraub and Claassen 2017). Paraphilias, defined as intense urges or behaviors involving nonnormative sexual interests, have been associated with dopamine agonist use (Solla et al. 2015). Sometimes described as dopamine dysregulation syndrome, these behaviors affect up to 20% of patients with PD (Weintraub and Claassen 2017). Management includes dopamine agonist dose reduction and treatment of secondary psychotic, manic, or behavioral symptoms.

Anticonvulsants

Adverse psychiatric effects (including irritability, anger, and aggression) have been associated with the anticonvulsants topiramate and levetiracetam when used to manage epilepsy (Steinhoff et al. 2021). Data support the practice of switching from levetiracetam to another anticonvulsant (brivaracetam) to ameliorate these adverse effects (Steinhoff et al. 2021). Although there are reports of increased rates of completed suicide associated with anticonvulsants, one large registry study found this risk to be associated predominantly with drugs with narrower therapeutic indexes (i.e., phenobarbital, clonazepam), and when data were adjusted to remove overdose on the anticonvulsant as a mechanism of suicide, risk of suicide associated with these agents was significantly reduced (Dreier et al. 2019).

Interferon-β-1a

Although interferon-α is commonly associated with depression, the risk of depression from interferon-β-1a, used for relapsing-remitting MS, is not well established. One systematic review found no consistent relationship between the use of interferon-β-1a and depression, with the possible exception of patients with a history of major depressive disorder, for whom additional monitoring may be advised (Alba Palé et al. 2017). Psychosis and delirium also have been reported as adverse effects of this treatment (Goëb et al. 2003).

Drug-Drug Interactions

Pharmacokinetic and pharmacodynamic interactions between psychiatric and neurological medications are outlined in Tables 9–3 and 9–4. The pharmacokinetic interaction of greatest clinical significance is the induction of CYP1A2-, CYP2C9-, CYP2C19-, and CYP3A4-mediated metabolism by phenytoin, phenobarbital, carbamazepine, and ethosuximide, resulting in decreased levels of many psychotropics. Valproate also may alter metabolism through hepatotoxicity and complex effects on induction and inhibition of several CYP enzymes. It is prudent to monitor (when possible) the levels of all coadministered medications with potential for toxicity when prescribing anticonvulsant agents.

Many psychotropic medications (TCAs, bupropion [>450 mg/day], high-dose venlafaxine, maprotiline, lithium, low-potency typical antipsychotics, clozapine) may lower the seizure threshold, which can erode the therapeutic effects of anticonvulsants. Amantadine, fosphenytoin, and felbamate may rarely increase QTc interval prolongation when given with other QTc interval–prolonging psychotropic drugs such as antipsychotics, TCAs, and lithium (for a list, see CredibleMeds 2022). Triptans and selegiline (inhibition of monoamine oxidase A is significant at >10 mg/day) increase the risk of serotonin syndrome when used by patients receiving SSRIs, SNRIs, mirtazapine, or TCAs. The risk of serotonin syndrome with either selegiline or rasagiline when used concomitantly with serotonergic antidepressants is thought to be minimal, but cases have been reported (Aboukarr and Giudice 2018). Triptans have a black box warning of the risk of serotonin syndrome in combination with serotonergic antidepressants; however, the frequency and clinical significance of this potential interaction have been questioned (Orlova et al. 2018). Psychotogenic effects of dopamine agonists, topiramate, and levetiracetam may erode the therapeutic effects of antipsychotics in patients with schizophrenia.

Table 9–3. Neurological medication–psychotropic medication interactions

Medication	Interaction mechanism	Effects on psychotropic medications and management
Anticonvulsants		
Carbamazepine, phenobarbital, and phenytoin	Induction of CYP1A2, CYP2C9/19, and CYP3A4 and of uridine 5'-diphosphate glucuronosyl-transferase	Increased metabolism and decreased levels of clozapine, olanzapine, buspirone, benzodiazepines (except oxazepam, lorazepam, and temazepam), pimozide, trazodone, and zolpidem
Ethosuximide	Induction of CYP3A4	Increased metabolism and decreased levels of buspirone, benzodiazepines (except oxazepam, lorazepam, and temazepam), pimozide, trazodone, and zolpidem
Felbamate and fosphenytoin	QT prolongation	Increased risk of cardiac arrhythmias with other QT-prolonging agents, including TCAs, typical antipsychotics, pimozide, risperidone, paliperidone, iloperidone, quetiapine, ziprasidone, and lithium
Valproate	Inhibition of urea cycle	Hyperammonemia with topiramate (also a urea cycle inhibitor)
Antiparkinsonian medications		
Levodopa	Additive psychotogenic effect	Erosion of antipsychotic control of psychosis
Amantadine	QT prolongation	Increased risk of cardiac arrhythmias with other QT-prolonging agents, including TCAs, typical antipsychotics, pimozide, risperidone, paliperidone, iloperidone, quetiapine, ziprasidone, and lithium

Table 9–3. Neurological medication–psychotropic medication interactions *(continued)*

Medication	Interaction mechanism	Effects on psychotropic medications and management
Antiparkinsonian medications *(continued)*		
Amantadine *(continued)*	Additive psychotogenic effect	Erosion of antipsychotic control of psychosis
Selegiline and rasagiline	Monoamine oxidase A inhibition at high dosage (selegiline >10 mg/day)	Increased risk of serotonin syndrome when combined with selective serotonin reuptake inhibitors, serotonin-norepinephrine reuptake inhibitors, mirtazapine, MAOIs, lithium, or TCAs
Pramipexole and ropinirole	Additive hypotensive effects	Increased risk of hypotensive effects with antipsychotics, TCAs, and MAOIs
	Additive psychotogenic effect	Erosion of antipsychotic control of psychosis
Cognitive enhancers		
Donepezil, galantamine, and rivastigmine	Cholinesterase inhibition	Exacerbates extrapyramidal symptoms
Triptans	Serotonin receptor agonist	Serotonin syndrome (FDA black box warning)
Dextromethorphan/ quinidine	Inhibition of CYP2D6	Decreased metabolism and increased levels of risperidone, haloperidol, chlorpromazine, thioridazine, perphenazine, paroxetine, fluoxetine, nortriptyline, and desipramine

Note.　CYP=cytochrome P450; MAOIs=monoamine oxidase inhibitors; TCAs=tricyclic antidepressants.

Table 9–4. Psychotropic medication–neurological medication interactions

Medication	Interaction mechanism	Effects on neurological medications and management
Antidepressants		
Selective serotonin reuptake inhibitors		
Fluoxetine and fluvoxamine	Inhibit CYP1A2, CYP2C9/19, CYP3A4	Inhibited metabolism and increased levels and toxicities of CYP1A2 substrates (rasagiline, frovatriptan, zolmitriptan, ropinirole), CYP2C9 and CYP2C19 substrates (mephenytoin, phenytoin, tiagabine), and CYP3A4 substrates (ergotamine, carbamazepine, ethosuximide, phenytoin, phenobarbital, tiagabine, zonisamide)
Serotonin-norepinephrine reuptake inhibitors and novel-action agents		
Bupropion, venlafaxine, and desvenlafaxine	Reduced seizure threshold	Increased risk of seizures and erosion of therapeutic effect of anticonvulsants. Avoid bupropion at dosages >450 mg/day and high-dose venlafaxine.
Tricyclic antidepressants	Reduced seizure threshold	Increased risk of seizures and erosion of therapeutic effect of anticonvulsants. Avoid clomipramine and maprotiline, especially at high dosages.
	QT prolongation	Additive QT prolongation in combination with amantadine, felbamate, and fosphenytoin. Consider QT-prolonging effects when selecting psychiatric and neurological medications.

Table 9–4. Psychotropic medication–neurological medication interactions *(continued)*

Medication	Interaction mechanism	Effects on neurological medications and management
Antidepressants *(continued)*		
MAOIs		
Moclobemide, phenelzine, tranylcypromine, and isocarboxazid	MAO inhibition	Inhibition of triptans metabolized by MAO, including sumatriptan, rizatriptan, and zolmitriptan. Avoid combining these triptans with MAOIs. Consider almotriptan, eletriptan, frovatriptan, or naratriptan, which are metabolized by CYP enzymes.
Mood stabilizers		
Valproic acid	CYP2C9 inhibition	Increased levels of phenytoin, carbamazepine, phenobarbital, and primidone
	Uridine 5′-diphosphate glucuronosyl-transferase inhibition	Reduced metabolism and increased levels of entacapone and tolcapone
Lithium	Reduced seizure threshold	Increased risk of seizures and erosion of therapeutic effect of anticonvulsants
	QT prolongation	Additive QT prolongation in combination with amantadine, felbamate, and fosphenytoin. Consider QT-prolonging effects when selecting psychiatric and neurological medications.
Antipsychotics		
Atypical and typical agents	Dopamine receptor blockade	Extrapyramidal symptoms; worsening of Parkinson's disease (except possibly with low-dose clozapine)

Table 9–4.   Psychotropic medication–neurological medication interactions *(continued)*

Medication	Interaction mechanism	Effects on neurological medications and management
Antipsychotics *(continued)*		
Atypical and typical agents *(continued)*	Reduced seizure threshold	Increased risk of seizures and erosion of therapeutic effect of anticonvulsants. Avoid clozapine and low-potency typical agents.
	QT prolongation	Additive QT prolongation in combination with amantadine, felbamate, and fosphenytoin. Consider QT-prolonging effects when selecting psychiatric and neurological medications.
Clozapine	Additive hematological toxicity	Increased risk of bone marrow suppression and agranulocytosis with carbamazepine
	Reduced seizure threshold	Increased risk of seizures and erosion of therapeutic effect of anticonvulsants
Psychostimulants		
Amphetamine and methylphenidate	Additive vasoconstriction	Excessive vasoconstriction, hypertension, and "ergotism" with triptans and ergot alkaloids
	Dopamine receptor agonism	Increased risk of psychosis with levodopa, amantadine, pramipexole, and ropinirole

Note.   CYP = cytochrome P450; MAO = monoamine oxidase; MAOIs = monoamine oxidase inhibitors.

Key Points

- Patients with cognitive impairment are at increased risk for noncompliance and often inaccurately report symptoms and side effects. Patient and collateral family and caregiver engagement and education improve assessment, medication compliance, and side-effect reporting.

- A comprehensive neuropsychiatric evaluation should define the nature of the CNS disease, disease stage or time since injury, and any neuropsychiatric disturbances.

- Treatment selection should consider whether a single intervention could address disparate symptoms (e.g., dopaminergic agents for mild depression in Parkinson's disease, antiepileptic drugs for the treatment of ictal or peri-ictal psychiatric symptoms). Patients with neurological disease are often taking multiple medications, and the "two birds, one stone" approach may help in lowering both clinical and financial burdens of unnecessary polypharmacy.

- The "start low, go slow" approach should be used, especially when the agent being added may mechanistically exacerbate other symptoms. On occasion, consideration should be given to augmentation with a different agent rather than dose escalation in order to minimize exacerbation of extant neurological symptoms.

- Clinical response, side effects, and therapeutic drug levels (when available) should be assessed frequently.

- Off-label use of medications in neuropsychiatry is the rule rather than the exception when addressing behavioral disturbances such as agitation, aggression, or sexual disinhibition. Mechanism of action and side-effect profile are often more pertinent considerations in a choice of agent than an approved indication.

- Clinicians should stay abreast of the latest developments in the treatment of primary neurological illnesses. New drugs and novel mechanisms of action continue to make their way to our pharmacological armamentarium.

References

Aboukarr A, Giudice M: Interaction between monoamine oxidase B inhibitors and selective serotonin reuptake inhibitors. Can J Hosp Pharm 71(3):196–207, 2018 29955193

Adams J, Alipio-Jocson V, Inoyama K, et al: Methylphenidate, cognition, and epilepsy: a double-blind, placebo-controlled, single-dose study. Neurology 88(5):470–476, 2017 28031390

Alba Palé L, León Caballero J, Samsó Buxareu B, et al: Systematic review of depression in patients with multiple sclerosis and its relationship to interferonβ treatment. Mult Scler Relat Disord 17:138–143, 2017 29055445

Arvanitakis Z, Shah RC, Bennett DA: Diagnosis and management of dementia: review. JAMA 322(16):1589–1599, 2019 31638686

Ayerbe L, Ayis S, Wolfe CD, et al: Natural history, predictors and outcomes of depression after stroke: systematic review and meta-analysis. Br J Psychiatry 202(1):14–21, 2013 23284148

Azhar L, Kusumo RW, Marotta G, et al: Pharmacological management of apathy in dementia. CNS Drugs 36(2):143–165, 2022 35006557

Bachoud-Lévi A-C, Ferreira J, Massart R, et al: International guidelines for the treatment of Huntington's disease. Front Neurol 10:710, 2019 31333565

Bardell A, Lau T, Fedoroff JP: Inappropriate sexual behavior in a geriatric population. Int Psychogeriatr 23(7):1182–1188, 2011 21554796

Bassett SS: Cognitive impairment in Parkinson's disease. Prim Psychiatry 12:50–55, 2005

Battle CE, Abdul-Rahim AH, Shenkin SD, et al: Cholinesterase inhibitors for vascular dementia and other vascular cognitive impairments: a network meta-analysis. Cochrane Database Syst Rev 2(2):CD013306, 2021 33704781

Bernardo CG, Singh V, Thompson PM: Safety and efficacy of psychopharmacological agents used to treat the psychiatric sequelae of common neurological disorders. Expert Opin Drug Saf 7(4):435–445, 2008 18613807

Birks JS, Chong LY, Grimley-Evans J: Rivastigmine for Alzheimer's disease. Cochrane Database Syst Rev (9):CD001191, 2015 26393402

Boeschoten RE, Braamse AMJ, Beekman ATF, et al: Prevalence of depression and anxiety in multiple sclerosis: a systematic review and meta-analysis. J Neurol Sci 372:331–341, 2017 28017241

Bosnjak Kuharic D, Markovic D, Brkovic T, et al: Cannabinoids for the treatment of dementia. Cochrane Database Syst Rev 9(9):CD012820, 2021 34532852

Boxer AL, Knopman DS, Kaufer DI, et al: Memantine in patients with frontotemporal lobar degeneration: a multicentre, randomised, double-blind, placebo-controlled trial. Lancet Neurol 12(2):149–156, 2013 23290598

Brooks BR, Crumpacker D, Fellus J, et al: PRISM: a novel research tool to assess the prevalence of pseudobulbar affect symptoms across neurological conditions. PLoS One 8(8):e72232, 2013 23991068

Brusa L, Bassi A, Stefani A, et al: Pramipexole in comparison to l-dopa: a neuropsychological study. J Neural Transm (Vienna) 110(4):373–380, 2003 12658365

Brusa L, Tiraboschi P, Koch G, et al: Pergolide effect on cognitive functions in early mild Parkinson's disease. J Neural Transm (Vienna) 112(2):231–237, 2005 15365788

Brusa L, Pavino V, Massimetti MC, et al: The effect of dopamine agonists on cognitive functions in non-demented early mild Parkinson's disease patients. Funct Neurol 28(1):13–17, 2013 23731911

Burn D, Emre M, McKeith I, et al: Effects of rivastigmine in patients with and without visual hallucinations in dementia associated with Parkinson's disease. Mov Disord 21(11):1899–1907, 2006 16960863

Cavazzoni P: FDA's decision to approve new treatment for Alzheimer's disease. 2021. Available at: www.fda.gov/drugs/news-events-human-drugs/fdas-decision-approve-new-treatment-alzheimers-disease. Accessed September 21, 2022.

Chen H, Song Z, Dennis JA: Hypertonic saline versus other intracranial pressure-lowering agents for people with acute traumatic brain injury. Cochrane Database Syst Rev 1(1):CD010904, 2020 31978260

Chen JJ: Pharmacotherapeutic management of pseudobulbar affect. Am J Manag Care 23(18 Suppl):S345–S350, 2017 29297657

Chen S, Wu H, Klebe D, et al: Valproic acid: a new candidate of therapeutic application for the acute central nervous system injuries. Neurochem Res 39(9):1621–1633, 2014 24482021

Chiong W, Tolchin BD, Bonnie RJ, et al: Decisions with patients and families regarding aducanumab in Alzheimer disease, with recommendations for consent: AAN position statement. Neurology 98(4):154–159, 2021 34789544

Chiu CT, Wang Z, Hunsberger JG, et al: Therapeutic potential of mood stabilizers lithium and valproic acid: beyond bipolar disorder. Pharmacol Rev 65(1):105–142, 2013 23300133

Choi-Kwon S, Kim JS: Anger, a result and cause of stroke: a narrative review. J Stroke 24(3):311–322, 2022 36221934

Choi-Kwon S, Han SW, Kwon SU, et al: Fluoxetine treatment in poststroke depression, emotional incontinence, and anger proneness: a double-blind, placebo-controlled study. Stroke 37(1):156–161, 2006 16306470

Chu CS, Yang FC, Tseng PT, et al: Treatment efficacy and acceptability of pharmacotherapies for dementia with Lewy bodies: a systematic review and network meta-analysis. Arch Gerontol Geriatr 96:104474, 2021 34256210

Clancy MJ, Clarke MC, Connor DJ, et al: The prevalence of psychosis in epilepsy; a systematic review and meta-analysis. BMC Psychiatry 14:75, 2014 24625201

CredibleMeds: Risk categories for drugs that prolong QT and induce torsades de pointes (TDP). 2022. Available at: https://crediblemeds.org. Accessed January 30, 2022.

Cummings J, Isaacson S, Mills R, et al: Pimavanserin for patients with Parkinson's disease psychosis: a randomised, placebo-controlled phase 3 trial. Lancet 383(9916):533–540, 2014 24183563

Cummings JL, Lyketsos CG, Peskind ER, et al: Effect of dextromethorphan-quinidine on agitation in patients with Alzheimer disease dementia: a randomized clinical trial. JAMA 314(12):1242–1254, 2015 26393847

Diaz-Arrastia R, Kochanek PM, Bergold P, et al: Pharmacotherapy of traumatic brain injury: state of the science and the road forward: report of the Department of Defense Neurotrauma Pharmacology Workgroup. J Neurotrauma 31(2):135–158, 2014 23968241

Divac N, Stojanović R, Savić Vujović K, et al: The efficacy and safety of antipsychotic medications in the treatment of psychosis in patients with Parkinson's disease. Behav Neurol 2016:4938154, 2016 27504054

Dreier JW, Pedersen CB, Gasse C, et al: Antiepileptic drugs and suicide: role of prior suicidal behavior and parental psychiatric disorder. Ann Neurol 86(6):951–961, 2019 31621936

Dudas R, Malouf R, McCleery J, et al: Antidepressants for treating depression in dementia. Cochrane Database Syst Rev 8(8):CD003944, 2018 30168578

Falk WE, Mahnke MW, Poskanzer DC: Lithium prophylaxis of corticotropin-induced psychosis. JAMA 241(10):1011–1012, 1979 216818

Fann JR, Quinn DK, Hart T: Treatment of psychiatric problems after traumatic brain injury. Biol Psychiatry 91(5):508–521, 2022 34511181

Feldman L, Lapin B, Busch RM, et al: Evaluating subjective cognitive impairment in the adult epilepsy clinic: effects of depression, number of antiepileptic medications, and seizure frequency. Epilepsy Behav 81:18–24, 2018 29455082

Ferreira JJ, Rodrigues FB, Duarte GS, et al: An MDS evidence-based review on treatments for Huntington's disease. Mov Disord 37(1):25–35, 2022 34842303

Fiest KM, Walker JR, Bernstein CN, et al: Systematic review and meta-analysis of interventions for depression and anxiety in persons with multiple sclerosis. Mult Scler Relat Disord 5:12–26, 2016 26856938

Fleminger S, Greenwood RJ, Oliver DL: Pharmacological management for agitation and aggression in people with acquired brain injury. Cochrane Database Syst Rev (4):CD003299, 2006 17054165

Forester BP, Vahia I: Behavioral and psychological symptoms: an emerging crisis of the Alzheimer dementia epidemic. JAMA Netw Open 2(3):e190790, 2019 30901037

Frakey LL, Salloway S, Buelow M, et al: A randomized, double-blind, placebo-controlled trial of modafinil for the treatment of apathy in individuals with mild-to-moderate Alzheimer's disease. J Clin Psychiatry 73(6):796–801, 2012 22687392

Gasim M, Bernstein CN, Graff LA, et al: Adverse psychiatric effects of disease-modifying therapies in multiple sclerosis: a systematic review. Mult Scler Relat Disord 26:124–156, 2018 30248593

Godschalx-Dekker JA, Siegers HP: Reduction of parkinsonism and psychosis with mirtazapine: a case report. Pharmacopsychiatry 47(3):81–83, 2014 24504487

Goëb JL, Cailleau A, Lainé P, et al: Acute delirium, delusion, and depression during IFN-beta-1a therapy for multiple sclerosis: a case report. Clin Neuropharmacol 26(1):5–7, 2003 12567157

Gonzalez-Heydrich J, Dodds A, Whitney J, et al: Psychiatric disorders and behavioral characteristics of pediatric patients with both epilepsy and attention-deficit hyperactivity disorder. Epilepsy Behav 10(3):384–388, 2007 17368109

Gross A, Devinsky O, Westbrook LE, et al: Psychotropic medication use in patients with epilepsy: effect on seizure frequency. J Neuropsychiatry Clin Neurosci 12(4):458–464, 2000 11083162

Guarnieri R, Hallak JE, Walz R, et al: Pharmacological treatment of psychosis in epilepsy [in Portuguese]. Br J Psychiatry 26(1):57–61, 2004 15057842

Guerreiro DF, Navarro R, Silva M, et al: Psychosis secondary to traumatic brain injury. Brain Inj 23(4):358–361, 2009 19274520

Guo J, Wang Z, Liu R, et al: Memantine, donepezil, or combination therapy: what is the best therapy for Alzheimer's disease? A network meta-analysis. Brain Behav 10(11):e01831, 2020 32914577

Hamberger MJ, Palmese CA, Scarmeas N, et al: A randomized, double-blind, placebo-controlled trial of donepezil to improve memory in epilepsy. Epilepsia 48(7):1283–1291, 2007 17484756

Hammond FM, Bickett AK, Norton JH, et al: Effectiveness of amantadine hydrochloride in the reduction of chronic traumatic brain injury irritability and aggression. J Head Trauma Rehabil 29(5):391–399, 2014 24263176

Hanagasi HA, Gurvit H, Unsalan P, et al: The effects of rasagiline on cognitive deficits in Parkinson's disease patients without dementia: a randomized, double-blind, placebo-controlled, multicenter study. Mov Disord 26(10):1851–1858, 2011 21500280

Hauser RA, Slawek J, Barone P, et al: Evaluation of rotigotine transdermal patch for the treatment of apathy and motor symptoms in Parkinson's disease. BMC Neurol 16:90, 2016 27267880

Hesdorffer DC, Ishihara L, Mynepalli L, et al: Epilepsy, suicidality, and psychiatric disorders: a bidirectional association. Ann Neurol 72(2):184–191, 2012 22887468

Hicks AJ, Clay FJ, Hopwood M, et al: The efficacy and harms of pharmacological interventions for aggression after traumatic brain injury—systematic review. Front Neurol 10:1169, 2019 31849802

Hoffmann T, Ownsworth T, Eames S, et al: Evaluation of brief interventions for managing depression and anxiety symptoms during early discharge period after stroke: a pilot randomized controlled trial. Top Stroke Rehabil 22(2):116–126, 2015 25936543

Johansson B, Wentzel AP, Andréll P, et al: Methylphenidate reduces mental fatigue and improves processing speed in persons suffered a traumatic brain injury. Brain Inj 29(6):758–765, 2015 25794299

Joseph B, Nandakumar AL, Ahmed AT, et al: Prevalence of bipolar disorder in multiple sclerosis: a systematic review and meta-analysis. Evid Based Ment Health 24(2):88–94, 2021 33328183

Kandil EA, Abdelkader NF, El-Sayeh BM, et al: Imipramine and amitriptyline ameliorate the rotenone model of Parkinson's disease in rats. Neuroscience 332:26–37, 2016 27365173

Kanner AM: The use of psychotropic drugs in epilepsy: what every neurologist should know. Semin Neurol 28(3):379–388, 2008 18777484

Kaplin A: Depression in multiple sclerosis, in Multiple Sclerosis Therapeutics. Edited by Cohen JA, Rudick R. London, Informa Healthcare, 2007, pp 823–840

Karaiskos D, Tzavellas E, Spengos K, et al: Duloxetine versus citalopram and sertraline in the treatment of poststroke depression, anxiety, and fatigue. J Neuropsychiatry Clin Neurosci 24(3):349–353, 2012 23037649

Kavirajan H, Schneider LS: Efficacy and adverse effects of cholinesterase inhibitors and memantine in vascular dementia: a meta-analysis of randomised controlled trials. Lancet Neurol 6(9):782–792, 2007 17689146

Kelsen J, Karlsson M, Hansson MJ, et al: Copenhagen Head Injury Ciclosporin study: a Phase IIa safety, pharmacokinetics, and biomarker study of ciclosporin in severe traumatic brain injury patients. J Neurotrauma 36(23):3253–3263, 2019 31210099

Khellaf A, Khan DZ, Helmy A: Recent advances in traumatic brain injury. J Neurol 266(11):2878–2889, 2019 31563989

Klein P, Devinsky O, French J, et al: Suicidality risk of newer antiseizure medications: a meta-analysis. JAMA Neurol 78(9):1118–1127, 2021 34338718

Kostić V, Dzoljić E, Todorović Z, et al: Fluoxetine does not impair motor function in patients with Parkinson's disease: correlation between mood and motor functions with plasma concentrations of fluoxetine/norfluoxetine. Vojnosanit Pregl 69(12):1067–1075, 2012 23424961

Kreitzer N, Ancona R, McCullumsmith C, et al: The effect of antidepressants on depression after traumatic brain injury: a meta-analysis. J Head Trauma Rehabil 34(3):E47–E54, 2019 30169440

Kyle K, Bronstein JM: Treatment of psychosis in Parkinson's disease and dementia with Lewy bodies: a review. Parkinsonism Relat Disord 75:55–62, 2020 32480308

Kyomen HH, Satlin A, Hennen J, et al: Estrogen therapy and aggressive behavior in elderly patients with moderate-to-severe dementia: results from a short-term, randomized, double-blind trial. Am J Geriatr Psychiatry 7(4):339–348, 1999 10521168

Landmeyer NC, Bürkner PC, Wiendl H, et al: Disease-modifying treatments and cognition in relapsing-remitting multiple sclerosis: a meta-analysis. Neurology 94(22):e2373–e2383, 2020 32430312

Lane-Brown A, Tate R: Interventions for apathy after traumatic brain injury. Cochrane Database Syst Rev (2):CD006341, 2009 19370632

Laux G: Parkinson and depression: review and outlook. J Neural Transm (Vienna) 129(5–6):601–608, 2022 34982207

Leeds PR, Yu F, Wang Z, et al: A new avenue for lithium: intervention in traumatic brain injury. ACS Chem Neurosci 5(6):422–433, 2014 24697257

Leeman-Markowski BA, Meador KJ, Moo LR, et al: Does memantine improve memory in subjects with focal-onset epilepsy and memory dysfunction? A randomized, double-blind, placebo-controlled trial. Epilepsy Behav 88:315–324, 2018 30449328

Liu L, Fuller M, Behymer TP, et al: Selective serotonin reuptake inhibitors and intracerebral hemorrhage risk and outcome. Stroke 51(4):1135–1141, 2020 32126942

Maier F, Spottke A, Bach JJP, et al: Bupropion for the treatment of apathy in Alzheimer disease: a randomized clinical trial. JAMA Netw Open 3(5):e206027, 2020 32463470

Matsunaga S, Kishi T, Yasue I, et al: Cholinesterase inhibitors for Lewy body disorders: a meta-analysis. Int J Neuropsychopharmacol 19(2):pyv086, 2015 26221005

McCleery J, Sharpley AL: Pharmacotherapies for sleep disturbances in dementia. Cochrane Database Syst Rev 11(11):CD009178, 2020 33189083

Mehraram R, Peraza LR, Murphy NRE, et al: Functional and structural brain network correlates of visual hallucinations in Lewy body dementia. Brain 145(6):2190–2205, 2022 35262667

Mehta S, McIntyre A, Janzen S, et al: Pharmacological management of agitation among individuals with moderate to severe acquired brain injury: a systematic review. Brain Inj 32(3):287–296, 2018 29359952

Mendonça DA, Menezes K, Jog MS: Methylphenidate improves fatigue scores in Parkinson disease: a randomized controlled trial. Mov Disord 22(14):2070–2076, 2007 17674415

Menn SJ, Yang R, Lankford A: Armodafinil for the treatment of excessive sleepiness associated with mild or moderate closed traumatic brain injury: a 12-week, randomized, double-blind study followed by a 12-month open-label extension. J Clin Sleep Med 10(11):1181–1191, 2014 25325609

Mikami K, Jorge RE, Moser DJ, et al: Prevention of poststroke apathy using escitalopram or problem-solving therapy. Am J Geriatr Psychiatry 21(9):855–862, 2013 23930743

Mintzer J, Lanctôt KL, Scherer RW, et al: Effect of methylphenidate on apathy in patients with Alzheimer disease: the ADMET 2 randomized clinical trial. JAMA Neurol 78(11):1324–1332, 2021 34570180

Mori E, Ikeda M, Nagai R, et al: Long-term donepezil use for dementia with Lewy bodies: results from an open-label extension of Phase III trial. Alzheimers Res Ther 7(1):5, 2015 25713600

Mortensen JK, Andersen G: Pharmacological management of post-stroke depression: an update of the evidence and clinical guidance. Expert Opin Pharmacother 22(9):1157–1166, 2021 33530765

Motavalli A, Majdi A, Hosseini L, et al: Pharmacotherapy in multiple sclerosis-induced cognitive impairment: a systematic review and meta-analysis. Mult Scler Relat Disord 46:102478, 2020 32896820

Moulton CD, Hopkins CWP, Bevan-Jones WR: Systematic review of pharmacological treatments for depressive symptoms in Huntington's disease. Mov Disord 29(12):1556–1561, 2014 25111961

Mühlbauer V, Möhler R, Dichter MN, et al: Antipsychotics for agitation and psychosis in people with Alzheimer's disease and vascular dementia. Cochrane Database Syst Rev 12(12):CD013304, 2021 34918337

Mula M, Brodie MJ, de Toffol B, et al: ILAE clinical practice recommendations for the medical treatment of depression in adults with epilepsy. Epilepsia 63(2):316–334, 2022 34866176

Murphy R, O'Donoghue S, Counihan T, et al: Neuropsychiatric syndromes of multiple sclerosis. J Neurol Neurosurg Psychiatry 88(8):697–708, 2017 28285265

Nathoo N, Mackie A: Treating depression in multiple sclerosis with antidepressants: a brief review of clinical trials and exploration of clinical symptoms to guide treatment decisions. Mult Scler Relat Disord 18:177–180, 2017 29141805

Niedermaier N, Bohrer E, Schulte K, et al: Prevention and treatment of poststroke depression with mirtazapine in patients with acute stroke. J Clin Psychiatry 65(12):1619–1623, 2004 15641866

Nourbakhsh B, Revirajan N, Morris B, et al: Safety and efficacy of amantadine, modafinil, and methylphenidate for fatigue in multiple sclerosis: a randomised, placebo-controlled, crossover, double-blind trial. Lancet Neurol 20(1):38–48, 2021 33242419

Olney NT, Spina S, Miller BL: Frontotemporal dementia. Neurol Clin 35(2):339–374, 2017 28410663

Orgeta V, Tabet N, Nilforooshan R, et al: Efficacy of antidepressants for depression in Alzheimer's disease: systematic review and meta-analysis. J Alzheimers Dis 58(3):725–733, 2017 28505970

Orlova Y, Rizzoli P, Loder E: Association of coprescription of triptan antimigraine drugs and selective serotonin reuptake inhibitor or selective norepinephrine reuptake inhibitor antidepressants with serotonin syndrome. JAMA Neurol 75(5):566–572, 2018 29482205

Ozkan B, Wilkins K, Muralee S, et al: Pharmacotherapy for inappropriate sexual behaviors in dementia: a systematic review of literature. Am J Alzheimers Dis Other Demen 23(4):344–354, 2008 18509106

Padala PR, Padala KP, Lensing SY, et al: Methylphenidate for apathy in community-dwelling older veterans with mild Alzheimer's disease: a double-blind, randomized, placebo-controlled trial. Am J Psychiatry 175(2):159–168, 2018 28945120

Patten SB, Marrie RA, Carta MG: Depression in multiple sclerosis. Int Rev Psychiatry 29(5):463–472, 2017 28681616

Pioro EP, Brooks BR, Cummings J, et al: Dextromethorphan plus ultra low-dose quinidine reduces pseudobulbar affect. Ann Neurol 68(5):693–702, 2010 20839238

Porsteinsson AP, Drye LT, Pollock BG, et al: Effect of citalopram on agitation in Alzheimer disease: the CitAD randomized clinical trial. JAMA 311(7):682–691, 2014 24549548

Prueter C, Norra C: Mood disorders and their treatment in patients with epilepsy. J Neuropsychiatry Clin Neurosci 17(1):20–28, 2005 15746479

Quinn GR, Singer DE, Chang Y, et al: Effect of selective serotonin reuptake inhibitors on bleeding risk in patients with atrial fibrillation taking warfarin. Am J Cardiol 114(4):583–586, 2014 25001151

Revet A, Montastruc F, Roussin A, et al: Antidepressants and movement disorders: a postmarketing study in the world pharmacovigilance database. BMC Psychiatry 20(1):308, 2020 32546134

Richter D, Charles James J, Ebert A, et al: Selective serotonin reuptake inhibitors for the prevention of post-stroke depression: a systematic review and meta-analysis. J Clin Med 10(24):5912, 2021 34945207

Rodrigues TM, Castro Caldas A, Ferreira JJ: Pharmacological interventions for daytime sleepiness and sleep disorders in Parkinson's disease: systematic review and meta-analysis. Parkinsonism Relat Disord 27:25–34, 2016 27010071

Rosenberg PB, Lanctôt KL, Drye LT, et al: Safety and efficacy of methylphenidate for apathy in Alzheimer's disease: a randomized, placebo-controlled trial. J Clin Psychiatry 74(8):810–816, 2013 24021498

Rosenblatt A: Neuropsychiatry of Huntington's disease. Dialogues Clin Neurosci 9(2):191–197, 2007 17726917

Ruffmann C, Bogliun G, Beghi E: Epileptogenic drugs: a systematic review. Expert Rev Neurother 6(4):575–589, 2006 16623656

Ruthirakuhan MT, Herrmann N, Abraham EH, et al: Pharmacological interventions for apathy in Alzheimer's disease. Cochrane Database Syst Rev 5(5):CD012197, 2018 29727467

Salter KL, McClure JA, Foley NC, et al: Pharmacotherapy for depression posttraumatic brain injury: a meta-analysis. J Head Trauma Rehabil 31(4):E21–E32, 2016 26479398

Santos CO, Caeiro L, Ferro JM, et al: Mania and stroke: a systematic review. Cerebrovasc Dis 32(1):11–21, 2011 21576938

Sarangi A, Jones H, Bangash F, et al: Treatment and management of sexual disinhibition in elderly patients with neurocognitive disorders. Cureus 13(10):e18463, 2021 34745786

Schneider LS, Tariot PN, Dagerman KS, et al: Effectiveness of atypical antipsychotic drugs in patients with Alzheimer's disease. N Engl J Med 355(15):1525–1538, 2006 17035647

Schneider LS, Frangakis C, Drye LT, et al: Heterogeneity of treatment response to citalopram for patients with Alzheimer's disease with aggression or agitation: the CitAD randomized clinical trial. Am J Psychiatry 173(5):465–472, 2016 26771737

Schreiber S, Klag E, Gross Y, et al: Beneficial effect of risperidone on sleep disturbance and psychosis following traumatic brain injury. Int Clin Psychopharmacol 13(6):273–275, 1998 9861578

Segal GS, Xie SJ, Paracha SU, et al: Psychosis in Parkinson's disease: current treatment options and impact on patients and caregivers. J Geriatr Psychiatry Neurol 34(4):274–279, 2021 34219522

Seibert M, Mühlbauer V, Holbrook J, et al: Efficacy and safety of pharmacotherapy for Alzheimer's disease and for behavioural and psychological symptoms of dementia in older patients with moderate and severe functional impairments: a systematic review of controlled trials. Alzheimers Res Ther 13(1):131, 2021 34271969

Seitz DP, Adunuri N, Gill SS, et al: Antidepressants for agitation and psychosis in dementia. Cochrane Database Syst Rev (2):CD008191, 2011 21328305

Seppi K, Ray Chaudhuri K, Coelho M, et al: Update on treatments for nonmotor symptoms of Parkinson's disease—an evidence-based medicine review. Mov Disord 34(2):180–198, 2019 30653247

Smyrke N, Dunn N, Murley C, et al: Standardized mortality ratios in multiple sclerosis: systematic review with meta-analysis. Acta Neurol Scand 145(3):360–370, 2022 34820847

Solla P, Bortolato M, Cannas A, et al: Paraphilias and paraphilic disorders in Parkinson's disease: a systematic review of the literature. Mov Disord 30(5):604–613, 2015 25759330

Solmi M, Pigato G, Kane JM, et al: Treatment of tardive dyskinesia with VMAT-2 inhibitors: a systematic review and meta-analysis of randomized controlled trials. Drug Des Devel Ther 12:1215–1238, 2018 29795977

Steinhoff BJ, Klein P, Klitgaard H, et al: Behavioral adverse events with brivaracetam, levetiracetam, perampanel, and topiramate: a systematic review. Epilepsy Behav 118:107939, 2021 33839453

Stocchi F, ADAGIO investigators: Benefits of treatment with rasagiline for fatigue symptoms in patients with early Parkinson's disease. Eur J Neurol 21(2):357–360, 2014 23790011

Sumsuzzman DM, Choi J, Jin Y, et al: Neurocognitive effects of melatonin treatment in healthy adults and individuals with Alzheimer's disease and insomnia: a systematic review and meta-analysis of randomized controlled trials. Neurosci Biobehav Rev 127:459–473, 2021 33957167

Takahashi M, Tabu H, Ozaki A, et al: Antidepressants for depression, apathy, and gait instability in Parkinson's disease: a multicenter randomized study. Intern Med 58(3):361–368, 2019 30146591

Takemoto M, Ohta Y, Hishikawa N, et al: The efficacy of sertraline, escitalopram, and nicergoline in the treatment of depression and apathy in Alzheimer's disease: the Okayama Depression and Apathy Project (ODAP). J Alzheimers Dis 76(2):769–772, 2020 32568205

Tampi RR, Tampi DJ: Efficacy and tolerability of benzodiazepines for the treatment of behavioral and psychological symptoms of dementia: a systematic review of randomized controlled trials. Am J Alzheimers Dis Other Demen 29(7):565–574, 2014 25551131

Tampi RR, Forester BP, Agronin M: Aducanumab: evidence from clinical trial data and controversies (editorial). Drugs Context 10:2021-7-3, 2021 34650610

Tolchin B, Hirsch LJ, LaFrance WC Jr: Neuropsychiatric aspects of epilepsy. Psychiatr Clin North Am 43(2):275–290, 2020 32439022

Tramontana MG, Cowan RL, Zald D, et al: Traumatic brain injury-related attention deficits: treatment outcomes with lisdexamfetamine dimesylate (Vyvanse). Brain Inj 28(11):1461–1472, 2014 24988121

Ward KM, Citrome L: Antipsychotic-related movement disorders: drug-induced parkinsonism vs. tardive dyskinesia—key differences in pathophysiology and clinical management. Neurol Ther 7(2):233–248, 2018 30027457

Watt JA, Goodarzi Z, Veroniki A, et al: Comparative efficacy of interventions for reducing symptoms of depression in people with dementia: systematic review and network meta-analysis. BMJ 372:n532, 2021 33762262

Weintraub D, Claassen DO: Impulse control and related disorders in Parkinson's disease. Int Rev Neurobiol 133:679–717, 2017 28802938

Wood LD, Neumiller JJ, Setter SM, et al: Clinical review of treatment options for select nonmotor symptoms of Parkinson's disease. Am J Geriatr Pharmacother 8(4):294–315, 2010 20869620

Yeh YC, Ouyang WC: Mood stabilizers for the treatment of behavioral and psychological symptoms of dementia: an update review. Kaohsiung J Med Sci 28(4):185–193, 2012 22453066

Zhang J, Cortese R, De Stefano N, et al: Structural and functional connectivity substrates of cognitive impairment in multiple sclerosis. Front Neurol 12:671894, 2021 34305785

Zhao J, Hylin MJ, Kobori N, et al: Post-injury administration of galantamine reduces traumatic brain injury pathology and improves outcome. J Neurotrauma 35(2):362–374, 2018 29088998

Zielińska-Nowak E, Włodarczyk L, Kostka J, et al: New strategies for the rehabilitation and pharmacological treatment of fatigue syndrome in multiple sclerosis. J Clin Med 9(11):3592, 2020 33171768

10

Endocrine and Metabolic Disorders

Stephen J. Ferrando, M.D.
Sahil Munjal, M.D.
Jennifer Kraker, M.D., M.S.

Disorders of the endocrine system are well known for their prominent psychiatric manifestations resulting from their interrelationship with the nervous system. Generally, correction of the underlying endocrine disorder will lead to improvement in psychiatric symptoms; however, symptoms may persist beyond the restoration of normal serum hormone levels, in which case psychopharmacological agents are often prescribed.

Three important clinical dimensions are covered in this chapter: 1) primary endocrine disorders and their treatments may cause or exacerbate psychiatric symptoms via alterations of serum hormone levels (Table 10–1; see also Table 10–4 later in this chapter), 2) psychiatric disorders may play a role

Table 10–1. Psychiatric symptoms of endocrine and metabolic disorders

Endocrine or metabolic condition	Psychiatric symptoms
Acromegaly (overproduction of growth hormone)	Mood lability, personality change
Addison's disease	Apathy, depression, fatigue
Cushing's disease/syndrome	Depression, anxiety, mania, psychosis
Diabetes	Depression, anxiety, cognitive dysfunction
Hyperparathyroidism	Depression, apathy, psychosis, delirium
Hyperprolactinemia	Depression, anxiety, sexual dysfunction
Hyperthyroidism	Anxiety, irritability, mania, apathy, depression, psychosis
Hypogonadism	Decreased libido, low energy, low mood
Hypothyroidism	Depression, psychosis, delirium, "myxedema madness"
Pheochromocytoma	Anxiety, panic

in endocrine dysregulation (e.g., depression exacerbates insulin resistance and impairs glycemic control in diabetes), and 3) psychiatric medications often cause endocrine side effects (see Table 10–2 later in this chapter).

In general, psychopharmacological treatment in the patient with endocrine dysfunction must accompany correction of the underlying hormone disorder. Psychopharmacological agents are generally prescribed when 1) psychiatric symptoms predate the endocrine disorder, 2) the patient presents with acute behavioral dysregulation during endocrine treatment, or 3) psychiatric symptoms persist after the endocrine disorder is treated. No psychopharmacological treatment literature exists for several endocrine disorders with psychiatric manifestations; the psychiatric symptom treatment literature focuses on correction of the hormonal dysfunction. These disorders—Cushing's disease, Addison's disease, and growth hormone disorders—are not covered explicitly in this chapter, and the reader is referred to standard endocrinology texts.

Diabetes Mellitus

Diabetes mellitus has significant associations with psychiatric disorders. About one in three to four patients with diabetes mellitus has depression at any point in time (Khaledi et al. 2019). Rates of overall mental disorders, particularly anxiety disorders, PTSD, and depression, are 1.5–2 times higher among people with either type 1 or type 2 diabetes than in the general population (Boden 2018). These disorders are more likely to be found in women and younger patients and are associated with diminished physical function (Boden 2018). Patients with schizophrenia, independent of antipsychotic medication use, are two to three times more likely than the general population to have type 2 diabetes (Stubbs et al. 2015), and up to 50% of patients with bipolar disorder and 26% of patients with schizoaffective disorder have type 2 diabetes (Regenold et al. 2002; Stubbs et al. 2015). Psychopharmacological treatments of psychiatric comorbidities may cause diabetes (see subsection "Psychotropic-Induced Metabolic Syndrome" later in this chapter).

Differential diagnostic considerations for psychiatric symptoms in diabetes include history of psychiatric disorder, acute mood and cognitive effects of hyperglycemia and hypoglycemia, cognitive and behavioral impairment resulting from CNS microvascular disease, and common medical comorbidities (e.g., cardiovascular or renal disease) and their treatments that cause or exacerbate neuropsychiatric symptoms.

In general, the psychopharmacological management of patients with diabetes must take into consideration potential end-organ damage (i.e., renal impairment, cardiovascular and cerebrovascular disease; see Chapters 5, "Renal and Urological Disorders," 6, "Cardiovascular Disorders," 9, "Central Nervous System Disorders," and 16, "Organ Transplantation") that may produce neuropsychiatric disorders and affect pharmacokinetics, as well as pharmacodynamic considerations, in terms of both desired (i.e., treatment of painful diabetic neuropathy) and undesired (i.e., exacerbation of poor glycemic control) effects.

Depression

Depression in diabetes is associated with poor adherence to dietary and medication treatment; functional impairment; poor glycemic control; increased risk of diabetic complications, such as microvascular and macrovascular disease; increased medical costs; and mortality (Ahola et al. 2020; Boden 2018).

Studies have examined whether treatment of depression is associated with improved glycemic control, possibly through 1) improvement in adherence to diabetes treatment, 2) reversal of depression-induced physiological changes such as hypercortisolism, or 3) the potential direct euglycemic effects of antidepressant medication. Some research has suggested a relationship between antidepressant use in depressed patients and glycemic abnormalities and new-onset diabetes mellitus, whereas other research has not found such an association. One pharmacovigilance pharmacodynamic study using the U.S. FDA spontaneous adverse events database found that six antidepressants—nortriptyline, doxepin, imipramine, amitriptyline, mirtazapine, and sertraline (listed from highest to lowest frequency)—were associated with reports of new-onset diabetes mellitus, with adjusted ORs of 1.3–2.0 compared with other antidepressants (Siafis and Papazisis 2018). In this study, there was a strong association with drug affinity for muscarinic receptor types 1, 3, 4, and 5 and histamine type 1 receptors. On the contrary, analysis of data from the U.S. National Health and Nutrition Examination Survey from 2005 to 2010 did not find an association between antidepressant use and abnormalities in glycemic control or diabetes mellitus (Mojtabai 2013). Furthermore, naturalistic studies generally have found that well-adhered-to antidepressant treatment, particularly with selective serotonin reuptake inhibitors (SSRIs), is associated with improved depression, improved glycemic control, and decreased adverse outcomes such as microvascular complications and all-cause mortality in diabetes mellitus (Wu et al. 2021).

Although the focus of this volume is on psychopharmacological treatment, it is important to note that diabetes mellitus is one of the most extensively studied disease models for collaborative care treatment of depression, which entails depression screening and follow-up, structural and psychotherapeutic supports, and medication components. The best known of these studies is the Pathways Study. This study, and its multiple successors, examined whether improving quality of care for depression in primary care improved both depression and diabetes outcomes (Katon et al. 2004, 2010). Patients with diabetes and persistent depressive disorder (dysthymia) were randomly assigned to a stepped case management intervention or usual care. The intervention provided enhanced education and support of antidepressant medication treatment or problem-solving therapy. After 1 year, patients in the intervention group showed greater improvement in adequacy of dosage of antidepressant medication, lower depression severity, a higher rating of patient-rated global improvement, and higher satisfaction with care. Subsequent studies found that collaborative care management of depression and diabetes improved both depression and glycemic outcomes in these patients (Diaz Bustamante et al. 2020), with the mechanism being improved adherence to medications for both diabetes mellitus and depression.

In terms of specific medication classes, SSRIs are the most studied and preferred medications for acute and maintenance treatment of depression in diabetes mellitus. Meta-analyses investigating the effects of SSRIs on depression and glycemic control indicate that SSRIs, particularly fluoxetine, citalopram, and escitalopram, at standard doses, were effective for improving depression and glycemic control (Roopan and Larsen 2017; Tharmaraja et al. 2019). For fluoxetine in particular, a meta-analysis of five placebo-controlled trials in adults with type 2 diabetes mellitus found fluoxetine to be more associated with weight loss (–4.3 kg) and improvement of fasting glucose and triglyceride levels compared with placebo (Ye et al. 2011).

The serotonin-norepinephrine reuptake inhibitor (SNRI) duloxetine has been approved by the FDA for the treatment of painful diabetic peripheral neuropathy, with or without depression. In preclinical studies, dosages of 60 mg/day and 120 mg/day were equally efficacious for diabetic peripheral neuropathy; however, dosing guidelines for comorbid depression and diabetic peripheral neuropathy have not been established (Sultan et al. 2008). Duloxetine was not shown to alter glycemic control or cardiovascular events. Duloxetine should be used with caution or avoided in patients with diabetes mellitus, uncontrolled hypertension, or substantial liver or renal impairment.

Tricyclic antidepressants (TCAs), particularly those with mixed serotonergic and noradrenergic effects, may be helpful for patients with depression as well as painful diabetic peripheral neuropathy. However, the risks of weight gain, exacerbation of autonomic neuropathy (e.g., gastroparesis, postural hypotension), and cardiac conduction problems have significantly limited their use, in favor of SSRIs and SNRIs.

Anxiety

Anxiety disorders in general, and PTSD in particular, are highly prevalent in patients with diabetes mellitus, are often comorbid with depression, and are associated with poor glucose control (Boden 2018; Roberts et al. 2015). Patients with diabetes mellitus and anxiety should be screened for depression, and intervention should mirror that used for depression, including collaborative care, SSRIs, and SNRIs (especially with comorbid pain).

Thyroid Disorders

Hypothyroidism

Clinical hypothyroidism is often associated with depressive symptoms, including depressed mood, fatigue, hypersomnolence, cognitive impairment, difficulty concentrating, and weight gain. However, the study of the relationship between clinical depression and hypothyroidism has yielded conflicting results. A recent meta-analysis indicated that overt hypothyroidism is associated with clinical depression, with an OR of 1.77 (Bode et al. 2021). An association between depression and subclinical hypothyroidism (defined biochemically as a normal serum free thyroxine [T_4] concentration in the presence of an elevated serum thyroid-stimulating hormone [TSH] concentration) is less clear and probably less powerful, if present at all (Airaksinen et al. 2021; Blum et al. 2016; Bode et al. 2021). Subclinical thyroid dysfunction is largely a laboratory diagnosis that merits follow-up but not necessarily treatment. Guidelines recommend that after these abnormal laboratory values are initially detected, TSH and T_4 as well as thyroid peroxidase antibodies be drawn after 2–3 months (Pearce et al. 2013). Watchful waiting is preferable in patients age 65 years or older with mild subclinical hypothyroidism (TSH < 10 mU/L) unless they have prominent mood, cognitive, or medical conditions—such as congestive heart failure or hyperlipidemia—that could benefit from early thyroid replacement. In adults younger than 65 years, clinicians should consider a TSH of 4.5–10 mU/L as a threshold for initiating thyroid replacement, particularly if anti–thyroid peroxidase antibodies are present (Pearce et al. 2013). Multiple studies have shown no evidence to support an association between subclinical hypothyroidism and cognitive impairment in relatively healthy older adults (van Vliet et al. 2021). Profound hypothyroidism can produce psychosis ("myxedema madness"), delirium, and catatonia. A corticosteroid-responsive encephalopathy has been reported with autoimmune thyroiditis, characterized by normal TSH and persistent anti–thyroid peroxidase and antithyroglobulin antibodies (Laurent et al. 2016). Symptomatic management with psychotropics may be necessary in these conditions; however, there is no guidance in the literature.

Some patients with treated hypothyroidism experience residual symptoms of low mood, fatigue, and cognitive impairment while receiving stable T_4 monotherapy. Some debate exists over the benefit of supplementing T_4 with low doses of triiodothyronine (T_3). Most randomized controlled trials (RCTs) show no additional benefit to combination T_4/T_3 treatment, with the additional disadvantage of thyrotoxic side effects (most commonly palpitations and anxiety) (Okosieme et al. 2016); however, there may be a subset of patients with genetic factors conferring diminished T_4 to T_3 conversion and more severe residual symptoms with T_4 monotherapy who may benefit from T_3 supplementation (Salvatore et al. 2022).

Little literature is available on antidepressant treatment in patients with hypothyroidism. One classic case series of psychiatrically hospitalized depressed hypothyroid patients compellingly documented poor response to antidepressants and electroconvulsive therapy without correction of serum T_4 (Russ and Ackerman 1989). In addition, bipolar disorder itself, rapid cycling in bipolar disorder, and lithium refractoriness have been associated with clinical and subclinical hypothyroidism and thyroid autoimmunity, underscoring the need for thyroid monitoring and treatment in the setting of mood disorders (Barbuti et al. 2017). A novel study of levothyroxine compared with T_3 compared with placebo as an adjunct for patients with rapid-cycling bipolar disorder found levothyroxine (but not T_3) to be superior to placebo in alleviating depression, reducing time in mixed states, and increasing time euthymic (Walshaw et al. 2018) (see subsection "Lithium-Induced Hypothyroidism" later in this chapter).

Hyperthyroidism

Psychiatric symptoms of overt and subclinical hyperthyroidism include heightened anxiety and mood symptoms and diminished quality of life (Gulseren et al. 2006). Patients with hyperthyroidism have significant psychiatric comorbidity. A population-based study reported that 14%, 33%, and 39% of the patients were treated with antipsychotics, antidepressants, and anxiolytics, respectively, and hyperthyroid patients had an increased risk of psychiatric hospitalization (Brandt et al. 2013). Hyperthyroidism has also been shown to increase the risk of developing bipolar disorder (Hu et al. 2013). As with subclinical hypothyroidism, subclinical hyperthyroidism (suppressed TSH with normal T_4) may have little (Kvetny et al. 2015) or no (de Jongh et al. 2011) effect on risk of depression. Apathetic hyperthyroidism, characterized by apathy, somnolence, psychomotor retardation, and cognitive impairment, also has been reported, particularly in elderly patients (Jurado-Flores et al. 2022). Finally, psychosis and acute encephalopathy can occur, perhaps related to high antithyroid antibody concentrations in the CNS (Jurado-Flores et al. 2022).

Anxiety, affective symptoms, and cognitive symptoms usually remit within weeks to months after normalization of thyroid function; however, at times symptoms persist that may necessitate psychopharmacological treatment (Bednarczuk et al. 2021).

β-Blockers, particularly propranolol, are part of standard therapy for hyperthyroidism, targeting adrenergic symptoms of anxiety, tremor, palpitations, and tachycardia. High-dose propranolol (and perhaps some other, but not all, β-blockers) reduces the transformation of T_4 to T_3 (Kumar et al. 2020), but this is probably not a major contribution to the drug's clinical benefits. Lithium is an effective adjunct to antithyroid drugs and propranolol in the treatment of hyperthyroid-induced mania (Brownlie et al. 2000). Benzodiazepines are not recommended for long-term use but may be useful over the short term, alone or in combination with other agents for acute anxiety, agitation, and manic symptoms. Antipsychotic medications are used for severe agitation, mania, and psychosis, but no systematic data are available regarding their use in thyrotoxicosis. Antidepressants for patients with Graves' disease have received little attention and should probably be reserved for persistent anxiety and depression after antithyroid treatment with normal serum thyroid levels.

Hyperparathyroidism

Psychiatric symptoms associated with hyperparathyroidism include fatigue, depression, and cognitive impairment; in rare cases, delirium, psychosis, and mania occur (Serdenes et al. 2021). Generally, older women are at greatest risk. Some studies of parathyroidectomy for patients with asymptomatic hyperparathyroidism have documented improvements in health-related quality of life, depression, and neuropsychological testing (Serdenes et al. 2021). Pooled data from randomized trials suggest that surgical treatment is superior to surveillance in the domain of emotional role functioning for patients with primary asymptomatic hyperparathyroidism (Cheng et al. 2015). In one study, 27% of patients taking antidepressants presurgically were able to discontinue antidepressant treatment, suggesting that although some patients improve, a substantial number continue to need antidepressant treatment after surgery (Wilhelm et al. 2004). Lithium can also induce hyperparathyroidism, as discussed later in the chapter.

Pheochromocytoma

Pheochromocytoma has been associated with depression, anxiety, and panic symptoms, and patients may present with these symptoms before diagnosis (Jia et al. 2021). TCAs, SSRIs, and some antipsychotics have been documented to unmask silent pheochromocytomas, probably through inhibition of neuronal uptake of high circulating levels of catecholamines and synergistic effects of serotonin. Monoamine oxidase inhibitors may be expected to be even more hazardous. Importantly, TCAs that increase norepinephrine levels can result in false-positive laboratory test results for pheochromocytoma (Eisenhofer et al. 2003).

Antidiuretic Hormone

The syndrome of inappropriate antidiuretic hormone (vasopressin) secretion is discussed in Chapter 2, "Severe Drug Reactions," and Chapter 5. A discussion of lithium-induced nephrogenic diabetes insipidus (NDI) appears in Chapter 5 and in the section "Endocrinological Side Effects of Psychiatric Medications" later in this chapter.

Reproductive Endocrine System Disorders

Disorders of the female reproductive endocrine system are discussed in Chapter 11, "Obstetrics and Gynecology." Hyperprolactinemia is discussed in the section "Endocrinological Side Effects of Psychiatric Medications" later in this chapter.

Hypogonadal Disorders

Low serum testosterone, or hypogonadism, in men is associated with aging and many chronic illnesses. Hypogonadism may cause depressed mood, low energy, and sexual and cognitive dysfunction. Testosterone replacement therapy (TRT) in aging men is controversial; however, it has become common in some illnesses, such as HIV/AIDS (see Chapter 12, "Infectious Diseases").

In a meta-analysis of 87 RCTs and 51 nonrandomized trials of TRT in hypogonadal men, TRT overall (all products included; i.e., gel, transdermal patch, intramuscular), compared with placebo, produced significant improvements in quality of life, libido, depression, and erectile dysfunction, with no significant increase in risk of adverse events (Elliott et al. 2017). Importantly, these clinical trials were short in duration, so they were biased toward detecting benefit but against longer-term adverse effects. Early studies of testosterone augmentation of antidepressants for treatment-refractory depression in men and women (low dose for women) appeared promising; however, subsequent large-scale clinical trials have not found benefit for depression response (Dichtel et al. 2020; Pope et al. 2010). In one RCT in depressed men with low or low-normal testosterone levels who continued to take serotonergic antidepressants, treatment with exogenous testosterone (regardless of baseline level) was associated with a significant improvement in sexual function, including ejaculatory ability (Amiaz et al. 2011). Despite concern about long-term cardiovascular risk of TRT in men, particularly those with underlying cardiac disease, small trials have shown improvement in mood (Malkin et al. 2004), whereas others have not (Malkin et al. 2006). In terms of concern about cardiac risk in this group of patients, however, a recent meta-analysis of multiple small randomized placebo-controlled trials found delayed time to ischemia and lowered heart rate in TRT- versus placebo-treated patients and no adverse cardiac events over the short term (Cannarella et al. 2022).

TRT also has been shown to have modest positive effects over the short term on various measures of cognitive function in hypogonadal men, especially when combined with active lifestyle modifications (Gregori et al. 2021); however, these benefits are not necessarily achieved over the longer term (Huang et al. 2016).

Overall, evidence for the benefits of TRT for symptoms of hypogonadism, including depression and impaired sexual function and cognition, is modest at best. Furthermore, the evidence base is limited regarding the long-term adverse effects of TRT, so that long-term safety, even in the setting of some clinical benefits, has not been established.

Psychiatric adverse effects of testosterone therapy are covered in the section "Psychiatric Side Effects of Endocrine Treatments" later in this chapter.

Endocrinological Side Effects of Psychiatric Medications

The endocrinological adverse effects of psychotropic medications, including antidepressants, antipsychotics, and mood stabilizers, are summarized in Table 10–2.

Table 10–2. Endocrinological adverse effects of psychotropic medications

Medication	Endocrinological adverse effects
Antidepressants	
SSRIs or SNRIs	Hyperprolactinemia, hypoglycemia (rare), hypothyroidism (rare)
TCAs	Hyperglycemia
Tertiary-amine TCAs (e.g., imipramine, amitriptyline, clomipramine)	Hyperprolactinemia
Antipsychotics	
Atypical and typical antipsychotics	Hyperglycemia, hyperprolactinemia, hypogonadism
Mood stabilizers	
Lithium	Hypothyroidism, hyperthyroidism, hyperparathyroidism, nephrogenic diabetes insipidus
Carbamazepine	Hypothyroidism, decreased FSH and LH, hypogonadism
Valproic acid	Hypothyroidism, decreased FSH and LH, hyperandrogenism (women)

Note.   FSH=follicle-stimulating hormone;   LH=luteinizing hormone;   SNRIs=serotonin-norepinephrine reuptake inhibitors; SSRIs=selective serotonin reuptake inhibitors; TCAs=tricyclic antidepressants.

Lithium Effects on the Thyroid

Lithium has multifaceted effects on the thyroid axis. Lithium may cause the development of hypothyroidism, goiter, and, rarely, hyperthyroidism. Lithium is actively transported into the thyroid gland and is three to four times more concentrated in the thyroid than in plasma. It interferes with thyroid uptake of iodine and the iodination of tyrosine, alters thyroglobulin structure, and inhibits release of T_4 (Czarnywojtek et al. 2020). These effects of lithium have been used clinically, albeit rarely, to increase the effectiveness of radioactive iodine when treating thyrotoxicosis (Ahmed et al. 2021). Lithium increases TSH by decreasing T_4 and T_3 and by independently evoking an exaggerated TSH response to thyrotropin-releasing hormone. Exaggerated elevation of TSH is probably the main cause of goiter formation, reported in 3%–60% of lithium-treated patients (Czarnywojtek et al. 2020). Lithium-associated thyrotoxicosis and thyromegaly are rare but important adverse effects of lithium therapy. Surgery is an effective and preferred treatment for thyroid enlargement that causes airway compression, especially for substernal goiter (Verma et al. 2012).

Lithium-Induced Hypothyroidism

Lithium has been shown to increase the risk of developing hypothyroidism, up to sixfold (McKnight et al. 2012). Both clinical and subclinical hypothyroidism are prevalent in lithium-treated patients. Rates vary greatly across studies, with up to 10% of patients developing one of these conditions (Bou Khalil and Richa 2011). However, most of these patients are asymptomatic, and the diagnosis is purely biochemical. There is no evidence as to whether stopping lithium tends to lead to a recovery of thyroid function when function is abnormal (McKnight et al. 2012). Among people taking lithium, the risk for hypothyroidism is higher in both women (14%) and men (4.5%) compared with the incidence in the general population. Women older than 40 and at risk for autoimmune thyroid disease are probably at greatest risk, in addition to people with diabetes (Johnston and Eagles 1999; Shine et al. 2015).

Thyroid function tests (serum TSH, free thyroid hormone T_4 and T_3 concentrations, and thyroid autoantibodies) and clinical assessment of thyroid size (on clinical examination and via ultrasound) are recommended for patients initiating lithium therapy, at baseline and annually thereafter (Kibirige et al. 2013). A higher index of suspicion should be maintained for women and patients with a personal or family history of autoimmune disease. A mild increase in TSH and a decrease in T_4 may be seen during the first few months of treatment; these effects are usually self-limited, and T_4 replacement is unwarranted. If clinically significant hypothyroidism develops or subclinical effects persist after 4 months of lithium treatment, T_4 replacement or a switch to an alternative mood stabilizer (e.g., valproate) is recommended (Kleiner et al. 1999).

Lithium-Induced Hyperthyroidism

Cases of hyperthyroidism have occurred with lithium treatment, particularly with long-term treatment (Bou Khalil and Richa 2011; Fairbrother et al. 2019), but much less commonly than have cases of hypothyroidism and goiter. One study with 15-year follow-up found only one case of hyperthyroidism among 976 patients (Bocchetta et al. 2007). Because lithium is best known for inducing hypothyroidism and has even been used to treat refractory hyperthyroidism (Kessler et al. 2014), it seems paradoxical that it can induce hyperthyroidism.

Lithium-induced or exacerbated autoimmune thyroiditis is the likely explanation for hyperthyroidism. Also, because lithium is concentrated in the thyroid, it is postulated that lithium might directly damage thyroid follicular cells, triggering temporary release of thyroglobulin into the circulation and causing thyrotoxicosis (Bou Khalil and Richa 2011), ultimately followed by hypothyroidism. Lithium-induced hyperthyroidism may be missed because it is often transient, asymptomatic, and followed by hypothyroidism (Stowell and Barnhill 2005).

Although no treatment guidelines are available for lithium-induced hyperthyroidism, a switch from lithium to an alternative mood stabilizer is generally necessary. In the interim, sedative-hypnotics, benzodiazepines, β-blockers, and antipsychotic medications may be used to treat the spectrum of activation symptoms.

Lithium and Hyperparathyroidism

Hyperparathyroidism is an underrecognized and frequent side effect of long-term lithium therapy. Primary hyperparathyroidism in patients taking lithium has an absolute risk of 10% (vs. 0.1% of the general population). The risk of hyperparathyroidism is probably attributable to lithium's inactivation of the calcium-sensing receptor and interference with intracellular second-messenger signaling, including glycogen synthase kinase 3 signaling. This effect leads to an increased release of parathyroid hormone, which raises calcium concentrations in serum and urine (Mifsud et al. 2020). Considering that thyroid and parathyroid abnormalities can occur in about 25% of patients receiving lithium therapy, clinical monitoring should reflect this finding, and routine screening for hypercalcemia should be done along with the thyroid tests (Saunders et al. 2009). However, although increases in parathyroid hormone during lithium treatment are common (14% of patients during the first 18 months in one study), clinically significant increases in calcium are much less common (Albert et al. 2015). Other studies have found higher rates of hyperparathyroidism with elevated calcium levels, especially in lithium-treated patients who were also vitamin D deficient (Meehan et al. 2015). Cessation of lithium often does not correct the hyperparathyroidism, necessitating parathyroidectomy. From a pharmacological standpoint, there are case reports of cinacalcet reversing the lithium-induced hypercalcemia, permitting continuation of lithium (Dixon et al. 2018). Although hyperparathyroidism is a risk factor for osteoporosis, patients taking lithium who have normal calcium and parathyroid hormone levels do not have an increased risk of osteoporosis. Maintenance therapy with lithium carbonate may actually preserve or increase bone mass (Zamani et al. 2009) and was found to be associated with a dose-proportional reduction in the risk of osteoporosis (Köhler-Forsberg et al. 2022).

Lithium and Nephrogenic Diabetes Insipidus

Lithium impairs antidiuretic hormone–induced water reabsorption in the cortical and medullary collecting tubules of the kidney, resulting in NDI. Lithium-induced NDI occurs in approximately 12% of lithium-treated patients and is more likely to occur with higher dosages and longer treatment duration (Davis et al. 2018). Polydipsia and polyuria are observed clinically in 19%–54% of cases. In severe cases, dehydration, renal failure, and lithium toxicity may occur because of a combination of water diuresis and lithium-induced natriuresis. Confirmation of NDI requires a water deprivation test, followed by a vasopressin challenge. Inability to concentrate urine (more than twofold increase in urine osmolality after 8-hour water deprivation) is suggestive of diabetes insipidus. NDI is confirmed by no change in urine osmolality over 1–2 hours after subcutaneous administration of 5 U of vasopressin. The syndrome generally remits days to weeks after discontinuation of lithium but may be irreversible with longer-term treatment. If lithium is continued, ample fluid intake is indicated. The potassium-sparing diuretic amiloride may be used to treat lithium-induced NDI (Schoot et al. 2020). In addition to sparing potassium, amiloride causes less natriuresis, lithium reabsorption, and volume contraction compared with other diuretics, thus reducing the risks for lithium toxicity, dehydration, and renal failure.

Psychotropic-Induced Metabolic Syndrome

Schizophrenia, bipolar disorder, major depressive disorder, and other disorders as well as antipsychotic medications, both typical and atypical, are associated with metabolic syndrome. Collectively, metabolic syndrome in psychiatric patients is 58% higher than in the general population and has a prevalence of 30%–50% (Penninx and Lange 2018; Vancampfort et al. 2015). There is additive risk associated with the neurobiology and lifestyle complications of psychiatric disorders as well as the pharmacodynamics of antipsychotics. In one meta-analysis (Vancampfort et al. 2015), olanzapine and clozapine were found to pose the greatest risk compared with other antipsychotics. Aripiprazole and amisulpride significantly decrease risk; however, this report did not include some newer agents. Other drug classes, including tricyclics, valproic acid, and lithium, also have been implicated. Although there are varying definitions, metabolic syndrome is generally defined by five criteria: abdominal obesity, triglycerides greater than 150 mg/dL (>1.7 mmol/L), high-density lipoprotein less than 40 mg/dL (<1.03 mmol/L) for men or less than 50 mg/dL (<1.28 mmol/L) for women, blood pressure higher than 130/85 mm Hg, and fasting glucose greater than 110 mg/dL (>6.0 mmol/L) (Penninx and Lange 2018). Metabolic syndrome is an independent risk factor for diabetes (including ketoacidosis) and for cardiovascular, cerebrovascular, and peripheral vascular disease (Penninx and Lange 2018).

All typical and atypical antipsychotics have an FDA black box warning that they may cause metabolic syndrome. The extent to which metabolic syndrome is solely a function of antipsychotic treatment is not entirely established. Overall, the development of metabolic syndrome is probably caused by inherent susceptibility, lifestyle, diet, and medication effects (Penninx and Lange 2018; Vancampfort et al. 2015).

Generally, antipsychotic-induced metabolic changes are proportional to weight gain, which has been related to blockade of histamine H_2 and serotonin type 2C receptors and to increased levels of insulin and leptin (Nasrallah 2003). Prospective data show mean weight increases during the first year of therapy of 6–12 kg for patients taking clozapine, 3–12 kg for olanzapine, 2–4 kg for quetiapine, and 2–3 kg for risperidone. Aripiprazole generally has been considered low risk but can cause significant weight gain in some patients (Parmar et al. 2022). Ziprasidone is weight neutral. Second-generation antipsychotics as a class have been associated with weight gain, abdominal obesity, lipid and glucose metabolism alterations, and insulin resistance, all of which may increase risk for diabetes and cardiac complications (Rojo et al. 2015).

Patients taking antipsychotics should be monitored for weight gain, hypertension, glucose intolerance, and lipid derangements. Guidelines for patient monitoring are summarized in Table 10–3.

Treatment of metabolic syndrome begins with dosage adjustment when this has been shown to be beneficial (e.g., olanzapine) or cross-tapering to a more weight-neutral medication (e.g., aripiprazole, ziprasidone). Clinical experience with newer second-generation agents is accruing; however, lurasidone, cariprazine, and lumateperone appear to have low risk for weight gain, so they may be suitable alternative agents, whereas brexpiprazole has somewhat higher risk in the acute phase of treatment (Corponi et al. 2019). Techniques including dietary education, exercise, and cognitive-behavioral interventions have been found in RCTs to be effective for either maintaining or losing weight in patients receiving an atypical antipsychotic. Meta-analysis suggests that adjunctive metformin (750 mg/day or even lower) is an effective, safe, and reasonable choice for antipsychotic-induced weight gain and metabolic abnormalities (de Silva et al. 2016). There is also evidence for benefit with topiramate (Wang et al. 2020).

Hyperprolactinemia

Hyperprolactinemia is a common side effect of antipsychotics. The main physiological action of prolactin is to initiate and maintain lactation. Dopamine D_2 receptors of the pituitary lactotrophs, when activated by dopamine, suppress prolactin gene expression and lactotroph proliferation. Normal ranges of serum prolactin have an upper limit of 10 ng/mL for men and 15 ng/mL for women. Hyperprolactinemia is generally defined as prolactin greater than 20 ng/mL (20 μg/L SI units) and may be physiological or pathogenic.

Hyperprolactinemia may cause impotence, menstrual dysregulation, infertility, and sexual dysfunction, primarily via inhibition of the pulsatile secretion of gonadotropin-releasing hormone (Bostwick et al. 2009). Symptoms of sexual dysfunction for men include loss of libido and erectile and ejaculatory

Table 10–3.   Consensus guidelines for monitoring metabolic status in patients taking antipsychotic medications

Metabolic risk parameter	Baseline	4 weeks	8 weeks	12 weeks	Quarterly	Annually	Every 5 years
Personal or family history of diabetes mellitus or cardiovascular disease	X					X	
Weight (body mass index)	X	X	X	X	X		
Waist circumference	X					X	
Blood pressure	X			X		X	
Fasting plasma glucose	X			X		X	
Fasting lipid profile	X			X			X

Source.   Adapted from American Diabetes Association et al. 2004.

dysfunction (Holtmann et al. 2003); for women, symptoms include loss of libido and anorgasmia (Canuso et al. 2002). Elevated prolactin levels may give rise to galactorrhea and gynecomastia; they also may cause loss of bone mineral density and increased risk for osteoporosis (Byerly et al. 2007), although evidence for this is mixed (Lally et al. 2019). Increased tumorigenesis and breast cancer (Taipale et al. 2021) and cardiovascular disease (Serri et al. 2006) also have been documented. Because bone loss may result from hyperprolactinemia-mediated hypogonadism, bone mineral density should be evaluated in patients with persistent high prolactin levels and reproductive dysfunction (Ajmal et al. 2014).

Antipsychotics are the most common drug-induced cause of hyperprolactinemia, but antidepressants, opioids, antiemetics, and antihypertensives also may be causal. An increase in serum prolactin levels usually occurs within hours of initiation of antipsychotic medication (Goode et al. 1981). Evidence indicates that hyperprolactinemia may be present in up to 39% of patients with schizophrenia independent of antipsychotic medication (Riecher-Rössler et al. 2013). Although there are reports of drug-induced hyperprolactinemia with serum concentrations of prolactin exceeding 200 ng/mL, this degree of elevation is rare, and other causes of hyperprolactinemia should be explored. Risk factors for drug-induced hyperprolactinemia include increased potency of D_2 blockade (Tsuboi et al. 2013), female sex, increased age (Kinon et al. 2003), and perhaps schizophrenia itself (Riecher-Rössler et al. 2013). Additionally, an increased risk is identified in those with the cytochrome P450 2D6*10 allele (Ozdemir et al. 2007).

Risk for hyperprolactinemia is reported with all antipsychotics; however, it is generally proportional to the potency of D_2 receptor blockade. The phenothiazine and butyrophenone first-generation antipsychotics risperidone and paliperidone carry the greatest risk (Bushe and Shaw 2007; Peuskens et al. 2014). Haloperidol raises the serum prolactin concentration by an average of 17 ng/mL, whereas risperidone may raise it by 45–80 ng/mL, with larger increases in women than in men (David et al. 2000). The atypical antipsychotics clozapine, olanzapine, and quetiapine carry modest risk for hyperprolactinemia, and ziprasidone, aripiprazole, brexpiprazole, cariprazine, and lumateperone are lower risk (Cutler et al. 2018; Ivkovic et al. 2019; Peuskens et al. 2014; Vanover et al. 2019). Antiemetics, such as prochlorperazine, metoclopramide, and trimethobenzamide, also have been reported to cause hyperprolactinemia and galactorrhea. Serotonergic antidepressants, including SSRIs, SNRIs, trazodone, tertiary-amine TCAs, and monoamine oxidase inhibitors, also have been reported to cause hyperprolactinemia and galactorrhea, probably because of serotonin-mediated dopamine antagonism (Molitch 2008).

Little emphasis has been placed on monitoring and management of psychotropic-induced hyperprolactinemia. American Psychiatric Association guidelines recommend screening for symptoms of hyperprolactinemia in patients at baseline before antipsychotic treatment and monitoring of prolactin level only on the basis of clinical history. However, patients may not be aware of their symptoms or may be unable or reluctant to describe them. In light of emerging evidence of long-term risk for adverse outcomes such as breast cancer, osteoporosis, and cardiovascular disease, the prudent course is to initiate antipsychotic treatment with lower-prolactin-risk medications and to monitor chronically treated patients for symptoms and serological evidence of hyperprolactinemia, perhaps in conjunction with other metabolic parameters, as outlined earlier in the subsection "Psychotropic-Induced Metabolic Syndrome."

Currently, limited data are available to offer insight on an optimal approach to the management of hyperprolactinemia. Treatment strategies include 1) decreasing the dosage of the offending agent, 2) changing medication to an agent less likely to affect prolactin, 3) using a dopamine agonist such as bromocriptine or a partial agonist such as aripiprazole, and 4) preventing long-term complications of hyperprolactinemia such as bone demineralization. Labad et al. (2020) and Rusgis et al. (2021) systematically reviewed and evaluated relevant RCTs for lowering prolactin levels in antipsychotic-treated patients and concluded that the addition of aripiprazole to the antipsychotic regimen is effective and safe and should be the first-line strategy for antipsychotic-induced hyperprolactinemia. Treatment with a dopamine agonist such as cabergoline or bromocriptine may be effective in lowering prolactin but carries risk for exacerbation of psychosis and cardiac valvular abnormalities with cabergoline. (Some evidence shows that dopamine agonists may reduce antipsychotic-induced hyperprolactinemia [Bo et al. 2016], but the effect is modest compared with that of other interventions [Rusgis et al. 2021].) No reports have been published on the effects of hormone replacement on bone mineral density in patients taking antipsychotics long term, but preliminary data suggest that active management of bone loss in those with antipsychotic-associated bone disease may halt or even reverse this process (O'Keane 2008).

Psychiatric Side Effects of Endocrine Treatments

Psychiatric symptoms of endocrine disorders are manifestations of hormone toxicity or deficiency syndromes described previously in this chapter. However, hormone treatments and endocrine treatments used for reasons other than mere correction of deficiency (e.g., corticosteroids, nonhormonal medications that treat endocrine disorders) also may cause psychiatric side effects (Table 10–4).

Oral Hypoglycemic Medications

The psychiatric side effects of oral hypoglycemic medications are secondary to their hypoglycemic effect. Prominent psychiatric symptoms include anxiety, dysphoria, irritability, and confusion. Such effects can be exacerbated in severely depressed patients with anorexia.

Table 10–4. Psychiatric adverse effects of endocrinological and hormonal treatments

Medication	Psychiatric adverse effects
Steroid hormones	
Corticosteroids	Mania, anxiety, irritability, psychosis (acute), depression (chronic), delirium, suicidal ideation
Testosterone and other anabolic or androgenic steroids (especially supraphysiological levels)	Irritability, mania, psychosis
Oral hypoglycemics	
Sulfonylureas, biguanides, α-glucosidase inhibitors, thiazolidinediones, and meglitinides	Anxiety, depression, irritability, cognitive impairment (secondary to hypoglycemia)
Antithyroid medications	
Carbimazole, methimazole, and propylthiouracil	None reported
Dopamine agonists	
Bromocriptine and cabergoline	Psychosis, hallucinations
Growth hormone–inhibiting hormones	
Somatostatin, octreotide, and lanreotide	Sleep disruption
Pegvisomant	None reported
Growth hormone	
Recombinant human growth hormone	Insomnia, fatigue

Antithyroid Medications

Carbimazole, methimazole, and propylthiouracil have *not* been documented to cause psychiatric side effects.

Corticosteroids

Exogenous corticosteroids (e.g., hydrocortisone, cortisone, prednisone, methylprednisolone, dexamethasone) and adrenocorticotropic hormone are well known to cause a range of neuropsychiatric side effects (Dubovsky et al. 2012). Adverse psychiatric reactions to corticosteroids have been reported in children as young as neonates (Drozdowicz and Bostwick 2014). Although many patients experience transient mild to moderate neuropsychiatric symptoms that do not meet severity or duration criteria for psychiatric disorder, approximately 6% of corticosteroid-treated patients have serious neuropsychiatric complications (Dubovsky et al. 2012). These include activation symptoms such as anxiety, insomnia, and irritability; mood symptoms such as dysphoria, euphoria, and mania; and psychotic symptoms.

Severe neuropsychiatric consequences have been reported to occur at a rate of 15.7/100 person-years at risk for all glucocorticoid courses and 22.2/100 person-years at risk for first courses (Judd et al. 2014). Greater risk of glucocorticoid-induced neuropsychiatric problems is associated with higher dosage, long-term treatment, older patient age, and history of a neuropsychiatric disorder during glucocorticoid treatment. Although mood disorders are most common, about one in six patients seen psychiatrically experiences delirium or psychosis (Dubovsky et al. 2012). Suicidal ideation can occur. High-dose, short-term administration is most often associated with mania and hypomania, whereas chronic therapy is most often associated with depression (Bolanos et al. 2004). Impairments in long-term recall of verbal information have been reported in patients with optic neuritis and multiple sclerosis who are receiving high-dose glucocorticoids; however, attentional and working memory function remain intact, and impairments reverse within 5 days of cessation of treatment (Brunner et al. 2005). Discontinuation of long-term glucocorticoid therapy is associated with an increased risk of both depression and delirium or confusion (Fardet et al. 2013). People treated with long-acting glucocorticoids are particularly at risk. Although psychiatric history, particularly mania, and prior steroid-induced psychiatric disorders are generally considered clinical risk factors, these have not been adequately addressed in the literature.

Prophylaxis against steroid-induced neuropsychiatric reactions may be considered for patients at risk; however, little literature is available to guide risk stratification or treatment recommendations. Success has been reported for lithium (Falk et al. 1979), valproic acid (Abbas and Styra 1994), lamotrigine (Preda et al. 1999), and chlorpromazine (Bloch et al. 1994). In a patient with an active corticosteroid-induced mood disorder, tapered discontinuation, reduction to minimal effective dosage, or switching to an alternative corticosteroid is recommended on the basis of status of the underlying illness (Dubovsky et al. 2012; Judd et al. 2014). For corticosteroid-induced depression and mania, case reports have supported the use of antipsychotics, lithium, valproic acid, and carbamazepine (Judd et al. 2014; Kenna et al. 2011; Roxanas and Hunt 2012). Corticosteroid-treated patients taking lithium should be monitored closely for fluid and electrolyte status and lithium levels because of mineralocorticoid effects.

In a systematic review (Dubovsky et al. 2012), steroid-induced manic and psychotic symptoms responded to low-dose typical antipsychotics, with cessation of symptoms in 83% of patients, 60% of whom responded in less than 1 week and 80% in less than 2 weeks. Olanzapine at dosages of 2.5–15 mg/day has been reported in a case series (Goldman and Goveas 2002) and an open-label trial (Brown et al. 2004) to be beneficial for patients with multiple underlying illnesses and steroid-induced mixed and manic episodes. With olanzapine, exacerbation of weight gain and insulin resistance in conjunction with corticosteroid use should be monitored. Another recent case series indicated that haloperidol and risperidone were the most prescribed agents, being well tolerated and effective (Huynh and Reinert 2021). A case series showed that sodium valproate rapidly and safely reversed maniclike symptoms within a few days without corticosteroids needing to be stopped, thus allowing the medical treatment to continue (Roxanas and Hunt 2012). Prophylactic lamotrigine can reduce memory problems, and prophylactic treatment should also be considered for patients with neurological disorders involving mood or cognitive disturbance (Judd et al. 2014).

Rapid tapering or discontinuation of corticosteroids can also induce corticosteroid withdrawal syndrome. Corticosteroid withdrawal syndrome is manifested by headache, fever, myalgias, arthralgias, weakness, anorexia, nausea, weight loss, and orthostatic hypotension and sometimes by depression, anxiety, agitation, or psychosis (Wolkowitz 1989). Symptoms respond to an increase or resumption of corticosteroid dosage. Adjunctive treatment with antipsychotics, antidepressants, or mood stabilizers can be helpful, depending on the particular psychiatric symptom constellation.

Testosterone

The most common adverse effects of TRT are acne and mild activation symptoms. Chronic administration may result in testicular atrophy and watery ejaculate. Although aggression ("steroid rage") is a highly publicized effect of anabolic-androgenic steroid administration, it most often occurs in the context of supraphysiological dosing common among athletes (Albano et al. 2021; Piacentino et al. 2015). Other neuropsychiatric effects can include depression, anxiety, and diminished cognitive performance, probably mediated through neurotoxic effects. Only a small portion of eugonadal and hypogonadal men receiving TRT develop increased aggressiveness, but this may be due to positive improvements in energy and vigor (O'Connor et al. 2001). Anabolic-androgenic steroids also have been associated with psychosis, although this may reflect triggering of underlying psychosis risk (Piacentino et al. 2015).

Although not an adverse psychiatric effect, prostate cancer risk is a theoretical concern among aging men receiving TRT. In a meta-analysis, TRT did not appear to increase prostate cancer risk in men with no history (Lenfant et al. 2020). Among men with active or prior prostate cancer, evidence is insufficient to draw a firm conclusion about risk. Likewise, regarding androgen replacement in women, there is concern about elevation of breast and endometrial cancer risk; however, some studies have found that testosterone treatment of premenopausal and postmenopausal endocrine disorders may actually reduce breast cancer risk (Donovitz and Cotten 2021). In general, adverse effects of testosterone replacement in women are mild and generally involve acne and body hair growth (Islam et al. 2019).

Growth Hormone (Somatotropin)

Psychiatric adverse effects with growth hormone treatment are infrequent. Pooled data from trials of growth hormone in HIV-associated adipose redistribution syndrome indicate higher rates of insomnia and fatigue compared with placebo (EMD Serono 2016).

Growth Hormone–Inhibiting Hormones

Both somatostatin and its long-acting analogue, octreotide, may disrupt sleep architecture and total sleep time (Ziegenbein et al. 2004), but neuropsychiatric side effects are seldom reported (Whyand et al. 2018).

Dopamine Agonists

The dopamine agonists bromocriptine and cabergoline may cause psychosis and hallucinations. This topic is covered in Chapter 9 (see especially Table 9–2).

Drug-Drug Interactions

Potential clinically significant interactions between psychotropic drugs and medications used for endocrine disorders are listed in Tables 10–5 and 10–6. Clinically significant drug interactions are rarely reported in the literature, and many are speculative in nature (e.g., DeVane and Markowitz 2002). Data presented are largely derived from information in product monographs.

Key Points

- Hormone deficiency and excess states are most likely to be associated with depression, anxiety, and cognitive impairment.

- Mania and hypomania occur predominantly with hyperthyroidism and with acute high-dose corticosteroid therapy.

- Although psychosis is rare, it occurs with severe hypothyroidism and hyperthyroidism, hyperparathyroidism, and acute high-dose corticosteroid therapy.

- For many endocrinological disorders, correction of the underlying hormone deficiency or excess generally improves psychiatric symptoms.

- Psychiatric symptoms may persist beyond normalization of laboratory parameters.

- Successful psychopharmacological treatment generally requires prior or concurrent correction of the underlying endocrinological disorder.

- Psychotropic-induced endocrinological dysfunction is common and should be routinely screened for via symptom assessment and laboratory testing. Examples of such dysfunction include

Table 10–5. Psychotropic medication–endocrine medication interactions

Psychotropic medication	Interaction mechanism	Endocrine medications and classes affected	Clinical effects
Antidepressants			
Fluvoxamine and sertraline	CYP2C9 inhibition	Glimepiride, glipizide, glyburide, nateglinide, rosiglitazone, and tolbutamide	Reduced clearance of oral hypoglycemics; potential enhanced hypoglycemic effect
Fluoxetine, fluvoxamine, and nefazodone	CYP3A4 inhibition	Nateglinide, pioglitazone, and repaglinide	Reduced clearance of oral hypoglycemics; potential enhanced hypoglycemic effect
Monoamine oxidase inhibitors	Stimulation of insulin release	Corticosteroids	Increased steroid levels and adverse effects
Tricyclic antidepressants	Weight gain, insulin resistance	Insulin and oral hypoglycemics	Possibly enhanced hyperglycemic effect
All antidepressants	Unknown mechanism	Augmentation of vasopressin effects	Enhanced antidiuretic effect
	Increased receptor sensitivity to catecholamines	T_3 and T_4 supplementation	Increased activation, sympathetic autonomic symptoms

Table 10–5. Psychotropic medication–endocrine medication interactions (*continued*)

Psychotropic medication	Interaction mechanism	Endocrine medications and classes affected	Clinical effects
Mood stabilizers			
Lithium	Nephrogenic diabetes insipidus via antidiuretic hormone inhibition in kidney	Corticosteroids, mineralocorticoids, and vasopressin	Increased urination, serum osmolality, sodium, and thirst
	Antithyroid effects	Thyroid hormone	Undercorrection of hypothyroidism
Carbamazepine, phenobarbital, and phenytoin	CYP2C9 induction	Glimepiride, glipizide, glyburide, nateglinide, rosiglitazone, and tolbutamide	Possibly reduced levels and effectiveness of oral hypoglycemics
	CYP3A4 induction	Nateglinide, pioglitazone, and repaglinide	Possibly reduced levels and effectiveness of oral hypoglycemics
	Induction of Phase II metabolism (uridine 5'-diphosphate glucuronosyltransferase sulfation)	T_4	Increased hepatic T_4 metabolism and decreased effect
	Unknown mechanism	Augmentation of vasopressin effects	Enhanced antidiuretic effect

Table 10–5.   Psychotropic medication–endocrine medication interactions *(continued)*

Psychotropic medication	Interaction mechanism	Endocrine medications and classes affected	Clinical effects
Antipsychotics			
Typical and atypical	Weight gain, insulin resistance	Antagonism of insulin and oral hypoglycemic	Possibly enhanced hyperglycemic effects
	Blockade of dopamine D_2 receptors	Hyperprolactinemia	Sexual dysfunction, galactorrhea, gynecomastia
Opioids	Unknown mechanism	Pegvisomant	Reduced pegvisomant levels and clinical effect; increase dosage with concurrent opioids

Note.   CYP = cytochrome P450; T_3 = triiodothyronine; T_4 = thyroxine.

Table 10–6. Endocrine medication–psychotropic medication interactions

Endocrine medication	Interaction mechanism	Psychotropic medication and classes affected	Clinical effects
Growth hormone			
Recombinant human growth hormone	CYP3A4 induction	Anticonvulsants, antidepressants, antipsychotics, benzodiazepines, and opioids	Possibly reduced serum psychotropic levels and reduced therapeutic effects
Growth hormone inhibitors			
Octreotide	General reduction in CYP-mediated metabolism via growth hormone inhibition	All drugs undergoing oxidative metabolism	Possibly increased serum psychotropic levels and increased aftereffects

Note.   CYP = cytochrome P450.

lithium-induced hypothyroidism or nephrogenic diabetes insipidus and antipsychotic-induced metabolic syndrome or hyperprolactinemia.

• Because clinically significant psychotropic drug–endocrine drug or hormone interactions occur infrequently, these agents generally can be combined safely.

References

Abbas A, Styra R: Valproate prophylaxis against steroid induced psychosis. Can J Psychiatry 39(3):188–189, 1994 8033028

Ahmed FW, Kirresh OZ, Majeed MS, et al: Meta-analysis of randomized controlled trials comparing the efficacy of radioactive iodine monotherapy versus radioactive iodine therapy and adjunctive lithium for the treatment of hyperthyroidism. Endocr Res 46(4):160–169, 2021 34028325

Ahola AJ, Radzeviciene L, Zaharenko L, et al: Association between symptoms of depression, diabetes complications and vascular risk factors in four European cohorts of individuals with type 1 diabetes—InterDiane Consortium. Diabetes Res Clin Pract 170:108495, 2020 33058955

Airaksinen J, Komulainen K, García-Velázquez R, et al: Subclinical hypothyroidism and symptoms of depression: evidence from the National Health and Nutrition Examination Surveys (NHANES). Compr Psychiatry 109:152253, 2021 34147730

Ajmal A, Joffe H, Nachtigall LB: Psychotropic-induced hyperprolactinemia: a clinical review. Psychosomatics 55(1):29–36, 2014 24140188

Albano GD, Amico F, Cocimano G, et al: Adverse effects of anabolic-androgenic steroids: a literature review. Healthcare (Basel) 9(1):97, 2021 33477800

Albert U, De Cori D, Aguglia A, et al: Effects of maintenance lithium treatment on serum parathyroid hormone and calcium levels: a retrospective longitudinal naturalistic study. Neuropsychiatr Dis Treat 11:1785–1791, 2015 26229473

American Diabetes Association; American Psychiatric Association; American Association of Clinical Endocrinologists; et al: Consensus development conference on antipsychotic drugs and obesity and diabetes. Diabetes Care 27(2):596–601, 2004 14747245

Amiaz R, Pope HG Jr, Mahne T, et al: Testosterone gel replacement improves sexual function in depressed men taking serotonergic antidepressants: a randomized, placebo-controlled clinical trial. J Sex Marital Ther 37(4):243–254, 2011 21707327

Barbuti M, Carvalho AF, Köhler CA, et al: Thyroid autoimmunity in bipolar disorder: a systematic review. J Affect Disord 221:97–106, 2017 28641149

Bednarczuk T, Attanasio R, Hegedüs L, et al: Use of thyroid hormones in hypothyroid and euthyroid patients: a THESIS* questionnaire survey of Polish physicians. *THESIS: Treatment of Hypothyroidism in Europe by Specialists: an International Survey. Endokrynol Pol 72(4):357–365, 2021 34010443

Bloch M, Gur E, Shalev A: Chlorpromazine prophylaxis of steroid-induced psychosis. Gen Hosp Psychiatry 16(1):42–44, 1994 8039683

Blum MR, Wijsman LW, Virgini VS, et al: Subclinical thyroid dysfunction and depressive symptoms among the elderly: a prospective cohort study. Neuroendocrinology. 103(3-4):291–299, 2016 26202797

Bo Q-J, Wang ZM, Li XB, et al: Adjunctive metformin for antipsychotic-induced hyperprolactinemia: a systematic review. Psychiatry Res 237:257–263, 2016 26822064

Bocchetta A, Cocco F, Velluzzi F, et al: Fifteen-year follow-up of thyroid function in lithium patients. J Endocrinol Invest 30(5):363–366, 2007 17598966

Bode H, Ivens B, Bschor T, et al: Association of hypothyroidism and clinical depression: a systematic review and meta-analysis. JAMA Psychiatry 78(12):1375–1383, 2021 34524390

Boden MT: Prevalence of mental disorders and related functioning and treatment engagement among people with diabetes. J Psychosom Res 106:62–69, 2018 29455901

Bolanos SH, Khan DA, Hanczyc M, et al: Assessment of mood states in patients receiving long-term corticosteroid therapy and in controls with patient-rated and clinician-rated scales. Ann Allergy Asthma Immunol 92(5):500–505, 2004 15191017

Bostwick JR, Guthrie SK, Ellingrod VL: Antipsychotic-induced hyperprolactinemia. Pharmacotherapy 29(1):64–73, 2009 19113797

Bou Khalil R, Richa S: Thyroid adverse effects of psychotropic drugs: a review. Clin Neuropharmacol 34(6):248–255, 2011 21996646

Brandt F, Thvilum M, Almind D, et al: Hyperthyroidism and psychiatric morbidity: evidence from a Danish nationwide register study. Eur J Endocrinol 170(2):341–348, 2013 24282192

Brown ES, Chamberlain W, Dhanani N, et al: An open-label trial of olanzapine for corticosteroid-induced mood symptoms. J Affect Disord 83(2–3):277–281, 2004 15555725

Brownlie BE, Rae AM, Walshe JW, et al: Psychoses associated with thyrotoxicosis—"thyrotoxic psychosis": a report of 18 cases, with statistical analysis of incidence. Eur J Endocrinol 142(5):438–444, 2000 10802519

Brunner R, Schaefer D, Hess K, et al: Effect of corticosteroids on short-term and long-term memory. Neurology 64(2):335–337, 2005 15668434

Bushe C, Shaw M: Prevalence of hyperprolactinaemia in a naturalistic cohort of schizophrenia and bipolar outpatients during treatment with typical and atypical antipsychotics. J Psychopharmacol 21(7):768–773, 2007 17606473

Byerly M, Suppes T, Tran Q-V, et al: Clinical implications of antipsychotic-induced hyperprolactinemia in patients with schizophrenia spectrum or bipolar spectrum disorders: recent developments and current perspectives. J Clin Psychopharmacol 27(6):639–661, 2007 18004132

Cannarella R, Barbagallo F, Cafa A, et al: Testosterone replacement therapy in hypogonadal male patients with hypogonadism and heart failure: a meta-analysis of randomized controlled studies. Minerva Urol Nephrol 74(4):418–427, 2022 33781026

Canuso CM, Goldstein JM, Wojcik J, et al: Antipsychotic medication, prolactin elevation, and ovarian function in women with schizophrenia and schizoaffective disorder. Psychiatry Res 111(1):11–20, 2002 12140115

Cheng SP, Lee JJ, Liu TP, et al: Quality of life after surgery or surveillance for asymptomatic primary hyperparathyroidism: a meta-analysis of randomized controlled trials. Medicine (Baltimore) 94(23):e931, 2015 26061318

Corponi F, Fabbri C, Bitter I, et al: Novel antipsychotics specificity profile: a clinically oriented review of lurasidone, brexpiprazole, cariprazine and lumateperone. Eur Neuropsychopharmacol 29(9):971–985, 2019 31255396

Cutler AJ, Durgam S, Wang Y, et al: Evaluation of the long-term safety and tolerability of cariprazine in patients with schizophrenia: results from a 1-year open-label study. CNS Spectr 23(1):39–50, 2018 28478771

Czarnywojtek A, Zgorzalewicz-Stachowiak M, Czarnocka B, et al: Effect of lithium carbonate on the function of the thyroid gland: mechanism of action and clinical implications. J Physiol Pharmacol 71(2), 2020 32633237

David SR, Taylor CC, Kinon BJ, et al: The effects of olanzapine, risperidone, and haloperidol on plasma prolactin levels in patients with schizophrenia. Clin Ther 22(9):1085–1096, 2000 11048906

Davis J, Desmond M, Berk M: Lithium and nephrotoxicity: a literature review of approaches to clinical management and risk stratification. BMC Nephrol 19(1):305, 2018 30390660

de Jongh RT, Lips P, van Schoor NM, et al: Endogenous subclinical thyroid disorders, physical and cognitive function, depression, and mortality in older individuals. Eur J Endocrinol 165(4):545–554, 2011 21768248

de Silva VA, Suraweera C, Ratnatunga SS, et al: Metformin in prevention and treatment of antipsychotic induced weight gain: a systematic review and meta-analysis. BMC Psychiatry 16(1):341, 2016 27716110

DeVane CL, Markowitz JS: Psychoactive drug interactions with pharmacotherapy for diabetes. Psychopharmacol Bull 36(2):40–52, 2002 12397839

Diaz Bustamante L, Ghattas KN, Ilyas S, et al: Does treatment for depression with collaborative care improve the glycemic levels in diabetic patients with depression? A systematic review. Cureus 12(9):e10551, 2020 33101799

Dichtel LE, Carpenter LL, Nyer M, et al: Low-dose testosterone augmentation for antidepressant-resistant major depressive disorder in women: an 8-week, two-site, randomized, placebo-controlled study. Am J Psychiatry 177(10):965–973, 2020 32660299

Dixon M, Luthra V, Todd C: Use of cinacalcet in lithium-induced hyperparathyroidism. BMJ Case Rep 2018:bcr2018225154, 2018 30158262

Donovitz G, Cotten M: Breast cancer incidence reduction in women treated with subcutaneous testosterone: Testosterone Therapy and Breast Cancer Incidence Study. Eur J Breast Health 17(2):150–156, 2021 33870115

Drozdowicz LB, Bostwick JM: Psychiatric adverse effects of pediatric corticosteroid use. Mayo Clin Proc 89(6):817–834, 2014 24943696

Dubovsky AN, Arvikar S, Stern TA, et al: The neuropsychiatric complications of glucocorticoid use: steroid psychosis revisited. Psychosomatics 53(2):103–115, 2012 22424158

Eisenhofer G, Goldstein DS, Walther MM, et al: Biochemical diagnosis of pheochromocytoma: how to distinguish true- from false-positive test results. J Clin Endocrinol Metab 88(6):2656–2666, 2003 12788870

Elliott J, Kelly SE, Millar AC, et al: Testosterone therapy in hypogonadal men: a systematic review and network meta-analysis. BMJ Open 7(11):e015284, 2017 29150464

EMD Serono: Serostim (somatropin). 2016. Available at: https://dailymed.nlm.nih.gov/dailymed/drugInfo.cfm?setid=62b01d29-90f0-45b2-a0c4-3a750ba36c8a. Accessed April 19, 2016.

Fairbrother F, Petzl N, Scott JG, et al: Lithium can cause hyperthyroidism as well as hypothyroidism: a systematic review of an under-recognised association. Aust N Z J Psychiatry 53(5):384–402, 2019 30841715

Falk WE, Mahnke MW, Poskanzer DC: Lithium prophylaxis of corticotropin-induced psychosis. JAMA 241(10):1011–1012, 1979 216818

Fardet L, Nazareth I, Whitaker HJ, et al: Severe neuropsychiatric outcomes following discontinuation of long-term glucocorticoid therapy: a cohort study. J Clin Psychiatry 74(4):e281–e286, 2013 23656853

Goldman LS, Goveas J: Olanzapine treatment of corticosteroid-induced mood disorders. Psychosomatics 43(6):495–497, 2002 12444234

Goode DJ, Meltzer HY, Fang VS: Daytime variation in serum prolactin level in patients receiving oral and depot antipsychotic medication. Biol Psychiatry 16(7):653–662, 1981 7196775

Gregori G, Celli A, Barnouin Y, et al: Cognitive response to testosterone replacement added to intensive lifestyle intervention in older men with obesity and hypogonadism: prespecified secondary analyses of a randomized clinical trial. Am J Clin Nutr 114(5):1590–1599, 2021 34375393

Gulseren S, Gulseren L, Hekimsoy Z, et al: Depression, anxiety, health-related quality of life, and disability in patients with overt and subclinical thyroid dysfunction. Arch Med Res 37(1):133–139, 2006 16314199

Holtmann M, Gerstner S, Schmidt MH: Risperidone-associated ejaculatory and urinary dysfunction in male adolescents. J Child Adolesc Psychopharmacol 13(1):107–109, 2003 12804132

Hu LY, Shen CC, Hu YW, et al: Hyperthyroidism and risk for bipolar disorders: a nationwide population-based study. PLoS One 8(8):e73057, 2013 24023669

Huang G, Wharton W, Bhasin S, et al: Effects of long-term testosterone administration on cognition in older men with low or low-to-normal testosterone concentrations: a prespecified secondary analysis of data from the randomised, double-blind, placebo-controlled TEAAM trial. Lancet Diabetes Endocrinol 4(8):657–665, 2016 27377542

Huynh G, Reinert JP: Pharmacological management of steroid-induced psychosis: a review of patient cases. J Pharm Technol 37(2):120–126, 2021 34752563

Islam RM, Bell RJ, Green S, et al: Safety and efficacy of testosterone for women: a systematic review and meta-analysis of randomised controlled trial data. Lancet Diabetes Endocrinol 7(10):754–766, 2019 31353194

Ivkovic J, Lindsten A, George V, et al: Effect of brexpiprazole on prolactin: an analysis of short- and long-term studies in schizophrenia. J Clin Psychopharmacol 39(1):13–19, 2019 30566415

Jia S, Li C, Lei Z, et al: Determinants of anxiety and depression among pheochromocytoma patients: a case-control study. Medicine (Baltimore) 100(3):e24335, 2021 33546066

Johnston AM, Eagles JM: Lithium-associated clinical hypothyroidism: prevalence and risk factors. Br J Psychiatry 175(4):336–339, 1999 10789300

Judd LL, Schettler PJ, Brown ES, et al: Adverse consequences of glucocorticoid medication: psychological, cognitive, and behavioral effects. Am J Psychiatry 171(10):1045–1051, 2014 25272344

Jurado-Flores M, Warda F, Mooradian ES: Pathophysiology and clinical features of neuropsychiatric manifestations of thyroid disease. J Endocr Soc 6(2):bvab194, 2022 35059548

Katon WJ, Von Korff M, Lin EH, et al: The Pathways Study: a randomized trial of collaborative care in patients with diabetes and depression. Arch Gen Psychiatry 61(10):1042–1049, 2004 15466678

Katon WJ, Lin EH, Von Korff M, et al: Collaborative care for patients with depression and chronic illnesses. N Engl J Med 363(27):2611–2620, 2010 21190455

Kenna HA, Poon AW, de los Angeles CP, et al: Psychiatric complications of treatment with corticosteroids: review with case report. Psychiatry Clin Neurosci 65(6):549–560, 2011 22003987

Kessler L, Palla J, Baru JS, et al: Lithium as an adjunct to radioactive iodine for the treatment of hyperthyroidism: a systematic review and meta-analysis. Endocr Pract 20(7):737–745, 2014 24793920

Khaledi M, Haghighatdoost F, Feizi A, et al: The prevalence of comorbid depression in patients with type 2 diabetes: an updated systematic review and meta-analysis on huge number of observational studies. Acta Diabetol 56(6):631–650, 2019 30903433

Kibirige D, Luzinda K, Ssekitoleko R: Spectrum of lithium induced thyroid abnormalities: a current perspective. Thyroid Res 6(1):3, 2013 23391071

Kinon BJ, Gilmore JA, Liu H, et al: Prevalence of hyperprolactinemia in schizophrenic patients treated with conventional antipsychotic medications or risperidone. Psychoneuroendocrinology 28(Suppl 2):55–68, 2003 12650681

Kleiner J, Altshuler L, Hendrick V, et al: Lithium-induced subclinical hypothyroidism: review of the literature and guidelines for treatment. J Clin Psychiatry 60(4):249–255, 1999 10221287

Köhler-Forsberg O, Rohde C, Nierenberg AA, et al: Association of lithium treatment with the risk of osteoporosis in patients with bipolar disorder. JAMA Psychiatry 79(5):454–463, 2022 35353126

Kumar KCK, Ghimire N, Limbu T, et al: Levothyroxine overdose in a hypothyroid patient with adjustment disorder: a case report. Ann Med Surg (Lond) 59:234–236, 2020 33088498

Kvetny J, Ellervik C, Bech P: Is suppressed thyroid-stimulating hormone (TSH) associated with subclinical depression in the Danish General Suburban Population Study? Nord J Psychiatry 69(4):282–286, 2015 25377023

Labad J, Montalvo I, González-Rodríguez A, et al: Pharmacological treatment strategies for lowering prolactin in people with a psychotic disorder and hyperprolactinaemia: a systematic review and meta-analysis. Schizophr Res 222:88–96, 2020 32507371

Lally J, Sahl AB, Murphy KC, et al: Serum prolactin and bone mineral density in schizophrenia: a systematic review. Clin Psychopharmacol Neurosci 17(3):333–342, 2019 31352700

Laurent C, Capron J, Quillerou B, et al: Steroid-responsive encephalopathy associated with autoimmune thyroiditis (SREAT): characteristics, treatment and outcome in 251 cases from the literature. Autoimmun Rev 15(12):1129–1133, 2016 27639840

Lenfant L, Leon P, Cancel-Tassin G, et al: Testosterone replacement therapy (TRT) and prostate cancer: an updated systematic review with a focus on previous or active localized prostate cancer. Urol Oncol 38(8):661–670, 2020 32409202

Malkin CJ, Pugh PJ, Morris PD, et al: Testosterone replacement in hypogonadal men with angina improves ischaemic threshold and quality of life. Heart 90(8):871–876, 2004 15253956

Malkin CJ, Pugh PJ, West JN, et al: Testosterone therapy in men with moderate severity heart failure: a double-blind randomized placebo controlled trial. Eur Heart J 27(1):57–64, 2006 16093267

McKnight RF, Adida M, Budge K, et al: Lithium toxicity profile: a systematic review and meta-analysis. Lancet 379(9817):721–728, 2012

Meehan AD, Humble MB, Yazarloo P, et al: The prevalence of lithium-associated hyperparathyroidism in a large Swedish population attending psychiatric outpatient units. J Clin Psychopharmacol 35(3):279–285, 2015 25853371

Mifsud S, Cilia K, Mifsud EL, et al: Lithium-associated hyperparathyroidism. Br J Hosp Med (Lond) 81(11):1–9, 2020 33263481

Mojtabai R: Antidepressant use and glycemic control. Psychopharmacology (Berl) 227(3):467–477, 2013 23334176

Molitch ME: Drugs and prolactin. Pituitary 11(2):209–218, 2008 18404390

Nasrallah H: A review of the effect of atypical antipsychotics on weight. Psychoneuroendocrinology 28(Suppl 1):83–96, 2003 12504074

O'Connor DB, Archer J, Hair WM, et al: Activational effects of testosterone on cognitive function in men. Neuropsychologia 39(13):1385–1394, 2001 11585606

O'Keane V: Antipsychotic-induced hyperprolactinaemia, hypogonadism and osteoporosis in the treatment of schizophrenia. J Psychopharmacol 22(2 Suppl):70–75, 2008 18477623

Okosieme O, Gilbert J, Abraham P, et al: Management of primary hypothyroidism: statement by the British Thyroid Association Executive Committee. Clin Endocrinol (Oxf) 84(6):799–808, 2016 26010808

Ozdemir V, Bertilsson L, Miura J, et al: CYP2D6 genotype in relation to perphenazine concentration and pituitary pharmacodynamic tissue sensitivity in Asians: CYP2D6-serotonin-dopamine crosstalk revisited. Pharmacogenet Genomics 17(5):339–347, 2007 17429316

Parmar A, Hulme D, Hacking D, et al: Aripiprazole in young people with early psychosis: a systematic review and meta-analysis of weight gain. Australas Psychiatry 30(1):90–94, 2022 35001673

Pearce SH, Brabant G, Duntas LH, et al: 2013 ETA guideline: management of subclinical hypothyroidism. Eur Thyroid J 2(4):215–228, 2013 24783053

Penninx BWJH, Lange SMM: Metabolic syndrome in psychiatric patients: overview, mechanisms and implications. Dialogues Clin Neurosci 20(1):63–73, 2018 29946213

Peuskens J, Pani L, Detraux J, et al: The effects of novel and newly approved antipsychotics on serum prolactin levels: a comprehensive review. CNS Drugs 28(5):421–453, 2014 24677189

Piacentino D, Kotzalidis GD, Del Casale A, et al: Anabolic-androgenic steroid use and psychopathology in athletes: a systematic review. Curr Neuropharmacol 13(1):101–121, 2015 26074746

Pope HG Jr, Amiaz R, Brennan BP, et al: Parallel-group placebo-controlled trial of testosterone gel in men with major depressive disorder displaying an incomplete response to standard antidepressant treatment. J Clin Psychopharmacol 30(2):126–134, 2010 20520285

Preda A, Fazeli A, McKay BG, et al: Lamotrigine as prophylaxis against steroid-induced mania. J Clin Psychiatry 60(10):708–709, 1999 10549692

Regenold WT, Thapar RK, Marano C, et al: Increased prevalence of type 2 diabetes mellitus among psychiatric inpatients with bipolar I affective and schizoaffective disorders independent of psychotropic drug use. J Affect Disord 70(1):19–26, 2002 12113916

Riecher-Rössler A, Rybakowski JK, Pflueger MO, et al: Hyperprolactinemia in antipsychotic-naive patients with first-episode psychosis. Psychol Med 43(12):2571–2582, 2013 23590895

Roberts AL, Agnew-Blais JC, Spiegelman D, et al: Posttraumatic stress disorder and incidence of type 2 diabetes mellitus in a sample of women: a 22-year longitudinal study. JAMA Psychiatry 72(3):203–210, 2015 25565410

Rojo LE, Gaspar PA, Silva H, et al: Metabolic syndrome and obesity among users of second generation antipsychotics: a global challenge for modern psychopharmacology. Pharmacol Res 101:74–85, 2015 26218604

Roopan S, Larsen ER: Use of antidepressants in patients with depression and comorbid diabetes mellitus: a systematic review. Acta Neuropsychiatr 29(3):127–139, 2017 27776567

Roxanas MG, Hunt GE: Rapid reversal of corticosteroid-induced mania with sodium valproate: a case series of 20 patients. Psychosomatics 53(6):575–581, 2012 23157995

Rusgis MM, Alabbasi AY, Nelson LA: Guidance on the treatment of antipsychotic-induced hyperprolactinemia when switching the antipsychotic is not an option. Am J Health Syst Pharm 78(10):862–871, 2021 33954421

Russ MJ, Ackerman SH: Antidepressant treatment response in depressed hypothyroid patients. Hosp Community Psychiatry 40(9):954–956, 1989 2793101

Salvatore D, Porcelli T, Ettleson MD, et al: The relevance of T3 in the management of hypothyroidism. Lancet Diabetes Endocrinol 10(5):366–372, 2022 35240052

Saunders BD, Saunders EF, Gauger PG: Lithium therapy and hyperparathyroidism: an evidence-based assessment. World J Surg 33(11):2314–2323, 2009 19252941

Schoot TS, Molmans THJ, Grootens KP, et al: Systematic review and practical guideline for the prevention and management of the renal side effects of lithium therapy. Eur Neuropsychopharmacol 31:16–32, 2020 31837914

Serdenes R, Lewis M, Chandrasekhara S: Clinical review of the psychiatric sequelae of primary hyperparathyroidism. Cureus 13(10):e19078, 2021 34722014

Serri O, Li L, Mamputu JC, et al: The influences of hyperprolactinemia and obesity on cardiovascular risk markers: effects of cabergoline therapy. Clin Endocrinol (Oxf) 64(4):366–370, 2006 16584506

Shine B, McKnight RF, Leaver L, et al: Long-term effects of lithium on renal, thyroid, and parathyroid function: a retrospective analysis of laboratory data. Lancet 386(9992):461–468, 2015 26003379

Siafis S, Papazisis G: Detecting a potential safety signal of antidepressants and type 2 diabetes: a pharmacovigilance-pharmacodynamic study. Br J Clin Pharmacol 84(10):2405–2414, 2018 29953643

Stowell CP, Barnhill JW: Acute mania in the setting of severe hypothyroidism. Psychosomatics 46(3):259–261, 2005 15883148

Stubbs B, Vancampfort D, De Hert M, et al: The prevalence and predictors of type two diabetes mellitus in people with schizophrenia: a systematic review and comparative meta-analysis. Acta Psychiatr Scand 132(2):144–157, 2015 25943829

Sultan A, Gaskell H, Derry S, et al: Duloxetine for painful diabetic neuropathy and fibromyalgia pain: systematic review of randomised trials. BMC Neurol 8:29, 2008 18673529

Taipale H, Solmi M, Lähteenvuo M, et al: Antipsychotic use and risk of breast cancer in women with schizophrenia: a nationwide nested case-control study in Finland. Lancet Psychiatry 8(10):883–891, 2021 34474013

Tharmaraja T, Stahl D, Hopkins CWP, et al: The association between selective serotonin-reuptake inhibitors and glycemia: a systematic review and meta-analysis of randomized controlled trials. Psychosom Med 81(7):570–583, 2019 31136376

Tsuboi T, Bies RR, Suzuki T, et al: Hyperprolactinemia and estimated dopamine D2 receptor occupancy in patients with schizophrenia: analysis of the CATIE data. Prog Neuropsychopharmacol Biol Psychiatry 45:178–182, 2013 23727135

Vancampfort D, Stubbs B, Mitchell AJ, et al: Risk of metabolic syndrome and its components in people with schizophrenia and related psychotic disorders, bipolar disorder and major depressive disorder: a systematic review and meta-analysis. World Psychiatry 14(3):339–347, 2015 26407790

Vanover KE, Davis RE, Zhou Y, et al: Dopamine D2 receptor occupancy of lumateperone (ITI-007): a positron emission tomography study in patients with schizophrenia. Neuropsychopharmacology 44(3):598–605, 2019 30449883

van Vliet NA, van Heemst D, Almeida OP, et al: Association of thyroid dysfunction with cognitive function: an individual participant data analysis. JAMA Intern Med 181(11):1440–1450, 2021 34491268

Verma A, Wartak S, Tidswell M: Lithium-associated thyromegaly: an unusual cause of airway obstruction. Case Rep Med 2012:627415, 2012 22991519

Walshaw PD, Gyulai L, Bauer M, et al: Adjunctive thyroid hormone treatment in rapid cycling bipolar disorder: a double-blind placebo-controlled trial of levothyroxine (L-T4) and triiodothyronine (T3). Bipolar Disord 20(7):594–603, 2018 29869405

Wang C, Shi W, Xu J, et al: Outcomes and safety of concomitant topiramate or metformin for antipsychotics-induced obesity: a randomized-controlled trial. Ann
Gen Psychiatry 19(1):68, 2020 33302986

Whyand T, Bouvier C, Davies P: Prevalence of self-reported side effects in neuro-
endocrine tumour patients prescribed somatostatin analogues. Br J Nurs
27(13):738–744, 2018 29995506

Wilhelm SM, Lee J, Prinz RA: Major depression due to primary hyperparathyroidism:
a frequent and correctable disorder. Am Surg 70(2):175–179, discussion 179–
180, 2004 15011923

Wolkowitz OM: Long-lasting behavioral changes following prednisone withdrawal.
JAMA 261(12):1731–1732, 1989 2918667

Wu C-S, Hsu LY, Pan YJ, et al: Associations between antidepressant use and advanced
diabetes outcomes in patients with depression and diabetes mellitus. J Clin Endocrinol Metab 106(12):e5136–e5146, 2021 34259856

Ye Z, Chen L, Yang Z, et al: Metabolic effects of fluoxetine in adults with type 2 diabetes mellitus: a meta-analysis of randomized placebo-controlled trials. PLoS
One 6(7):e21551, 2011 21829436

Zamani A, Omrani GR, Nasab MM: Lithium's effect on bone mineral density. Bone
44(2):331–334, 2009 18992857

Ziegenbein M, Held K, Kuenzel HE, et al: The somatostatin analogue octreotide impairs sleep and decreases EEG sigma power in young male subjects. Neuropsychopharmacology 29(1):146–151, 2004 12955096

11

Obstetrics and Gynecology

Margaret Altemus, M.D.

Mallay Occhiogrosso, M.D.

The course of psychiatric illnesses in women is often modulated by reproductive events, including the menstrual cycle, pregnancy, lactation, and menopause. In addition, physiological changes during pregnancy, the postpartum period, and menopause can mimic psychiatric symptoms and should be considered in a differential diagnosis. Several gynecological disorders and treatments can also affect psychiatric status. Conversely, psychiatric disorders and psychopharmacological treatments can have an effect on reproductive functions. It can be difficult to interpret research findings regarding adverse medication effects in infants exposed during pregnancy or lactation because infant morbidity associated with maternal psychiatric conditions is itself a significant confounding factor. Because half of pregnancies are unintended and organ development occurs during the first trimester, it is often too late to avoid teratogenic drug effects by the time the pregnancy is identified. Treatment of any woman of reproductive age should include a plan for birth control and consideration of possible drug effects in the event of pregnancy.

Differential Diagnosis

Psychiatric Manifestations of Reproductive Conditions and Disorders

Psychiatric Manifestations of Menstrual Cycle and Fertility Disorders

Premenstrual dysphoric disorder (PMDD), which affects 3%–8% of menstruating women, is diagnosed if distinct mood and physical symptoms appear only during the luteal phase of the menstrual cycle and cause significant impairment. PMDD must be distinguished from perimenstrual exacerbation of another psychiatric disorder and premenstrual physical symptoms without a significant mood component. Irritability, other affective symptoms, anxiety, intrusive memories, and binge eating typically intensify during the luteal phase, whereas the subjective reward and craving for alcohol, cocaine, and tobacco are blunted in the luteal phase. In contrast, nonaffective symptoms of psychosis, completed suicide, and suicide attempts are exacerbated in the few days before and the week after onset of menses, when estrogen and progesterone levels are lowest (Handy et al. 2022). Among nonclinical and clinical samples, there is substantial variability in mood responses to the menstrual cycle. Multiple case reports describe an apparently rare syndrome with recurrent psychotic symptoms limited to the late luteal or menstrual phase of the cycle (Ahern et al. 2022).

Polycystic ovary syndrome, which affects 10%–18% of women of reproductive age, is associated with hyperandrogenism and an increased risk of a wide range of psychiatric disorders, including anxiety, depression, personality disorders, bipolar disorder, schizophrenia, and suicide attempts (Cesta et al. 2016; Månsson et al. 2008). It is yet not known whether correction of hormonal abnormalities could improve symptoms of comorbid psychiatric disorders.

Psychiatric Issues Related to Pregnancy

It is unclear whether rates of major depression are increased during pregnancy or postpartum. The demands of infant care do exacerbate the functional impairment and distress associated with depression. During the postpartum period, there is a clear increased risk of onset or relapse of bipolar disorder (Viguera et al. 2000). Therefore, it is crucial to carefully manage perinatal bipolar illness by scheduling frequent follow-up appointments, avoiding antidepressant monotherapy, and minimizing sleep disruption. Partial or total formula feeding may be preferable to breastfeeding to permit assistance with night feedings and decrease stress. Careful screening for past episodes of mania or hypomania is important for identifying women with previously undiagnosed bipolar disorder. For women undergoing treatment, serum levels of lithium and lamotrigine can decline substantially during pregnancy, beginning in the first trimester and continuing throughout pregnancy. There is great variability among pregnant women in the degree of change across pregnancy, but lithium levels typically decrease 20%–30% per trimester, and the lamotrigine dose may need to be increased as much as threefold by the end of pregnancy to maintain the prepregnancy blood levels. It is unclear whether dosage changes should be based on symptoms or an effort to maintain the prepregnancy blood levels.

Postpartum psychosis typically begins in the first 6 weeks postpartum. It is characterized by insomnia, agitation, paranoia, manic symptoms, and, in some cases, delirium. The strongest risk factors are personal and family histories of bipolar disorder or postpartum psychosis. Postpartum psychosis is a psychiatric emergency and usually warrants hospitalization because of behavioral dyscontrol, confusion, and risk of suicide and infanticide. There is a 50% incidence of recurrence after future deliveries (Blackmore et al. 2013). Although postpartum psychosis has a high association with chronic bipolar or psychotic illness, a substantial minority of women (20%–40%) will have recurrence only postpartum (Wesseloo et al. 2016). There is generally a favorable prognosis for rapid remission after treatment with mood stabilizers, antipsychotics, benzodiazepines, or a combination of these agents (Bergink et al. 2015). Prophylactic treatment with mood stabilizers, either atypical antipsychotics or lithium, is recommended in future pregnancies for patients with a history of postpartum psychosis (Wesseloo et al. 2016).

A large proportion of women with eating disorders have symptom remission during pregnancy (Micali et al. 2007).

Women with antithyroid antibodies (up to 11% of reproductive-age women) have a 33%–50% risk of postpartum thyroiditis (Nicholson et al. 2006; Wesseloo et al. 2018), which manifests as hyperthyroidism or hypothyroidism and can precipitate or worsen mood dysregulation and anxiety. Free thyroxine and thyroid-stimulating hormone levels should be checked in women presenting with postpartum onset of mood dysregulation or anxiety.

Restless legs syndrome, which causes insomnia and daytime fatigue, often begins or worsens during pregnancy. Restless legs syndrome that begins before pregnancy is associated with more severe symptoms and an increased risk of depression during pregnancy and postpartum (Wesström et al. 2014). Treatment options include correction of iron deficiency, benzodiazepines, gabapentin, and dopamine agonists (carbidopa/levodopa), but safety data for these medications during pregnancy are limited.

Hyperemesis occurs in up to 2% of pregnant women. No psychiatric risk factors have been identified, but the condition itself is a severe stressor, causing insomnia, fatigue, anticipatory anxiety, and elevated risk for depression, even in the setting of no history of depression (Kjeldgaard et al. 2017). Typical treatments include a doxylamine and pyridoxine combination, ondansetron, and the dopamine antagonists metoclopramide and promethazine. Growing anecdotal evidence suggests that mirtazapine also may be effective (Abramowitz et al. 2017). Benzodiazepines and tricyclic antidepressants (TCAs) have been suggested to target the associated anticipatory anxiety, but there is little evidence of efficacy.

Psychiatric Manifestations of Menopause

Perimenopause, the years from the onset of menstrual irregularity until a year past the last menstrual period, is associated with increased risk for several psychiatric symptoms. Some perimenopause symptoms overlap with depression, including fatigue, cognitive difficulties, insomnia, and loss of libido. Vasomotor symptoms are associated with increased risk for depression and insomnia, although insomnia often emerges during perimenopause independent of hot flashes. There is less evidence that vasomotor symptoms increase the risk of major depression (Maki et al. 2019).

The risk for major depression during perimenopause is elevated two- to fourfold. Perimenopausal depression occurs much more commonly in women with a history of depression (Maki et al. 2019). Suicidal ideation is also several times more common during perimenopause (Usall et al. 2009). Women with bipolar I or bipolar II disorder have more mood episodes during perimenopause, particularly depressive episodes (Perich et al. 2017; Truong and Marsh 2019). One study reported that bipolar women who used hormone replacement therapy (HRT) had less worsening of mood during perimenopause (Freeman et al. 2002). The risk of major depression is also increased after hysterectomy and more so after hysterectomy with ovariectomy (Maki et al. 2019).

There is a second wave of onset of schizophrenia in women ages 45–54, and women with earlier-onset schizophrenia often have symptom exacerbation during these years (Riecher-Rössler et al. 2018).

Obstetrical and Gynecological Manifestations of Psychiatric Disorders

Effects of Psychiatric Disorders on Menstrual Cycle and Fertility

Childhood sexual abuse is associated with earlier onset of puberty in girls (Hamlat et al. 2022). Perceived stress has been shown to reduce estradiol and progesterone levels, to increase risk of anovulatory cycles (Schliep et al. 2015) and irregular cycles (Nillni et al. 2018), and to increase time to pregnancy (Schliep et al. 2019). Severe depression is also associated with irregular cycle length (Nillni et al. 2018). In addition, reduced sleep duration and shift work have been linked to menstrual irregularity, polycystic ovary syndrome, infertility, and early pregnancy loss (Beroukhim et al. 2022). Several psychotherapy treatments have been associated with higher rates of conception for infertile women, including women undergoing in vitro fertilization (Zhou et al. 2021). Eating disorders disrupt menstrual cyclicity and fertility in proportion to energy deficits brought on by dieting and exercise.

Among other major psychiatric disorders, autism spectrum disorder, schizophrenia, depression, anxiety, anorexia nervosa, and substance use disorders have been associated with having fewer children (Jacobson 2016; Power et al. 2013). Factors contributing to reduced fertility in major psychiatric disorders probably include social function deficits and medication side effects that have an effect on the gonadal hormone axis and sexual function.

Effects of Psychiatric Disorders on Pregnancy and Fetus

Untreated mental illness can lead to maternal behaviors that can have adverse effects on the fetus, including substance use, insomnia, suboptimal nutrition, and poor compliance with prenatal care. These behaviors, as well as physiological sequelae of maternal stress and anxiety during pregnancy, contribute to shortened gestations and low birth weight (Traylor et al. 2020). Reduced fetal weight gain and shortened gestation have long-term effects on the endocrine stress response system, cognition, and mental health of offspring (Monk et al. 2019; Orri et al. 2021).

Depression during pregnancy seems to increase the risk of premature birth and low birth weight one- to twofold, depending on the severity of depression (Jarde et al. 2016). PTSD also has been associated with shortened gestation, preterm birth, and low birth weight (Sanjuan et al. 2021). Compared with pregnant women without a psychiatric diagnosis, pregnant women with schizophrenia show higher rates of placental abruption, gestational diabetes and hypertension, prematurity, low birth weight, low Apgar scores, and congenital anomalies in offspring (Jablensky et al. 2005; Simoila et al. 2020; Webb et al. 2005). Pregnant women with schizophrenia have high rates of smoking and obesity, which probably mediate some of these adverse outcomes.

Maternal anorexia nervosa is associated with smaller birth length, and binge-eating disorder is associated with large for gestational age newborns (Watson et al. 2017). The risk of ADHD may be elevated in offspring of women who had active bulimia or anorexia nervosa during pregnancy, and the risk of autism spectrum disorders seems to be elevated in offspring of women with active anorexia nervosa during pregnancy (Mantel et al. 2022).

Effects of Psychiatric Disorders on Perimenopause

Premorbid somatic anxiety symptoms predict higher risk of vasomotor symptoms during the menopausal transition (Freeman et al. 2005). Women with a history of depression have earlier onset of menopause (Harlow et al. 2003).

Pharmacotherapy for Premenstrual Mood Symptoms

Premenstrual Dysphoric Disorder

Selective serotonin reuptake inhibitors (SSRIs) and serotonin-norepinephrine reuptake inhibitors (SNRIs) are first-line agents for treatment of PMDD and have been shown to be effective when taken either throughout the cycle or during the 2 weeks preceding menstruation and when administered during only symptomatic premenstrual days (Marjoribanks et al. 2013; Yonkers et al. 2015). Approximately 30% of women who have PMDD do not respond to SSRI treatment. Oral contraceptives containing the progestin drospirenone have shown efficacy for treatment of PMDD (Lopez et al. 2012). However, drospirenone-containing oral contraceptives have a U.S. FDA black box warning because of the higher risk of serious cardiovascular events compared with other hormonal contraceptives. The relative efficacy of these oral contraceptives for treatment of PMDD compared with oral contraceptives containing other progestins is unclear (Lopez et al. 2012). Continuous dosing of oral contraceptives is commonly used for control of PMDD symptoms, but this is not yet supported by controlled trials. Although some women experience reduction in premenstrual mood symptoms during oral contraceptive treatment, other women experience exacerbation of mood symptoms (Edwards et al. 2022; Kulkarni 2007). Gonadotropin-releasing hormone agonists, which shut down the gonadal axis, are effective treatments for PMDD, but use is complicated by menopausal side effects. A progesterone receptor antagonist, ulipristal acetate, which also suppresses ovulation, was effective in an initial study (Comasco et al. 2021). Calcium supplements (600 mg bid) have shown some benefit for PMDD, but efficacy is less than that seen with SSRI treatment (Yonkers et al. 2013). There is also limited support for treatment with clomipramine, alprazolam, or spironolactone; quetiapine augmentation of an SSRI; and cognitive therapy. Combined treatments are commonly used when response to a single agent is inadequate.

Premenstrual Exacerbations of Depression and Anxiety

Despite strong evidence of premenstrual exacerbation of affective illness, effective treatment approaches have not been established (Kuehner and Nayman 2021). For a few medications, changes in metabolism have been found across the menstrual cycle and during oral contraceptive treatment. Lithium levels are reduced in the luteal phase and linked to premenstrual symptom exacerbation (Carmassi et al. 2019). Lamotrigine and valproic acid levels do not change significantly across the menstrual cycle but are suppressed during oral contraceptive use, with 40% and 20% reductions in clearance, respectively, during days without active pills (Herzog et al. 2009; Wegner et al. 2014).

Pharmacotherapy for Menopause-Related Depression, Anxiety, and Insomnia

Standard treatments for depression, anxiety, and insomnia are recommended as first line during the menopause transition (Maki et al. 2019). SSRIs, SNRIs, and mirtazapine can also improve vasomotor symptoms in addition to treating affective symptoms.

Several psychotropic agents, including desvenlafaxine (50–200 mg/day), paroxetine (7.5–10 mg/day), escitalopram (10–20 mg/day), gabapentin (900–2,400 mg/day), pregabalin (150–300 mg/day), and clonidine (0.1–1.5 mg/day), can relieve hot flashes, although efficacy is less than with hormonal treatments (Genazzani et al. 2021). Targeting insomnia with the nonbenzodiazepine hypnotic eszopiclone produced improvement in depression and vasomotor symptoms (Soares et al. 2006). In a large multicenter trial, yoga, exercise, and omega-3 fatty acid supplements did not relieve hot flashes more than placebo (Guthrie et al. 2015). There have been no controlled studies of psychotherapy for treatment of perimenopausal depression, but an effective cognitive therapy has been developed to relieve vasomotor symptoms (Hunter 2021).

Short-term transdermal estradiol treatment can relieve unipolar major depression in perimenopausal but not postmenopausal women (Morrison et al. 2004; Schmidt et al. 2000; Soares et al. 2001). Transdermal estradiol has been found to be effective for major and minor depression at dosages of 50–100 μg/day for 8–12 weeks; response rate was independent of comorbid hot flashes (Joffe et al. 2011; Schmidt et al. 2000; Soares et al. 2001). Estrogen augmentation of antidepressant medication also may be effective during perimenopause (Maki et al. 2019; Morgan et al. 2005). One study found that yearlong treatment with transdermal estradiol with 10 days of oral progesterone every 3 months prevented depression in perimenopausal women (Gordon et al. 2018). Estradiol treatment in perimenopause and early postmenopause can also improve insomnia and urogenital function, which affect mood and quality of life.

Although the Women's Health Initiative and other early trials found increased risk of breast cancer, heart disease, stroke, dementia, and pulmonary embolism with HRT, more recent studies have shown that these risks are not elevated in women who start HRT within 10 years of menopause, use transdermal estrogen delivery, or use micronized progesterone rather than medroxyprogesterone acetate (Langer et al. 2021).

Many women also experience impairment of memory, attention, or executive function during the menopause transition (Weber et al. 2014). If cognitive symptoms persist after affective and vasomotor symptoms have been treated, stimulant treatment can be beneficial (Epperson et al. 2015).

Psychopharmacology During Pregnancy and Breastfeeding

Approach to Pharmacotherapy During Pregnancy and the Postpartum Period

Management of any psychiatric disorder during pregnancy and lactation is complicated by the need to consider the effects of psychiatric medication on the fetus and newborn (Table 11–1) and the potential effects of untreated illness on fetal development and maternal health. Pregnant and lactating women should use the minimal number of medications at the lowest effective dosage. Medications with more reproductive safety data are preferred. When interpreting findings regarding medication use during breastfeeding, infant serum levels are a better indication of exposure than drug levels in milk.

Current reviews of the reproductive safety of different classes of medication and of specific drugs are available online at the Massachusetts General Hospital Center for Women's Mental Health (https://womensmentalhealth.org); Reprotox, a subscription-based resource (https://reprotox.org); and LactMed, a resource maintained by the National Library of Medicine (Drugs and Lactation Database 2022).

In 2015, the FDA published a new pregnancy and lactation labeling rule that removes the letter rating system (A, B, C, D, X), replacing it with more detailed summaries of available evidence regarding risks of drug exposure during pregnancy and lactation (https://www.fda.gov/drugs/labeling-information-drug-products/pregnancy-and-lactation-labeling-drugs-final-rule). The rule is being phased in gradually for existing medications and applies to all new medications. Under the letter system, some drugs received more favorable ratings because fewer data were available, and some drugs received less favorable ratings because of similarities to drugs with reported risks.

Prospective studies have found that 68% of pregnant women with recurrent depression who discontinued antidepressant use because of pregnancy relapsed during the first or second trimester (Cohen et al. 2006), and 80% of bipolar women who discontinued mood stabilizers relapsed during pregnancy (Viguera et al. 2007b). In contrast, no increased risk of relapse was seen in a community sample of women who discontinued antidepressant medication during pregnancy, probably because of inclusion of women with less severe ill-

Table 11–1. Effects of psychiatric medications on the fetus or infant

Medication	Pregnancy	Neonatal	Lactation
Anxiolytics and sleep aids			
Benzodiazepines	No risk of congenital abnormalities	Premature birth, low Apgar score, neonatal ICU admission	Limited information indicates low exposure. Use short-half-life agents (e.g., lorazepam or oxazepam).
Buspirone	Very limited human data	Very limited human data	Limited data indicate low levels in infant serum.
Hydroxyzine	Very limited human data	Very limited human data	Very limited human data
Melatonin	Very limited human data	Very limited human data	Very limited human data
Trazodone	Very limited human data	Very limited human data	Low levels in milk
Zolpidem	Very limited human data	Very limited human data	Low levels in milk

Table 11–1. Effects of psychiatric medications on the fetus or infant (*continued*)

Medication	Pregnancy	Neonatal	Lactation
Antidepressants			
SSRIs and SNRIs	Small increased risk of prematurity, similar to rates in untreated depression Not teratogenic No increased risk of miscarriage, possible reduced rates of conception Placental transfer lowest for sertraline and paroxetine and highest for citalopram, escitalopram, and fluoxetine Small increased risk of postpartum hemorrhage Less robust data for venlafaxine and duloxetine Up to 50% drop in serum levels during pregnancy	Neonatal syndrome (irritability, high-pitched cry) for 2–7 days postpartum in up to 30% described in a small observational study Transient respiratory difficulty (rare) Pulmonary hypertension risk increased by 30% but still very low	Infant generally has low exposure to SSRIs. Lowest infant serum levels with paroxetine and sertraline Fluoxetine produces infant serum levels >10% of maternal levels in 10% of infants. Infant levels of venlafaxine are usually low, and lower levels are found with desvenlafaxine.
Vortioxetine	Very limited information	No information	Very limited information indicates low exposure.

Table 11–1. Effects of psychiatric medications on the fetus or infant *(continued)*

Medication	Pregnancy	Neonatal	Lactation
Antidepressants *(continued)*			
Vilazodone	Very limited information	No information	No information
Bupropion	Limited human data show no evidence of teratogenicity; could exacerbate seizure risk in preeclampsia	Limited data	Generally undetectable levels in infant serum, but two cases of infant seizures have been reported
Mirtazapine	Limited data show no evidence of teratogenicity; reports of relief of nausea and hyperemesis	No adverse effects	Very low levels in breast milk
Tricyclic antidepressants	Limited data; no evidence of teratogenicity; can exacerbate orthostatic hypotension	More safety data and less side-effect burden with nortriptyline; lack of effect on postnatal development with nortriptyline	Limited data indicate very low infant serum levels.
Electroconvulsive therapy	Generally safe and well tolerated in first and second trimester of pregnancy; case reports of premature labor and placental abruption in third trimester		

Table 11–1.   Effects of psychiatric medications on the fetus or infant (*continued*)

Medication	Pregnancy	Neonatal	Lactation
Antipsychotics	Teratogenic risk low for most second-generation antipsychotics; more limited evidence for first-generation antipsychotics and ziprasidone and none for lurasidone or asenapine; increased risk of gestational diabetes with olanzapine and quetiapine	Newborn extrapyramidal symptoms, may be prolonged	Little evidence: quetiapine and olanzapine are preferred because of low infant serum levels; risk of agranulocytosis with clozapine
Mood stabilizers			
Lithium	Increased risk of heart defect: 2%–8% for any heart defect, 0.1% for Ebstein's anomaly; increased risk of noncardiac birth defects Clearance increases 30%–50% during pregnancy	Case reports of neonatal hypothyroidism and polyhydramnios Increased risk of premature delivery Lower Apgar scores and increased CNS and neuromuscular complications with lithium level >0.64 mEq/L at delivery	Infant serum levels 10%–50% of maternal levels; monitor for dehydration and thyroid function
Carbamazepine	Increased risk of neural tube defects, facial dysmorphism, genitourinary defects, and fingernail hypoplasia		Infant serum levels 5%–44% of maternal levels; no adverse effects reported

Table 11–1. Effects of psychiatric medications on the fetus or infant *(continued)*

Medication	Pregnancy	Neonatal	Lactation
Mood stabilizers *(continued)*			
Oxcarbazepine	No human data	No human data	Infant serum levels 5% of maternal levels
Lamotrigine	No teratogenicity; clearance increases up to 300% during pregnancy		Infant serum levels 18%–46% of maternal levels
Valproic acid	Dose-dependent risks of neural tube defect (1%–4%) and overall 5%–11% risk of congenital abnormalities, including cardiac, limb, genitourinary, and craniofacial abnormalities	Risk of neonatal hepatic toxicity	Low concentration in breast milk
Psychostimulants	Limited data; no evidence of teratogenicity with methylphenidate and amphetamine; mixed results regarding association of modafinil with congenital malformations		Infant serum levels of amphetamine and methylphenidate are very low; very limited data regarding modafinil or armodafinil exposure through breast milk

Note.   SNRIs=serotonin-norepinephrine reuptake inhibitors; SSRIs=selective serotonin reuptake inhibitors.

ness (Yonkers et al. 2011). Women with severe disease should continue their mood stabilizer or antidepressant treatments during the first trimester and throughout pregnancy. In women with mild disease and low relapse risk, the mood stabilizer or antidepressant may be tapered off entirely or continued until pregnancy is achieved.

Use of the lowest effective dose of psychotropics will lessen the adverse effects of an abrupt taper. Abrupt cessation of mood stabilizers greatly increases the risk of relapse (50% within 2 weeks) compared with a gradual taper (Viguera et al. 2007b). In women with moderate disease or relapse risk who respond best to lithium, which has a teratogenic risk, an option is to slowly discontinue lithium for conception and then restart lithium at 12 weeks, after the structural development of the fetal heart is complete.

Maternal metabolic changes over the course of pregnancy can lead to substantial declines in psychiatric medication plasma levels. This effect has been documented for SSRIs (40%–50%), SNRIs, lithium (30%–50%), lamotrigine (up to 300%), quetiapine, and aripiprazole. If symptoms are exacerbated during pregnancy, an increase in dose should be considered. If that is not successful, augmenting agents should be considered, with a preference for agents that have been successful in the past.

Electroconvulsive therapy is a safe, effective, and generally well-tolerated treatment option for acute episodes of mania and severe depression during pregnancy. During pregnancy, electroconvulsive therapy requires some modification of standard techniques (Rose et al. 2020). Response rates to electroconvulsive therapy for depression and psychosis may be particularly high in the postpartum period (Rundgren et al. 2018).

Anxiolytics and Sedative-Hypnotics

Teratogenicity. Benzodiazepine prescribing practices in pregnancy vary widely from country to country, with highest prevalence in the third trimester (3.1%) and in Eastern Europe (14%) (Bais et al. 2020). Despite their common use, the data are limited to guide clinicians regarding the safety of the use of benzodiazepines in pregnancy and even more limited regarding the use of nonbenzodiazepine sedative-hypnotics.

Although small retrospective case-control studies from the 1970s raised concerns that first-trimester exposure to benzodiazepines may be associated with an increased risk of cleft lip or cleft palate, more recent studies that used large administrative databases have not found increased teratogenic risk with the use of benzodiazepines or nonbenzodiazepine z-drug hypnotics (Ban et al. 2014; Jensen et al. 2022; Wang et al. 2022; Wikner and Källén 2011).

For treatment of insomnia during pregnancy, the over-the-counter antihistamine diphenhydramine is frequently recommended. Extremely limited research exists on safety, but North American case-control registry data and a meta-analysis identified no associated increase in malformation risk with first-trimester exposure to antihistamines (Etwel et al. 2017; Li et al. 2013).

Restless legs syndrome occurs in up to 30% of pregnant women (Wesström et al. 2014). In addition to insomnia, restless legs have been associated with increased risk of depression during pregnancy and premature birth. Treatment options include correction of iron deficiency, benzodiazepines, gabapentin, and dopamine agonists (carbidopa/levodopa), but safety data for these medications during pregnancy are limited (Picchietti et al. 2015). Gabapentin exposure during pregnancy has been associated with possible increased risk of cardiac defects, preterm birth, and neonatal intensive care unit (NICU) admission (Patorno et al. 2020). Dopamine agonists, normally a first-line treatment for restless legs syndrome, should be avoided during pregnancy because little is known about potential effects on the fetus.

Neonatal symptoms.   A large prospective cohort study found a 2-day reduction in gestational age and 40% increased risk of premature birth associated with benzodiazepine or z-drug exposure in utero (Huitfeldt et al. 2020). In a meta-analysis, antenatal benzodiazepine exposure was associated with preterm birth, low birth weight, low Apgar score, and NICU admission (Grigoriadis et al. 2020).

If benzodiazepines are used regularly late in pregnancy, infants should be closely monitored for neonatal adverse effects, including irritability, tremor, withdrawal seizures, floppy baby syndrome, and apnea and other respiratory difficulties. Short-half-life agents with no active metabolites, such as lorazepam and oxazepam, are less likely to accumulate in the fetus.

Postnatal development.   In a large prospective cohort study, including 283 women who used benzodiazepines or z-hypnotic medications during pregnancy, offspring at 5 years old did not show elevated rates of ADHD or fine motor deficits (Lupattelli et al. 2019). A 2022 meta-analysis of 19 studies conducted between 1958 and 2016 (Wang et al. 2022) showed no consistent findings of adverse neurodevelopmental outcomes, but the investigators cautioned that the data were limited, and no definitive conclusions could be drawn. However, because little is known about the effects of in utero benzodiazepine exposure on neurobehavioral development, low doses and time-limited use are recommended during pregnancy. In addition, the combination of benzodiazepines and SSRIs should be avoided if possible, in light of evidence that the combination has greater adverse effects on infant arousal and regulation across the first month postpartum (Salisbury et al. 2016).

Antidepressants

Fertility.   SSRIs as a group are not associated with elevated risk of spontaneous abortion (Sjaarda et al. 2020; Wu et al. 2019), although a few studies have noted an elevated rate of spontaneous abortion in women taking fluoxetine (Sjaarda et al. 2020). SSRI exposure has been associated with 25% lower rates of conception (Casilla-Lennon et al. 2016; Sjaarda et al. 2020), but it is unclear whether reduced conception rates are linked to drug effects or reduced sexual activity. A retrospective study found no effect of SSRIs on success of in vitro fertilization (Friedman et al. 2009).

Teratogenicity.   SSRIs are the most extensively studied class of medication regarding safety in pregnancy, with a particularly large body of research data available for fluoxetine and sertraline, which are the two most commonly prescribed. Numerous studies have shown no association of SSRIs with teratogenicity. Although initial reports suggested increased risk of cardiac defects with prenatal paroxetine exposure, more recent studies do not support a teratogenic effect of paroxetine.

Data on duloxetine are reassuring in terms of cardiac risk and pregnancy complications (Ankarfeldt et al. 2021; Huybrechts et al. 2020). More limited data suggest that mirtazapine and bupropion are not associated with birth defects or pregnancy complications (Ostenfeld et al. 2022; Turner et al. 2019). Teratogenic effects have not been found for venlafaxine, nefazodone, or trazodone, but studies have been underpowered. Little is known about the new antidepressant agents vortioxetine and vilazodone, so their use in pregnancy should be avoided if possible.

Although less formally studied, TCAs do not seem to be associated with birth defects.

In utero development.   Treatment of maternal psychiatric disorders with SSRIs in pregnancy appears to reduce rates of preterm birth and cesarean delivery relative to the offspring of mothers with psychiatric disorders who are unexposed to medications. On the other hand, SSRI exposure may raise the risk of other complications, including neonatal abstinence syndrome and NICU admission (Malm et al. 2015). Exposure to SSRIs in the third trimester of pregnancy, when lung maturation occurs, also appears to increase the risk of persistent pulmonary hypertension of the newborn (PPHN). Baseline risk of PPHN is estimated at 1.9 per 1,000 live births. With SSRI exposure, risk has been estimated to rise 1.2- to 3.5-fold, depending on the analysis methods (Grigoriadis et al. 2014; Huybrechts et al. 2015). However, the absolute risk remains very low. To date, there have been no reported cases of PPHN associated with SSRI exposure resulting in death of an infant. Several risk factors for PPHN, including obesity, premature delivery, and cesarean delivery, are also associated with depression, making it difficult to sort out the degree of risk associated with SSRI exposure and depression itself (Occhiogrosso et al. 2012). Among the TCAs, nortriptyline and desipramine are preferred in order to minimize risk of maternal orthostatic hypotension, which could compromise placental perfusion. A 30% increased risk of postpartum hemorrhage is associated with SSRIs and other antidepressants (Andrade 2022). Because this risk is found across all antidepressant categories, it suggests that this outcome is more likely to be secondary to illness-related confounds than to antidepressants.

Neonatal syndromes.   A neonatal syndrome has been associated with SSRI exposure in the third trimester. Symptoms include difficulty feeding, tremor, high-pitched cry, irritability, muscle rigidity or low muscle tone, respiratory distress, tachypnea, jitteriness, and convulsions. This syndrome, most common with paroxetine and fluoxetine, occurs in approximately 20% of SSRI-exposed infants but usually lasts only a few days (Moses-Kolko et al. 2005; Oberlander et al. 2006; Sanz et al. 2005), although one study found that symptoms of hyperarousal persisted for up to 14 days postpartum (Salisbury et al. 2016). A similar neonatal syndrome has been described with in utero clomipramine exposure but not with exposure to other TCAs.

Postnatal development.   Infants exposed to SSRIs in utero appear to have normal neurocognitive outcomes, although data are limited. Cognitive function, temperament, and general behavior were similar in children exposed prenatally to TCAs or fluoxetine and in unexposed comparison children in two studies (Nulman et al. 1997, 2002).

Small studies seem to indicate that infants exposed to SSRIs in utero may have mild transient motor delays in the first year of life (e.g., Pedersen et al. 2010). However, these delays do not appear to be clinically significant (Santucci et al. 2014). SSRI exposure was not found to be linked with an increased risk of autism spectrum disorder in several large registry studies when maternal psychiatric illness and other potential confounders were controlled for (Vega et al. 2020).

Summary. Sertraline is a first-line antidepressant for use during pregnancy, as supported by a large amount of reassuring teratogenicity data for SSRIs, evidence of less placental transfer for sertraline than for other SSRIs (Loughhead et al. 2006), and a benign safety profile during lactation (see the "Approach to Psychopharmacotherapy During Breastfeeding" subsection later in this chapter).

Antipsychotics

In utero development. Although all second-generation antipsychotics examined in a 2007 study passed into the placental circulation, quetiapine had the least and olanzapine the most placental transfer (Newport et al. 2007). Recent studies that used large clinical databases found no teratogenic risk of commonly used typical and atypical antipsychotics, although a small increased risk of overall birth defects and cardiac defects was found for risperidone (Huybrechts et al. 2016). There is an increased risk of gestational diabetes with olanzapine and quetiapine exposure during pregnancy (Park et al. 2018), presumed to be mediated by weight gain and metabolic side effects associated with these drugs. Obesity itself is associated with an increased rate of multiple birth defects and eclampsia (Waller et al. 2007).

Postnatal development. Two large birth cohort studies found increased rates of ADHD, autism spectrum disorder, and other neurodevelopmental disorders among children exposed to antipsychotics in utero. However, there was no difference in adjusted analyses, suggesting that other characteristics of the women who used antipsychotic medications accounted for the increased rates of neurodevelopmental disorders (Hálfdánarson et al. 2022; Straub et al. 2022). In utero exposure to antipsychotic medication did not affect risk for development of other psychiatric disorders in offspring (Momen et al. 2022).

Mood Stabilizers

Teratogenicity.   Lithium completely equilibrates across the placenta. Studies have found a 0.6- to 2-fold increased rate of major malformations and a 0.5- to 4-fold increased rate of cardiac malformations, although many of the cardiac malformations resolve spontaneously (Diav-Citrin et al. 2014; Hastie et al. 2021; Munk-Olsen et al. 2018). The risk for the potentially severe Ebstein's anomaly is elevated 20-fold but is still low (1 in 1,000 infants) (Giles and Bannigan 2006). With fetal exposure to lithium in the first trimester, ultrasonography or fetal echocardiography to assess fetal cardiac development and level 2 ultrasound to screen for other abnormalities are advised. Use of sustained-release lithium preparations minimizes peak lithium levels, which may be protective (Yonkers et al. 2004).

Use of antiepileptic agents in pregnancy has been studied mainly for patients with epilepsy. Valproic acid is associated with a significantly higher risk of incomplete neural tube closure (1%–4%), cardiac defects, craniofacial abnormalities, and limb defects. Valproate exposure increases the rate of any congenital malformation to 9.3%. It has also been associated with neurodevelopmental delays and increased risk of autism. Risk increases with dosage and with combined anticonvulsant therapy. Carbamazepine is also teratogenic, increasing the risk of neural tube defects, facial dysmorphism, and fingernail hypoplasia, but the risk of malformations is much lower (3% in a large database study) than with valproate (Hernández-Díaz et al. 2012). Folate supplementation decreases the incidence of neural tube defects in carbamazepine-exposed pregnancies (Hernández-Díaz et al. 2001) but not in valproate-exposed pregnancies (Wyszynski et al. 2005).

Lamotrigine registry data indicate no increased risk of congenital malformations, although some database studies have found a risk of oral clefts slightly above population baseline (Hernández-Díaz et al. 2012). Topiramate also has been associated with an increased risk of oral cleft (Hernández-Díaz et al. 2012). Insufficient data are available to assess the teratogenicity of levetiracetam, gabapentin, or oxcarbazepine, but the few existing data are reassuring (Hernández-Díaz et al. 2012).

In utero development.   Valproic acid exposure is associated with fetal growth restriction. Preliminary evidence suggests that topiramate reduces birth weight but does not increase the risk of prematurity (Ornoy et al. 2008).

Neonatal syndromes.   A study of 727 lithium-exposed pregnancies found a 60% higher rate of admission to neonatal intensive care (Munk-Olsen et al. 2018) and two- to threefold elevated rates of premature delivery (Diav-Citrin et al. 2014; Hastie et al. 2021). In a separate study, infants with higher lithium concentrations (>0.64 mEq/L) at delivery had lower Apgar scores, longer hospital stays, and higher rates of CNS and neuromuscular complications compared with neonates with lower lithium levels (Newport et al. 2005). Symptoms of neonatal lithium toxicity include flaccidity, lethargy, and poor reflexes. For the mother, intravenous fluids are indicated at delivery to counterbalance maternal blood volume contraction during delivery. After delivery, the prepregnancy dosage should be resumed, with close monitoring for dosage adjustments as maternal fluid volume contracts.

Postnatal development.   Follow-up studies of children and adolescents exposed to lithium in utero did not find evidence of neurobehavioral toxicity (Forsberg et al. 2018; Poels et al. 2022). In utero valproic acid exposure has been clearly linked to dose-dependent cognitive impairment, with IQ at 3 years reduced by 9 points and 6 points compared with children exposed to lamotrigine and carbamazepine, respectively (Meador et al. 2009).

Summary.   Because of the significant risks to the fetus of valproic acid exposure during pregnancy, for women needing mood stabilizer treatment, a switch to lithium, lamotrigine, or an antipsychotic should be considered.

Psychostimulants

A large clinical database study found no increased risk of congenital malformations for amphetamine and a possible small increased risk of cardiac malformations with exposure to methylphenidate (Huybrechts et al. 2018). Amphetamine exposure in utero did not affect birth weight (Rose et al. 2021).

Small studies have reported mixed results regarding risk of congenital malformations during in utero exposure to modafinil (Cesta et al. 2020; Kaplan et al. 2021). Insufficient data are available to evaluate the teratogenic effects of the therapeutic use of atomoxetine during pregnancy.

Approach to Pharmacotherapy During Breastfeeding

Concern about the exposure of breastfeeding infants to maternal medications leads women and their physicians to avoid medications, at times unnecessarily, and to avoid lactation. Although breastfeeding is strongly recommended by the medical community, the clinician should put breastfeeding in context, supporting the mother's decision to forgo breastfeeding if she needs a medication that poses a risk to the infant or if the demands of breastfeeding are impeding her recovery. Well-controlled studies show only a few differences in health outcome between breastfed and bottle-fed children (Colen and Ramey 2014; Sanefuji et al. 2021; Yang et al. 2018). Long-term outcome data from medication exposure during lactation are not available, but the long-term risks of maternal depression for infants and older siblings are substantial and well documented (Pilowsky et al. 2008).

Although the quantitative data on infant exposure to drugs through breast milk are limited, with some exceptions the exposure is at least an order of magnitude less than the exposure during pregnancy. Exceptions are lamotrigine (9%–18% of maternal serum levels) and lithium (12%–30% of maternal serum levels). In general, breast milk concentrations of medications and active metabolites are in equilibrium with maternal serum concentrations. Infant exposure is also determined by maturation of the infant's metabolic systems, gut-blood barrier, and blood-brain barrier. For example, lamotrigine levels are relatively high in infant serum because the glucuronidation metabolic pathway is inefficient in infants. For medications taken infrequently on an as-needed basis, shorter half-life can reduce exposure. Maternal serum and milk concentrations will be reduced by 75% after two half-lives. Therapeutic drug level monitoring in infants is of limited clinical use because serum levels associated with toxicity have not been established for infants. Infant exposure to medication can be reduced by replacing breast milk with formula at some feedings. The U.S. National Library of Medicine's LactMed database contains information on the levels of drugs and other chemicals in breast milk and infant blood and the possible adverse effects in the nursing infant (Drugs and Lactation Database 2022).

Anxiolytics and Sedative-Hypnotics

Limited information is available on the safety of benzodiazepines and the newer nonbenzodiazepine hypnotics in lactating women, and no long-term exposure data are available. Exposed infants should be monitored for sedation, weight gain, and developmental milestones. If benzodiazepines are necessary for mothers, agents with short half-lives (e.g., lorazepam, oxazepam) are preferred. Nortriptyline and mirtazapine, which have low serum levels in breastfed infants, also can be used to promote sleep in lactating women. There are no data on infant serum levels of zolpidem or eszopiclone and limited safety data. Zolpidem is preferred because of its shorter half-life and low levels in milk.

Antidepressants

Paroxetine and sertraline have minimal or undetectable circulating levels in breastfed infants. Citalopram, mirtazapine, and nortriptyline also have very low blood levels in breastfed infants. A few medications, including venlafaxine, fluoxetine, and doxepin, occasionally produce infant serum levels of parent drug plus active metabolites that are greater than 10% of maternal serum levels, although these higher levels have not been linked to adverse outcomes (Uguz 2021). Although infant levels of bupropion and its active metabolite are low, authors of two case reports described seizures in infants exposed to bupropion ("Bupropion" 2005; Chaudron and Schoenecker 2004). Little is known about newer antidepressant agents vortioxetine and vilazodone, so their use in pregnancy should be avoided if possible. Brexanolone, an allopregnanolone analogue approved for treatment of postpartum depression, is delivered in a 90-minute intravenous infusion. Predicted infant dosage based on maternal milk and plasma levels of brexanolone was 1%–2%. Maternal blood levels declined below detection limits within 3 days after completion of the infusion.

Antipsychotics

Little research has focused on infants exposed to antipsychotic medications through breastfeeding. On the basis of case reports of very low infant serum levels, olanzapine, quetiapine, and risperidone are first choices for lactating women who need antipsychotic treatment. Observational studies of breastfeeding women using second-generation antipsychotics have not found higher rates of adverse events in exposed infants compared with nonexposed comparison groups (Gilad et al. 2011; Viguera et al. 2022). If possible, the use of antipsychotics with fewer safety data should be avoided. The only antipsychotic contraindicated for breastfeeding is clozapine because of the risk of agranulocytosis. Among first-generation antipsychotics, haloperidol has limited evidence of low infant serum levels and lack of adverse effects (Drugs and Lactation Database 2022).

Mood Stabilizers

Lithium levels in breastfed infants average 30%–50% of maternal levels, raising concerns of lithium toxicity should the infant become dehydrated or febrile (Viguera et al. 2007a). Signs of lithium toxicity in an infant are lethargy, poor feeding, and hypotonia. Monitoring of lithium levels, serum urea nitrogen, creatinine, and thyroid-stimulating hormone is indicated for exposed infants at 6-week intervals after the in utero contribution has been cleared. Use of infant blood sampling equipment containing lithium heparin may produce spuriously high lithium levels (Arslan et al. 2016).

Studies suggest very limited diffusion of valproic acid into breast milk. Liver function, platelets, and valproic acid levels should be monitored in exposed infants.

Carbamazepine is present in infant plasma at concentrations averaging 31% of maternal levels, and a few reports have described adverse events, including hepatic toxicity and poor feeding, in breastfed infants. Use of carbamazepine while breastfeeding should be approached with caution, and infant serum levels, liver function, and complete blood count should be monitored.

Infant serum levels of lamotrigine have been found to be 18%–33% of maternal concentrations. No adverse effects, other than a case of mild thrombocytopenia, have been reported in infants (Newport et al. 2008). Complete blood count and liver function should be monitored.

Psychostimulants

Amphetamine and methylphenidate can suppress prolactin release by 20%–40%, but there is no evidence that this has an adverse effect on lactation. Few data are available to evaluate infant exposure to methylphenidate or other stimulants through breast milk. Infant serum levels of racemic amphetamine in one case report were 5%–15% of maternal serum levels (Öhman et al. 2015). No data have been published to guide use of modafinil or atomoxetine during lactation.

Adverse Obstetrical and Gynecological Reactions to Psychotropic Drugs

Hyperprolactinemia and Prolactin Suppression

Hyperprolactinemia is a relatively common side effect of psychotropic medications, particularly antipsychotic medications and SSRIs, and can interfere with the menstrual cycle and fertility. Aripiprazole inhibits prolactin release and has been anecdotally associated with lactation failure (Komaroff 2021).

A full discussion of this topic is provided in Chapter 10, "Endocrine and Metabolic Disorders."

Polycystic Ovary Syndrome

Women taking valproate have a 10% risk of developing polycystic ovary syndrome, which often corrects on medication discontinuation (Zhang et al. 2016). For premenopausal women starting to take valproate, menstrual cycle pattern, hirsutism, acne, and weight should be assessed at baseline and monitored closely, particularly during the first year of treatment, to detect development of polycystic ovary syndrome.

Effects of Psychotropic Drugs on Sexual Function

SSRIs and SNRIs produce sexual side effects in 30%–70% of users. Women experience impairments in libido, genital sensitivity, and the ability to experience orgasm. The biological mechanism responsible for these side effects is not clear, but dose reduction can be helpful. Limited evidence in women, consistent with studies in men, indicates that bupropion can increase desire, lubrication, and ability to reach orgasm in women with SSRI-induced sexual dysfunction (Safarinejad 2011). Sildenafil was also effective for improvement of arousal, orgasm, and enjoyment in women with antidepressant-associated sexual dysfunction (Nurnberg et al. 2008). SSRI-induced sexual dysfunction also improved with buspirone, and this effect was stronger in women than in men (Landén et al. 1999). Antipsychotics, TCAs, and monoamine oxidase inhibitors also can impair sexual function. No pharmacological antidotes for these agents have been identified in controlled studies. Rates of sexual side effects are lower with the antidepressants bupropion, mirtazapine, vortioxetine, and vilazodone. Among the antipsychotic medications, sexual side effects are lower with olanzapine, quetiapine, and ziprasidone and least with aripiprazole and lurasidone (Clayton et al. 2018; Montejo et al. 2021).

Psychiatric Effects of Obstetrical and Gynecological Agents and Procedures

As discussed in the following subsections, a variety of obstetrical and gynecological medications and procedures have negative psychiatric effects. Table 11–2 lists the psychiatric adverse effects of the medications.

Table 11–2. Psychiatric adverse effects of obstetrical and gynecological medications

Medication	Psychiatric adverse effects
Hormonal contraceptives	Increased mood lability and depressive symptoms
β-Adrenergic agonists (systemic)	
Terbutaline, salbutamol, and ritodrine	Anxiety
Galactagogues	
Metoclopramide	Anxiety, depression, extrapyramidal symptoms
Gonadotropins	Mood lability and irritability
Estrogen receptor modulators	
Clomiphene	Mood lability, irritability
Gonadotropin-releasing hormone agonists	
Buserelin, goserelin, histrelin, leuprolide, and nafarelin	Depression

Hormonal Contraceptives

Little systematic study has been done on the effects of hormonal contraceptives on mood. Some estimates suggest that 10%–21% of patients experience adverse mood symptoms (Lundin et al. 2017; Segebladh et al. 2009), although meta-analyses do not support this finding, and some women experience improved mood, particularly premenstrually (de Wit et al. 2021; Lundin et al. 2017). Risk factors associated with negative mood reactions are younger age, history of adverse mood reaction to oral contraception, and history of mood disorders (Segebladh et al. 2009). Higher rates of initiation of antidepressant treatment and suicide attempts were found within months after starting contraception in adolescents but not adults. The highest rates of suicide attempts and suicide were with non-oral progestin-only methods in adolescents (Skovlund et al. 2016, 2018). Hormonal contraceptives lower free testosterone levels and may thereby reduce libido in some women (Both et al. 2019; Greco et al. 2007).

Infertility Treatment

Often during artificial insemination, intrauterine insemination, and in vitro fertilization, medications are administered to stimulate ovarian follicle development, producing supraphysiological levels of circulating estrogen. A review of reports of healthy women undergoing ovarian stimulation found mild mood worsening, particularly with gonadotropin-releasing hormone agonists (González-Rodríguez et al. 2020). Little systematic study has been done of the effects of ovarian stimulation on psychiatric disorders. Women with a history of depression or anxiety are more likely to have exacerbation of anxiety and depression symptoms during in vitro fertilization treatment than are women with no history of mood disorders (Zaig et al. 2013). One study found a 40% relapse rate in women with major depression and a 30% relapse rate in women with bipolar depression during infertility treatment (Freeman et al. 2018). In addition, there are case reports of manic and psychotic reactions to clomiphene and gonadotropins, often in women with preexisting mood disorders (Choi et al. 2005; Grimm and Hubrich 2008). Gonadotropin-releasing hormone agonists, often used to stop endogenous cycling for treatment of endometriosis and for in vitro fertilization protocols, also can cause depression (Warnock et al. 2000). However, depression induction is much rarer in women who have no history of psychiatric illness (Ben Dor et al. 2013). Considering these reports, women prone to mood destabilization who are undergoing gonadal suppression or ovarian stimulation may consider continuing antidepressant medication or a mood stabilizer at least until pregnancy is achieved. However, in one prospective study, maintaining antidepressant treatment was not protective (Freeman et al. 2018).

Tocolytics

β-Adrenergic agonists prescribed to halt premature labor can be anxiogenic, and among these, salbutamol is most likely to cause anxiety (Neilson et al. 2014).

Galactagogues

Agents commonly used to increase breast milk production include the herbal supplement fenugreek and the dopamine antagonists metoclopramide and domperidone, both of which could improve lactation by increasing prolactin release. Evidence supporting efficacy of any of these agents is very limited

(Forinash et al. 2012). Domperidone (not available in the United States) has very limited CNS access and is without psychoactive effects (Osadchy et al. 2012) but has been linked to prolonged QT syndrome and sudden cardiac death, and efficacy is not well established (Paul et al. 2015). Metoclopramide acts centrally and peripherally and may cause clinically significant anxiety and depression and extrapyramidal symptoms (Anfinson 2002; Kluge et al. 2007).

Surgical or Medication-Induced Menopause

Ovariectomy or medical precipitation of menopause during treatment of endometriosis, fibroids, or breast cancer increases risk for hot flashes, depression, anxiety, pain, and sexual dysfunction compared with natural menopause and its more gradual drop in hormone levels. Surgical menopause increases lifelong risk for anxiety, depression, and dementia (Faubion et al. 2015), probably because of a longer lifetime exposure to reduced hormone levels. The increased risk of dementia, depression, and anxiety in women with surgical menopause may be attenuated by HRT initiated before age 50 (Faubion et al. 2015).

Menopausal phenomenology and treatment were also discussed earlier in the section "Pharmacotherapy for Menopause-Related Depression, Anxiety, and Insomnia."

Hormone Replacement Therapy

Estrogen and progesterone are often administered at menopause for a range of physical symptoms, including hot flashes, osteoporosis, and vaginal dryness. Although short-term estradiol can be an effective treatment for perimenopausal depression, longer-term treatment with progesterone or progestins to prevent uterine hyperplasia may have a negative effect on mood. A proportion of healthy women have adverse mood reactions to HRT, particularly the progestin components, and premorbid anxiety and premenstrual symptoms are a risk factor for adverse mood reactions to combined HRT (Björn et al. 2000, 2006; Scali et al. 2010). Cessation of HRT also may adversely affect mood in some women (Björn et al. 2000), but this possibility has not been well studied.

Testosterone supplementation by transdermal patch, spray, or cream can increase sexual desire in postmenopausal women (Wierman et al. 2014). However, because available formulations in the United States have much higher doses intended for men, low-dose preparations are suggested, which can be specially compounded (see also Chapter 10). Flibanserin, a 5-hydroxytryptamine type

1A agonist and 2A antagonist, was approved in 2015 for treatment of low libido only in premenopausal women, but there is evidence of efficacy in postmenopausal women as well (Simon et al. 2014).

Drug-Drug Interactions

Numerous complex pharmacokinetic and pharmacodynamic interactions can occur between psychotropic medications and obstetrical and gynecological medications (Tables 11–3 and 11–4). See Chapter 1, "Pharmacokinetics, Pharmacodynamics, and Principles of Drug-Drug Interactions," for a comprehensive discussion.

Pharmacokinetic Interactions

Several psychotropics, including carbamazepine, phenytoin, oxcarbazepine, topiramate, armodafinil, modafinil, and St. John's wort, induce cytochrome P450 3A4, the principal enzyme involved in sex steroid metabolism. This increased metabolism may reduce the efficacy of oral contraceptives and the vaginal ring and cause breakthrough bleeding. Carbamazepine reduces estradiol and levonorgestrel levels by 50% (Dutton and Foldvary-Schaefer 2008). Lamotrigine and carbamazepine also increase production of sex hormone–binding globulin, which binds progestins, thereby potentially reducing contraceptive efficacy of progestin-only oral and implant formulations. There are several case reports of pregnancy despite progestin implants in women also taking anticonvulsants (Dutton and Foldvary-Schaefer 2008).

Estrogen increases glucuronidation reactions through induction of uridine 5′-diphosphate glucuronosyltransferase. For psychotropic drugs eliminated primarily through conjugation (lamotrigine, valproic acid, oxazepam, lorazepam, temazepam, desvenlafaxine, and olanzapine), increased clearance has been observed with estrogen coexposure. Estrogen-containing hormonal contraceptives reduce serum levels of lamotrigine by 30%–50% and valproic acid levels by 23% (Christensen et al. 2007; Herzog et al. 2009). By increasing estradiol to supraphysiological levels, infertility treatments that stimulate ovulation may also increase glucuronidation. Lamotrigine levels are known to decline during HRT (Reimers 2017). However, it remains to be seen whether these changes in lamotrigine and valproic acid levels have a negative effect on mood. The effect of lower estradiol dosages in HRT on lamotrigine metabolism has not been studied.

Table 11–3.   Obstetrical and gynecological medication–
psychotropic medication interactions

Medication	Interaction mechanism	Effects on psychotropic medications and management
β-Adrenergic agonists (systemic), such as terbutaline	Additive hypertensive effect	Increased risk of hypertension with monoamine oxidase inhibitors; avoid concurrent use
Estradiol	Induction of uridine 5′-diphosphate glucuronosyl-transferase enzymes	Increased clearance and reduced therapeutic effect of drugs eliminated primarily through conjugation (e.g., desvenlafaxine, lamotrigine, valproic acid, lorazepam, olanzapine, oxazepam, temazepam)
Estradiol and levonorgestrel	Reduced activity of cytochrome P450 1A2, 2C19, and 3A4	Reduced clearance of clozapine; plasma levels increase two- to threefold during active hormone phase of oral contraceptives
Domperidone and terbutaline	QT prolongation	Increased QT prolongation in combination with other QT-prolonging drugs, such as tricyclic antidepressants, typical antipsychotics, lithium, pimozide, iloperidone, paliperidone, quetiapine, risperidone, and ziprasidone
Domperidone	Peripheral dopamine receptor antagonism	Increased hyperprolactinemia and galactorrhea with antipsychotics
Metoclopramide	Peripheral and central dopamine receptor antagonism	Increased extrapyramidal symptoms with antipsychotics, serotonin-norepinephrine reuptake inhibitors, and selective serotonin reuptake inhibitors Increased hyperprolactinemia and galactorrhea with antipsychotics

Table 11–4. Psychotropic medication–obstetrical and gynecological medication interactions

Medication	Interaction mechanism	Effects on obstetrical and gynecological medications and management
Carbamazepine, oxcarbazepine, phenytoin, and topiramate; armodafinil and modafinil; and St. John's wort	Induction of CYP3A4	Increased metabolism of estradiol and progesterone and possible reduced efficacy of oral contraceptives and vaginal ring
Carbamazepine and lamotrigine	Increased sex hormone–binding globulin	Reduced free progestin and estradiol levels
Atomoxetine, bupropion, duloxetine, fluoxetine, moclobemide, and paroxetine	Inhibition of CYP2D6	Reduced bioactivation of prodrug tamoxifen and decreased therapeutic effect
Atypical antipsychotics iloperidone, paliperidone, quetiapine, risperidone, and ziprasidone; lithium; pimozide; tricyclic antidepressants; citalopram; typical antipsychotics	QT prolongation	Increased QT prolongation in combination with other QT-prolonging drugs such as terbutaline and domperidone

Note. CYP=cytochrome P450.

Oral contraceptives containing estradiol or levonorgestrel also reduce activity of the cytochrome P450 enzymes 1A2, 2C19, and 3A4, which can increase plasma clozapine concentrations two- to threefold. Clozapine dosage needs to be reduced during the active hormone phase of the contraceptive preparation. For this reason, non-oral contraceptive preparations that bypass first-pass metabolism in the liver are preferred for women taking clozapine (Bookholt and Bogers 2014).

Pharmacodynamic Interactions

Several drugs used in obstetrics and gynecology, including terbutaline and domperidone, prolong the QT interval. These agents should be used with caution in the presence of other drugs that have QT-prolonging effects, such as TCAs, typical antipsychotics, pimozide, risperidone, paliperidone, iloperidone, quetiapine, ziprasidone, and lithium. Systemic β-adrenergic agonist tocolytics, such as terbutaline, may precipitate a hypertensive crisis in combination with monoamine oxidase inhibitors. Metoclopramide may increase extrapyramidal symptoms when coadministered with antipsychotics, SSRIs, or SNRIs.

Key Points

- All psychotropic medications must be selected in light of the possibility of pregnancy, and patients should be counseled about the risks and benefits of medication (and untreated psychopathology) during pregnancy and lactation.

- To distinguish premenstrual dysphoric disorder (PMDD) from premenstrual exacerbation of another psychiatric disorder, PMDD should be diagnosed with two cycles of prospective ratings before treatment is initiated.

- Selective serotonin reuptake inhibitors (SSRIs), serotonin-norepinephrine reuptake inhibitors (SNRIs), and the drospirenone-containing oral contraceptives are effective treatments for PMDD.

- Untreated psychiatric illness carries a risk to mother and fetus, dependent on severity of illness.

- Valproic acid and carbamazepine should be avoided if possible because of high risk of teratogenic and neurodevelopmental effects.

- Generally, infant exposure to psychotropic drugs through breast milk is substantially lower than levels of exposure in utero. Lithium, carbamazepine, and lamotrigine are exceptions.

- Among antidepressants, sertraline and paroxetine have the most data supportive of safety during lactation.

- Risk of depressive symptoms and major depression recurrence is elevated during perimenopause but not after menopause.

- Hormone replacement therapy can relieve depression during perimenopause but not after menopause.

- Vasomotor symptoms respond to SSRIs, SNRIs, and gabapentin in some women, but response rates are lower than with estradiol treatment.

References

Abramowitz A, Miller ES, Wisner KL: Treatment options for hyperemesis gravidarum. Arch Womens Ment Health 20(3):363–372, 2017 28070660

Ahern E, Cohen D, Prior C, et al: Menstrual psychosis. Ir J Psychol Med 39(1):103–105, 2022 31500681

Andrade C: Selective serotonin reuptake inhibitor use in pregnancy and risk of postpartum hemorrhage. J Clin Psychiatry 83(2):22f14455, 2022 35390232

Anfinson TJ: Akathisia, panic, agoraphobia, and major depression following brief exposure to metoclopramide. Psychopharmacol Bull 36(1):82–93, 2002 12397849

Ankarfeldt MZ, Petersen J, Andersen JT, et al: Exposure to duloxetine during pregnancy and risk of congenital malformations and stillbirth: a nationwide cohort study in Denmark and Sweden. PLoS Med 18(11):e1003851, 2021 34807906

Arslan Z, Athiraman NK, Clark SJ: Lithium toxicity in a neonate owing to false elevation of blood lithium levels caused by contamination in a lithium heparin container: case report and review of the literature. Paediatr Int Child Health 36(3):240–242, 2016 26249250

Bais B, Munk-Olsen T, Bergink V, et al: Prescription patterns of benzodiazepine and benzodiazepine-related drugs in the peripartum period: a population-based study. Psychiatry Res 288:112993, 2020 32334277

Ban L, West J, Gibson JE, et al: First trimester exposure to anxiolytic and hypnotic drugs and the risks of major congenital anomalies: a United Kingdom population-based cohort study. PLoS One 9(6):e100996, 2014 24963627

Ben Dor R, Harsh VL, Fortinsky P, et al: Effects of pharmacologically induced hypogonadism on mood and behavior in healthy young women. Am J Psychiatry 170(4):426–433, 2013 23545794

Bergink V, Burgerhout KM, Koorengevel KM, et al: Treatment of psychosis and mania in the postpartum period. Am J Psychiatry 172(2):115–123, 2015 25640930

Beroukhim G, Esencan E, Seifer DB: Impact of sleep patterns upon female neuroendocrinology and reproductive outcomes: a comprehensive review. Reprod Biol Endocrinol 20(1):16, 2022 35042515

Björn I, Bixo M, Nöjd KS, et al: Negative mood changes during hormone replacement therapy: a comparison between two progestogens. Am J Obstet Gynecol 183(6):1419–1426, 2000 11120505

Björn I, Bäckström T, Lalos A, et al: Adverse mood effects during postmenopausal hormone treatment in relation to personality traits. Climacteric 9(4):290–297, 2006 16857659

Blackmore ER, Rubinow DR, O'Connor TG, et al: Reproductive outcomes and risk of subsequent illness in women diagnosed with postpartum psychosis. Bipolar Disord 15(4):394–404, 2013 23651079

Bookholt DE, Bogers JP: Oral contraceptives raise plasma clozapine concentrations. J Clin Psychopharmacol 34(3):389–390, 2014 24717251

Both S, Lew-Starowicz M, Luria M, et al: Hormonal contraception and female sexuality: position statements from the European Society of Sexual Medicine (ESSM). J Sex Med 16(11):1681–1695, 2019 31521571

Bupropion: seizures in an infant exposed through breast-feeding. Prescrire Int 14(78):144, 2005 16108101

Carmassi C, Del Grande C, Masci I, et al: Lithium and valproate serum level fluctuations within the menstrual cycle: a systematic review. Int Clin Psychopharmacol 34(3):143–150, 2019 30907774

Casilla-Lennon MM, Meltzer-Brody S, Steiner AZ: The effect of antidepressants on fertility. Am J Obstet Gynecol 215(3):314.e1–314.e5, 2016 26827878

Cesta CE, Månsson M, Palm C, et al: Polycystic ovary syndrome and psychiatric disorders: co-morbidity and heritability in a nationwide Swedish cohort. Psychoneuroendocrinology 73:196–203, 2016 27513883

Cesta CE, Engeland A, Karlsson P, et al: Incidence of malformations after early pregnancy exposure to modafinil in Sweden and Norway. JAMA 324(9):895–897, 2020 32870289

Chaudron LH, Schoenecker CJ: Bupropion and breastfeeding: a case of a possible infant seizure. J Clin Psychiatry 65(6):881–882, 2004 15291673

Choi SH, Shapiro H, Robinson GE, et al: Psychological side-effects of clomiphene citrate and human menopausal gonadotrophin. J Psychosom Obstet Gynaecol 26(2):93–100, 2005 16050534

Christensen J, Petrenaite V, Atterman J, et al: Oral contraceptives induce lamotrigine metabolism: evidence from a double-blind, placebo-controlled trial. Epilepsia 48(3):484–489, 2007 17346247

Clayton AH, Tsai J, Mao Y, et al: Effect of lurasidone on sexual function in major depressive disorder patients with subthreshold hypomanic symptoms (mixed features): results from a placebo-controlled trial. J Clin Psychiatry 79(5):18m12132, 2018 30086213

Cohen LS, Altshuler LL, Harlow BL, et al: Relapse of major depression during pregnancy in women who maintain or discontinue antidepressant treatment. JAMA 295(5):499–507, 2006 16449615

Colen CG, Ramey DM: Is breast truly best? Estimating the effects of breastfeeding on long-term child health and wellbeing in the United States using sibling comparisons. Soc Sci Med 109:55–65, 2014 24698713

Comasco E, Kopp Kallner H, Bixo M, et al: Ulipristal acetate for treatment of premenstrual dysphoric disorder: a proof-of-concept randomized controlled trial. Am J Psychiatry 178(3):256–265, 2021 33297719

de Wit AE, de Vries YA, de Boer MK, et al: Hormonal contraceptive use and depressive symptoms: systematic review and network meta-analysis of randomised trials. BJPsych Open 7(4):e110, 2021 34099098

Diav-Citrin O, Shechtman S, Tahover E, et al: Pregnancy outcome following in utero exposure to lithium: a prospective, comparative, observational study. Am J Psychiatry 171(7):785–794, 2014 24781368

Drugs and Lactation Database: Methylphenidate. 2022. Available at: www.ncbi.nlm.nih.gov/books/NBK501310/#:~:text=Summary%20of%20Use%20during%20Lactation&text=If%20methylphenidate%20is%20required%20by,lactation%20is%20not%20well%20established. Accessed September 29, 2022.

Dutton C, Foldvary-Schaefer N: Contraception in women with epilepsy: pharmacokinetic interactions, contraceptive options, and management. Int Rev Neurobiol 83:113–134, 2008 18929078

Edwards AC, Lonn SL, Crump C, et al: Oral contraceptive use and risk of suicidal behavior among young women. Psychol Med 52(9):1710–1717, 2022 33084550

Epperson CN, Shanmugan S, Kim DR, et al: New onset executive function difficulties at menopause: a possible role for lisdexamfetamine. Psychopharmacology (Berl) 232(16):3091–3100, 2015 26063677

Etwel F, Faught LH, Rieder MJ, et al: The risk of adverse pregnancy outcome after first trimester exposure to H1 antihistamines: a systematic review and meta-analysis. Drug Saf 40(2):121–132, 2017 27878468

Faubion SS, Kuhle CL, Shuster LT, et al: Long-term health consequences of premature or early menopause and considerations for management. Climacteric 18(4):483–491, 2015 25845383

Forinash AB, Yancey AM, Barnes KN, et al: The use of galactogogues in the breast-feeding mother. Ann Pharmacother 46(10):1392–1404, 2012 23012383

Forsberg L, Adler M, Römer Ek I, et al: Maternal mood disorders and lithium exposure in utero were not associated with poor cognitive development during childhood. Acta Paediatr 107(8):1379–1388, 2018 29150869

Freeman EW, Sammel MD, Lin H, et al: The role of anxiety and hormonal changes in menopausal hot flashes. Menopause 12(3):258–266, 2005 15879914

Freeman MP, Smith KW, Freeman SA, et al: The impact of reproductive events on the course of bipolar disorder in women. J Clin Psychiatry 63(4):284–287, 2002 12004800

Freeman MP, Lee H, Savella GM, et al: Predictors of depressive relapse in women undergoing infertility treatment. J Womens Health (Larchmt) 27(11):1408–1414, 2018 30067141

Friedman BE, Rogers JL, Shahine LK, et al: Effect of selective serotonin reuptake inhibitors on in vitro fertilization outcome. Fertil Steril 92(4):1312–1314, 2009 19423105

Genazzani AR, Monteleone P, Giannini A, et al: Pharmacotherapeutic options for the treatment of menopausal symptoms. Expert Opin Pharmacother 22(13):1773–1791, 2021 33980106

Gilad O, Merlob P, Stahl B, et al: Outcome of infants exposed to olanzapine during breastfeeding. Breastfeed Med 6(2):55–58, 2011 21034242

Giles JJ, Bannigan JG: Teratogenic and developmental effects of lithium. Curr Pharm Des 12(12):1531–1541, 2006 16611133

González-Rodríguez A, Cobo J, Soria V, et al: Women undergoing hormonal treatments for infertility: a systematic review on psychopathology and newly diagnosed mood and psychotic disorders. Front Psychiatry 11:479, 2020 32528332

Gordon JL, Rubinow DR, Eisenlohr-Moul TA, et al: Efficacy of transdermal estradiol and micronized progesterone in the prevention of depressive symptoms in the menopause transition: a randomized clinical trial. JAMA Psychiatry 75(2):149–157, 2018 29322164

Greco T, Graham CA, Bancroft J, et al: The effects of oral contraceptives on androgen levels and their relevance to premenstrual mood and sexual interest: a comparison of two triphasic formulations containing norgestimate and either 35 or 25 microg of ethinyl estradiol. Contraception 76(1):8–17, 2007 17586130

Grigoriadis S, Vonderporten EH, Mamisashvili L, et al: Prenatal exposure to antidepressants and persistent pulmonary hypertension of the newborn: systematic review and meta-analysis. BMJ 348:f6932, 2014 24429387

Grigoriadis S, Graves L, Peer M, et al: Pregnancy and delivery outcomes following benzodiazepine exposure: a systematic review and meta-analysis. Can J Psychiatry 65(12):821–834, 2020 32148076

Grimm O, Hubrich P: Delusional belief induced by clomiphene treatment. Prog Neuropsychopharmacol Biol Psychiatry 32(5):1338–1339, 2008 18538909

Guthrie KA, LaCroix AZ, Ensrud KE, et al: Pooled analysis of six pharmacologic and nonpharmacologic interventions for vasomotor symptoms. Obstet Gynecol 126(2):413–422, 2015 26241433

Hálfdánarson Ó, Cohen JM, Karlstad Ø, et al: Antipsychotic use in pregnancy and risk of attention/deficit-hyperactivity disorder and autism spectrum disorder: a Nordic cohort study. Evid Based Ment Health 25(2):54–62, 2022 34810174

Hamlat EJ, Laraia B, Bleil ME, et al: Effects of early life adversity on pubertal timing and tempo in Black and White girls: the National Growth and Health Study. Psychosom Med 84(3):297–305, 2022 35067653

Handy AB, Greenfield SF, Yonkers KA, et al: Psychiatric symptoms across the menstrual cycle in adult women: a comprehensive review. Harv Rev Psychiatry 30(2):100–117, 2022 35267252

Harlow BL, Wise LA, Otto MW, et al: Depression and its influence on reproductive endocrine and menstrual cycle markers associated with perimenopause: the Harvard Study of Moods and Cycles. Arch Gen Psychiatry 60(1):29–36, 2003 12511170

Hastie R, Tong S, Hiscock R, et al: Maternal lithium use and the risk of adverse pregnancy and neonatal outcomes: a Swedish population-based cohort study. BMC Med 19(1):291, 2021 34856987

Hernández-Díaz S, Werler MM, Walker AM, et al: Neural tube defects in relation to use of folic acid antagonists during pregnancy. Am J Epidemiol 153(10):961–968, 2001 11384952

Hernández-Díaz S, Smith CR, Shen A, et al: Comparative safety of antiepileptic drugs during pregnancy. Neurology 78(21):1692–1699, 2012 22551726

Herzog AG, Blum AS, Farina EL, et al: Valproate and lamotrigine level variation with menstrual cycle phase and oral contraceptive use. Neurology 72(10):911–914, 2009 19273825

Huitfeldt A, Sundbakk LM, Skurtveit S, et al: Associations of maternal use of benzodiazepines or benzodiazepine-like hypnotics during pregnancy with immediate pregnancy outcomes in Norway. JAMA Netw Open 3(6):e205860, 2020 32568398

Hunter MS: Cognitive behavioral therapy for menopausal symptoms. Climacteric 24(1):51–56, 2021 32627593

Huybrechts KF, Bateman BT, Palmsten K, et al: Antidepressant use late in pregnancy and risk of persistent pulmonary hypertension of the newborn. JAMA 313(21):2142–2151, 2015 26034955

Huybrechts KF, Hernández-Díaz S, Patorno E, et al: Antipsychotic use in pregnancy and the risk for congenital malformations. JAMA Psychiatry 73(9):938–946, 2016 27540849

Huybrechts KF, Bröms G, Christensen LB, et al: Association between methylphenidate and amphetamine use in pregnancy and risk of congenital malformations: a cohort study from the International Pregnancy Safety Study Consortium. JAMA Psychiatry 75(2):167–175, 2018 29238795

Huybrechts KF, Bateman BT, Pawar A, et al: Maternal and fetal outcomes following exposure to duloxetine in pregnancy: cohort study. BMJ 368:m237, 2020 32075794

Jablensky AV, Morgan V, Zubrick SR, et al: Pregnancy, delivery, and neonatal complications in a population cohort of women with schizophrenia and major affective disorders. Am J Psychiatry 162(1):79–91, 2005 15625205

Jacobson NC: Current evolutionary adaptiveness of psychiatric disorders: fertility rates, parent-child relationship quality, and psychiatric disorders across the lifespan. J Abnorm Psychol 125(6):824–839, 2016 27362490

Jarde A, Morais M, Kingston D, et al: Neonatal outcomes in women with untreated antenatal depression compared with women without depression: a systematic review and meta-analysis. JAMA Psychiatry 73(8):826–837, 2016 27276520

Jensen AG, Knudsen SS, Bech BH: Prenatal exposure to benzodiazepines and the development of the offspring: a systematic review. Neurotoxicol Teratol 91:107078, 2022 35189281

Joffe H, Petrillo LF, Koukopoulos A, et al: Increased estradiol and improved sleep, but not hot flashes, predict enhanced mood during the menopausal transition. J Clin Endocrinol Metab 96(7):E1044–E1054, 2011 21525161

Kaplan S, Braverman DL, Frishman I, et al: Pregnancy and fetal outcomes following exposure to modafinil and armodafinil during pregnancy. JAMA Intern Med 181(2):275–277, 2021 33074297

Kjeldgaard HK, Eberhard-Gran M, Benth JS, et al: History of depression and risk of hyperemesis gravidarum: a population-based cohort study. Arch Womens Ment Health 20(3):397–404, 2017 28064341

Kluge M, Schüssler P, Steiger A: Persistent generalized anxiety after brief exposure to the dopamine antagonist metoclopramide. Psychiatry Clin Neurosci 61(2):193–195, 2007 17362439

Komaroff A: Aripiprazole and lactation failure: the importance of shared decision making. A case report. Case Rep Womens Health 30:e00308, 2021 33796446

Kuehner C, Nayman S: Premenstrual exacerbations of mood disorders: findings and knowledge gaps. Curr Psychiatry Rep 23(11):78, 2021 34626258

Kulkarni J: Depression as a side effect of the contraceptive pill. Expert Opin Drug Saf 6(4):371–374, 2007 17688380

Landén M, Eriksson E, Agren H, et al: Effect of buspirone on sexual dysfunction in depressed patients treated with selective serotonin reuptake inhibitors. J Clin Psychopharmacol 19(3):268–271, 1999 10350034

Langer RD, Hodis HN, Lobo RA, et al: Hormone replacement therapy: where are we now? Climacteric 24(1):3–10, 2021 33403881

Li Q, Mitchell AA, Werler MM, et al: Assessment of antihistamine use in early pregnancy and birth defects. J Allergy Clin Immunol Pract 1(6):666.e1–674.e1, 2013 24565715

Lopez LM, Kaptein AA, Helmerhorst FM: Oral contraceptives containing drospirenone for premenstrual syndrome. Cochrane Database Syst Rev(2):CD006586, 2012 22336820

Loughhead AM, Fisher AD, Newport DJ, et al: Antidepressants in amniotic fluid: another route of fetal exposure. Am J Psychiatry 163(1):145–147, 2006 16390902

Lundin C, Danielsson KG, Bixo M, et al: Combined oral contraceptive use is associated with both improvement and worsening of mood in the different phases of the treatment cycle—a double-blind, placebo-controlled randomized trial. Psychoneuroendocrinology 76:135–143, 2017 27923181

Lupattelli A, Chambers CD, Bandoli G, et al: Association of maternal use of benzodiazepines and Z-hypnotics during pregnancy with motor and communication skills and attention-deficit/hyperactivity disorder symptoms in preschoolers. JAMA Netw Open 2(4):e191435, 2019 30951155

Maki PM, Kornstein SG, Joffe H, et al: Guidelines for the evaluation and treatment of perimenopausal depression: summary and recommendations. J Womens Health (Larchmt) 28(2):117–134, 2019 30182804

Malm H, Sourander A, Gissler M, et al: Pregnancy complications following prenatal exposure to SSRIs or maternal psychiatric disorders: results from population-based National Register data. Am J Psychiatry 172(12):1224–1232, 2015 26238606

Månsson M, Holte J, Landin-Wilhelmsen K, et al: Women with polycystic ovary syndrome are often depressed or anxious: a case control study. Psychoneuroendocrinology 33(8):1132–1138, 2008 18672334

Mantel Ä, Örtqvist AK, Hirschberg AL, et al: Analysis of neurodevelopmental disorders in offspring of mothers with eating disorders in Sweden. JAMA Netw Open 5(1):e2143947, 2022 35040968

Marjoribanks J, Brown J, O'Brien PM, et al: Selective serotonin reuptake inhibitors for premenstrual syndrome. Cochrane Database Syst Rev (6):CD001396, 2013 23744611

Meador KJ, Baker GA, Browning N, et al: Cognitive function at 3 years of age after fetal exposure to antiepileptic drugs. N Engl J Med 360(16):1597–1605, 2009 19369666

Micali N, Treasure J, Simonoff E: Eating disorders symptoms in pregnancy: a longitudinal study of women with recent and past eating disorders and obesity. J Psychosom Res 63(3):297–303, 2007 17719368

Momen NC, Robakis T, Liu X, et al: In utero exposure to antipsychotic medication and psychiatric outcomes in the offspring. Neuropsychopharmacology 47(3):759–766, 2022 34750566

Monk C, Lugo-Candelas C, Trumpff C: Prenatal developmental origins of future psychopathology: mechanisms and pathways. Annu Rev Clin Psychol 15:317–344, 2019 30795695

Montejo AL, de Alarcón R, Prieto N, et al: Management strategies for antipsychotic-related sexual dysfunction: a clinical approach. J Clin Med 10(2):308, 2021 33467621

Morgan ML, Cook IA, Rapkin AJ, et al: Estrogen augmentation of antidepressants in perimenopausal depression: a pilot study. J Clin Psychiatry 66(6):774–780, 2005 15960574

Morrison MF, Kallan MJ, Ten Have T, et al: Lack of efficacy of estradiol for depression in postmenopausal women: a randomized, controlled trial. Biol Psychiatry 55(4):406–412, 2004 14960294

Moses-Kolko EL, Bogen D, Perel J, et al: Neonatal signs after late in utero exposure to serotonin reuptake inhibitors: literature review and implications for clinical applications. JAMA 293(19):2372–2383, 2005 15900008

Munk-Olsen T, Liu X, Viktorin A, et al: Maternal and infant outcomes associated with lithium use in pregnancy: an international collaborative meta-analysis of six cohort studies. Lancet Psychiatry 5(8):644–652, 2018 29929874

Neilson JP, West HM, Dowswell T: Betamimetics for inhibiting preterm labour. Cochrane Database Syst Rev (2):CD004352, 2014 24500892

Newport DJ, Viguera AC, Beach AJ, et al: Lithium placental passage and obstetrical outcome: implications for clinical management during late pregnancy. Am J Psychiatry 162(11):2162–2170, 2005 16263858

Newport DJ, Calamaras MR, DeVane CL, et al: Atypical antipsychotic administration during late pregnancy: placental passage and obstetrical outcomes. Am J Psychiatry 164(8):1214–1220, 2007 17671284

Newport DJ, Pennell PB, Calamaras MR, et al: Lamotrigine in breast milk and nursing infants: determination of exposure. Pediatrics 122(1):e223–e231, 2008 18591203

Nicholson WK, Robinson KA, Smallridge RC, et al: Prevalence of postpartum thyroid dysfunction: a quantitative review. Thyroid 16(6):573–582, 2006 16839259

Nillni YI, Wesselink AK, Hatch EE, et al: Mental health, psychotropic medication use, and menstrual cycle characteristics. Clin Epidemiol 10:1073–1082, 2018 30214312

Nulman I, Rovet J, Stewart DE, et al: Neurodevelopment of children exposed in utero to antidepressant drugs. N Engl J Med 336(4):258–262, 1997 8995088

Nulman I, Rovet J, Stewart DE, et al: Child development following exposure to tricyclic antidepressants or fluoxetine throughout fetal life: a prospective, controlled study. Am J Psychiatry 159(11):1889–1895, 2002 12411224

Nurnberg HG, Hensley PL, Heiman JR, et al: Sildenafil treatment of women with antidepressant-associated sexual dysfunction: a randomized controlled trial. JAMA 300(4):395–404, 2008 18647982

Oberlander TF, Warburton W, Misri S, et al: Neonatal outcomes after prenatal exposure to selective serotonin reuptake inhibitor antidepressants and maternal depression using population-based linked health data. Arch Gen Psychiatry 63(8):898–906, 2006 16894066

Occhiogrosso M, Omran SS, Altemus M: Persistent pulmonary hypertension of the newborn and selective serotonin reuptake inhibitors: lessons from clinical and translational studies. Am J Psychiatry 169(2):134–140, 2012 22420034

Öhman I, Wikner BN, Beck O, et al: Narcolepsy treated with racemic amphetamine during pregnancy and breastfeeding. J Hum Lact 31(3):374–376, 2015 25948577

Ornoy A, Zvi N, Arnon J, et al: The outcome of pregnancy following topiramate treatment: a study on 52 pregnancies. Reprod Toxicol 25(3):388–389, 2008 18424066

Orri M, Pingault JB, Turecki G, et al: Contribution of birth weight to mental health, cognitive and socioeconomic outcomes: two-sample Mendelian randomisation. Br J Psychiatry 219(3):507–514, 2021 33583444

Osadchy A, Moretti ME, Koren G: Effect of domperidone on insufficient lactation in puerperal women: a systematic review and meta-analysis of randomized controlled trials. Obstet Gynecol Int 2012:642893, 2012 22461793

Ostenfeld A, Petersen TS, Pedersen LH, et al: Mirtazapine exposure in pregnancy and fetal safety: a nationwide cohort study. Acta Psychiatr Scand 145(6):557–567, 2022 35320582

Park Y, Hernandez-Diaz S, Bateman BT, et al: Continuation of atypical antipsychotic medication during early pregnancy and the risk of gestational diabetes. Am J Psychiatry 175(6):564–574, 2018 29730938

Patorno E, Hernandez-Diaz S, Huybrechts KF, et al: Gabapentin in pregnancy and the risk of adverse neonatal and maternal outcomes: a population-based cohort study nested in the US Medicaid Analytic eXtract dataset. PLoS Med 17(9):e1003322, 2020 32870921

Paul C, Zénut M, Dorut A, et al: Use of domperidone as a galactagogue drug: a systematic review of the benefit-risk ratio. J Hum Lact 31(1):57–63, 2015 25475074

Pedersen LH, Henriksen TB, Olsen J: Fetal exposure to antidepressants and normal milestone development at 6 and 19 months of age. Pediatrics 125(3):e600–e608, 2010 20176667

Perich T, Ussher J, Meade T: Menopause and illness course in bipolar disorder: a systematic review. Bipolar Disord 19(6):434–443, 2017 28796389

Picchietti DL, Hensley JG, Bainbridge JL, et al: Consensus clinical practice guidelines for the diagnosis and treatment of restless legs syndrome/Willis-Ekbom disease during pregnancy and lactation. Sleep Med Rev 22:64–77, 2015 25553600

Pilowsky DJ, Wickramaratne P, Talati A, et al: Children of depressed mothers 1 year after the initiation of maternal treatment: findings from the STAR*D-Child Study. Am J Psychiatry 165(9):1136–1147, 2008 18558646

Poels EMP, Schrijver L, White TJH, et al: The effect of prenatal lithium exposure on the neuropsychological development of the child. Bipolar Disord 24(3):310–319, 2022 34585812

Power RA, Kyaga S, Uher R, et al: Fecundity of patients with schizophrenia, autism, bipolar disorder, depression, anorexia nervosa, or substance abuse vs their unaffected siblings. JAMA Psychiatry 70(1):22–30, 2013 23147713

Reimers A: Hormone replacement therapy with estrogens may reduce lamotrigine serum concentrations: a matched case-control study. Epilepsia 58(1):e6–e9, 2017 27805259

Riecher-Rössler A, Butler S, Kulkarni J: Sex and gender differences in schizophrenic psychoses—a critical review. Arch Womens Ment Health 21(6):627–648, 2018 29766281

Rose S, Dotters-Katz SK, Kuller JA: Electroconvulsive therapy in pregnancy: safety, best practices, and barriers to care. Obstet Gynecol Surv 75(3):199–203, 2020 32232498

Rose SJ, Hathcock MA, White WM, et al: Amphetamine-dextroamphetamine and pregnancy: neonatal outcomes after prenatal prescription mixed amphetamine exposure. J Atten Disord 25(9):1295–1301, 2021 31931669

Rundgren S, Brus O, Båve U, et al: Improvement of postpartum depression and psychosis after electroconvulsive therapy: a population-based study with a matched comparison group. J Affect Disord 235:258–264, 2018 29660641

Safarinejad MR: Reversal of SSRI-induced female sexual dysfunction by adjunctive bupropion in menstruating women: a double-blind, placebo-controlled and randomized study. J Psychopharmacol 25(3):370–378, 2011 20080928

Salisbury AL, O'Grady KE, Battle CL, et al: The roles of maternal depression, serotonin reuptake inhibitor treatment, and concomitant benzodiazepine use on infant neurobehavioral functioning over the first postnatal month. Am J Psychiatry 173(2):147–157, 2016 26514656

Sanefuji M, Senju A, Shimono M, et al: Breast feeding and infant development in a cohort with sibling pair analysis: the Japan Environment and Children's Study. BMJ Open 11(8):e043202, 2021 34380712

Sanjuan PM, Fokas K, Tonigan JS, et al: Prenatal maternal posttraumatic stress disorder as a risk factor for adverse birth weight and gestational age outcomes: a systematic review and meta-analysis. J Affect Disord 295:530–540, 2021 34509068

Santucci AK, Singer LT, Wisniewski SR, et al: Impact of prenatal exposure to serotonin reuptake inhibitors or maternal major depressive disorder on infant developmental outcomes. J Clin Psychiatry 75(10):1088–1095, 2014 25373117

Sanz EJ, De-las-Cuevas C, Kiuru A, et al: Selective serotonin reuptake inhibitors in pregnant women and neonatal withdrawal syndrome: a database analysis. Lancet 365(9458):482–487, 2005 15705457

Scali J, Ryan J, Carrière I, et al: A prospective study of hormone therapy and depression in community-dwelling elderly women: the Three City Study. J Clin Psychiatry 71(12):1673–1679, 2010 20816026

Schliep KC, Mumford SL, Vladutiu CJ, et al: Perceived stress, reproductive hormones, and ovulatory function: a prospective cohort study. Epidemiology 26(2):177–184, 2015 25643098

Schliep KC, Mumford SL, Silver RM, et al: Preconception perceived stress is associated with reproductive hormone levels and longer time to pregnancy. Epidemiology 30(Suppl 2):S76–S84, 2019 31569156

Schmidt PJ, Nieman L, Danaceau MA, et al: Estrogen replacement in perimenopause-related depression: a preliminary report. Am J Obstet Gynecol 183(2):414–420, 2000 10942479

Segebladh B, Borgström A, Odlind V, et al: Prevalence of psychiatric disorders and premenstrual dysphoric symptoms in patients with experience of adverse mood during treatment with combined oral contraceptives. Contraception 79(1):50–55, 2009 19041441

Simoila L, Isometsä E, Gissler M, et al: Schizophrenia and pregnancy: a national register-based follow-up study among Finnish women born between 1965 and 1980. Arch Womens Ment Health 23(1):91–100, 2020 30762149

Simon JA, Kingsberg SA, Shumel B, et al: Efficacy and safety of flibanserin in post-menopausal women with hypoactive sexual desire disorder: results of the SNOWDROP trial. Menopause 21(6):633–640, 2014 24281236

Sjaarda LA, Radoc JG, Flannagan KS, et al: Urinary selective serotonin reuptake inhibitors across critical windows of pregnancy establishment: a prospective cohort study of fecundability and pregnancy loss. Fertil Steril 114(6):1278–1287, 2020 33066974

Skovlund CW, Mørch LS, Kessing LV, et al: Association of hormonal contraception with depression. JAMA Psychiatry 73(11):1154–1162, 2016 27680324

Skovlund CW, Mørch LS, Kessing LV, et al: Association of hormonal contraception with suicide attempts and suicides. Am J Psychiatry 175(4):336–342, 2018 29145752

Soares CN, Almeida OP, Joffe H, et al: Efficacy of estradiol for the treatment of depressive disorders in perimenopausal women: a double-blind, randomized, placebo-controlled trial. Arch Gen Psychiatry 58(6):529–534, 2001 11386980

Soares CN, Joffe H, Rubens R, et al: Eszopiclone in patients with insomnia during perimenopause and early postmenopause: a randomized controlled trial. Obstet Gynecol 108(6):1402–1410, 2006 17138773

Straub L, Hernández-Díaz S, Bateman BT, et al: Association of antipsychotic drug exposure in pregnancy with risk of neurodevelopmental disorders: a National Birth Cohort Study. JAMA Intern Med 182(5):522–533, 2022 35343998

Traylor CS, Johnson JD, Kimmel MC, et al: Effects of psychological stress on adverse pregnancy outcomes and nonpharmacologic approaches for reduction: an expert review. Am J Obstet Gynecol MFM 2(4):100229, 2020 32995736

Truong D, Marsh W: Bipolar disorder in the menopausal transition. Curr Psychiatry Rep 21(12):130, 2019 31768664

Turner E, Jones M, Vaz LR, et al: Systematic review and meta-analysis to assess the safety of bupropion and varenicline in pregnancy. Nicotine Tob Res 21(8):1001–1010, 2019 29579233

Uguz F: A new safety scoring system for the use of psychotropic drugs during lactation. Am J Ther 28(1):e118–e126, 2021 30601177

Usall J, Pinto-Meza A, Fernández A, et al: Suicide ideation across reproductive life cycle of women: results from a European epidemiological study. J Affect Disord 116(1–2):144–147, 2009 19155069

Vega ML, Newport GC, Bozhdaraj D, et al: Implementation of advanced methods for reproductive pharmacovigilance in autism: a meta-analysis of the effects of prenatal antidepressant exposure. Am J Psychiatry 177(6):506–517, 2020 32375539

Viguera AC, Nonacs R, Cohen LS, et al: Risk of recurrence of bipolar disorder in pregnant and nonpregnant women after discontinuing lithium maintenance. Am J Psychiatry 157(2):179–184, 2000 10671384

Viguera AC, Newport DJ, Ritchie J, et al: Lithium in breast milk and nursing infants: clinical implications. Am J Psychiatry 164(2):342–345, 2007a 17267800

Viguera AC, Whitfield T, Baldessarini RJ, et al: Risk of recurrence in women with bipolar disorder during pregnancy: prospective study of mood stabilizer discontinuation. Am J Psychiatry 164(12):1817–1824, quiz 1923, 2007b 18056236

Viguera AC, Vanderkruik R, Gaccione P, et al: Breastfeeding practices among women taking second-generation antipsychotics: findings from the National Pregnancy Registry for Atypical Antipsychotics. Arch Womens Ment Health 25(2):511–516, 2022 34318375

Waller DK, Shaw GM, Rasmussen SA, et al: Prepregnancy obesity as a risk factor for structural birth defects. Arch Pediatr Adolesc Med 161(8):745–750, 2007 17679655

Wang X, Zhang T, Ekheden I, et al: Prenatal exposure to benzodiazepines and Z-drugs in humans and risk of adverse neurodevelopmental outcomes in offspring: a systematic review. Neurosci Biobehav Rev 137:104647, 2022 35367514

Warnock JK, Bundren JC, Morris DW: Depressive mood symptoms associated with ovarian suppression. Fertil Steril 74(5):984–986, 2000 11056245

Watson HJ, Zerwas S, Torgersen L, et al: Maternal eating disorders and perinatal outcomes: a three-generation study in the Norwegian Mother and Child Cohort Study. J Abnorm Psychol 126(5):552–564, 2017 28691845

Webb R, Abel K, Pickles A, et al: Mortality in offspring of parents with psychotic disorders: a critical review and meta-analysis. Am J Psychiatry 162(6):1045–1056, 2005 15930050

Weber MT, Maki PM, McDermott MP: Cognition and mood in perimenopause: a systematic review and meta-analysis. J Steroid Biochem Mol Biol 142:90–98, 2014 23770320

Wegner I, Wilhelm AJ, Lambrechts DA, et al: Effect of oral contraceptives on lamotrigine levels depends on comedication. Acta Neurol Scand 129(6):393–398, 2014 24571554

Wesseloo R, Kamperman AM, Munk-Olsen T, et al: Risk of postpartum relapse in bipolar disorder and postpartum psychosis: a systematic review and meta-analysis. Am J Psychiatry 173(2):117–127, 2016 26514657

Wesseloo R, Kamperman AM, Bergink V, et al: Thyroid peroxidase antibodies during early gestation and the subsequent risk of first-onset postpartum depression: a prospective cohort study. J Affect Disord 225:399–403, 2018 28850854

Wesström J, Skalkidou A, Manconi M, et al: Pre-pregnancy restless legs syndrome (Willis-Ekbom disease) is associated with perinatal depression. J Clin Sleep Med 10(5):527–533, 2014 24812538

Wierman ME, Arlt W, Basson R, et al: Androgen therapy in women: a reappraisal: an Endocrine Society clinical practice guideline. J Clin Endocrinol Metab 99(10):3489–3510, 2014 25279570

Wikner BN, Källén B: Are hypnotic benzodiazepine receptor agonists teratogenic in humans? J Clin Psychopharmacol 31(3):356–359, 2011 21508851

Wu P, Velez Edwards DR, Gorrindo P, et al: Association between first trimester antidepressant use and risk of spontaneous abortion. Pharmacotherapy 39(9):889–898, 2019 31278762

Wyszynski DF, Nambisan M, Surve T, et al: Increased rate of major malformations in offspring exposed to valproate during pregnancy. Neurology 64(6):961–965, 2005 15781808

Yang S, Martin RM, Oken E, et al: Breastfeeding during infancy and neurocognitive function in adolescence: 16-year follow-up of the PROBIT cluster-randomized trial. PLoS Med 15(4):e1002554, 2018 29677187

Yonkers KA, Wisner KL, Stowe Z, et al: Management of bipolar disorder during pregnancy and the postpartum period. Am J Psychiatry 161(4):608–620, 2004 15056503

Yonkers KA, Gotman N, Smith MV, et al: Does antidepressant use attenuate the risk of a major depressive episode in pregnancy? Epidemiology 22(6):848–854, 2011 21900825

Yonkers KA, Pearlstein TB, Gotman N: A pilot study to compare fluoxetine, calcium, and placebo in the treatment of premenstrual syndrome. J Clin Psychopharmacol 33(5):614–620, 2013 23963058

Yonkers KA, Kornstein SG, Gueorguieva R, et al: Symptom-onset dosing of sertraline for the treatment of premenstrual dysphoric disorder: a randomized clinical trial. JAMA Psychiatry 72(10):1037–1044, 2015 26351969

Zaig I, Azem F, Schreiber S, et al: Psychological response and cortisol reactivity to in vitro fertilization treatment in women with a lifetime anxiety or unipolar mood disorder diagnosis. J Clin Psychiatry 74(4):386–392, 2013 23656846

Zhang L, Li H, Li S, et al: Reproductive and metabolic abnormalities in women taking valproate for bipolar disorder: a meta-analysis. Eur J Obstet Gynecol Reprod Biol 202:26–31, 2016 27160812

Zhou R, Cao YM, Liu D, et al: Pregnancy or psychological outcomes of psychotherapy interventions for infertility: a meta-analysis. Front Psychol 12:643395, 2021 33868114

12

Infectious Diseases

James L. Levenson, M.D.
Stephen J. Ferrando, M.D.

Psychiatric symptoms are part of many systemic and CNS infections. Even limited infections may cause neuropsychiatric symptoms in vulnerable patients, such as those who are elderly or who have preexisting brain disease. In this chapter, we discuss bacterial, viral, and parasitic infections with prominent neuropsychiatric involvement, with a focus on HIV and AIDS. (Hepatitis C is covered in Chapter 4, "Gastrointestinal Disorders.") Neuropsychiatric side effects of commonly used antibiotics, as well as drug-disease and drug-drug interactions, are reviewed (see also Chapter 1, "Pharmacokinetics, Pharmacodynamics, and Principles of Drug-Drug Interactions").

Bacterial Infections

Pediatric Autoimmune Neuropsychiatric Disorders Associated With Streptococcal Infections

Pediatric autoimmune neuropsychiatric disorders associated with streptococcal infections (PANDAS) are a subset of obsessive-compulsive and tic disorders that appear to be triggered by an infection with group A β-hemolytic streptococci (GABHS). PANDAS are defined by onset of symptoms during early childhood; an episodic course characterized by abrupt onset of symptoms with frequent relapses and remissions; associated neurological signs, especially tics; and temporal association with GABHS infections (most commonly pharyngitis). The diagnosis of PANDAS is controversial, and higher rates of temporally associated GABHS infections and exacerbations of neuropsychiatric symptoms in children with PANDAS have not been clearly established (Nielsen et al. 2019). Children who have uncomplicated streptococcal infections treated with antibiotics appear to have no increased risk for PANDAS (Perrin et al. 2004).

Although PANDAS are conceptualized as autoimmune disorders, antibiotics active against GABHS may be beneficial in reducing current symptoms (Snider et al. 2005). In children with recurrent streptococcal infections, antibiotic prophylaxis to prevent neuropsychiatric exacerbations has yielded mixed results. Whereas one double-blind, placebo-controlled trial found no benefit of penicillin over placebo in preventing PANDAS exacerbations (Garvey et al. 1999), another trial found that either penicillin or azithromycin was able to lower rates of recurrent streptococcal infections and to decrease PANDAS symptom exacerbations (Snider et al. 2005). A more recent small trial found improvement in acute-onset pediatric OCD with azithromycin compared with placebo (Murphy et al. 2017). Improvements in PANDAS symptoms have also been seen in patients after use of plasma exchange and intravenous immunoglobulin (IVIG). In one small open-label study, severity of OCD symptoms decreased by 45%–58% after treatment with either plasma exchange or IVIG (Perlmutter et al. 1999). However, a more recent double-blind study by the same group with 35 patients failed to establish superiority of IVIG to placebo (Williams et al. 2016). The bottom line is that all clinical trials to date have been very small, and neither immunomodulatory therapies nor antibiotics can be clearly recommended as a routine treatment for PANDAS.

Neuroborreliosis

Lyme disease is caused by the spirochete *Borrelia burgdorferi*. If untreated, patients may develop chronic neuroborreliosis, including a mild sensory radiculopathy, difficulty with concentration and memory, fatigue, daytime hypersomnolence, irritability, and depression. These chronic symptoms are not distinctive but are almost always preceded by the classic early symptoms of Lyme disease. The differential diagnosis of neuroborreliosis in a patient presenting with poorly explained fatigue, depression, or impaired cognition includes fibromyalgia, chronic fatigue syndrome, other infections, somatoform disorders, depression, autoimmune diseases, and multiple sclerosis.

Neither serological testing nor antibiotic treatment is cost-effective for patients who have a low probability of having the disease (i.e., nonspecific symptoms, low-incidence region). A meta-analysis of antibiotic treatment for acute Lyme disease found no differences between doxycycline and β-lactam antibiotics regarding residual neurological symptoms at 4–12 months (Dersch et al. 2015). Multiple controlled trials have found no benefit of extended intravenous or oral antibiotics in patients with well-documented previously treated Lyme disease who had persistent pain, neurocognitive symptoms, dysesthesia, or fatigue (Dersch et al. 2015; Kaplan et al. 2003; Klempner et al. 2001; Krupp et al. 2003; Oksi et al. 2007). Most recently, a double-blind, randomized controlled trial (RCT; $N=280$) for chronic symptoms attributed to Lyme found no benefit from prolonged antibiotic treatment with doxycycline or clarithromycin plus hydroxychloroquine compared with placebo (Berende et al. 2016). The consensus of experts is that chronic antibiotic therapy is not indicated for persistent neuropsychiatric symptoms in patients previously adequately treated for Lyme disease (Cadavid et al. 2016; Dersch et al. 2015; Lantos et al. 2021).

Neurosyphilis

Neurosyphilis is now the predominant form of tertiary syphilis and most frequently occurs in immunocompromised patients. Symptoms include cognitive dysfunction, including dementia, changes in personality, psychosis, and seizures. Intravenous penicillin G is the recommended treatment for all forms of neurosyphilis (Buitrago-Garcia et al. 2019; Ropper 2019). In some patients with dementia due to neurosyphilis, the infection appears to have "burned out," and they show no clinical response to penicillin G. A recent review concluded that penicillin probably does not improve late neurosyphilitic syndromes but may halt their progression (Ropper 2019). Data are insufficient to support the long-term benefit of penicillin therapy for cognitive function (Moulton and Koychev 2015). Multiple case reports but no controlled trials have addressed treatment of psychiatric symptoms associated with neurosyphilis. One review recommended treatment of psychosis in patients with neurosyphilis by using the typical antipsychotic haloperidol or the atypical agents quetiapine or risperidone (Sanchez and Zisselman 2007). An anticonvulsant such as divalproex sodium was also recommended for agitation and mood stabilization. Case reports have supported atypical antipsychotics (Taycan et al. 2006; Turan et al. 2007) or memantine (Chen et al. 2019) in the treatment of neurosyphilis-associated psychosis, electroconvulsive therapy in treatment-refractory cases (Pecenak et al. 2015), and donepezil for residual neurocognitive symptoms (Wu et al. 2015).

Tuberculosis in the CNS

Tuberculosis of the brain, spinal cord, or meninges (CNS TB) is caused primarily by *Mycobacterium tuberculosis* and most often occurs in immunocompromised patients. CNS TB may manifest with meningitis, cerebritis, tuberculomas, and abscesses. Seizures are common, and psychiatric symptoms include delirium, delusions, hallucinations, and affective lability. Corticosteroids used to reduce inflammation and edema may exacerbate these symptoms (see Chapter 10, "Endocrine and Metabolic Disorders"). Antitubercular agents have been reported to cause multiple psychiatric adverse effects (Table 12–1) and may be associated with significant interactions with psychotropic drugs (Table 12–2). Literature on psychopharmacological treatment of CNS TB is scant. Anticonvulsants are used for seizures and may treat affective instability, whereas antipsychotics may be used for psychotic symptoms, with caution exercised because of the risk of developing extrapyramidal side effects (EPS) and lowering of the seizure threshold (Woodroof and Gleason 2002).

Viral Infections: HIV/AIDS

Substantial research data demonstrate the safety and efficacy of psychopharmacological treatments in patients with HIV/AIDS. Knowledge about differential diagnosis, neuropsychiatric adverse effects of antiretroviral drugs, and

Table 12–1. Psychiatric adverse effects of antibiotic therapy

Medication	Neuropsychiatric adverse effects
Antibacterials	
Aminoglycosides	Delirium, psychosis
Antitubercular agents	
Cycloserine	Agitated depression, mania, psychosis, delirium, confusion, insomnia, anxiety
Ethambutol	Confusion, psychosis
Ethionamide (thiocarbamides)	Depression, psychosis, sedation
Isoniazid (hydrazides)	Insomnia, cognitive dysfunction, hallucinations, delusions, OCD symptoms, depression, agitation, anxiety, mania, suicidal ideation and behavior
Rifampin	Drowsiness, cognitive dysfunction, delusions, hallucinations, dizziness
β-Lactam agents	
Cephalosporins	Euphoria, delusions, depersonalization, visual illusions
Imipenem	Encephalopathy
β-Lactam antibiotics	Confusion, paranoia, hallucinations, mania
Penicillins	Anxiety, illusions and hallucinations, depersonalization, agitation, insomnia, delirium, mania (amoxicillin), psychosis and delirium (procaine penicillin)
Fluoroquinolones	
Ciprofloxacin, levofloxacin, moxifloxacin, and ofloxacin	Class effects: psychosis, insomnia, delirium, mania, depression

Table 12–1. Psychiatric adverse effects of antibiotic
therapy *(continued)*

Medication	Neuropsychiatric adverse effects
Antibacterials *(continued)*	
Macrolides	
Clarithromycin and erythromycin	Nightmares, confusion, anxiety, mood lability, psychosis, mania
Metronidazole	Agitated depression, insomnia, confusion, panic, delusions, hallucinations, mania, disulfiram-like reaction
Quinolones	Class effects: restlessness, hallucinations, delusions, irritability, delirium, anxiety, insomnia, depression, psychosis
Sulfonamides	
Trimethoprim/ sulfamethoxazole, dapsone	Class effects: depression, mania, restlessness, irritability, panic, hallucinations, delusions, delirium, confusion, anorexia
Tetracyclines	Class effects: memory disturbance
Antivirals	
Nucleoside reverse transcriptase inhibitors	
Abacavir	Depression, mania, suicidal ideation, anxiety, psychosis, insomnia, nightmares, fatigue
Didanosine	Nervousness, agitation, mania, insomnia, dizziness, lethargy
Emtricitabine	Depression, abnormal dreams, insomnia, dizziness, confusion, irritability
Interferon-α-2a	Depression, suicidal ideation, anxiety, mania, psychosis, sleep disturbance, fatigue, delirium, cognitive dysfunction
Lamivudine	Depression, insomnia, dizziness, dystonia

Table 12–1.   Psychiatric adverse effects of antibiotic therapy *(continued)*

Medication	Neuropsychiatric adverse effects
Antivirals *(continued)*	
Nucleoside reverse transcriptase inhibitors (continued)	
Zidovudine	Anxiety, agitation, restlessness, insomnia, mild confusion, mania, psychosis
Delavirdine	Anxiety, agitation, amnesia, confusion, dizziness
Efavirenz	Anxiety, insomnia, irritability, depression, suicidal ideation and behavior, psychosis, vivid dreams or nightmares, cognitive dysfunction, dizziness
Nevirapine	Vivid dreams or nightmares, visual hallucinations, delusions, mood changes
Etravirine	Sleep changes, dizziness
Rilpivirine[a]	Abnormal dreams, insomnia, dizziness
Protease inhibitors	
Atazanavir	Depression, insomnia
Fosamprenavir	Depression
Indinavir	Anxiety, agitation, insomnia
Lopinavir and ritonavir	Insomnia
Nelfinavir	Depression, anxiety, insomnia
Ritonavir	Anxiety, agitation, insomnia, confusion, amnesia, emotional lability, euphoria, hallucinations, decreased libido, metallic taste
Saquinavir	Anxiety, agitation, irritability, depression, excessive dreaming, hallucinations, euphoria, confusion, amnesia
Tipranavir	Depression

Table 12–1. Psychiatric adverse effects of antibiotic therapy *(continued)*

Medication	Neuropsychiatric adverse effects
Antivirals *(continued)*	
Integrase inhibitors	
Raltegravir	Depression, suicidal ideation, psychosis, vivid dreams or nightmares, vertigo, dizziness
Elvitegravir	Depression, insomnia, suicidal ideation
Dolutegravir	Insomnia, fatigue, anxiety, depression, diminished concentration
Bictegravir	Headache
Cabotegravir[a]	Immediate postinjection anxiety, light-headedness; ongoing anxiety, restlessness, insomnia, abnormal dreams, depression
Fusion inhibitors	
Enfuvirtide	Depression, insomnia
Maraviroc	Dizziness, insomnia
Antiherpetics	
Acyclovir and valacyclovir	Visual hallucinations, depersonalization, mood lability, delusions, insomnia, lethargy, agitation, delirium
Other antivirals	
Amantadine	Insomnia, anxiety, irritability, nightmares, depression, confusion, psychosis
Foscarnet	Irritability, hallucinations
Ganciclovir	Nightmares, hallucinations, agitation
Antifungals	
Amphotericin B	Delirium, lethargy
Ketoconazole	Somnolence, dizziness, asthenia, hallucinations

Table 12–1. Psychiatric adverse effects of antibiotic
therapy *(continued)*

Medication	Neuropsychiatric adverse effects
Antifungals *(continued)*	
Pentamidine	Confusion, anxiety, mood lability, hallucinations
Anthelmintics	
Thiabendazole	Hallucinations

[a]Cabotegravir and rilpivirine can be coadministered in a long-acting injectable monthly formulation. There are reports of immediate postinjection transient side effects of anxiety and light-headedness and ongoing side effects of anxiety, insomnia, abnormal dreams, and depression.
Source.   Compiled in part from Abers et al. 2014; Abouesh et al. 2002; Celano et al. 2011; "Drugs That May Cause Psychiatric Symptoms" 2002; Hoffmann and Llibre 2019; Sternbach and State 1997; Warnke et al. 2007; Witkowski et al. 2007.

drug-drug interactions is particularly important in the psychopharmacological treatment of these patients.

Differential Diagnosis

The differential diagnosis of psychiatric symptoms in patients with HIV/AIDS is extensive. HIV-infected patients have a higher prevalence of psychiatric disorders than the general population, with mood and anxiety disorders, substance abuse, and cognitive disorders predominating (Bing et al. 2001; Ferrando 2000). Delirium, dementia, and bipolar spectrum disorders are common in medically hospitalized patients with HIV/AIDS (Ferrando and Lyketsos 2006).

Even though 60%–70% of patients with HIV have a history of psychiatric disorder before contracting HIV illness (Williams et al. 1991), and HIV diagnosis or disease exacerbation may trigger relapse, it is essential to consider potential medical etiologies. HIV-associated neuropsychiatric disorders can have multiple cognitive and behavioral symptoms, including apathy, depression, sleep disturbances, mania, and psychosis (Ferrando 2000). Patients with CNS opportunistic infections (including cryptococcal meningitis, toxoplasmosis, and progressive multifocal leukoencephalopathy) and cancers can also present with a wide range of behavioral symptoms, as a result of focal or generalized neuropathological processes. Substance intoxication and withdrawal

Table 12–2.   Antibiotic medication–psychotropic medication interactions

Medication	Interaction mechanism	Effects on psychotropic medication levels	Potential clinical effects
Antibacterials			
Antitubercular agents			
Isoniazid	Inhibition of MAO-A	Increased potential for serotonin syndrome with SSRIs, SNRIs	Serotonin syndrome
		Hypertensive crisis possible with TCAs, meperidine, tyramine-containing foods, OTC sympathomimetics, and stimulants	Hypertensive crisis
	Inhibition of CYP2C19 and CYP3A4	Phenytoin levels increased	Increased phenytoin effects and adverse effects
		Carbamazepine levels increased	Increased carbamazepine adverse effects
		Benzodiazepine serum levels increased, except for oxazepam, lorazepam, and temazepam	May increase benzodiazepine effects

Table 12–2. Antibiotic medication–psychotropic medication interactions *(continued)*

Medication	Interaction mechanism	Effects on psychotropic medication levels	Potential clinical effects
Antibacterials *(continued)*			
Antitubercular agents (continued)			
Rifampin and rifabutin (to a lesser degree)	Induction of CYP3A4	Risperidone levels reduced	Reduced risperidone effect
		Sertraline levels reduced	Sertraline withdrawal symptoms
		Benzodiazepine (especially midazolam and triazolam) serum levels reduced, except for oxazepam, lorazepam, and temazepam	May reduce benzodiazepine effects
		Phenytoin levels reduced	Reduced phenytoin effects
		Methadone levels reduced	Reduced methadone effects and opioid withdrawal
		Clozapine levels reduced	Reduced clozapine therapeutic effects
		Morphine and codeine levels reduced	Reduced analgesic effect

Table 12–2.   Antibiotic medication–psychotropic medication interactions *(continued)*

Medication	Interaction mechanism	Effects on psychotropic medication levels	Potential clinical effects
Antibacterials *(continued)*			
Antitubercular agents (continued)			
Rifampin and rifabutin (to a lesser degree) *(continued)*		Zolpidem levels reduced (AUC reduced 73%)	Reduced hypnotic effect
		Carbamazepine induces its own metabolism; coadministration can significantly reduce carbamazepine levels	Diminished therapeutic effect
Clarithromycin, erythromycin, telithromycin, and troleandomycin	Inhibition of CYP3A4	Benzodiazepine serum levels may increase, except for oxazepam, lorazepam, and temazepam	May increase benzodiazepine levels and effects (sedation, confusion, respiratory depression)
		Buspirone levels increased (AUC increased sixfold)	May increase psychomotor impairment and buspirone adverse effects
		Carbamazepine levels increased	Increased carbamazepine adverse effects

Table 12–2. Antibiotic medication–psychotropic medication interactions (*continued*)

Medication	Interaction mechanism	Effects on psychotropic medication levels	Potential clinical effects
Antibacterials (*continued*)			
Antitubercular agents (*continued*)			
Clarithromycin, erythromycin, telithromycin, and troleandomycin (*continued*)		Pimozide, haloperidol, aripiprazole, and quetiapine levels increased	Increased drug effects, including hypotension, arrhythmias, sedation
Ciprofloxacin and norfloxacin	Inhibition of CYP1A2 and CYP3A4	Benzodiazepine serum levels increased, except for oxazepam, lorazepam, and temazepam	May increase benzodiazepine levels and effects (sedation, confusion, respiratory depression)
		Methadone levels increased	Increased methadone effects (sedation, respiratory depression)
		Clozapine levels increased	Increased clozapine effects
		Olanzapine levels increased	Increased olanzapine effects
Enoxacin	Inhibition of CYP1A2	Clozapine levels increased	Increased clozapine effects
		Olanzapine levels increased	Increased olanzapine effects

Table 12–2.   Antibiotic medication–psychotropic medication interactions (*continued*)

Medication	Interaction mechanism	Effects on psychotropic medication levels	Potential clinical effects
Antibacterials (continued)			
Antitubercular agents (continued)			
Linezolid	Inhibition of MAO-A	Increased potential for serotonin syndrome with SSRIs and SNRIs	Serotonin syndrome
		Hypertensive crisis possible with TCAs, meperidine, tyramine-containing foods, OTC sympathomimetics, and stimulants	Hypertensive crisis
Antivirals			
Nonnucleoside reverse transcriptase inhibitors			
Delavirdine	Inhibition of CYP3A4 and CYP2C9	Benzodiazepine serum levels increased, except for oxazepam, lorazepam, and temazepam	May increase benzodiazepine levels and effects (sedation, confusion, respiratory depression)
Efavirenz	Induction of CYP2B6	Bupropion levels reduced (AUC reduced 55%)	Reduced bupropion effects

Table 12–2. Antibiotic medication–psychotropic medication interactions *(continued)*

Medication	Interaction mechanism	Effects on psychotropic medication levels	Potential clinical effects
Antivirals *(continued)*			
Nonnucleoside reverse transcriptase inhibitors (continued)			
Efavirenz *(continued)*	Induction of CYP3A4	Phenytoin levels reduced	Reduced phenytoin effects
		Carbamazepine levels reduced (AUC reduced 26%)	Reduced carbamazepine efficacy
		Buprenorphine levels reduced (AUC reduced 49%)	Possible reduced buprenorphine effects
		Methadone levels reduced 30%–60%	Reduced methadone effects and opioid withdrawal
Nevirapine	Induction of CYP3A4	Carbamazepine levels reduced	Reduced carbamazepine efficacy
		Methadone levels reduced 30%–60%	Reduced methadone effects and opioid withdrawal

Table 12–2. Antibiotic medication–psychotropic medication interactions (*continued*)

Medication	Interaction mechanism	Effects on psychotropic medication levels	Potential clinical effects
Antivirals (continued)			
Nonnucleoside reverse transcriptase inhibitors (continued)			
Rilpivirine	Inducer of CYP3A4, 2C19, 1A2 (potent)	May decrease levels of SSRIs, SNRIs, monoamine oxidase inhibitors, antipsychotics, trazodone, stimulants, modafinil, armodafinil	Decreased psychotropic levels and clinical effects
Protease inhibitors			
General protease inhibitor interactions	Most protease inhibitors inhibit CYP2D6 and CYP3A4. Exceptions include darunavir, fosamprenavir, and ritonavir, which induce CYP2D6 and inhibit CYP3A4, and tipranavir, which in itself is a CYP3A4 inducer (see below).	Benzodiazepine serum levels increased, except for oxazepam, lorazepam, and temazepam	Increased benzodiazepine levels and effects (sedation, confusion, respiratory depression)
		Pimozide levels increased	Increased pimozide effects, including hypotension, arrhythmias

Table 12–2. Antibiotic medication–psychotropic medication interactions *(continued)*

Medication	Interaction mechanism	Effects on psychotropic medication levels	Potential clinical effects
Antivirals *(continued)*			
Protease inhibitors (continued)			
General protease inhibitor interactions *(continued)*		Clozapine levels increased	Increased clozapine effects and adverse effects
		Methadone levels reduced 16%–53%	Reduced methadone effects and opioid withdrawal
Amprenavir	Inhibition of CYP3A4	Carbamazepine levels increased	Increased carbamazepine adverse effects
Darunavir	Mechanism unclear	Paroxetine levels reduced (AUC reduced 39%)	Reduced paroxetine effects
		Sertraline levels reduced (AUC reduced 49%)	Reduced sertraline effects
	Inhibition of CYP3A4	Trazodone levels increased (AUC increased 240%)	Increased trazodone adverse effects (nausea, dizziness, hypotension, syncope)

Table 12–2. Antibiotic medication–psychotropic medication interactions (*continued*)

Antivirals (*continued*)

Protease inhibitors (*continued*)

Medication	Interaction mechanism	Effects on psychotropic medication levels	Potential clinical effects
Fosamprenavir	Induction of CYP3A4 Inhibition of CYP3A4	Paroxetine levels reduced (AUC reduced 55%)	Reduced paroxetine effect
Indinavir	Inhibition of CYP3A4	Trazodone levels increased	Increased trazodone adverse effects (nausea, dizziness, hypotension, syncope)
		Carbamazepine levels increased	Increased carbamazepine adverse effects
Lopinavir	Inhibition of CYP3A4	Trazodone levels increased (AUC increased 240%)	Increased trazodone adverse effects (nausea, dizziness, hypotension, syncope)
	Possible induction of CYP2C9	Phenytoin levels reduced	Reduced phenytoin effects
	Possible induction of UGT-mediated glucuronidation by lopinavir/ritonavir	Lamotrigine levels reduced (AUC reduced 50%)	Reduced lamotrigine effects
Nelfinavir	Inhibition of CYP2D6 and CYP3A4	Carbamazepine levels increased	Increased carbamazepine adverse effects

Table 12–2. Antibiotic medication–psychotropic medication interactions *(continued)*

Medication	Interaction mechanism	Effects on psychotropic medication levels	Potential clinical effects
Antivirals (continued)			
Protease inhibitors (continued)			
Ritonavir	Inhibition of CYP3A4	Trazodone levels increased (AUC increased 240%)	Increased trazodone adverse effects (nausea, dizziness, hypotension, syncope)
		Carbamazepine levels increased	Increased carbamazepine adverse effects
		Quetiapine levels increased	Increased quetiapine adverse effects
	Induction of CYP1A2	Olanzapine levels reduced (AUC reduced 53%)	Reduced olanzapine effects
		Clozapine levels reduced	Reduced clozapine effects
	Induction of CYP2B6	Bupropion levels reduced	Reduced bupropion effects
Tipranavir	Alone, tipranavir is an inducer of CYP3A4; however, the combination with ritonavir is a CYP3A4 inhibitor.	Tipranavir alone: reduced bupropion (AUC reduced 46%) and carbamazepine levels	Increased or reduced bupropion and carbamazepine effects and adverse effects

Table 12–2. Antibiotic medication–psychotropic medication interactions (*continued*)

Medication	Interaction mechanism	Effects on psychotropic medication levels	Potential clinical effects
Antivirals (*continued*)			
Protease inhibitors (*continued*)			
Tipranavir (*continued*)		Tipranavir and ritonavir combination: increased bupropion and carbamazepine (AUC increased 24%) levels	
Integrase strand transfer inhibitors			
Raltegravir	Substrate at UGT1A1	No CYP interactions	—
Elvitegravir	Substrate at CYP3A, UGT1A1/3	CYP2C9 inducer, coformulated with cobicistat, may inhibit CYP3A metabolized drugs, SSRIs, SNRIs, mirtazapine, TCAs, maprotiline, reboxetine, trazodone	May elevate valproic acid and antidepressant levels and adverse effects
Dolutegravir	Substrate at CYP3A, UGT1A1/3/9, breast cancer resistance protein, P-glycoprotein	Organic cation transporter Multidrug toxin extrusion	No effects on psychotropics; levels may be reduced by carbamazepine, phenytoin, valproic acid

Table 12–2. Antibiotic medication–psychotropic medication interactions *(continued)*

Medication	Interaction mechanism	Effects on psychotropic medication levels	Potential clinical effects
Integrase strand transfer inhibitors *(continued)*			
Bictegravir	Substrate at CYP3A, UGT1A1	Organic cation transporter Multidrug toxin extrusion	
Cabotegravir (long-acting injectable with rilpivirine)	Substrate at UGT1A1	Drug interactions minimal, mostly due to rilpivirine	Avoids gut-level drug interactions, hepatic level still possible
Antifungals			
Fluconazole	Inhibition of CYP2C19	Amitriptyline and nortriptyline levels increased	Increased adverse effects (behavioral changes and toxicity)
		Phenytoin levels increased	Increased phenytoin effects and adverse effects
		Triazolam and midazolam serum levels increased	Increased triazolam and midazolam levels and effects, including adverse effects (sedation, confusion, respiratory depression)

Table 12–2. Antibiotic medication–psychotropic medication interactions *(continued)*

Medication	Interaction mechanism	Effects on psychotropic medication levels	Potential clinical effects
Antifungals (continued)			
Itraconazole	Inhibition of CYP3A4	Benzodiazepine serum levels increased, except for oxazepam, lorazepam, and temazepam	Increased benzodiazepine levels and effects (sedation, confusion, respiratory depression)
Ketoconazole	Inhibition of CYP3A4	Benzodiazepine serum levels increased, except for oxazepam, lorazepam, and temazepam	Increased benzodiazepine levels and effects (sedation, confusion, respiratory depression)
		Buspirone levels possibly increased	May increase psychomotor impairment and buspirone adverse effects
Miconazole and sulfamethoxazole	Inhibition of CYP2C9	Phenytoin levels increased	Increased phenytoin effects and adverse effects

Note.   AUC=area under the curve; CYP=cytochrome P450; MAO-A=monoamine oxidase A; OTC=over-the-counter; SNRIs=serotonin-norepinephrine reuptake inhibitors; SSRIs=selective serotonin reuptake inhibitors; TCAs=tricyclic antidepressants; UGT=uridine 5′-diphosphate glucuronosyltransferase.

Source.   Compiled in part from Bruce et al. 2006; Cozza et al. 2003; Desta et al. 2001; Finch et al. 2002; Flockhart et al. 2000; Foisy and Tseng 2015; Jacobs et al. 2014; Kharasch et al. 2008; Kuper and D'Aprile 2000; Lu et al. 2021; Ma et al. 2005; Mahatthanatrakul et al. 2007; Repetto and Petitto 2008; Venkatakrishnan et al. 2000; Warnke et al. 2007; Witkowski et al. 2007; Yew 2002.

states are also common, and preexisting psychopathology may be exacerbated by ongoing substance use (Batki et al. 1996). The high rate of polysubstance abuse complicates the assessment of behavioral symptoms and presents the challenge of treating mixed withdrawal states.

Antiretroviral and other medications used in the context of HIV have been associated with neuropsychiatric adverse effects (see Table 12–1). Most of these effects are infrequent, and causal relationships are often difficult to establish. Clinical concern resulted from early reports of sudden-onset depression and suicidal ideation associated with interferon-α-2a (see Chapter 4) and neuropsychiatric adverse effects of efavirenz. Efavirenz is a serotonin type 2A receptor antagonist, a serotonin-dopamine reuptake inhibitor, an inhibitor of monoamine oxidase, and a vesicular monoamine transporter 2 inhibitor, which are mechanisms common with many psychotropic drugs (Zareifopoulos et al. 2020). Although the overall rate of severe neuropsychiatric adverse effects of efavirenz is low (Ford et al. 2015) and symptoms have been shown to decrease after switching to an alternative regimen (Mothapo et al. 2015), vigilance is recommended when efavirenz is initiated for patients with prior psychiatric disorders.

Patients with HIV/AIDS often experience endocrinopathies that may produce psychiatric symptoms. These include clinical and subclinical hypothyroidism (16% of patients) (Beltran et al. 2003; Chen et al. 2005), hypogonadism (50% of males) (Mylonakis et al. 2001; Rabkin et al. 1999; Rochira and Guaraldi 2014), and hypothalamic-pituitary-adrenal axis dysfunction (Chrousos and Zapanti 2014), including adrenal insufficiency (50% of patients) (Marik et al. 2002; Mayo et al. 2002). These endocrinopathies can be associated with fatigue, low mood, low libido, and loss of lean body mass. Patients with Graves' disease (autoimmune thyroiditis) present with anxiety, irritability, insomnia, weight loss, mania, and agitation when the disease occurs in the setting of immune reconstitution (Chen et al. 2005).

Treatment of Psychiatric Symptoms in Patients With HIV/AIDS

Depression

Conventional antidepressants.   Multiple open-label and double-blind, placebo-controlled clinical trials of antidepressant treatment of depression in patients living with HIV/AIDS have been conducted. In general, women, injection drug users, and people in resource-poor countries have been underrepresented in RCTs of antidepressants, studies are of variable quality and methodology, and most occurred before the year 2000. With these caveats, a Cochrane systematic review (Eshun-Wilson et al. 2018) of 10 RCTs concluded that antidepressants are superior to placebo for patients living with HIV/AIDS with no major adverse outcomes. For brevity, the following discussion is derived from a critical review with extensive literature references (Ferrando and Freyberg 2008). References for more recent studies are cited here.

Early RCTs demonstrated the efficacy of imipramine for depression in patients with HIV. However, imipramine-treated patients experienced anticholinergic, antihistaminic, and antiadrenergic side effects that contributed to significant attrition. Response rates and adverse effects did not vary as a function of CD4+ lymphocyte count.

Early open-label trials and later RCTs of selective serotonin reuptake inhibitors (SSRIs) alone or compared with tricyclic antidepressants (TCAs) demonstrated efficacy of SSRIs with few adverse effects, supporting use of SSRIs as first-line treatment for depression in patients with HIV. However, fixed-dose escitalopram, 10 mg/day, was not more efficacious than placebo over 6 weeks (Hoare et al. 2014). Weekly directly observed fluoxetine, 90 mg, was found to be more effective in treating depression than standard care in homeless and marginally housed patients with HIV/AIDS (Tsai et al. 2013).

Mirtazapine, venlafaxine, and sustained-release bupropion have been studied in small open-label trials in patients with major depression and HIV infection. All of the medications were associated with favorable response rates (>60%–70%) and few adverse effects.

The few published studies on comparative efficacy and effectiveness of antidepressants in patients living with HIV/AIDS have had inconclusive results. There has been particular interest in comparing dual-acting (i.e., mirtazapine) with single-acting (i.e., SSRIs) medications, with the hypothesis that multiple-neurotransmitter activity may be beneficial for mood and somatic or cognitive symptoms. Patel et al. (2013) found no difference in response and remission rates in mirtazapine- and escitalopram-treated patients but some indication of greater symptom reduction with mirtazapine. Mills et al. (2017) found no group differences between dual- and single-acting agents, with low remission rates (32% overall).

Studies that included group or individual therapy in combination with antidepressant medication have suggested that combining psychotherapy with medication may be the optimal approach to treating depression in patients with HIV, as in other patient groups.

Psychostimulants and wakefulness agents. Psychostimulants have shown efficacy in the treatment of depressed mood, fatigue, and cognitive impairment in both open-label (Holmes et al. 1989; Wagner et al. 1997) and placebo-controlled (Breitbart et al. 2001; Wagner and Rabkin 2000) studies in patients with HIV. For patients in both RCTs, overstimulation was more common with psychostimulants than with placebo. Concern over abuse liability may limit the use of psychostimulants, particularly for substance abusers with early HIV infection. In two RCTs in which fatigue was the primary outcome measure, the wakefulness agents modafinil and armodafinil significantly reduced depression compared with placebo only in the presence of improved fatigue (Rabkin et al. 2010, 2011).

Nonconventional agents with antidepressant efficacy. Testosterone deficiency with clinical symptoms of hypogonadism (depressed mood, fatigue, diminished libido, decreased appetite, and loss of lean body mass) is present in up to 50% of men with symptomatic HIV/AIDS. Deficiency of adrenal androgens, particularly dehydroepiandrosterone, is also common in both men and women with HIV. These abnormalities have led to clinical interest in administering anabolic androgenic steroids, most commonly testosterone, to patients with HIV infection. (Studies are referenced in the critical review by Ferrando and Freyberg 2008.)

Open-label trials and RCTs have demonstrated efficacy of weekly to biweekly testosterone decanoate injections for HIV-infected men with low serum testosterone levels and low libido, low energy, and subclinical depressive symptoms. A prospective observational registry also confirmed efficacy of testosterone replacement in men with HIV (Blick et al. 2013). In these studies, fewer than 5% of patients dropped out of treatment because of adverse effects (irritability, tension, reduced energy, bossiness, hair loss, and acne). Extreme irritability and assaultiveness ("roid rage") did not occur at replacement dosages (usually 400 mg), unlike the supraphysiological dosing used illicitly for anabolic effects. Long-term adverse effects include testicular atrophy, decreased volume of ejaculate, and watery ejaculate. Long-term testosterone replacement was also efficacious for depression and body composition measures in HIV-infected women (Dolan Looby et al. 2009). No studies have reported serious hepatotoxicity or prostate cancer associated with chronic treatment.

Testosterone replacement preparations include esterified oral testosterone (undecanoate capsules, available in Canada only) and intramuscular depot testosterone (propionate, enanthate, and cypionate), skin patches, and testosterone gel. Intramuscular depot preparations are the least expensive and most studied. Patch and gel formulations may produce less variability in serum testosterone levels and therefore in target symptoms.

Dehydroepiandrosterone, an adrenal androgen, has mild androgenic and anabolic effects and is a precursor to testosterone. It has been studied in an RCT, and efficacy was shown at dosages of 100–400 mg/day in patients with HIV and dysthymia or subsyndromal depression. Other steroid hormones, including nandrolone and oxandrolone, are widely used but have not been studied for their mood effects in patients with HIV.

St. John's wort is not recommended for use by patients with HIV because it is a cytochrome P450 3A4 (CYP3A4) inducer and may reduce levels of protease inhibitors. *S*-adenosylmethionine improved mood in an open-label trial of HIV-infected patients with major depression.

Anxiety

Anxiety is present in 11%–25% of patients with HIV, is often comorbid with depression, and is associated with fatigue and physical functional limitations (Sewell et al. 2000). The most common manifestations are PTSD, social phobia, agoraphobia, generalized anxiety disorder, and panic disorder.

SSRIs are first-line agents for the treatment of anxiety disorders; however, there are no published trials in patients with HIV in which anxiety is the primary end point. In SSRI depression trials, anxiety symptoms appear to decrease. Buspirone has been shown to be effective for treating anxiety symptoms in asymptomatic gay men and intravenous drug users with HIV and is well tolerated, with a low risk for drug interactions (Batki 1990). Buspirone also may improve immune reconstitution through adenosine 3′,5′-cyclic monophosphate/protein kinase A type 1 pathway modulation (Eugen-Olsen et al. 2000). Benzodiazepines should be used with caution because of their risk for drug interactions (see Table 12–2), excessive sedation, cognitive impairment, and abuse. Lorazepam has the advantage of having no active metabolites and nonoxidative metabolism, but disadvantages include a shorter half-life and more frequent dosing. Benzodiazepines should be avoided in patients with HIV/AIDS and cognitive impairment or delirium (Breitbart et al. 1996). Nonaddictive alternatives to benzodiazepines for acute anxiety include the antihistamines diphenhydramine and hydroxyzine, sedating TCAs, and trazodone. Excessive sedation and anticholinergic-induced cognitive impairment should be monitored.

Mania

Manic symptoms in patients with HIV may be found in conjunction with primary bipolar illness or with HIV infection of the brain (HIV-associated mania) (Lyketsos et al. 1997). When compared with primary bipolar mania, HIV-associated mania is less associated with a personal or family history of mood disorder and may include more irritability, less hypertalkativeness, and more cognitive impairment. Given that HIV-associated mania is directly related to HIV brain infection, antiretroviral agents may offer protection from incident mania and later dementia (Karstaedt et al. 2015). Despite some reports of manic or hypomanic symptoms being associated with antiretroviral medications, particularly efavirenz, since the advent of highly active antiretroviral therapy, HIV-associated mania appears to be declining in incidence, consistent with the reduction in HIV-associated dementia.

Practice guidelines recommend lithium, valproic acid, or carbamazepine as standard therapy for bipolar mania (American Psychiatric Association 2002). However, there are concerns about their use in patients with HIV infection, especially those with later-stage illness. Lithium has a low therapeutic index but may have favorable immunomodulatory and neuroprotective effects in HIV and was well tolerated in an RCT for HIV-associated neurocognitive impairment (Decloedt et al. 2016). Valproate is associated with hepatotoxicity (Cozza et al. 2000) and has been found to stimulate HIV-1 replication in vitro (Jennings and Romanelli 1999). Carbamazepine may cause blood dyscrasias and may lower serum levels of protease inhibitors. The use of these medications is further complicated by the need for serum drug level monitoring.

Little research has been published on the psychopharmacological treatment of HIV-associated mania. A case report of lithium for HIV-associated mania in a patient with AIDS showed control of symptoms at a dosage of

1,200 mg/day; however, significant neurotoxicity (cognitive slowing, fine tremor) occurred, leading to discontinuation (Tanquary 1993). One study showed that valproic acid, up to 1,750 mg/day, led to significant improvement in acute manic symptoms, with few adverse effects, at serum levels of 50–110 µg/L (Halman et al. 1993; RachBeisel and Weintraub 1997). There have been reports that valproic acid increases HIV replication in vitro in a dose-dependent manner (Jennings and Romanelli 1999) and that it both increases cytomegalovirus replication and reduces the effectiveness of antiviral drugs used to treat cytomegalovirus (Michaelis et al. 2008). The clinical relevance of these findings remains controversial, and to date no reports have been published of valproic acid causing elevations in viral load in vivo.

The anticonvulsant lamotrigine, which has been approved by the U.S. FDA for maintenance therapy in bipolar illness, particularly for patients with prominent depression, may also be useful for treating mania in patients with HIV. A study of lamotrigine treatment for peripheral neuropathy in patients with HIV suggested its safety; however, careful upward dose titration is necessary because of the risk of severe hypersensitivity (Simpson et al. 2003). Gabapentin, an anticonvulsant commonly used to treat HIV-associated peripheral neuropathy, has not demonstrated mood-stabilizing properties in controlled trials (Evins 2003).

Atypical antipsychotics may improve HIV-associated mania. Risperidone treatment significantly decreased patients' Young Mania Rating Scale scores in a case report of four patients with HIV-related manic psychosis (Singh and Catalan 1994) and successfully treated mania with catatonia when used in conjunction with lorazepam (Prakash and Bagepally 2012). Ziprasidone was effective in treating acute mania in a series of patients with HIV without a history of bipolar disorder (Spiegel et al. 2010).

A case report of clonazepam treatment of HIV-associated manic symptoms described rapid clinical response, reduction of concurrent antipsychotic dosage, and few adverse effects (Budman and Vandersall 1990). However, given the cognitive impairment associated with HIV mania, as well as comorbid substance abuse, benzodiazepines should be used only for acute stabilization.

Psychosis

New-onset psychosis in patients with HIV, which has a prevalence ranging from 0.5% to 15% (McDaniel 2000), is most often seen in neurocognitive disorders, such as delirium, HIV-associated dementia, or HIV-associated minor cognitive motor disorder. One study comparing new-onset psychotic with nonpsychotic HIV patients with similar demographic and illness profiles showed a trend toward greater global neuropsychological impairment, history of substance abuse, and higher mortality in the psychosis group (Sewell et al. 1994a). Psychosis presumed secondary to antiretroviral medications has been reported (Foster et al. 2003); however, as with HIV-associated mania, antiretroviral agents are much more likely to be protective in this regard (de Ronchi et al. 2000).

Antipsychotic treatment is complicated by HIV-infected patients' susceptibility to drug-related EPS as a result of HIV-induced damage to the basal ganglia. Movement disorders (acute dystonia, parkinsonism, ataxia) can be seen in advanced HIV disease in the absence of antipsychotic exposure. General recommendations include avoidance of high-potency typical antipsychotics (e.g., haloperidol) and depot antipsychotics and brief treatment when possible. Another concern is the possibility of metabolic syndrome with antipsychotics, particularly second-generation antipsychotics, in combination with antiretrovirals, particularly protease inhibitors. One study found increased BMI in HIV-infected adolescents receiving second-generation antipsychotics, particularly with protease inhibitors (Kapetanovic et al. 2009).

Studies of treatment of psychosis in patients with HIV are rare and have generally focused on psychosis occurring in encephalopathic, schizophrenic, and manic patients. The typical antipsychotics haloperidol and thioridazine were effective in treating positive psychotic symptoms associated with HIV and schizophrenia. Haloperidol, but not thioridazine, was associated with a high incidence of EPS (Mauri et al. 1997; Sewell et al. 1994b). Thioridazine was used as last resort because of risk for QTc interval prolongation. Molindone was beneficial for HIV-associated psychosis and agitation, with minimal EPS (Fernandez and Levy 1993).

Clozapine was found to be effective and generally safe in treating HIV-associated psychosis (including negative symptoms) in patients with prior drug-induced parkinsonism (Lera and Zirulnik 1999) and in HIV-infected patients with schizophrenia (Nejad et al. 2009). However, clozapine must be used with caution in HIV-infected patients because of the risk of agranulocytosis, and it is contraindicated with ritonavir. Risperidone improved HIV-related psychotic and manic symptoms and was associated with mild sedation and sialorrhea but few EPS (Singh et al. 1997; Zilikis et al. 1998). Olanzapine treatment of a patient with AIDS and psychosis who developed EPS with risperidone and other antipsychotics is described in a case report; however, this patient experienced akathisia, necessitating propranolol (Meyer et al. 1998). Adverse reactions have been reported from quetiapine in patients taking atazanavir or ritonavir, probably because of ritonavir's inhibition of CYP3A4 (Pollack et al. 2009). Lorazepam was reported to be useful in the treatment of AIDS-associated psychosis with catatonia (Scamvougeras and Rosebush 1992).

Delirium

Delirium is diagnosed in 11%–29% of hospitalized patients with HIV/AIDS, is generally multifactorial in etiology, and is often superimposed on HIV-associated neurocognitive disorders (Ferrando et al. 1998). In a study of delirium in AIDS, patients had an average of 12.6 medical complications, with the most common being hematological (anemia, leukopenia, thrombocytopenia) and infectious (e.g., septicemia, systemic fungal infections, *Pneumocystis carinii* pneumonia, TB, disseminated viral infections) diseases (Breitbart et al. 1996).

Pharmacological treatment of delirium in HIV is generally with atypical antipsychotics because of concern about EPS. However, the only double-blind clinical trial of delirium treatment in AIDS compared low-dose haloperidol, chlorpromazine, and lorazepam (Breitbart et al. 1996). There were three important findings in that study: 1) haloperidol and chlorpromazine were equally effective; 2) lorazepam worsened delirium symptoms, including oversedation, disinhibition, ataxia, and increased confusion; and 3) antipsychotic adverse effects were limited and included mild EPS. Benzodiazepines should be reserved for delirium secondary to the withdrawal of alcohol or another CNS-depressant agent or for severe agitation that does not respond to antipsychotics.

Sleep Disorders

Sleep disorders, primarily insomnia, are prevalent in the HIV-infected population. In a survey study of 115 HIV clinic patients, 73% endorsed insomnia (Wiegand et al. 1991). Poor sleep quality in HIV-infected patients accompanies higher levels of depressive, anxiety, and physical symptoms; daytime sleepiness; and cognitive and functional impairment (Nokes and Kendrew 2001). High efavirenz serum levels have been associated with the development of insomnia and with transient vivid dreams during the early stages of treatment and neuropsychological impairment (Clifford 2003; Shikuma et al. 2018).

Psychopharmacological treatment of insomnia should take a hierarchical approach based on safety, abuse liability, and chronicity of symptoms, similar to treatment of anxiety disorders. Generally, benzodiazepines are indicated for short-term use only and should be avoided in patients with substance abuse histories. Trazodone, 50 mg alone or in combination with sleep hygiene training, was found effective for sleep, daytime sleepiness, and cognitive function in injection drug users in methadone treatment (Alikhani et al. 2020). The nonbenzodiazepine sedative-hypnotics eszopiclone, zopiclone (available in Canada), and zolpidem may have low abuse potential; however, patients with substance use histories should be monitored because abuse of these drugs has been reported (Jaffe et al. 2004). The melatonin receptor agonist ramelteon and the orexin antagonist suvorexant have not been studied in HIV. Other agents, such as sedating antidepressants, atypical antipsychotics, and anticonvulsants, may be used for comorbid psychiatric symptoms.

Viral Infections Other Than HIV

Viruses can produce psychiatric symptoms through primary CNS involvement, through secondary effects of immune activation, or indirectly from systemic effects. One serious sequela of several viral infections is acute disseminated encephalomyelitis, which can present with encephalopathy, acute psychosis, seizures, and other CNS dysfunction.

Systemic Viral Infections

Patients who have chronic viral infections (e.g., Epstein-Barr virus, cytomegalovirus) may report overwhelming fatigue, malaise, depression, low-grade fever, lymphadenopathy, and other nonspecific symptoms. Although viral infections may resemble chronic fatigue syndrome, only a small fraction of chronic fatigue symptoms are attributable to specific viral infection, and the differential diagnosis should also include depression and other common causes of fatigue. Epstein-Barr virus infection is most common in adolescents and young adults. Cytomegalovirus should be considered when acute depression or cognitive dysfunction appears in immunocompromised patients (e.g., during the first few months after transplantation). Although controlled trials are lacking, both antidepressants and stimulants have been reported as beneficial in patients with depressive symptoms and fatigue following recovery from acute viral infection or accompanying chronic viral infection.

Herpes Encephalitis

Herpes simplex virus type 1 causes herpes simplex encephalitis (HSE), which is the most common source of acute viral encephalitis in the United States and the most common identified cause of viral encephalitis simulating a primary psychiatric disorder (Arciniegas and Anderson 2004; Caroff et al. 2001; Chaudhuri and Kennedy 2002). HSE can cause personality change, dysphasia, seizures, olfactory hallucinations, autonomic dysfunction, ataxia, delirium, psychosis, and focal neurological symptoms. One possible sequela is Klüver-Bucy syndrome, which includes oral touching compulsions, hypersexuality, amnesia, placidity, agnosia, and hyperphagia. Early antiviral treatment may ameliorate some of these symptoms; however, especially in young and elderly people, cognitive impairment secondary to HSE may lead to postencephalitic dementia.

HSE is treated with intravenous acyclovir. Recovery is related to the speed of treatment, with increased morbidity and mortality associated with delays in treatment. Acyclovir may cause neuropsychiatric adverse effects, including lethargy, agitation, delirium, and hallucinations (see Table 12–1). These effects may be difficult to distinguish from HSE itself but are generally self-limited and dose dependent. Patients who are elderly, who have renal impairment, or who are taking other neurotoxic medications are at heightened risk for neuropsychiatric effects of acyclovir. Although no well-defined treatments are available for the associated cognitive and neuropsychiatric symptoms of HSE, case reports describe success with anticonvulsants, such as carbamazepine (Vallini and Burns 1987), atypical antipsychotics (Guaiana and Markova 2006), atypical antipsychotics combined with anticonvulsants (Vasconcelos-Moreno et al. 2011), SSRIs (Mendhekar and Duggal 2005), stimulants, clonidine (Begum et al. 2006), and cholinesterase inhibitors (Catsman-Berrevoets et al. 1986).

Coronavirus SARS-CoV-2 Disease

Mental health disorders, and especially schizophrenia and other severe mental illnesses, are associated with a significantly increased risk for coronavirus SARS-CoV-2 disease (COVID-19) and morbidity and mortality from COVID-19

(Fond et al. 2021). One small study reported increased mortality in geriatric patients with acute COVID-19 infection who had been receiving antipsychotics (Austria et al. 2021). A large electronic database study (*n* = 474,432) found that antipsychotic drugs were associated with severe COVID-19 morbidity (OR = 2.79; 95% CI = 2.23–3.49) and increased risk of death among COVID-19–infected men (OR = 1.71; 95% CI = 1.18–2.48) and women (OR = 1.96; 95% CI = 1.41–2.73) (Iloanusi et al. 2021). In contrast, several reports found that antidepressants were associated with lower morbidity and mortality (speculatively attributed to anti-inflammatory effects), with one RCT that observed a lower likelihood of clinical deterioration in fluvoxamine-versus placebo-treated outpatients with mild COVID-19 illness (Lenze et al. 2020). One subsequent U.S. RCT concluded that fluvoxamine did not prevent the occurrence of hypoxemia, emergency department visits, hospitalization, or death associated with COVID-19 (Bramante et al. 2022), whereas a summary of a Brazilian RCT reported that it did prevent hospitalization (Reis et al. 2022). Several meta-analyses have examined these three studies but did not reach the same conclusions regarding fluvoxamine's benefits for COVID. Because we now have clearly more effective drugs for reducing symptoms in early COVID-19 infection (e.g., nirmatrelvir plus ritonavir), there is no clear role for fluvoxamine. There has been similar interest in melatonin's potential prophylactic effects on the acquisition and progression of COVID-19 through beneficial sleep-wake, antioxidant, and anti-inflammatory effects. Several systematic reviews and meta-analyses (e.g., Lan et al. 2022) have concluded that melatonin also may improve clinical outcomes.

A variety of somatic and neuropsychiatric symptoms have been reported after acute COVID-19 infection. "Long COVID" probably includes a variety of medical and psychiatric disorders, the latter including PTSD, somatic symptom disorder, depression, functional neurological symptom disorder, and cognitive disorders. Chronic fatigue has been reported as a frequent sequela of COVID-19, as it has following other viral infections (Sandler et al. 2021). There are no published randomized trials of antidepressants for post-COVID depression or fatigue. One open trial reported that 55 of 60 patients with post-COVID depression showed a good clinical response to antidepressant therapy (Mazza et al. 2022).

Treatment of COVID-related delirium is discussed in Chapter 15, "Critical Care and Surgery." Several medications have been used to treat COVID-

19, some with emergency use authorization (EUA) and many of them off label. Psychotropic drug–disease and drug-drug interactions may be a consideration (Bilbul et al. 2020). Remdesivir, an adenosine analogue with COVID EUA, has broad-spectrum antiviral activity. This agent appears to have minimal neuropsychiatric adverse effects but can elevate liver enzymes and cause nausea, which may affect the concurrent use of some psychotropics. Monoclonal antibody infusion therapies (sotrovimab, bamlanivimab/etesevimab, casirivimab/imdevimab, tixagevimab/cilgavimab), targeting the SARS-CoV-2 spike protein, have EUAs for treatment and postexposure prophylaxis. Neuropsychiatric adverse effects are limited to fatigue and altered mental status immediately after injection (U.S. Food and Drug Administration 2022). The oral protease inhibitor combination nirmatrelvir/ritonavir has EUA for mild to moderate COVID-19 illness. Neuropsychiatric adverse effects are not common; however, interactions with psychotropics are possible given the CYP3A inhibitory effects of ritonavir (U.S. Food and Drug Administration 2023). Other agents used off label with limited evidence to treat (or prevent) COVID, including hydroxychloroquine, chloroquine, and azithromycin, have potential interactions with psychotropics, including risk of QT prolongation. Lopinavir/ritonavir has effects on many CYP enzymes (Plasencia-García et al. 2022). Ivermectin has been associated with multiple adverse neuropsychiatric side effects, including delirium, amnesia, psychosis, and encephalitis (O'Higgins et al. 2021).

Parasitic Infections: Neurocysticercosis

Neurocysticercosis, caused by the tapeworm *Taenia solium*, acquired from undercooked pork, is the most common parasitic disease of the CNS, particularly in Asia, Latin America, and Africa. It is now appearing more frequently in the southwestern United States. Neurocysticercosis is the major etiology for acquired epilepsy in affected areas, and patients are often left with chronic neurocognitive and psychiatric problems, most commonly depression, but psychosis and dementia are possible sequelae (El-Kady et al. 2021; Srivastava et al. 2013). Neurocysticercosis is treated with anthelmintic agents, such as praziquantel and albendazole, which are relatively free of neuropsychiatric side effects and drug-drug interactions (Nash et al. 2006). Other agents given with these drugs include systemic corticosteroids (see Chapter 10) to treat pericystic inflammation and encephalitis, as well as anticonvulsants to treat seizures. Antipsychotics may be used to treat psychotic symptoms, but patients may be more susceptible to EPS, including tardive dyskinesia (Bills and Symon 1992).

Adverse Psychiatric Effects of Antibiotics

Antimicrobials can cause a multitude of psychiatric symptoms. Although many of these adverse effects are rare, clinical suspicion is warranted with new onset or exacerbation of preexisting psychiatric symptoms when these drugs are initiated. The best-documented psychiatric side effects of selected antibiotic drugs are listed in Table 12–1. Delirium and psychosis have been particularly associated with quinolones (e.g., ciprofloxacin), procaine penicillin, antimalarial and other antiparasitic drugs, and the antituberculous drug cycloserine. The most common adverse effect causing discontinuation of interferon is depression. Depression, anxiety, and insomnia are the most frequently reported neuropsychiatric adverse effects of antiretroviral medications for HIV infection, particularly efavirenz.

Drug-Drug Interactions

Acute infection results in the downregulation of multiple CYP enzymes and of uridine $5'$-diphosphate glucuronosyltransferase activity, potentially resulting in impaired drug metabolism and excretion and elevated toxicity (Morgan et al. 2008; Renton 2005). This effect appears to be mediated by proinflammatory cytokines, including interferon, interleukin-1, tumor necrosis factor, and interleukin-6. Inhibition of CYP1A2 and CYP3A4 appears to have the most potential clinical significance in humans. For example, elevated levels of clozapine, a CYP1A2 substrate, have been reported in the setting of acute respiratory and other infections, associated with excessive sedation in some cases (Clark et al. 2018). The clinical significance of this phenomenon for the metabolism of other psychotropic drugs is not known; however, in the setting of acute infection, careful dosage titration and serum level monitoring (when available) are prudent.

Some pharmacokinetic drug interactions may occur between antibiotics and psychotropic drugs. Selected well-established interactions are described in

Table 12–2. Drug interactions are discussed in more detail in Chapter 1. Many antibacterials, including macrolides and fluoroquinolones, conazole antifungals, and antiretrovirals, are potent inhibitors of one or more CYP isozymes, whereas the antitubercular agent rifampin and several nonnucleoside reverse transcriptase inhibitors and protease inhibitors induce multiple CYP enzymes. Isoniazid and linezolid are weak inhibitors of monoamine oxidase A. Erythromycin (and similar macrolide antibiotics, such as clarithromycin) and ketoconazole (and similar antifungals) may cause QT interval prolongation and ventricular arrhythmias when given to a patient taking other QT-prolonging drugs, including TCAs and many antipsychotics.

Multiple case reports have described serotonin syndrome associated with coadministration of linezolid, a weak, reversible monoamine oxidase type A inhibitor indicated for the treatment of methicillin-resistant *Staphylococcus aureus*, and SSRIs and serotonin-norepinephrine reuptake inhibitors, with an incidence of 1.8%–3% in retrospective studies (Lorenz et al. 2008; Taylor et al. 2006). An observational matched comparison study of acutely ill hospitalized veterans did not find an increased risk for serotonin toxicity or serotonin syndrome in patients receiving linezolid compared with vancomycin (Lodise et al. 2013). Another case-control study did not find a significant increased incidence of serotonin syndrome in SSRI/linezolid-treated patients compared with those receiving linezolid monotherapy (Karkow et al. 2017). The literature suggests that patients taking SSRIs and serotonin-norepinephrine reuptake inhibitors can safely receive linezolid as long as there is clinical vigilance for signs and symptoms of serotonin toxicity. Coadministration of linezolid with direct or indirect sympathomimetic drugs (e.g., psychostimulants, meperidine) may precipitate hypertensive crisis.

Use of the anticonvulsants carbamazepine, phenytoin, and phenobarbital is of concern in HIV infection. In addition to possible anticonvulsant toxicity caused by protease inhibitor–mediated inhibition of anticonvulsant metabolism, these anticonvulsants also induce protease inhibitor metabolism, which reduces protease inhibitor serum levels and leads to virological failure (Bartt 1998; Repetto and Petitto 2008).

Potentially dangerous cardiovascular side effects have occurred because of increased levels of sildenafil, commonly used for sexual dysfunction, after concurrent administration of ritonavir, saquinavir, and indinavir (Merry et al. 1999; Muirhead et al. 2000). Illicit drugs may have dangerous clinical interactions with protease inhibitors. Fatalities have been reported with concurrent use of 3,4-methylenedioxymethamphetamine (commonly called "ecstasy"), methamphetamine, and ritonavir (Hales et al. 2000; Mirken 1997).

Key Points

- Systemic and CNS infectious diseases may cause psychiatric and cognitive symptoms that persist despite antibiotic treatment and warrant psychopharmacological intervention.

- Acute infection may inhibit metabolism of psychotropic drugs, warranting caution with initial dosage and subsequent titration.

- There is significant potential for interaction between psychotropic drugs and antibiotics. Clinicians should query for potential interactions before combining these agents.

- Substantial evidence supports the efficacy of selective serotonin reuptake inhibitors and some novel agents for the treatment of depression in HIV/AIDS. However, the psychopharmacology literature is limited for other psychiatric disorders in the context of infectious diseases.

- Patients with HIV/AIDS and other infections with CNS involvement are susceptible to extrapyramidal side effects of antipsychotic drugs.

References

Abers MS, Shandera WX, Kass JS: Neurological and psychiatric adverse effects of antiretroviral drugs. CNS Drugs 28(2):131–145, 2014 24362768

Abouesh A, Stone C, Hobbs WR: Antimicrobial-induced mania (antibiomania): a review of spontaneous reports. J Clin Psychopharmacol 22(1):71–81, 2002 11799346

Alikhani M, Ebrahimi A, Farnia V, et al: Effects of treatment of sleep disorders on sleep, psychological and cognitive functioning and biomarkers in individuals with HIV/AIDS and under methadone maintenance therapy. J Psychiatr Res 130:260–272, 2020 32858346

American Psychiatric Association: Practice guideline for the treatment of patients with bipolar disorder (revision). Am J Psychiatry 159(4 Suppl):1–50, 2002 11958165

Arciniegas DB, Anderson CA: Viral encephalitis: neuropsychiatric and neurobehavioral aspects. Curr Psychiatry Rep 6(5):372–379, 2004 15355760

Austria B, Haque R, Mittal S, et al: Mortality in association with antipsychotic medication use and clinical outcomes among geriatric psychiatry outpatients with COVID-19. PLoS One 16(10):e0258916, 2021 34673821

Bartt R: An effect of anticonvulsants on antiretroviral therapy: neuroscience of HIV infection. J Neurovirol 4(Suppl):340, 1998

Batki SL: Buspirone in drug users with AIDS or AIDS-related complex. J Clin Psychopharmacol 10(3 Suppl):111S–115S, 1990 2376626

Batki S, Ferrando S, Manfredi L, et al: Psychiatric disorders, drug use, and HIV disease in 84 injection drug users. Am J Addict 5:249–258, 1996

Begum H, Nayek K, Khuntdar BK: Kluver-Bucy syndrome: a rare complication of herpes simplex encephalitis. J Indian Med Assoc 104(11):637–638, 2006 17444064

Beltran S, Lescure FX, Desailloud R, et al: Increased prevalence of hypothyroidism among human immunodeficiency virus-infected patients: a need for screening. Clin Infect Dis 37(4):579–583, 2003 12905143

Berende A, ter Hofstede HJM, Vos FJ, et al: Randomized trial of longer-term therapy for symptoms attributed to Lyme disease. N Engl J Med 374(13):1209–1220, 2016 27028911

Bilbul M, Paparone P, Kim AM, et al: Psychopharmacology of COVID-19. Psychosomatics 61(5):411–427, 2020 32425246

Bills DC, Symon L: Cysticercosis producing various neurological presentations in a patient: case report. Br J Neurosurg 6(4):365–369, 1992 1388832

Bing EG, Burnam MA, Longshore D, et al: Psychiatric disorders and drug use among human immunodeficiency virus-infected adults in the United States. Arch Gen Psychiatry 58(8):721–728, 2001 11483137

Blick G, Khera M, Bhattacharya RK, et al: Testosterone replacement therapy in men with hypogonadism and HIV/AIDS: results from the TRiUS registry. Postgrad Med 125(2):19–29, 2013 23816768

Bramante CT, Huling JD, Tignanelli CJ, et al: Randomized trial of metformin, ivermectin, and fluvoxamine for Covid-19. N Engl J Med 387(7):599–610, 2022 36070710

Breitbart W, Marotta R, Platt MM, et al: A double-blind trial of haloperidol, chlorpromazine, and lorazepam in the treatment of delirium in hospitalized AIDS patients. Am J Psychiatry 153(2):231–237, 1996 8561204

Breitbart W, Rosenfeld B, Kaim M, et al: A randomized, double-blind, placebo-controlled trial of psychostimulants for the treatment of fatigue in ambulatory patients with human immunodeficiency virus disease. Arch Intern Med 161(3):411–420, 2001 11176767

Bruce RD, McCance-Katz E, Kharasch ED, et al: Pharmacokinetic interactions between buprenorphine and antiretroviral medications. Clin Infect Dis 43(Suppl 4):S216–S223, 2006 17109308

Budman CL, Vandersall TA: Clonazepam treatment of acute mania in an AIDS patient (letter). J Clin Psychiatry 51(5):212, 1990 2335499

Buitrago-Garcia D, Martí-Carvajal AJ, Jimenez A, et al: Antibiotic therapy for adults with neurosyphilis. Cochrane Database Syst Rev 5(5):CD011399, 2019 31132142

Cadavid D, Auwaerter PG, Rumbaugh J, et al: Antibiotics for the neurological complications of Lyme disease. Cochrane Database Syst Rev 12(12):CD006978, 2016 27931077

Caroff SN, Mann SC, Glittoo MF, et al: Psychiatric manifestations of acute viral encephalitis. Psychiatr Ann 31:193–204, 2001 73103597

Catsman-Berrevoets CE, Van Harskamp F, Appelhof A: Beneficial effect of physostigmine on clinical amnesic behaviour and neuropsychological test results in a patient with a post-encephalitic amnesic syndrome. J Neurol Neurosurg Psychiatry 49(9):1088–1090, 1986 3760902

Celano CM, Freudenreich O, Fernandez-Robles C, et al: Depressogenic effects of medications: a review. Dialogues Clin Neurosci 13(1):109–125, 2011 21485751

Chaudhuri A, Kennedy PG: Diagnosis and treatment of viral encephalitis. Postgrad Med J 78(924):575–583, 2001 12415078

Chen F, Day SL, Metcalfe RA, et al: Characteristics of autoimmune thyroid disease occurring as a late complication of immune reconstitution in patients with advanced human immunodeficiency virus (HIV) disease. Medicine (Baltimore) 84(2):98–106, 2005 15758839

Chen WC, Wang HY, Chen PA, et al: Memantine rescues neurosyphilis-related schizophrenic-like features and cognitive deficit. Clin Neuropharmacol 42(4):133–135, 2019 31135390

Chrousos GP, Zapanti ED: Hypothalamic-pituitary-adrenal axis in HIV infection and disease. Endocrinol Metab Clin North Am 43(3):791–806, 2014 25169568

Clark SR, Warren NS, Kim G, et al: Elevated clozapine levels associated with infection: a systematic review. Schizophr Res 192:50–56, 2018 28392207

Clifford DB: ACTG 5097 Team: Impact of EF on neuropsychological performance, mood and sleep behavior in HIV-positive individuals. Paper presented at the 2nd International AIDS Society Conference on HIV Pathogenesis and Treatment, Paris, France, July 2003

Cozza KL, Swanton EJ, Humphreys CW: Hepatotoxicity with combination of valproic acid, ritonavir, and nevirapine: a case report. Psychosomatics 41(5):452–453, 2000 11015639

Cozza KL, Armstrong SC, Oesterheld JR: Concise Guide to the Cytochrome P450 System: Drug Interaction Principles for Medical Practice. Washington, DC, American Psychiatric Publishing, 2003

Decloedt EH, Freeman C, Howells F, et al: Moderate to severe HIV-associated neurocognitive impairment: a randomized placebo-controlled trial of lithium. Medicine (Baltimore) 95(46):e5401, 2016 27861379

de Ronchi D, Faranca I, Forti P, et al: Development of acute psychotic disorders and HIV-1 infection. Int J Psychiatry Med 30(2):173–183, 2000 11001280

Dersch R, Freitag MH, Schmidt S, et al: Efficacy and safety of pharmacological treatments for acute Lyme neuroborreliosis: a systematic review. Eur J Neurol 22(9):1249–1259, 2015 26058321

Desta Z, Soukhova NV, Flockhart DA: Inhibition of cytochrome P450 (CYP450) isoforms by isoniazid: potent inhibition of CYP2C19 and CYP3A. Antimicrob Agents Chemother 45(2):382–392, 2001 11158730

Dolan Looby SE, Collins M, Lee H, et al: Effects of long-term testosterone administration in HIV-infected women: a randomized, placebo-controlled trial. AIDS 23(8):951–959, 2009 19287303

Drugs that may cause psychiatric symptoms. Med Lett Drugs Ther 44(1134):59–62, 2002 12138379

El-Kady AM, Allemailem KS, Almatroudi A, et al: Psychiatric disorders of neurocysticercosis: narrative review. Neuropsychiatr Dis Treat 17:1599–1610, 2021 34079258

Eshun-Wilson I, Siegfried N, Akena DH, et al: Antidepressants for depression in adults with HIV infection. Cochrane Database Syst Rev 1(1):CD008525, 2018 29355886

Eugen-Olsen J, Benfield T, Axen TE, et al: Effect of the serotonin receptor agonist, buspirone, on immune function in HIV-infected individuals: a six-month randomized, double-blind, placebo-controlled trial. HIV Clin Trials 1(1):20–26, 2000 11590486

Evins AE: Efficacy of newer anticonvulsant medications in bipolar spectrum mood disorders. J Clin Psychiatry 64(Suppl 8):9–14, 2003 12892536

Fernandez F, Levy JK: The use of molindone in the treatment of psychotic and delirious patients infected with the human immunodeficiency virus: case reports. Gen Hosp Psychiatry 15(1):31–35, 1993 8094699

Ferrando SJ: Diagnosis and treatment of HIV-associated neurocognitive disorders. New Dir Ment Health Serv 87(87):25–35, 2000 11031798

Ferrando SJ, Freyberg Z: Treatment of depression in HIV positive individuals: a critical review. Int Rev Psychiatry 20(1):61–71, 2008 18240063

Ferrando SJ, Lyketsos CG: Psychiatric comorbidities in medically ill patients with HIV/AIDS, in Psychiatric Aspects of HIV/AIDS. Edited by Fernandez F, Ruiz P. Philadelphia, PA, Lippincott Williams & Wilkins, 2006, pp 198–211

Ferrando SJ, Rabkin JG, Rothenberg J: Psychiatric disorders and adjustment in HIV and AIDS patients during and after medical hospitalization. Psychosomatics 39:214–215, 1998

Finch CK, Chrisman CR, Baciewicz AM, et al: Rifampin and rifabutin drug interactions: an update. Arch Intern Med 162(9):985–992, 2002 11996607

Flockhart DA, Drici MD, Kerbusch T, et al: Studies on the mechanism of a fatal clarithromycin-pimozide interaction in a patient with Tourette syndrome. J Clin Psychopharmacol 20(3):317–324, 2000 10831018

Foisy M, Tseng A: Predicted interactions between psychotropics and antiretrovirals. 2015. Available at: www.hivclinic.ca/main/drugs_interact_files/psych-int.pdf. Accessed September 29, 2022.

Fond G, Nemani K, Etchecopar-Etchart D, et al: Association between mental health disorders and mortality among patients with COVID-19 in 7 countries: a systematic review and meta-analysis. JAMA Psychiatry 78(11):1208–1217, 2021 34313711

Ford N, Shubber Z, Pozniak A, et al: Comparative safety and neuropsychiatric adverse events associated with efavirenz use in first-line antiretroviral therapy: a systematic review and meta-analysis of randomized trials. J Acquir Immune Defic Syndr 69(4):422–429, 2015 25850607

Foster R, Olajide D, Everall IP: Antiretroviral therapy-induced psychosis: case report and brief review of the literature. HIV Med 4(2):139–144, 2003 12702135

Garvey MA, Perlmutter SJ, Allen AJ, et al: A pilot study of penicillin prophylaxis for neuropsychiatric exacerbations triggered by streptococcal infections. Biol Psychiatry 45(12):1564–1571, 1999 10376116

Guaiana G, Markova I: Antipsychotic treatment improves outcome in herpes simplex encephalitis: a case report (letter). J Neuropsychiatry Clin Neurosci 18(2):247, 2006 16720808

Hales G, Roth N, Smith D: Possible fatal interaction between protease inhibitors and methamphetamine (letter). Antivir Ther 5(1):19, 2000 10846588

Halman MH, Worth JL, Sanders KM, et al: Anticonvulsant use in the treatment of manic syndromes in patients with HIV-1 infection. J Neuropsychiatry Clin Neurosci 5(4):430–434, 1993 8286943

Hoare J, Carey P, Joska JA, et al: Escitalopram treatment of depression in human immunodeficiency virus/acquired immunodeficiency syndrome: a randomized, double-blind, placebo-controlled study. J Nerv Ment Dis 202(2):133–137, 2014 24469525

Hoffmann C, Llibre JM: Neuropsychiatric adverse events with dolutegravir and other integrase strand transfer inhibitors. AIDS Rev 21(1):4–10, 2019 30899113

Holmes VF, Fernandez F, Levy JK: Psychostimulant response in AIDS-related complex patients. J Clin Psychiatry 50(1):5–8, 1989 2642894

Iloanusi S, Mgbere O, Essien EJ: Polypharmacy among COVID-19 patients: a systematic review. J Am Pharm Assoc (2003) 61(5):e14–e25, 2021 34120855

Jacobs BS, Colbers AP, Velthoven-Graafland K, et al: Effect of fosamprenavir/ritonavir on the pharmacokinetics of single-dose olanzapine in healthy volunteers. Int J Antimicrob Agents 44(2):173–177, 2014 24929949

Jaffe JH, Bloor R, Crome I, et al: A postmarketing study of relative abuse liability of hypnotic sedative drugs. Addiction 99(2):165–173, 2004 14756709

Jennings HR, Romanelli F: The use of valproic acid in HIV-positive patients. Ann Pharmacother 33(10):1113–1116, 1999 10534224

Kapetanovic S, Aaron L, Montepiedra G, et al: The use of second-generation antipsychotics and the changes in physical growth in children and adolescents with perinatally acquired HIV. AIDS Patient Care STDS 23(11):939–947, 2009 19827949

Kaplan RF, Trevino RP, Johnson GM, et al: Cognitive function in post-treatment Lyme disease: do additional antibiotics help? Neurology 60(12):1916–1922, 2003 12821733

Karkow DC, Kauer JF, Ernst EJ: Incidence of serotonin syndrome with combined use of linezolid and serotonin reuptake inhibitors compared with linezolid monotherapy. J Clin Psychopharmacol 37(5):518–523, 2017 28796019

Karstaedt AS, Kooverjee S, Singh L, et al: Antiretroviral outcomes in patients with severe mental illness. J Int Assoc Provid AIDS Care 14(5):428–433, 2015 26173943

Kharasch ED, Mitchell D, Coles R, et al: Rapid clinical induction of hepatic cytochrome P4502B6 activity by ritonavir. Antimicrob Agents Chemother 52(5):1663–1669, 2008 18285471

Klempner MS, Hu LT, Evans J, et al: Two controlled trials of antibiotic treatment in patients with persistent symptoms and a history of Lyme disease. N Engl J Med 345(2):85–92, 2001 11450676

Krupp LB, Hyman LG, Grimson R, et al: Study and treatment of post Lyme disease (STOP-LD): a randomized double masked clinical trial. Neurology 60(12):1923–1930, 2003 12821734

Kuper JI, D'Aprile M: Drug-drug interactions of clinical significance in the treatment of patients with Mycobacterium avium complex disease. Clin Pharmacokinet 39(3):203–214, 2000 11020135

Lan SH, Lee HZ, Chao CM, et al: Efficacy of melatonin in the treatment of patients with COVID-19: a systematic review and meta-analysis of randomized controlled trials. J Med Virol 94(5):2102–2107, 2022 35032042

Lantos PM, Rumbaugh J, Bockenstedt LK, et al: Clinical practice guidelines by the Infectious Diseases Society of America, American Academy of Neurology, and American College of Rheumatology: 2020 guidelines for the prevention, diagnosis, and treatment of Lyme disease. Neurology 96(6):262–273, 2021 33257476

Lenze EJ, Mattar C, Zorumski CF, et al: Fluvoxamine vs placebo and clinical deterioration in outpatients with symptomatic COVID-19: a randomized clinical trial. JAMA 324(22):2292–2300, 2020 33180097

Lera G, Zirulnik J: Pilot study with clozapine in patients with HIV-associated psychosis and drug-induced parkinsonism. Mov Disord 14(1):128–131, 1999 9918355

Lodise TP, Patel N, Rivera A, et al: Comparative evaluation of serotonin toxicity among Veterans Affairs patients receiving linezolid and vancomycin. Antimicrob Agents Chemother 57(12):5901–5911, 2013 24041888

Lorenz RA, Vandenberg AM, Canepa EA: Serotonergic antidepressants and linezolid: a retrospective chart review and presentation of cases. Int J Psychiatry Med 38(1):81–90, 2008 18624020

Lu C-H, Bednarczyk EM, Catanzaro LM, et al: Pharmacokinetic drug interactions of integrase strand transfer inhibitors. Curr Res Pharmacol Drug Discov 2:100044, 2021 34909672

Lyketsos CG, Schwartz J, Fishman M, et al: AIDS mania. J Neuropsychiatry Clin Neurosci 9(2):277–279, 1997 9144109

Ma Q, Okusanya OO, Smith PF, et al: Pharmacokinetic drug interactions with nonnucleoside reverse transcriptase inhibitors. Expert Opin Drug Metab Toxicol 1(3):473–485, 2005 16863456

Mahatthanatrakul W, Nontaput T, Ridtitid W, et al: Rifampin, a cytochrome P450 3A inducer, decreases plasma concentrations of antipsychotic risperidone in healthy volunteers. J Clin Pharm Ther 32(2):161–167, 2007 17381666

Marik PE, Kiminyo K, Zaloga GP: Adrenal insufficiency in critically ill patients with human immunodeficiency virus. Crit Care Med 30(6):1267–1273, 2002 12072680

Mauri MC, Fabiano L, Bravin S, et al: Schizophrenic patients before and after HIV infection: a case-control study. Encephale 23(6):437–441, 1997 9488926

Mayo J, Collazos J, Martínez E, et al: Adrenal function in the human immunodeficiency virus-infected patient. Arch Intern Med 162(10):1095–1098, 2002 12020177

Mazza MG, Zanardi R, Palladini M, et al: Rapid response to selective serotonin reuptake inhibitors in post-COVID depression. Eur Neuropsychopharmacol 54:1–6, 2022 34634679

McDaniel JS: Working Group on HIV/AIDS: practice guideline for the treatment of patients with HIV/AIDS. Am J Psychiatry 157(11 Suppl):1–62, 2000 11085570

Mendhekar DN, Duggal HS: Sertraline for Klüver-Bucy syndrome in an adolescent. Eur Psychiatry 20(4):355–356, 2005 16018931

Merry C, Barry MG, Ryan M, et al: Interaction of sildenafil and indinavir when co-administered to HIV-positive patients. AIDS 13(15):F101–F107, 1999 10546851

Meyer JM, Marsh J, Simpson G: Differential sensitivities to risperidone and olanzapine in a human immunodeficiency virus patient. Biol Psychiatry 44(8):791–794, 1998 9798086

Michaelis M, Ha TA, Doerr HW, et al: Valproic acid interferes with antiviral treatment in human cytomegalovirus-infected endothelial cells. Cardiovasc Res 77(3):544–550, 2008 18006438

Mills JC, Harman JS, Cook RL, et al: Comparative effectiveness of dual-action versus single-action antidepressants for the treatment of depression in people living with HIV/AIDS. J Affect Disord 215:179–186, 2017 28340444

Mirken B: Danger: possibly fatal interactions between ritonavir and "ecstasy," some other psychoactive drugs. AIDS Treat News 265(265):5, 1997 11364241

Morgan ET, Goralski KB, Piquette-Miller M, et al: Regulation of drug-metabolizing enzymes and transporters in infection, inflammation, and cancer. Drug Metab Dispos 36(2):205–216, 2008 18218849

Mothapo KM, Schellekens A, van Crevel R, et al: Improvement of depression and anxiety after discontinuation of long-term efavirenz treatment. CNS Neurol Disord Drug Targets 14(6):811–818, 2015 25808896

Moulton CD, Koychev I: The effect of penicillin therapy on cognitive outcomes in neurosyphilis: a systematic review of the literature. Gen Hosp Psychiatry 37(1):49–52, 2015 25468254

Muirhead GJ, Wulff MB, Fielding A, et al: Pharmacokinetic interactions between sildenafil and saquinavir/ritonavir. Br J Clin Pharmacol 50(2):99–107, 2000 10930961

Murphy TK, Brennan EM, Johnco C, et al: A double-blind randomized placebo-controlled pilot study of azithromycin in youth with acute-onset obsessive-compulsive disorder. J Child Adolesc Psychopharmacol 27(7):640–651, 2017 28358599

Mylonakis E, Koutkia P, Grinspoon S: Diagnosis and treatment of androgen deficiency in human immunodeficiency virus-infected men and women. Clin Infect Dis 33(6):857–864, 2001 11512091

Nash TE, Singh G, White AC, et al: Treatment of neurocysticercosis: current status and future research needs. Neurology 67(7):1120–1127, 2006 17030744

Nejad SH, Gandhi RT, Freudenreich O: Clozapine use in HIV-infected schizophrenia patients: a case-based discussion and review. Psychosomatics 50(6):626–632, 2009 19996235

Nielsen MØ, Köhler-Forsberg O, Hjorthøj C, et al: Streptococcal infections and exacerbations in PANDAS: a systematic review and meta-analysis. Pediatr Infect Dis J 38(2):189–194, 2019 30325890

Nokes KM, Kendrew J: Correlates of sleep quality in persons with HIV disease. J Assoc Nurses AIDS Care 12(1):17–22, 2001 11211669

O'Higgins MG, Barrios JI, Almirón-Santacruz JD, et al: Off-label use of ivermectin for COVID-19: are there any neuropsychiatric effects to be aware of? Indian J Psychiatry 63(5):516–517, 2021 34789946

Oksi J, Nikoskelainen J, Hiekkanen H, et al: Duration of antibiotic treatment in disseminated Lyme borreliosis: a double-blind, randomized, placebo-controlled, multicenter clinical study. Eur J Clin Microbiol Infect Dis 26(8):571–581, 2007 17587070

Patel S, Kukreja S, Atram U, et al: Escitalopram and mirtazapine for the treatment of depression in HIV patients: a randomized controlled open label trial. ASEAN Journal of Psychiatry 14(1):141–149, 2013

Pecenak J, Janik P, Vaseckova B, et al: Electroconvulsive therapy treatment in a patient with neurosyphilis and psychotic disorder: case report and literature review. J ECT 31(4):268–270, 2015 25634568

Perlmutter SJ, Leitman SF, Garvey MA, et al: Therapeutic plasma exchange and intravenous immunoglobulin for obsessive-compulsive disorder and tic disorders in childhood. Lancet 354(9185):1153–1158, 1999 10513708

Perrin EM, Murphy ML, Casey JR, et al: Does group A beta-hemolytic streptococcal infection increase risk for behavioral and neuropsychiatric symptoms in children? Arch Pediatr Adolesc Med 158(9):848–856, 2004 15351749

Plasencia-García BO, Rico-Rangel MI, Rodríguez-Menéndez G, et al: Drug-drug interactions between COVID-19 treatments and antidepressants, mood stabilizers/anticonvulsants, and benzodiazepines: integrated evidence from 3 databases. Pharmacopsychiatry 55(1):40–47, 2022 34171927

Pollack TM, McCoy C, Stead W: Clinically significant adverse events from a drug interaction between quetiapine and atazanavir-ritonavir in two patients. Pharmacotherapy 29(11):1386–1391, 2009 19857154

Prakash O, Bagepally BS: Catatonia and mania in patient with AIDS: treatment with lorazepam and risperidone. Gen Hosp Psychiatry 34(3):321.e5–321.e6, 2012 22361355

Rabkin JG, Wagner GJ, Rabkin R: Testosterone therapy for human immunodeficiency virus-positive men with and without hypogonadism. J Clin Psychopharmacol 19(1):19–27, 1999 9934939

Rabkin JG, McElhiney MC, Rabkin R, et al: Modafinil treatment for fatigue in HIV/AIDS: a randomized placebo-controlled study. J Clin Psychiatry 71(6):707–715, 2010 20492840

Rabkin JG, McElhiney MC, Rabkin R: Treatment of HIV-related fatigue with ar-modafinil: a placebo-controlled randomized trial. Psychosomatics 52(4):328–336, 2011 21777715

RachBeisel JA, Weintraub E: Valproic acid treatment of AIDS-related mania. J Clin Psychiatry 58:406–407, 1997 9378697

Reis G, Dos Santos Moreira-Silva EA, Silva DCM, et al: Effect of early treatment with fluvoxamine on risk of emergency care and hospitalisation among patients with COVID-19: the TOGETHER randomised, platform clinical trial [Errata in: Lancet Glob Health 10(4):e481, 2022; Lancet Glob Health 10(9):e1246, 2022]. Lancet Glob Health 10(1):e42–e51, 2022 34717820

Renton KW: Regulation of drug metabolism and disposition during inflammation and infection. Expert Opin Drug Metab Toxicol 1(4):629–640, 2005 16863429

Repetto MJ, Petitto JM: Psychopharmacology in HIV-infected patients. Psychosom Med 70(5):585–592, 2008 18519881

Rochira V, Guaraldi G: Hypogonadism in the HIV-infected man. Endocrinol Metab Clin North Am 43(3):709–730, 2014 25169563

Ropper AH: Neurosyphilis. N Engl J Med 381(14):1358–1363, 2019 31577877

Sanchez FM, Zisselman MH: Treatment of psychiatric symptoms associated with neu-rosyphilis. Psychosomatics 48(5):440–445, 2007 17878505

Sandler CX, Wyller VBB, Moss-Morris R, et al: Long COVID and post-infective fatigue syndrome: a review. Open Forum Infect Dis 8(10):ofab440, 2021 34631916

Scamvougeras A, Rosebush PI: AIDS-related psychosis with catatonia responding to low-dose lorazepam. J Clin Psychiatry 53(11):414–415, 1992 1459974

Sewell DD, Jeste DV, Atkinson JH, et al: HIV-associated psychosis: a study of 20 cases. Am J Psychiatry 151(2):237–242, 1994a 8296896

Sewell DD, Jeste DV, McAdams LA, et al: Neuroleptic treatment of HIV-associated psychosis. HNRC group. Neuropsychopharmacology 10(4):223–229, 1994b 7945732

Sewell MC, Goggin KJ, Rabkin JG, et al: Anxiety syndromes and symptoms among men with AIDS: a longitudinal controlled study. Psychosomatics 41(4):294–300, 2000 10906351

Shikuma CM, Kohorn L, Paul R, et al: Sleep and neuropsychological performance in HIV+ subjects on efavirenz-based therapy and response to switch in therapy. HIV Clin Trials 19(4):139–147, 2018 30451595

Simpson DM, McArthur JC, Olney R, et al: Lamotrigine for HIV-associated painful sensory neuropathies: a placebo-controlled trial. Neurology 60(9):1508–1514, 2003 12743240

Singh AN, Catalan J: Risperidone in HIV-related manic psychosis. Lancet 344(8928):1029–1030, 1994 7523809

Singh AN, Golledge H, Catalan J: Treatment of HIV-related psychotic disorders with risperidone: a series of 21 cases. J Psychosom Res 42(5):489–493, 1997 9194023

Snider LA, Lougee L, Slattery M, et al: Antibiotic prophylaxis with azithromycin or penicillin for childhood-onset neuropsychiatric disorders. Biol Psychiatry 57(7):788–792, 2005 15820236

Spiegel DR, Weller AL, Pennell K, et al: The successful treatment of mania due to acquired immunodeficiency syndrome using ziprasidone: a case series. J Neuropsychiatry Clin Neurosci 22(1):111–114, 2010 20160218

Srivastava S, Chadda RK, Bala K, et al: A study of neuropsychiatric manifestations in patients of neurocysticercosis. Indian J Psychiatry 55(3):264–267, 2013 24082247

Sternbach H, State R: Antibiotics: neuropsychiatric effects and psychotropic interactions. Harv Rev Psychiatry 5(4):214–226, 1997 9427014

Tanquary J: Lithium neurotoxicity at therapeutic levels in an AIDS patient. J Nerv Ment Dis 181(8):518–519, 1993 8360645

Taycan O, Ugur M, Ozmen M: Quetiapine vs. risperidone in treating psychosis in neurosyphilis: a case report. Gen Hosp Psychiatry 28(4):359–361, 2006 16814638

Taylor JJ, Wilson JW, Estes LL: Linezolid and serotonergic drug interactions: a retrospective survey. Clin Infect Dis 43(2):180–187, 2006 16779744

Tsai AC, Karasic DH, Hammer GP, et al: Directly observed antidepressant medication treatment and HIV outcomes among homeless and marginally housed HIV-positive adults: a randomized controlled trial. Am J Public Health 103(2):308–315, 2013 22720766

Turan S, Emul M, Duran A, et al: Effectiveness of olanzapine in neurosyphilis related organic psychosis: a case report. J Psychopharmacol 21(5):556–558, 2007 17092977

U.S. Food and Drug Administration: Fact sheet for health care providers: emergency use authorization (EUA) of bamlanivimab and etesevimab. January 24, 2022. Available at: https://www.fda.gov/media/145802/download. Accessed September 29, 2022.

U.S. Food and Drug Administration: Fact sheet for healthcare providers: emergency use authorization for Paxlovid. February 2023. Available at: https://www.fda.gov/media/155050/download?ftag=MSF0951a8. Accessed September 29, 2022.

Vallini AD, Burns RL: Carbamazepine as therapy for psychiatric sequelae of herpes simplex encephalitis. South Med J 80(12):1590–1592, 1987 3423906

Vasconcelos-Moreno MP, Dargél AA, Goi PD, et al: Improvement of behavioural and manic-like symptoms secondary to herpes simplex virus encephalitis with mood stabilizers: a case report. Int J Neuropsychopharmacol 14(5):718–720, 2011 21294940

Venkatakrishnan K, von Moltke LL, Greenblatt DJ: Effects of the antifungal agents on oxidative drug metabolism: clinical relevance. Clin Pharmacokinet 38(2):111–180, 2000 10709776

Wagner GJ, Rabkin R: Effects of dextroamphetamine on depression and fatigue in men with HIV: a double-blind, placebo-controlled trial. J Clin Psychiatry 61(6):436–440, 2000 10901342

Wagner GJ, Rabkin JG, Rabkin R: Dextroamphetamine as a treatment for depression and low energy in AIDS patients: a pilot study. J Psychosom Res 42(4):407–411, 1997 9160280

Warnke D, Barreto J, Temesgen Z: Antiretroviral drugs. J Clin Pharmacol 47(12):1570–1579, 2007 18048575

Wiegand M, Möller AA, Schreiber W, et al: Alterations of nocturnal sleep in patients with HIV infection. Acta Neurol Scand 83(2):141–142, 1991 2017899

Williams JB, Rabkin JG, Remien RH, et al: Multidisciplinary baseline assessment of homosexual men with and without human immunodeficiency virus infection, II: standardized clinical assessment of current and lifetime psychopathology. Arch Gen Psychiatry 48(2):124–130, 1991 1671198

Williams KA, Swedo SE, Farmer CA, et al: Randomized, controlled trial of intravenous immunoglobulin for pediatric autoimmune neuropsychiatric disorders associated with streptococcal infections. J Am Acad Child Adolesc Psychiatry 55(10):860.e2–867.e2, 2016 27663941

Witkowski AE, Manabat CG, Bourgeois JA: Isoniazid-associated psychosis. Gen Hosp Psychiatry 29(1):85–86, 2007 17189755

Woodroof A, Gleason O: Psychiatric symptoms in a case of intracranial tuberculosis. Psychosomatics 43(1):82–84, 2002 11927766

Wu YS, Lane HY, Lin CH: Donepezil improved cognitive deficits in a patient with neurosyphilis. Clin Neuropharmacol 38(4):156–157, 2015 26166240

Yew WW: Clinically significant interactions with drugs used in the treatment of tuberculosis. Drug Saf 25(2):111–133, 2002 11888353

Zareifopoulos N, Lagadinou M, Karela A, et al: Efavirenz as a psychotropic drug. Eur Rev Med Pharmacol Sci 24(20):10729–10735, 2020 33155233

Zilikis N, Nimatoudis I, Kiosses V, et al: Treatment with risperidone of an acute psychotic episode in a patient with AIDS. Gen Hosp Psychiatry 20(6):384–385, 1998 9854654

13

Dermatological Disorders

Madhulika A. Gupta, M.D., M.Sc., FRCPC

James L. Levenson, M.D.

Psychiatric and psychosocial comorbidity is present among 25%–30% of patients with dermatological disorders (Gupta and Gupta 1996), and effective management of the condition also involves management of the associated psychiatric factors that can necessitate the use of psychotropic medications (Kuhn et al. 2017). Patients with dermatological disorders are often reluctant to see a psychiatrist; therefore, for effective treatment, a close collaboration between the psychiatrist and the dermatologist may be necessary (Shah and Levenson 2018). The skin is both a source and a target of immunomodulatory mediators of the psychological stress response (Arck et al. 2006). Acute psychological stress and sleep deprivation adversely affect skin barrier function recovery and may exacerbate barrier-mediated dermatoses such as psoriasis and atopic dermatitis (Choi et al. 2005). Various skin-related factors show circadian rhythmicity, including the stratum corneum barrier of the skin, transepidermal water loss (TEWL), skin surface pH, and skin temperature at most anatomical sites, with skin permeability being higher in the evening and night than in the morning (Yosipovitch et al.

1998). Higher TEWL in the evening suggests that the epidermal barrier function at this time is not optimal, and TEWL is associated with greater itch intensity, which typically tends to be higher in the evening, before bedtime. These circadian rhythms are maintained in healthy skin during treatment with high- and medium-potency corticosteroids (Yosipovitch et al. 2004). Clinically, this could be an important consideration in the use of moisturizers and timing of topical drug application (Patel et al. 2007; Yosipovitch et al. 1998, 2004).

The skin is also a large sensory organ with afferent sensory nerves conveying sensations of touch, itch, pain, temperature, and other physical stimuli to the CNS, with the efferent autonomic and mainly cholinergic sympathetic nerves regulating vasomotor and pilomotor functions and activity of the apocrine and eccrine sweat glands (Gupta and Gupta 2014). Unlike other organs, reactions of the skin therefore represent a primarily sympathetic nervous response. Sleep disorders such as obstructive sleep apnea (OSA) and insomnia are often associated with a heightened sympathetic tone. It is therefore important to assess the patient for comorbid sleep-wake disorders (Gupta and Gupta 2013b), especially OSA, which is encountered in a wide range of inflammatory skin conditions (Gupta et al. 2016, 2017b). Insomnia or an elevated periodic leg movement index in patients with atopic dermatitis may also be an indication of underlying sympathetic activation that needs to be addressed. Sympathetic activation can affect sudomotor activity, leading to sweat gland dysfunction, impaired barrier function of the stratum corneum in atopic dermatitis, and exacerbation of atopic dermatitis (Gupta and Gupta 2020). There can be a bidirectional relationship between certain sleep disorders (e.g., those associated with sympathetic activation) and inflammatory dermatological disorders. Comorbid sleep disorders (e.g., OSA) in the patient with a dermatological disorder, when untreated, can have an adverse effect on the response to psychiatric medications. Manipulation of the skin and its appendages (e.g., skin picking, hair pulling, nail peeling, scratching) can be used to manage high levels of anxiety and sympathetic activation in dissociative and obsessive-compulsive states and can result in self-induced dermatoses as a result of the body-focused repetitive behaviors (BFRBs) (American Psychiatric Association 2022).

Classification

Psychodermatological disorders are generally classified into two major categories (Gupta and Gupta 1996; Medansky and Handler 1981): 1) dermatological symptoms of psychiatric disorders and 2) psychiatric symptoms of dermatological disorders.

The dermatological symptoms of psychiatric disorders can be encountered in two DSM-5-TR (American Psychiatric Association 2022) diagnostic groups: 1) "Schizophrenia Spectrum and Other Psychotic Disorders," which includes delusional infestation, delusions of parasitosis, and delusions of bromhidrosis, conditions that are examples of delusional disorder, somatic type; and 2) "Obsessive-Compulsive and Related Disorders," including the BFRBs, consisting of excoriation (skin-picking) disorder, trichotillomania (hair-pulling disorder), and pathological onychophagia (nail biting), and body dysmorphic disorder (BDD), in which dermatological treatments and surgery are most commonly used. Excessive complaints about imagined or slight "flaws," which are a common feature of BDD, are encountered in 11%–13% of patients with dermatological disorders (American Psychiatric Association 2022). A third subcategory that represents dermatological symptoms of psychiatric disorders includes cutaneous reactions due to physiological changes associated with a wide range of psychiatric disorders (e.g., flushing of the skin and profuse daytime perspiration may be the presenting features of panic attacks; unexplained night sweats can be a feature of sympathetic nervous arousal in PTSD [Gupta et al. 2017a]; dramatic unexplained cutaneous sensory symptoms may represent a conversion reaction or a posttraumatic flashback [Gupta 2013a]).

Psychiatric symptoms of dermatological disorders (Gupta and Gupta 1996; Medansky and Handler 1981) can be further subdivided into 1) disorders that have a primary dermatopathological basis but may be influenced in part by psychological factors and often have an immune or inflammatory basis (e.g., psoriasis; atopic dermatitis; urticaria and angioedema; alopecia areata; acne; hidradenitis suppurativa; lichen planus, vitiligo, viral warts, rosacea); 2) disorders that are considered primary dermatological symptoms that represent an accentuated physiological response to psychological stress (e.g., hyperhidrosis, blushing) and may overlap with some of the dermatological symptoms of psychiatric disorders (discussed earlier); 3) disorders that result in an emotional reaction primarily as a result of cosmetic disfigurement or the social stigma associated with the disease; and 4) the cutaneous and mucosal sensory syndromes that represent a heterogeneous clinical situation in which the patient presents with a disagreeable sensation such as itching, burning, stinging, neuropathic pain or allodynia, or negative sensory symptoms such as numbness and hypoesthesia, with no apparently diagnosable dermatological or medical condition that explains the symptoms. Skin regions that normally have a greater density of epidermal innervation tend to be most susceptible. These syndromes tend to be referred to with region-specific terms such as *scalp dysesthesias*, *burning mouth syndrome* or *glossodynia*, and *vulvodynia* (Gupta and Gupta 2013a). These sensory syndromes represent a complex and often poorly understood interplay between local dermatological and neurobiological factors associated with neuropathic pain, neuropathic itch, and neurological or neuropsychiatric states (e.g., radiculopathies, stroke, depression, PTSD) (Gupta and Gupta 2013a). These subcategories are not mutually exclusive.

The skin is a highly visible organ that readily reacts to psychosocial stress and plays a vital role as a complex organ of communication throughout the life span (Gupta and Gupta 2014). A wide range of dermatological symptoms (which may include the disorders described earlier), depending on their presentation, may be classified under DSM-5-TR "Somatic Symptom and Related Disorders" (Levenson et al. 2017).

Clinically, treatment for most patients requires a comprehensive biopsychosocial approach that typically includes both psychopharmacological treatments and psychotherapeutic interventions (e.g., cognitive-behavioral therapy, including habit reversal therapy, and dialectical behavior therapy).

Currently, no orally administered drugs are approved by the U.S. FDA for the treatment of a primary dermatological disorder or a BFRB involving the skin; 5% topical doxepin cream is FDA approved for short-term management (up to 8 days) of moderate pruritus for adults with conditions such as atopic dermatitis.

Pharmacotherapy for Dermatological Symptoms of Psychiatric Disorders

Delusional Disorder, Somatic Type

Delusional disorder, somatic type, classified in DSM-5-TR under "Schizophrenia Spectrum and Other Psychotic Disorders," can manifest as a delusion that there is an infestation affecting the skin (delusional infestation, delusions of parasitosis) or that a foul odor is being emitted from the skin or mucous membranes (delusions of bromhidrosis). Tactile hallucinations are particularly common in delirium, drug intoxication, and drug withdrawal. In some cases of delusional infestation, activation of itch pathways may be the underlying cause of the skin sensations (Kimsey 2016), and treatments for pruritus may be effective.

The biggest challenge in the pharmacotherapy of delusional infestation is convincing patients to take a psychiatric drug, because they do not view themselves as having a psychiatric disorder. In such instances, a strong therapeutic alliance involving the dermatologist and primary care physician can become an essential prerequisite for effective pharmacotherapy, and treatment of the delusional infestation must be customized depending on the underlying cause of the delusion. In cases of secondary delusional infestation (e.g., other psychiatric disorder, sensory deprivation, multiple sclerosis, stroke, Parkinson's disease, early dementia, effects of prescription medication, feature of pruritus during dialysis or illicit drug use), the primary disorder must be managed (Heller et al. 2013). The clinician must maintain an index of suspicion, because delusional infestation can present as *folie à deux* (E.J. Yang et al. 2019) involving the marital partner (Rodríguez-Cerdeira et al. 2017). Patients who believe they are infested present with a broad range of symptoms that may be classified as an infection or a somatic delusion, in which case a low-dose antipsychotic agent may be helpful (Beuerlein et al. 2021).

Selective serotonin reuptake inhibitors (SSRIs) have sometimes been helpful for patients with delusional infestation whose parasite sensations are more obsessional than delusional. Pimozide has been referred to as the gold standard for treating delusional infestation (Heller et al. 2013); however, little evidence substantiates its use. The recommended starting dosage for pimozide is 0.5 mg/day, to a maximum of 4 mg/day, with a therapeutic range of 2–3 mg/day (Heller et al. 2013); this is not an FDA-approved indication for pimozide, and no clinical trials have reported superiority of pimozide over other typical or atypical antipsychotics. It has been recommended that pimozide not be used as a first-line drug because of its extensive side-effect profile (Lepping and Freudenmann 2008). Sudden unexpected deaths have been reported with pimozide, with the possible mechanism being ventricular arrhythmias caused by QTc interval prolongation.

In a study of 17 consecutive patients with delusional infestation, 88% were taking antipsychotics, and 71% reached full remission; the average duration of treatment was 3.8 years (Huber et al. 2011). In a series of 59 patients with delusional infestation who received treatment, 68% reported improvement or resolution of symptoms. Recurrence of symptoms occurred in 27% within 4 months of stopping; these patients may need long-term maintenance therapy (Wong and Bewley 2011). Both first-generation (haloperidol) and second-generation (risperidone, olanzapine, quetiapine) antipsychotic drugs and aripiprazole have been used in delusional infestation (Heller et al. 2013); risperidone and olanzapine have been reported to be the most commonly used second-generation antipsychotics, with about 70% efficacy with doses lower than those used in schizophrenia (Freudenmann and Lepping 2008). However, the experience of most dermatologists is much less positive than these reports, because most patients with delusional infestation refuse psychiatric referral or antipsychotic medication.

Body-Focused Repetitive Behaviors

The BFRBs are classified in DSM-5-TR under the obsessive-compulsive and related disorders. *N*-acetylcysteine (NAC), at a dosage of 2,400–3,000 mg/day for a course of 12 weeks, has resulted in a reduction in severity of BFRB symptoms with a good tolerability profile (Oliver et al. 2015). No medications are specifically FDA approved for the treatment of BFRBs involving the integument (excoriation disorder, trichotillomania). Psychiatric medications tend to be more helpful when the BFRB is significantly mediated by underlying depression or anxiety. The BFRBs may further exacerbate an underlying dermatological disorder (e.g., acne excoriée). Nonpharmacological interventions such as cognitive-behavioral therapy with a habit reversal training component tend to be more effective in the treatment of the behavioral component of BFRBs.

A meta-analysis of randomized controlled trials (RCTs) examining treatments for trichotillomania symptoms (Farhat et al. 2020) involving 24 trials and 857 participants found that those who underwent habit reversal training had a greater improvement than control participants; clomipramine (maximum dose=250 mg; duration=9 weeks), NAC (maximum dose=2,400 mg/day; duration=12 weeks), and olanzapine (maximum dose=20 mg/day; duration=12 weeks) showed significant benefits compared with placebo in the RCTs (Farhat et al. 2020). A Cochrane review that examined a wider range of trichotillomania treatments reported similar findings (Hoffman et al. 2021). Trichotillomania is associated with trichobezoars in up to 10% of cases, which can lead to bowel obstruction and necessitate surgical removal.

If the patient's grooming behaviors in trichotillomania are strictly to improve appearance, the patient may have BDD (American Psychiatric Association 2022); it is important to recognize and treat comorbid BDD. Excoriation disorder is present in up to 30% of patients with BDD (Odlaug and Grant 2012).

Excoriation disorder (American Psychiatric Association 2022) is a heterogeneous group of disorders (Gupta and Gupta 2019), from the typical patient who picks benign irregularities, pimples, or scabs to cases of dermatitis artefacta, in which the lesions are wholly self-inflicted, often when the patient is in a dissociated state. Patients with dermatitis artefacta typically deny the self-inflicted nature of their lesions, which are often bizarre looking and surrounded by normal-looking skin. Presentation of these lesions (e.g., blisters, purpura, ulcers, erythema, edema, sinuses, nodules) depends on the means used to create them, such as deep excoriation by fingernails or sharp object or chemical and thermal burns (Gupta et al. 1987). Dermatitis artefacta can result in full-thickness skin loss and severe scarring, necessitating extensive plastic surgery and even amputations (Gupta and Gupta 2019).

Various approaches to the treatment of excoriation disorder (Lochner et al. 2017) include cognitive-behavioral therapy (including habit reversal therapy), SSRIs (fluoxetine average dosage of 55 mg/day, citalopram 20 mg/day), NAC (Grant et al. 2009, 2012), and naltrexone. Lamotrigine, 25–300 mg/day, was shown to be effective in excoriation disorder in a 12-week open-label trial (Grant et al. 2007) but did not show greater benefit than placebo in a follow-up double-blind, placebo-controlled trial (Grant et al. 2010). Ten patients with DSM-5 (American Psychiatric Association 2013) excoriation disorder were treated with 12-week open-label topiramate (titrating upward dosage = 25–200 mg/day) (Jafferany and Osuagwu 2017). The mean time to respond to topiramate was 8–10 weeks, and topiramate was reported to reduce time spent skin picking from 85 to 30 minutes per day (Jafferany and Osuagwu 2017). A case study reported efficacy of augmentation with 15 mg of mirtazapine at bedtime in a 60-year-old patient for whom several other treatments had failed (Keshtkarjahromi et al. 2021). A systematic review and meta-analysis including 12 trials and excoriation disorder treatment moderators (Selles et al. 2016) found a large overall treatment effect size (Hedges' g = 1.13), comprising a large effect size for behavioral treatments (Hedges' g = 1.19), lamotrigine (Hedges' g = 0.98), and SSRIs (Hedges' g = 1.09). Overall, the meta-analysis did not provide strong evidence to support any specific treatment (Selles et al. 2016).

Dissociative states tend to be underrecognized in the BFRBs (Gupta 2013b; Gupta et al. 2017c); excoriation disorder manifesting as dermatitis artefacta typically is associated with high levels of dissociation (Gupta et al. 2018a). Case studies suggest that mood stabilizers (lamotrigine, divalproex) are effective in managing both the anxiety and the manipulation of the integument when high levels of dissociation are present (Gupta 2013b). High dissociation levels in patients with obsessive-compulsive and related disorders tend to be associated with a poor response to standard therapies (Belli et al. 2012; Semiz et al. 2014). Studies of mood stabilizers in the BFRBs—lamotrigine in excoriation disorder (Grant et al. 2007, 2010) and topiramate in trichotillomania (Lochner et al. 2006)—have reported essentially negative results; these studies included all patients with BFRBs and did not consider only the subgroup with high dissociation levels. Reports involving case studies and case series show some positive response of BFRBs to electroconvulsive therapy in 70% of cases (Dos Santos-Ribeiro et al. 2018).

Psychiatric Associations of Dermatological Disorders

Pruritus

Pruritus, including nocturnal pruritus, is transdiagnostically one of the most common symptoms of dermatological disease that contributes significantly to psychiatric morbidity. Psychiatric factors alone can play an important role in chronic pruritus in the absence of dermatological disease (Weisshaar et al. 2019). Scratching during sleep (DelRosso and Hoque 2012), which has been shown to be proportional to the overall level of sympathetic nervous activity during the respective sleep stages, usually occurs most frequently during non–rapid eye movement stages N1 and N2, when the sympathetic tone is the highest, and least frequently in stage N3, when the sympathetic tone is the lowest (Gupta and Gupta 2013b). Benzodiazepines suppress stage N3 sleep, and their long-term use can be associated with autonomic dysregulation as a result of withdrawal symptoms. Benzodiazepines are not recommended as a treatment for sleep disturbance due to pruritus.

Chronic pruritus in dermatological diseases can represent several clinical situations (Andrade et al. 2020): 1) the cause of pruritus is known and treatment of the underlying skin condition may be sufficient; 2) a comorbid psychiatric disorder such as depression mediates pruritus perception in patients with pruritic dermatoses (Gupta et al. 1994), in which case the psychiatric co-morbidity should be treated; and 3) the pruritus is of unknown origin, which has been reported in 8%–15% of affected patients (Andrade et al. 2020). Doxepin has been described by some (Myers et al. 2022) as "the most efficacious antipruritic available to dermatologists"; however, it is often associated with a suboptimal response because of interpatient variability in doxepin plasma levels and clinical response. The authors explore the possible role of genetic polymorphisms that affect doxepin metabolism and monitoring of doxepin blood levels in order to optimize the response to doxepin (Myers et al. 2022). A case report described a 67-year-old man whose intractable scalp itch was controlled for 3 years with high-dose doxepin at 280 mg/day (Chan et al. 2020); clinicians should familiarize themselves with the potentially serious side effects of high doses of tricyclic antidepressants (TCAs) (e.g., confusion and other anticholinergic side effects and cardiac side effects [slowing of cardiac conduction, orthostatic hypotension]) and carefully monitor the patient. A Cochrane review of treatments of pruritus of unknown origin in which the primary outcome measures were patient- or parent-reported pruritus severity found an absence of evidence for the main interventions of interest, which included topical antidepressants, systemic antihistamines, systemic antidepressants, and systemic anticonvulsants (Andrade et al. 2020). In some patients, pruritus of unknown origin may represent dissociation and conversion symptoms, with a background of severe trauma and PTSD (Gupta et al. 2017c). Such patients are usually complex, and their chronic pruritus often represents an interaction between local dermatological and neuropsychiatric factors; treatment usually involves psychotherapy and pharmacotherapy (Gupta et al. 2018a, 2018b) individualized for optimal symptom management.

The literature on psychosomatic dermatology has tended to focus on inflammatory or immune-mediated dermatological conditions that tend to be exacerbated by psychological stress. In a systematic review (Eskeland et al. 2017) involving 1,252 patients with a wide range of inflammatory dermatoses (atopic dermatitis and other eczema, psoriasis, chronic urticaria, alopecia areata) (from 28 clinical trials or case reports), treatment with monoaminergic antidepressants was unambiguously associated with reports of a reduced disease burden of dermatological symptoms; the authors attributed the improvement to the anti-inflammatory effect of antidepressants (Eskeland et al. 2017).

Atopic Dermatitis or Eczema

The management of atopic dermatitis requires a multifaceted approach that takes into consideration the psychiatric and psychosocial dimensions of the condition (Senra and Wollenberg 2014; Sidbury et al. 2014). In a meta-analysis (Patel et al. 2019) involving 36 observational studies, atopic dermatitis was associated with significantly higher depression scale scores, parental depression, antidepressant use, and suicidal ideation. A systematic review and meta-analysis involving 15 studies and 310,681 patients with atopic dermatitis found significant ORs for both suicidal ideation (OR = 1.44; 95% CI = 1.25–1.65) and suicide attempt (OR = 1.36; 95% CI = 1.09–1.70); studies of completed suicides in atopic dermatitis had inconsistent findings (Sandhu et al. 2019). Important goals in the pharmacotherapy for atopic dermatitis are interruption of the itch-scratch cycle and optimization of nighttime sleep (Levenson 2008a). In a longitudinal cohort study of 13,988 children, including 4,938 children (ages 2–16 years) with atopic dermatitis, maternal- or self-reported sleep quality (difficulty falling asleep, nighttime and early-morning awakenings, nightmares) but not maternal- or self-reported total sleep duration was affected in children with active atopic dermatitis (Ramirez et al. 2019). Sleep disruption in children as a result of pruritus can stress the entire family, exacerbate the atopic dermatitis as a result of the itch-scratch cycle, affect cognitive functioning, and lead to behaviors that simulate ADHD (Camfferman et al. 2010). A randomized double-blind, placebo-controlled study using melatonin, 6 mg/day, in 70 children with atopic dermatitis (ages 6–12 years) found that after 6 weeks of intervention, melatonin supplementation had no significant effect on pruritus scores but significantly improved the Scoring Atopic Dermatitis index, which assesses the extent and severity of eczema (Taghavi Ardakani et al. 2018).

Topical doxepin (5% cream) is effective in the treatment of pruritus in atopic dermatitis (Drake et al. 1995) and is FDA approved for short-term (up to 8 days) treatment of moderate pruritus in adults with atopic dermatitis but not in children because of the greater risk of systemic side effects such as drowsiness. Low-dose oral doxepin (e.g., starting at 10 mg at bedtime and titrated on the basis of efficacy and side effects) is helpful in adults because of its antihistaminic sedative properties (Kelsay 2006). Sedating antidepressants may be beneficial, in part through promoting sleep.

The strongly antihistaminic antidepressants doxepin, trimipramine, and amitriptyline also may be effective because of their strong anticholinergic properties, as the eccrine sweat glands in atopic dermatitis have been found to be hypersensitive to acetylcholine. When prescribing agents with strong anticholinergic properties, the clinician must monitor the adverse cognitive effects associated with their long-term use.

Bupropion has been reported to be beneficial in atopic dermatitis in case reports (González et al. 2006) and a small open-label study of bupropion sustained release, 150 mg/day for 3 weeks, followed by 150 mg bid for 3 weeks (Modell et al. 2002). There are also case reports of benefits from dextroamphetamine (Check and Chan 2014); mirtazapine, 15 mg/day (Hundley and Yosipovitch 2004); and mirtazapine, 30 mg/day, with olanzapine up to 7.5 mg at bedtime (Mahtani et al. 2005). No guidelines have been established for the treatment of sleep disturbance in atopic dermatitis (Kelsay 2006). In a small short-term, double-blind, placebo-controlled crossover trial, the benzodiazepine nitrazepam did not significantly reduce nocturnal scratching (Ebata et al. 1998). The lack of response of pruritus to nitrazepam is consistent with the observation that scratching from pruritus is least likely to occur during stage N3 sleep, which is suppressed by benzodiazepines (Gupta and Gupta 2013b). For the management of anxiety in atopic dermatitis, an antihistaminic TCA such as doxepin starting at 10 mg/day is recommended over benzodiazepines because benzodiazepine withdrawal may exacerbate pruritus.

Psoriasis

Among dermatological disorders, psoriasis and psoriatic arthritis are frequently associated with serious psychiatric comorbidity (Gupta and Gupta 1998). In a multicenter European study (Dalgard et al. 2015), suicidal ideation was significantly more common in patients with dermatological conditions than in control subjects (hospital employees) (adjusted OR=1.94; 95% CI=1.33–2.82); among the individual dermatological disorders, only psoriasis had a significant association with suicidal ideation (Dalgard et al. 2015). A systematic review and meta-analysis (Dowlatshahi et al. 2014) reported a 28% prevalence of clinical depression among patients with psoriasis in studies that used questionnaires and a 19% prevalence in studies that used DSM-IV criteria (American Psychiatric Association 1994); population-based studies showed that patients with psoriasis were more likely to experience depression

(OR = 1.57; 95% CI = 1.40–1.76) and to use more antidepressants (OR = 4.24; 95% CI = 1.53–11.76) than were control subjects. Inpatients with severe psoriasis were almost 2.5 times more likely than the general population to be receiving psychotropic medications (Gerdes et al. 2008). In a cohort study, 25,691 patients with psoriasis and 128,573 reference subjects were followed up for more than 9 years (Dowlatshahi et al. 2013). The adjusted hazard ratio (HR) of first antidepressant use in psoriasis was 1.55 (95% CI = 1.50–1.61); in the psoriasis cohort, the HR of receiving an antidepressant was significantly higher (1.07) after the first antipsoriatic treatment (95% CI = 1.02–1.12).

Improvement in the clinical severity of psoriasis is generally associated with an improvement in psychiatric comorbidity. However, in many cases clinically mild psoriasis that affects a small percentage of total body surface area in socially visible regions or the genital area (emotionally charged body regions) can carry a significant psychosocial burden. Psoriasis-related stress, most often associated with psoriasis in emotionally charged body regions, can lead to exacerbations of the psoriasis (Gupta et al. 1989). A review of the literature concluded that patients with psoriasis experience psychiatric and psychosocial morbidity that is not always commensurate with the extent of cutaneous lesions (Rieder and Tausk 2012). In a study of 414 patients with psoriasis, dermatological improvement was less likely to be associated with psychological improvement in female patients and those with localization of the psoriasis on the face (Sampogna et al. 2007).

SSRI antidepressant use in psoriasis has been associated with a decreased need for systemic psoriasis treatments. A Swedish population-based cohort study of 1,282 patients with plaque psoriasis (89% with mild psoriasis) who also had prescriptions for SSRIs twice during a 6-month period and 1,282 patients with psoriasis matched for demographics and psoriasis severity who were not exposed to SSRIs reported that the risk of switching from less aggressive topical therapies to systemic psoriasis treatments was significantly lower in the SSRI-exposed group (OR = 0.44; 95% CI = 0.28–0.68) (Thorslund et al. 2013). The authors discussed various possible factors, including an improvement in the SSRI-exposed subjects' mood, which increased compliance with nonsystemic psoriasis treatments, and a direct anti-inflammatory effect from the SSRIs (Thorslund et al. 2013).

SSRIs may have a role in augmenting the effect of a biological agent in psoriasis. In a study of 38 patients receiving anti–tumor necrosis factor-α biological drugs ("biologics") for their psoriasis, augmentation with citalopram, 10 mg/day, was associated at 6 months with a significant decline in pruritus ratings (patient rated via a visual analog scale) but not in the Psoriasis Area and Severity Index score (D'Erme et al. 2014). Several studies have reported a significant improvement in psychiatric comorbidity in patients with psoriasis who received biologics (Strober et al. 2018).

Two double-blind, controlled studies of monoamine oxidase inhibitors (MAOIs) have reported a significant improvement in Psoriasis Area and Severity Index score in patients compared with control participants. In one study (Di Prima and De Pasquale 1989), 13 patients with moderate to severe psoriasis received 8 weeks of tranylcypromine, 5 mg/day, and 8 weeks of placebo in a double-blind crossover design; in the second study (Alpsoy et al. 1998), involving patients with moderate or less severe psoriasis, 22 patients with psoriasis received the reversible MAOI moclobemide (300 mg qam and 150 mg qhs) for 6 weeks, compared with 20 control subjects who received only topical corticosteroids.

In a small open-label trial involving 10 patients, bupropion induced improvement in psoriasis, with return to baseline levels after its discontinuation (Modell et al. 2002), and paroxetine was reported to be effective in 2 patients with both depression and psoriasis (Luis Blay 2006). Overall, the evidence base is limited, and antidepressants, including bupropion (Cox et al. 2002), sometimes have been reported to cause or aggravate psoriasis (Warnock and Morris 2002a). A case study reported improvement of psoriasis with pregabalin or gabapentin (Boyd et al. 2008). In a case series, seven patients with psoriasis (six of whom also had a mood disorder) treated with topiramate for a minimum of 4 months at an average dosage of 56 mg/day had significant improvement in their psoriasis (Ryback 2002).

Meditation, relaxation training, and cognitive-behavioral stress management are some psychological therapies that have been reported to be effective for patients with psoriasis (Levenson 2008b). Obesity, moderately heavy alcohol use, and tobacco smoking should be addressed in the management of psoriasis because they have been associated with poor response to dermatological therapies (Gottlieb et al. 2008). The association between psoriasis and metabolic syndrome, obesity, hyperlipidemia, hypertension, and cardiovascular mortality (A. W. Armstrong et al. 2013; E. J. Armstrong et al. 2013; Gottlieb et al. 2008) has important implications in the choice of psychopharmacological agents, which may also be associated with glycemic dysregulation, dyslipidemias, and metabolic syndrome.

Urticaria and Angioedema

In interpreting the chronic idiopathic urticaria (CIU, also known as spontaneous urticaria) treatment literature, one must take into consideration the very high rate of response to placebo (Rudzki et al. 1970). CIU tends to be frequently associated with comorbid psychopathology (Konstantinou and Konstantinou 2019); treatment of the comorbid psychiatric disorder is an important component of the overall management of CIU (Gupta and Gupta 2012). A low dose of a sedating antihistaminic antidepressant, such as doxepin, is helpful in the management of pruritus in CIU, especially when pruritus interferes with sleep (Yosipovitch et al. 2002). Doxepin, 5–25 mg tid, may provide more than symptomatic relief, reducing the urticarial reaction itself (Goldsobel et al. 1986; Greene et al. 1985; Rao et al. 1988). Potent histaminic H_1 plus H_2 blockers, such as doxepin, trimipramine, and amitriptyline, are more effective than H_1 antihistamines alone for urticaria (Levenson 2008b). A retrospective cross-sectional study of 36 Turkish patients with CIU (72.2% had accompanying angioedema; duration of urticaria before doxepin was 2–288 months) who did not respond to various combinations of H_1 and H_2 antihistamines and received doxepin determined that doxepin was effective in 75% of patients, with 44.4% showing a complete response (Özkaya et al. 2019). Doxepin was started orally at 10–25 mg/day and gradually increased to 10–25 mg tid (Özkaya et al. 2019). There are also case reports of the benefits of quetiapine in H_1-antihistamine refractory CIU (Yang et al. 2019) and of mirtazapine (Bigatà et al. 2005) and SSRIs (Gupta and Gupta 1995) in CIU. A small open-label study (N= 16) of recalcitrant CIU reported a significant reduction in urticarial activity scores, with reserpine, 0.3–0.4 mg/day, as an add-on therapy to antihistamines at 1–2 weeks and 4–8 weeks (Demitsu et al. 2010). A mood stabilizer may be used when urticaria is a feature of the physiological effect of severe emotional dysregulation in PTSD (Gupta and Gupta 2012); patients with PTSD may develop cholinergic urticaria in response to extreme stress. Adrenergic urticaria (or "halo hives") typically arises in association with extreme stress and has been reported to respond to propranolol (Ollaik et al. 2020); it can arise during a heightened state of anxiety (e.g., during a traumatic flashback in PTSD) and also responds to a low dose of a sedating antipsychotic such as olanzapine.

Alopecia Areata

The literature on the use of psychotropic agents in treating alopecia areata is confounded by the fact that patients may experience spontaneous remission of their alopecia in the absence of any treatments (Levenson 2008b). Trichotillomania, which may coexist with alopecia areata, should be ruled out (Messenger et al. 2012). In a population-based retrospective cohort study in which patients were followed up for up to 26 years, major depressive disorder (MDD) was reported to increase the risk of developing alopecia areata by 90% (HR=1.90; 95% CI=1.67–2.15; $P<0.001$), antidepressants were associated with a protective effect on alopecia areata risk (HR=0.57; 95% CI=0.53–0.62; $P<0.001$), and having alopecia areata was associated with a 34% increased risk of developing MDD (HR=1.34; 95% CI=1.23–1.46; $P<0.001$) (Vallerand et al. 2019). In a study of 60 patients with alopecia areata (with <25% scalp involvement), 30 who also had a diagnosis of major depression received citalopram, 20 mg/day, plus triamcinolone injections every 4 weeks; the patients who received citalopram were compared with 30 patients without depression who received triamcinolone injections alone. After 6 months of therapy, the citalopram group had greater improvement in alopecia than the triamcinolone-alone group, suggesting that antidepressant treatment might help in improving alopecia areata in patients who also have major depression (Abedini et al. 2014). Small double-blind, placebo-controlled trials have reported benefit from imipramine, 75 mg/day ($N=13$) (Perini et al. 1994), and paroxetine, 20 mg/day ($N=13$) (Cipriani et al. 2001).

Acne

Psychiatric drug treatment for patients with acne should focus on any underlying psychiatric disorder (e.g., MDD, BDD, bulimia nervosa). Various antidepressants (clomipramine, fluoxetine, paroxetine) have been shown to be effective in treating depression in acne (Samuels et al. 2020). The patient should be evaluated for acne excoriée because excoriation of the acne lesion can exacerbate the underlying inflammation. The clinician should always maintain an index of suspicion for an underlying BFRB such as DSM-5-TR excoriation disorder in a patient with acne excoriée who may be experiencing trauma and dissociation and picking their skin in a dissociated state. Case studies suggest efficacy of olanzapine in treating self-excoriative behavior in acne excoriée (Gupta and Gupta 2000).

Isotretinoin, which is FDA approved for the treatment of nodulocystic acne, has been associated with multiple case reports of suicidal behaviors (Droitcourt et al. 2019, 2020; Eichenfield et al. 2021); however, a causal relationship has not been proven. An epidemiological study using the Nationwide French Health Insurance database reported that suicide attempts with isotretinoin are rare events, and most affected patients have a risk-prone profile that is detectable at the time of treatment initiation (Droitcourt et al. 2020). Droitcourt et al. (2020) further stated that the risk-benefit ratio of continuing isotretinoin after a suicide attempt warrants further research. A meta-analysis of 31 studies concluded that the prevalence of depression significantly declined after isotretinoin treatment (RR=0.588; 95% CI=0.382–0.904) (Huang and Cheng 2017). In some case studies, hormonal contraceptives have failed in patients who self-medicated their depression with St. John's wort (Hall et al. 2003). St. John's wort is a cytochrome P450 3A4 (CYP3A4) inducer that increases the metabolism of some hormonal contraceptives and decreases their efficacy; patients taking isotretinoin and hormonal contraceptives should be advised of this interaction.

Hidradenitis Suppurativa

Hidradenitis suppurativa (acne inversa) is a chronic inflammatory disorder, with a 0.05%–4.10% prevalence, that typically presents as recurrent or chronic painful suppurating lesions in the apocrine gland–bearing skin regions (axillae, inframammary folds, groin, and perigenital and perineal regions) (Saunte and Jemec 2017). Hidradenitis suppurativa has been associated with bipolar disorder (Benhadou et al. 2020), and lithium therapy has been associated with hidradenitis suppurativa (Gupta et al. 1995). A cohort study that used data from the Danish national registries (Thorlacius et al. 2018) reported an increased risk of completed suicide in patients with hidradenitis suppurativa (HR=2.42; 95% CI=1.07–5.45; P=0.0334) and an increased risk of antidepressant drug use (HR=1.30; 95% CI=1.17–1.45; P<0.0001). The results of a systematic review and meta-analysis of data from 27 studies indicated that the prevalence of depression (26.5% vs. 6.6%) and anxiety (18.1% vs 7.1%) was higher in patients with versus without hidradenitis suppurativa; hidradenitis suppurativa was also associated with higher rates of antidepressant drug use (OR = 1.85; 95% CI = 1.26–2.71) (in two studies) and anxiolytic medication use (based on one study) (29.7% in patients with hidradenitis suppurativa vs. 18.0% in the general population) (Patel et al. 2020). Hidradenitis suppurativa can profoundly reduce quality of life and can be associated with embarrassment and pain (Goldburg et al. 2020). Various psychotherapeutic interventions, including cognitive-behavioral therapy and acceptance and commitment therapy, and the possible beneficial effects of various serotonin-norepinephrine reuptake inhibitors and TCAs (e.g., duloxetine, venlafaxine, nortriptyline, desipramine, amitriptyline), have been discussed as part of a chronic pain management algorithm for hidradenitis suppurativa (Savage et al. 2021).

Cutaneous and Mucosal Dysesthesias

The cutaneous and mucosal dysesthesias are a heterogeneous and often multifactorial group of disorders; treatments used and their efficacy depend largely on the etiology of the cutaneous sensory syndrome (Gupta and Gupta 2013a). Burning mouth syndrome (BMS) is a complex, chronic disorder of orofacial sensation, commonly affecting perimenopausal and postmenopausal women, that is difficult to diagnose and to treat, with psychological or psychiatric factors present in up to 85% of patients with BMS (Charleston 2013). In a 10-week RCT, clonazepam, 0.5 mg/day, was more effective than placebo in treating pain of idiopathic BMS (Heckmann et al. 2012). A retrospective chart review of 51 patients with BMS seen over 10 years found that 42 patients (82.4%) had been prescribed antidepressants and 31 (60.8%) had been prescribed SSRIs. SSRIs tended to be more effective for patients who reported that stress was the major factor aggravating their BMS (Fleuret et al. 2014). An open-label study of 150 patients with BMS that compared vortioxetine, 15 mg/day, with other antidepressants (paroxetine, 20 mg/day; sertraline, 50 mg/day; escitalopram, 10 mg/day; or duloxetine, 60 mg/day) observed that all antidepressants were associated with a significant decrease in symptoms; vortioxetine had a significantly shorter latency of action and fewer adverse events than the other antidepressants (Adamo et al. 2021). An RCT of 20 patients with BMS (Varoni et al. 2018) who received melatonin (12 mg/day) or placebo in an 8-week crossover design showed that melatonin was not superior to placebo in relieving pain, and sleep quality did not change significantly during the trial. In a Cochrane review of 23 RCTs with 1,121 analyzed participants, the RCTs compared any drug with placebo in patients with BMS, with a primary outcome of symptom relief (burning or pain) and change in quality of life. The evidence about the effectiveness of systemic benzodiazepines, antidepressants, and cholinergics was insufficient or contradictory (McMillan et al. 2016). McMillan et al. (2016) further concluded that because of the limited number of clinical trials with low risk of bias, evidence was insufficient to support or refute the use of any treatment interventions in managing BMS.

Vulvodynia is a complex disorder in which patients typically present with complaints of burning, stinging, irritation, or rawness that is difficult to treat (Stockdale and Lawson 2014). The onset and maintenance involve a complex interplay of peripheral and central nervous system factors (e.g., anxiety, depression, childhood maltreatment) (Bergeron et al. 2020). A multicenter double-blind, placebo-controlled study of extended-release gabapentin (1,200–3,000 mg/day) involving 89 women found that gabapentin did not improve pain over placebo; the results did not support the recommendation of gabapentin alone as a treatment of vulvodynia (Brown et al. 2018). Treatment guidelines for vulvodynia based on expert consensus (Stockdale and Lawson 2014) include TCAs, such as amitriptyline, nortriptyline, and desipramine, starting at 10–25 mg at bedtime, which may be increased to 100–150 mg depending on the response; other antidepressants, including venlafaxine and SSRIs; and some anticonvulsants (Haefner et al. 2005). Rapid resolution of symptoms in vulvodynia is unusual even with appropriate therapy, and no single treatment is successful for all women (Stockdale and Lawson 2014). Evidence indicates a significant placebo effect in the treatment of vulvodynia (Miranda Varella Pereira et al. 2018).

Scalp dysesthesia tends to be underrecognized and misdiagnosed as seborrheic dermatitis (Kinoshita-Ise and Shear 2019). Case reports suggest that scalp dysesthesia may respond to low dosages of antihistaminic TCAs, such as amitriptyline, 10–50 mg/day, and doxepin, 20–50 mg/day (Hoss and Segal 1998), or pregabalin, 75–150 mg/day (Sarifakioglu and Onur 2013). A systematic review of studies of treatment for prurigo nodularis found that pregabalin, amitriptyline, paroxetine, fluvoxamine, and neurokinin 1 receptor antagonists have demonstrated promising evidence in five level 2b studies (level of evidence according to the Oxford Center for Evidence-Based Medicine) (Qureshi et al. 2019).

Adverse Cutaneous Drug Reactions to Psychotropic Agents

Adverse cutaneous drug reactions (Litt 2013; Warnock and Morris 2002a, 2002b, 2003) can be divided into common (usually relatively benign) reactions and rare life-threatening reactions (Stevens-Johnson syndrome [SJS]/toxic epidermal necrolysis [TEN, also known as Lyell's syndrome]; acute generalized exanthematous pustulosis, also referred to as drug reaction with eosinophilia and systemic symptoms [DRESS]). Adverse cutaneous drug reactions are reported to affect 2%–3% of hospitalized patients, and 2% of these cutaneous reactions are severe and life-threatening. Approximately 2%–5% of patients receiving psychotropic medications will develop adverse cutaneous drug reactions (Kimyai-Asadi et al. 1999).

Mild Adverse Cutaneous Drug Reactions

Mild adverse cutaneous drug reactions can occur with antipsychotics, antidepressants, and mood stabilizers. They include the following:

- *Pruritus* is the most common adverse cutaneous drug reaction, encountered with all antipsychotics, antidepressants, and mood stabilizers, and is usually secondary to other adverse cutaneous drug reactions.
- *Exanthematous rashes* (morbilliform or maculopapular eruptions) can occur with all antipsychotics, antidepressants, and mood stabilizers. The rash usually occurs within the first 3–14 days after the drug is started and may subside without discontinuation of the causative agent. In some cases, the rash, especially if it includes painful lesions, may represent the early stages of one of the more severe and life-threatening adverse cutaneous drug reactions, such as SJS.
- *Urticaria*, with or without angioedema, is the second most common adverse cutaneous drug reaction after pruritus. It occurs within minutes to a few hours but sometimes as late as several days after the drug is started and can lead to laryngeal angioedema and anaphylaxis. Urticaria can occur with all antipsychotics, antidepressants, and anticonvulsants.
- *Fixed drug eruptions* can theoretically occur with any drug. They characteristically appear as sharply demarcated, solitary, or occasionally multiple

lesions that occur within a few to 24 hours after ingestion of the drug and resolve within several weeks of drug discontinuation.

- *Photosensitivity reactions* are the result of an interaction of the drug with ultraviolet radiation and are limited to body regions exposed to light. Such reactions can be caused by any of the antipsychotics but are much more frequently associated with chlorpromazine (3% incidence) (Warnock and Morris 2002b). Photosensitivity also occurs with antidepressants, including the TCAs and SSRIs; some mood stabilizers, including carbamazepine, valproic acid, topiramate, gabapentin, and oxcarbazepine; and some sedatives and hypnotics, including amobarbital, phenobarbital, pentobarbital, alprazolam, estazolam, chlordiazepoxide, eszopiclone, zaleplon, and zolpidem. The incidence of photosensitivity for each of the medications from the three classes of drugs is 1% or less (Litt 2013). Patients should be advised about the use of sunscreen and minimization of sun exposure if the medication must be continued. Photosensitivity caused by psychotropic drugs may interfere with psoralen plus ultraviolet A and ultraviolet B light therapy for psoriasis and other pruritic dermatoses.

- *Drug-induced pigmentation*, which may involve the skin and eyes (retina, lens, and cornea), has been reported after long-term (>6 months), high-dose (>500 mg/day) use of low-potency typical antipsychotics, especially chlorpromazine and thioridazine. The cutaneous discoloration in some instances is secondary to dermal granules containing melanin bound to the drug or its metabolites; the discoloration can take months or years to completely resolve after discontinuation of the drug. Pigmentary changes have been associated with some antidepressants, including various TCAs, all SSRIs, and venlafaxine (hypopigmentation), and with some anticonvulsants, including lamotrigine (also associated with leukoderma), carbamazepine, topiramate, gabapentin, and valproic acid (also associated with changes in hair color and texture).

- *Alopecia*, which typically appears as diffuse, nonscarring, and localized or generalized hair loss from the scalp, is usually reversible after discontinuation of the offending drug. Hair loss may occur rapidly or a few months after the drug has been started, with recovery generally 2–5 months after drug discontinuation. Alopecia has been reported frequently with lithium (>5%) and valproic acid (>5%) and less frequently with the other mood stabilizers. Alopecia also has been associated with most antidepressants, including all

SSRIs, bupropion, venlafaxine, and duloxetine, and with several antipsychotics, including olanzapine, risperidone, ziprasidone, loxapine, and haloperidol.

Severe Adverse Cutaneous Drug Reactions

Severe and life-threatening skin reactions are most frequently associated with the aromatic antiepileptic drugs (e.g., lamotrigine, carbamazepine, phenytoin, oxcarbazepine, phenobarbital) and include erythema multiforme, SJS, TEN, drug hypersensitivity syndrome or DRESS, exfoliative dermatitis, and vasculitis (Litt 2013; Warnock and Morris 2002a, 2002b, 2003). Erythema multiforme, SJS, and TEN lie on a continuum of increasing severity. About 16% of cases of SJS or TEN have been associated with short-term use of antiepileptic drugs, with the greatest risk for development of TEN within the first 8 weeks of initiating therapy. Use of multiple anticonvulsants and higher doses increase the risk. Treatment of severe reactions should include immediate discontinuation of the drug and an emergency dermatology consultation. Patients typically need fluid and nutritional support, as well as infection and pain control, which may involve management in an intensive care or burn unit. Increased risk is associated with immunosuppression, especially when accompanied by primary or viral reactivation of herpesviruses (e.g., human herpesviruses 6 and 7) or infection with Epstein-Barr virus or HIV (Dodiuk-Gad et al. 2014; Husain et al. 2013). Adequate psychiatric supervision should also be provided when mood stabilizer antiepileptic drugs are abruptly discontinued because significant relapse of psychiatric symptoms may occur (Bliss and Warnock 2013).

Increased risk of developing SJS/TEN because of use of anticonvulsants, most commonly carbamazepine, has been attributed to several human leukocyte antigen (HLA) allele variants (Cheng et al. 2014; Grover and Kukreti 2014), specifically *HLA-B*1502* and *HLA-A*3101*. The *B*1502* variant is seen more often in Asian populations. The FDA suggests that patients of Asian (including South Asian Indian) ancestry be screened for the *B*1502* variant before commencing carbamazepine or phenytoin therapy (U.S. Food and Drug Administration 2007). This variant has also been associated with SJS/TEN induced by other anticonvulsants (Hung et al. 2010). The *A*3101* variant is seen in numerous populations, including white individuals, and is associated with several adverse cutaneous drug reactions, including SJS/TEN and DRESS. At present, the FDA does not explicitly suggest genotyping for the *A*3101* variant before commencing carbamazepine; however, some investigators (Amstutz et al. 2014) have recommended screening all carbamazepine-naive patients for the *A*3101* allele.

Erythema multiforme occurs within days of starting the drug and may present as a polymorphous eruption, with pathognomonic "target lesions" typically involving the extremities and palmoplantar surfaces. Progression of erythema multiforme to more serious SJS and TEN should always be considered a possibility. Although erythema multiforme is most commonly associated with carbamazepine, valproic acid, lamotrigine, gabapentin, and oxcarbazepine, it has also (albeit rarely) been associated with antipsychotics (e.g., clozapine, risperidone) and antidepressants (e.g., fluoxetine, paroxetine, bupropion) and occasionally with sedative-hypnotics (including barbiturates, some benzodiazepines, and eszopiclone).

SJS usually occurs within the first few weeks of drug exposure. Patients present with flulike symptoms, followed by mucocutaneous lesions and a mortality rate as high as 5% as a result of the loss of the cutaneous barrier and sepsis. Bullous lesions can involve mucosal surfaces, including the eyes, mouth, and genital tract. SJS is most frequently associated with the same anticonvulsants as erythema multiforme.

TEN is considered to be an extreme variant of SJS, resulting in epidermal detachment in more than 30% of patients, occurring within the first 2 months of treatment, with a mortality rate as high as 45% due to sepsis. In 80% of TEN cases, a strong association is made with specific medications (vs. a 50% association with specific medications in SJS), most often anticonvulsants (Litt 2013; Warnock and Morris 2002a, 2002b, 2003). Use of more than one anticonvulsant increases the risk of SJS/TEN. For lamotrigine, the risk of a serious rash may be increased by coadministration with divalproex sodium, exceeding the initial recommended dosage, or exceeding the recommended dosage escalation. Benign rashes also occur with lamotrigine, and it is not possible to reliably predict which rash will prove to be serious or life-threatening. Therefore, lamotrigine should be discontinued at the first sign of a rash unless the rash is clearly benign or not drug related.

Drug hypersensitivity syndrome, or DRESS, characteristically occurs 1–8 weeks after the start of drug treatment and manifests as a drug eruption, most commonly a morbilliform rash, with fever, eosinophilia, lymphadenopathy, and multiple organ involvement (including liver, kidney, lungs, and brain). Treatment involves immediate discontinuation of the suspected drug. Antihistamines and systemic corticosteroids may be needed. The mortality rate is 10% if symptoms are unrecognized or untreated. The rash can range from a simple exanthem to TEN. DRESS is most commonly associated with anticonvulsants and has been reported with bupropion and fluoxetine (Husain et al. 2013).

Exfoliative dermatitis appears as a widespread rash characterized by desquamation, pruritic erythema, fever, and lymphadenopathy within the first few weeks of drug therapy, with a good prognosis if the causative agent is withdrawn immediately. It has been reported with antipsychotics, most TCAs and other antidepressants, mood stabilizers, lithium, sedatives, and hypnotics.

Drug hypersensitivity vasculitis is characterized by inflammation and necrosis of the walls of blood vessels within a few weeks of starting a drug. Lesions (e.g., palpable purpura) are localized primarily on the lower third of the legs and ankles. It has been associated with clozapine, maprotiline, trazodone, carbamazepine, lithium, phenobarbital, pentobarbital, diazepam, and chlordiazepoxide.

Exacerbation of Dermatological Disorders by Psychotropic Medications

Psychotropic drugs may precipitate or exacerbate some primary dermatological disorders (Litt 2013; Warnock and Morris 2002a, 2002b, 2003), including acne, psoriasis, seborrheic dermatitis, hyperhidrosis, and porphyria. Acne has been associated with most TCAs, all SSRIs, and other antidepressants such as venlafaxine, duloxetine, and bupropion; lithium carbonate and occasionally other anticonvulsant mood stabilizers, including topiramate, lamotrigine, gabapentin, and oxcarbazepine; and antipsychotics such as quetiapine and haloperidol.

Lithium is well known to precipitate or exacerbate psoriasis (Brauchli et al. 2009). Lithium-induced psoriasis can occur within a few months but usually occurs within the first few years of treatment. Lithium has an inhibitory effect on intracellular cyclic adenosine monophosphate and the phosphoinositides. Inositol supplements have been shown to have a significant beneficial effect on psoriasis for patients taking lithium (Allan et al. 2004). The β-blocker propranolol, which is often used to treat lithium-induced tremors, has also been associated with psoriasis, but a population-based study by Brauchli et al. (2008) did not support this association. Psoriasis precipitated or exacerbated by lithium is typically resistant to conventional antipsoriatic treatments, and usually the patient has no family history of psoriasis. When psoriasis becomes intractable, lithium must be discontinued, and remission usually follows within a few months.

Anticonvulsants, atypical antipsychotics, and SSRIs have been reported less commonly to precipitate or aggravate psoriasis. Results of an epidemiological study suggest possible reduced psoriasis risk with atypical antipsychotics, mainly olanzapine (Brauchli et al. 2009), although case studies have reported onset or exacerbation of psoriasis by olanzapine (Latini and Carducci 2003).

Seborrheic dermatitis typically occurs in regions where the sebaceous glands are most active, such as the scalp, face, chest, and genitalia. Seborrheic dermatitis is very common in patients taking long-term phenothiazines and also has been reported with other antipsychotics, including olanzapine, quetiapine, and loxapine. Seborrheic eruptions have also been reported with lithium and anticonvulsants.

Hyperhidrosis, often manifested as night sweats, is common with SSRIs, serotonin-norepinephrine reuptake inhibitors, bupropion, and MAOIs. Sweating is mediated by the sympathetic cholinergic innervation of the eccrine sweat glands; however, the more anticholinergic TCAs have also caused hyperhidrosis, and therefore switching to a more anticholinergic antidepressant is not necessarily helpful. The mechanism underlying antidepressant-mediated hyperhidrosis is believed to be centrally mediated but is unclear. Hyperhidrosis has also been reported with antipsychotics (e.g., olanzapine, quetiapine, pimozide) and mood stabilizers (e.g., carbamazepine, topiramate [1% of patients], lamotrigine [2%], gabapentin, oxcarbazepine [3%]) (Litt 2013; Warnock and Morris 2002a, 2002b, 2003).

Porphyria may be exacerbated by certain drugs, such as carbamazepine, valproic acid, and many sedative-hypnotics (especially barbiturates and other sedative-hypnotics, excluding benzodiazepines), resulting in acute dermatological, neuropsychiatric, and abdominal pain symptoms. Chlorpromazine, although photosensitizing, is considered to be safe and actually was approved by the FDA for use in acute intermittent porphyria.

Adverse Psychiatric Effects of Dermatological Agents

Corticosteroids

Psychiatric side effects of systemic glucocorticoid therapy are reviewed in detail in Chapter 7, "Respiratory Disorders," and Chapter 10, "Endocrine and Metabolic Disorders." Topical corticosteroids may cause psychiatric adverse effects, especially in patients with extensive lesions who are using high-potency topical steroids (Hughes et al. 1983).

Retinoids

Isotretinoin is generally used to treat nodulocystic acne or acne that is refractory to other therapies and has been associated with depression, psychosis, suicide attempts, and suicide (Azoulay et al. 2008; Borovaya et al. 2013; Jick et al. 2000; Marqueling and Zane 2007; Marron et al. 2013; McGrath et al. 2010; Nevoralová and Dvořáková 2013; Rademaker 2010; Rehn et al. 2009; Sundström et al. 2010; Thomas et al. 2014). In an analysis of reports of depression and suicide to the FDA from the initial marketing of isotretinoin from 1982 to May 2000, the FDA received reports regarding 431 patients: 37 completed suicides (24 while using isotretinoin and 13 after stopping isotretinoin); 110 hospitalizations for depression, suicidal ideation, or suicide attempt; and 284 cases of nonhospitalized depression (Wysowski et al. 2001). Factors suggesting a possible association between isotretinoin and depression included a temporal association between isotretinoin use and depression, positive dechallenges (often necessitating psychiatric treatment), and positive rechallenges. Compared with all drugs in the FDA's Adverse Event Reporting System, isotretinoin ranked in the top 10 for number of reports of depression and suicide (Wysowski et al. 2001). The study concluded that "additional studies are needed to determine whether isotretinoin causes depression and to identify susceptible persons" (Wysowski et al. 2001, p. 518). The general consensus is that research on the possible causal effect of isotretinoin use on psychiatric morbidity, including suicide risk, is inconclusive.

The guidelines for prescribing isotretinoin (earlier trade name Accutane; only generic brands have been marketed since 2009) (Physicians' Desk Reference 2009) include the following warning:

> Accutane may cause depression, psychosis and, rarely, suicidal ideation, suicide attempts, suicide, and aggressive and/or violent behaviors. No mechanism of action has been established for these events....Therefore prior to initiation of Accutane therapy, patients and family members should be asked about any history of psychiatric disorder, and at each visit during therapy patients should be assessed for symptoms of depression, mood disturbance, psychosis, or aggression to determine if further evaluation may be necessary. (pp. 2607–2614)

The guidelines further indicate that if patients develop psychiatric symptoms, they should promptly stop the isotretinoin and contact the prescriber. Prescribing of isotretinoin must also follow an FDA-approved risk evaluation and mitigation strategy under the iPLEDGE Program, which closely monitors prescribing and dispensing of isotretinoin (U.S. Food and Drug Administration 2012). Prescribers should familiarize themselves with the current guidelines in their own respective jurisdictions. Discontinuation of isotretinoin does not always lead to remission of psychiatric symptoms, including suicide risk, and further evaluation and treatment may be necessary. The determination as to whether a patient should continue taking isotretinoin after having experienced a psychiatric reaction should be based on the risk-benefit ratio for that particular patient. Some investigators have proposed that the comorbidity of major psychiatric disorders (psychosis, mood disorders) and isotretinoin-associated psychiatric effects suggests a genetic vulnerability in isotretinoin users who experience psychiatric reactions (Kontaxakis et al. 2010). However, it is important to note that serious psychiatric reactions associated with isotretinoin such as suicide attempt can occur in patients without a personal or family history of psychiatric disorders (Goldsmith et al. 2004). A 2010 statement from the American Academy of Dermatology noted, "A correlation between isotretinoin use and depression/anxiety symptoms has been suggested but an evidence-based causal relationship has not been established" (American Academy of Dermatology 2010, p. 1). A study of 500 Israeli conscripts who were seen by a dermatologist for severe acne reported five cases of psychosis (two soldiers diagnosed with schizophreniform disorder and three with schizoaffective disorder) in patients taking isotretinoin whose psychiatric histories were negative before recruitment, with a mean lag time from intake of isotretinoin to occurrence of psychosis of 7.6 ± 4.2 months (Barak et al. 2005). Other retinoids such as etretinate and acitretin also have been reported to cause depression and suicidal thoughts (Arican et al. 2006; Henderson and Highet 1989).

Antihistamines

Sedating first-generation H_1 histamine receptor antagonists such as diphenhydramine and hydroxyzine readily cross the blood-brain barrier and have antianxiety and sedative effects. In diphenhydramine overdose, patients may present with a toxic psychosis with bizarre behavior and hallucinations (Jones et al. 1986), and there is a trend toward an increased risk of delirium (Clegg and Young 2011). The anticholinergic effects of these antihistamines may cause subtle cognitive impairment and, in overdose, an anticholinergic delirium. The H_2 histamine receptor antagonists cimetidine, ranitidine, and famotidine have been associated with mania (von Einsiedel et al. 2002), depression, and delirium (Catalano et al. 1996).

Antifungal and Antimicrobial Agents

The antifungal agent voriconazole has been associated with visual hallucinations in about 17% of cases, accompanied by auditory hallucinations in about 5% of patients (Zonios et al. 2014), within the first week of treatment. The hallucinations, which are a sign of neurotoxicity, are more common in the slow metabolizer phenotype of CYP2C19, and patients with this phenotype achieve significantly higher blood levels of voriconazole. The hallucinations resolve with decrease or discontinuation of voriconazole.

Minocycline, which is used in the treatment of acne and rosacea, may have beneficial effects in the treatment of schizophrenia (Chaudhry et al. 2012; Dodd et al. 2013; Keller et al. 2013) and depression (Miyaoka et al. 2012; Soczynska et al. 2012). Other antimicrobials can cause a variety of psychiatric symptoms. These medications are discussed in Chapter 12, "Infectious Diseases."

Biologics

There is an extensive emerging literature on possibly increased suicidal behaviors in association with certain drugs and biologics that are used to treat dermatological disorders. Clinicians should familiarize themselves with the current guidance on the suicide risk associated with a specific biologic or drug that the patient may be using, by checking the most current guidelines on the FDA website. The following is an example of the guidance for a biologic (brodalumab) that is used to treat severe plaque psoriasis and has a black box warning for "suicidal ideation and behavior": "Prior to prescribing, weigh potential risks and benefits in patients with a history of depression and/or suicidal ideation or behavior," "Patients with new or worsening suicidal thoughts and behavior should be referred to a mental health professional, as appropriate," and "Advise patients and caregivers to seek medical attention for manifestation of suicidal ideation or behavior, new onset or worsening depression, anxiety, or other mood changes." This approach places a great deal of responsibility on the prescribing physician's clinical judgment.

Most reports of suicidal behaviors with biologics are based on small case series; larger controlled studies typically indicate an improvement in mental health with improvement in the skin disorder after treatment with the biologic (Strober et al. 2018). No effective algorithm can be used currently to predict increased suicide risk (Turecki and Brent 2016) in patients with dermatological disorders. Each patient should be clinically assessed for psychiatric morbidity and suicide risk via the standard biopsychosocial approach.

Other Agents

Finasteride, a 5α-reductase inhibitor that is used for the treatment of benign prostatic hyperplasia and androgenetic alopecia, has been associated with suicidal behaviors (reporting OR = 1.63; 95% CI = 1.47–1.81) and psychological adverse events (reporting OR = 4.33; 95% CI = 4.17–4.49) when used for the treatment of alopecia in patients younger than 45 years (Nguyen et al. 2021). Cyclosporine, an immunosuppressant used in organ transplantation and also used in severe psoriasis, has been associated with organic mental disorders, with various symptoms—including mood disorders, anxiety disorders, hallucinations and delusions, cognitive difficulties, and delirium—usually observed within 2 weeks of beginning treatment (Craven 1991). Cyclosporine is covered in Chapter 16, "Organ Transplantation." Dapsone, used for a variety of dermatological conditions, has been associated with mania (Carmichael and Paul 1989) in several reports.

Drug-Drug Interactions

Most pharmacokinetic interactions (Litt 2013) between dermatological and psychotropic drugs result from inhibition of CYP-mediated drug metabolism, mainly the CYP2D6 and CYP3A4 isozymes. Some of the key interactions are listed in Table 13–1 (see also Chapter 1, "Pharmacokinetics, Pharmacodynamics, and Principles of Drug-Drug Interactions," for a comprehensive list of drug interactions; Chapter 12 for antimicrobials; and Chapter 10 for corticosteroids).

Table 13–1. Dermatological medication–psychotropic medication pharmacokinetic interactions

Medication	Interaction mechanism	Effects on psychotropic medication levels	Management
Azole antifungals (oral formulations only) Itraconazole Ketoconazole	Inhibition of CYP3A4	Benzodiazepine serum levels for agents undergoing hepatic oxidative metabolism, such as alprazolam and triazolam, may increase.	Consider alternative benzodiazepines, such as oxazepam, which is metabolized by glucuronidation.
Macrolide antibiotics Clarithromycin Erythromycin	Inhibition of CYP3A4	Buspirone levels increase. Carbamazepine levels increase.	Consider alternative anxiolytics. Use alternative anticonvulsants.
Cyclosporine	Substrate and inhibition of CYP3A4	Doxepin, amitriptyline, and imipramine levels increase, with risk of arrhythmias. Pimozide levels increase, with risk of arrhythmias.	Decrease dosage or use alternative antidepressants. Do not coadminister pimozide with these agents.[a]
Terbinafine	Inhibition of CYP2D6	Antidepressant serum levels may increase for CYP2D6 substrates, including tricyclic antidepressants, paroxetine, venlafaxine, and atomoxetine. Antipsychotic serum levels may increase for CYP2D6 substrates, including phenothiazines (risking arrhythmias), haloperidol, risperidone, olanzapine, clozapine, and aripiprazole.	Consider alternative agents such as citalopram or sertraline. Atomoxetine dosage usually must be reduced. Decrease dosage or consider alternatives such as paliperidone or quetiapine.

Table 13–1. Dermatological medication–psychotropic medication pharmacokinetic interactions (*continued*)

Medication	Interaction mechanism	Effects on psychotropic medication levels	Management
Antihistamines Chlorpheniramine Diphenhydramine Hydroxyzine	Substrate of CYP2D6	Potential for QTc interval prolongation at higher dosages if taken with CYP2D6 inhibitors (e.g., the selective serotonin reuptake inhibitors paroxetine, fluoxetine, sertraline).	Lower dosage of antihistamine or use alternative antidepressant (e.g., venlafaxine).

Note. CYP = cytochrome P450.
[a]Several atypical antipsychotics (e.g., clozapine, quetiapine, ziprasidone, aripiprazole) are also CYP3A4 substrates; if used with a CYP3A4 inhibitor, their dosage may need to be decreased.

Many drugs used in dermatological conditions are inhibitors of CYP3A4, including azole antifungals (e.g., itraconazole, ketoconazole), some macrolides (erythromycin, clarithromycin), and cyclosporine, which is also a CYP3A4 substrate. Use of these drugs can dramatically increase blood levels of psychotropic drugs that are CYP3A4 substrates, including anticonvulsants such as carbamazepine; antidepressants such as doxepin, amitriptyline, and imipramine; benzodiazepines such as alprazolam, triazolam, and diazepam; and the antipsychotic pimozide. Elevated levels of certain drugs such as antidepressants and pimozide can result in prolongation of the QTc interval and cardiac arrhythmias (Beach et al. 2013). The clinical importance of this interaction is exemplified by the fact that the antihistamines terfenadine and astemizole, both CYP3A4 substrates, have been withdrawn from the market because of potentially fatal interactions with CYP3A4 inhibitors, resulting in life-threatening ventricular arrhythmias.

The antifungal agent terbinafine is a CYP2D6 inhibitor and can result in drug toxicity, such as serious cardiac arrhythmias, when administered in conjunction with CYP2D6 substrates, such as the TCAs and the phenothiazine antipsychotics. Alternatively, elevated levels of the antihistamines chlorpheniramine, diphenhydramine, and hydroxyzine, all of which are CYP2D6 substrates, may occur when these drugs are used in conjunction with psychiatric agents that are CYP2D6 inhibitors (e.g., SSRI antidepressants; see Table 13–1).

In addition, significant adverse effects may occur as a result of elevated levels of CYP3A4 substrates such as cyclosporine and corticosteroids when they are coadministered with psychotropic agents that are CYP3A4 inhibitors, such as fluoxetine, fluvoxamine, and nefazodone. Cyclosporine is both substrate and inhibitor of CYP3A4, resulting in many potential drug-drug interactions. Carbamazepine and other CYP3A4 inducers lower cyclosporine and pimozide blood levels and may decrease their therapeutic effect.

The following dermatological medications are associated with a known risk of torsades de pointes (defined as "substantial evidence supports the conclusion that these drugs prolong the QTc interval and are clearly associated with a risk of torsades de pointes [TdP], even when taken as directed in official labelling"): fluconazole, azithromycin, ciprofloxacin, clarithromycin, erythromycin, levofloxacin, moxifloxacin, and pentamidine (Woosley and Romero 2015). There may be a synergistic effect when two drugs that are known to produce torsades de pointes are taken together.

Key Points

- Standard psychopharmacological agents may be used with adequate clinical monitoring to treat psychiatric comorbidity in dermatological disorders.

- Antidepressants are the most frequently studied class of psychotropic agents for patients with dermatological disorders.

- Antidepressants may be effective in a wide range of dermatological disorders because of their possible direct anti-inflammatory effect, in addition to their antidepressant effect.

- Pruritus and sleep difficulties contribute to dermatological and psychiatric morbidity, including increased suicide risk. Effective management of sleep difficulties and pruritus is important in the choice of a psychopharmacological agent.

- The strongly antihistaminic tricyclic antidepressant (TCA) doxepin is effective for pruritus and sleep difficulties in the pruritic dermatoses. Because the strongly antihistaminic TCAs also are typically anticholinergic, patients using them should be monitored for cognitive side effects.

- The high prevalence of suicidal behavior in patients with dermatological disorders is not always associated with more clinically severe skin disease (e.g., in the adolescent patient with acne). Covert body dysmorphic disorder or other psychiatric comorbidities (e.g., PTSD) can increase suicide risk and treatment resistance.

- Certain medications (e.g., isotretinoin, biologics) have been reported to be associated with increased suicidal behavior in small case series; however, results of controlled studies suggest that improvement in the dermatological disorder with the biologic is associated with an improvement in the patient's mental state.

- Severe and life-threatening dermatological reactions such as Stevens-Johnson syndrome (SJS), toxic epidermal necrolysis (TEN), and drug hypersensitivity syndrome are most frequently associated with the aromatic mood-stabilizer anticonvulsants (e.g., carbamazepine, lamotrigine), with greatest risk of development in the first 2 months of therapy.

- Increased risk of developing SJS/TEN due to anticonvulsants, most commonly carbamazepine, has been attributed to several human leukocyte antigen (HLA) allele variants, specifically *HLA-B*1502*, in people of Asian (including South Asian Indian) descent. Patients of Asian ancestry should be screened for the *B*1502* allele before commencing carbamazepine or phenytoin therapy.

- Most important dermatological drug–psychotropic drug interactions involve the use of cytochrome P450 (CYP) 3A4 inhibitors (e.g., azole antifungals, macrolide antibiotics) with CYP3A4 substrates such as pimozide, resulting in increased blood levels of these medications and increased risk of cardiac side effects secondary to QTc interval prolongation.

References

Abedini H, Farshi S, Mirabzadeh A, et al: Antidepressant effects of citalopram on treatment of alopecia areata in patients with major depressive disorder. J Dermatolog Treat 25(2):153–155, 2014 23339335

Adamo D, Pecoraro G, Coppola N, et al: Vortioxetine versus other antidepressants in the treatment of burning mouth syndrome: an open-label randomized trial. Oral Dis 27(4):1022–1041, 2021 32790904

Allan SJ, Kavanagh GM, Herd RM, et al: The effect of inositol supplements on the psoriasis of patients taking lithium: a randomized, placebo-controlled trial. Br J Dermatol 150(5):966–969, 2004 15149510

Alpsoy E, Ozcan E, Cetin L, et al: Is the efficacy of topical corticosteroid therapy for psoriasis vulgaris enhanced by concurrent moclobemide therapy? A double-blind, placebo-controlled study. J Am Acad Dermatol 38(2 Pt 1):197–200, 1998 9486674

American Academy of Dermatology: Position statement on isotretinoin, 2010. Available at: http://www.aad.org/Forms/Policies/Uploads/PS/PS-Isotretinoin.pdf. Accessed July 15, 2015.

American Psychiatric Association: Diagnostic and Statistical Manual of Mental Disorders, 4th Edition. Washington, DC, American Psychiatric Association, 1994

American Psychiatric Association: Diagnostic and Statistical Manual of Mental Disorders, 5th Edition. Arlington, VA, American Psychiatric Association, 2013

American Psychiatric Association: Diagnostic and Statistical Manual of Mental Disorders, 5th Edition, Text Revision. Washington, DC, American Psychiatric Association, 2022

Amstutz U, Shear NH, Rieder MJ, et al: Recommendations for HLA-B*15:02 and HLA-A*31:01 genetic testing to reduce the risk of carbamazepine-induced hypersensitivity reactions. Epilepsia 55(4):496–506, 2014 24597466

Andrade A, Kuah CY, Martin-Lopez JE, et al: Interventions for chronic pruritus of unknown origin. Cochrane Database Syst Rev 1(1):CD013128, 2020 31981369

Arck PC, Slominski A, Theoharides TC, et al: Neuroimmunology of stress: skin takes center stage. J Invest Dermatol 126(8):1697–1704, 2006 16845409

Arican O, Sasmaz S, Ozbulut O: Increased suicidal tendency in a case of psoriasis vulgaris under acitretin treatment. J Eur Acad Dermatol Venereol 20(4):464–465, 2006 16643152

Armstrong AW, Harskamp CT, Armstrong EJ: Psoriasis and metabolic syndrome: a systematic review and meta-analysis of observational studies. J Am Acad Dermatol 68(4):654–662, 2013 23360868

Armstrong EJ, Harskamp CT, Armstrong AW: Psoriasis and major adverse cardiovascular events: a systematic review and meta-analysis of observational studies. J Am Heart Assoc 2(2):e000062, 2013 23557749

Azoulay L, Blais L, Koren G, et al: Isotretinoin and the risk of depression in patients with acne vulgaris: a case-crossover study. J Clin Psychiatry 69(4):526–532, 2008 18363422

Barak Y, Wohl Y, Greenberg Y, et al: Affective psychosis following Accutane (isotretinoin) treatment. Int Clin Psychopharmacol 20(1):39–41, 2005 15602115

Beach SR, Celano CM, Noseworthy PA, et al: QTc prolongation, torsades de pointes, and psychotropic medications. Psychosomatics 54(1):1–13, 2013 23295003

Belli H, Ural C, Vardar MK, et al: Dissociative symptoms and dissociative disorder comorbidity in patients with obsessive-compulsive disorder. Compr Psychiatry 53(7):975–980, 2012 22425531

Benhadou F, Villani AP, Guillem P: Hidradenitis suppurativa and bipolar disorders: a role for lithium therapy? Dermatology 236(4):305–306, 2020 32036365

Bergeron S, Reed BD, Wesselmann U, et al: Vulvodynia. Nat Rev Dis Primers 6(1):36, 2020 32355269

Beuerlein KG, Balogh EA, Feldman SR: Morgellons disease etiology and therapeutic approach: a systematic review. Dermatol Online J 27(8), 2021 34755952

Bigatà X, Sais G, Soler F: Severe chronic urticaria: response to mirtazapine. J Am Acad Dermatol 53(5):916–917, 2005 16243165

Bliss SA, Warnock JK: Psychiatric medications: adverse cutaneous drug reactions. Clin Dermatol 31(1):101–109, 2013 23245981

Borovaya A, Olisova O, Ruzicka T, et al: Does isotretinoin therapy of acne cure or cause depression? Int J Dermatol 52(9):1040–1052, 2013 23962262

Boyd ST, Mihm L, Causey NW: Improvement in psoriasis following treatment with gabapentin and pregabalin (letter). Am J Clin Dermatol 9(6):419, 2008 18973412

Brauchli YB, Jick SS, Curtin F, et al: Association between beta-blockers, other antihypertensive drugs and psoriasis: population-based case-control study. Br J Dermatol 158(6):1299–1307, 2008 18410416

Brauchli YB, Jick SS, Curtin F, et al: Lithium, antipsychotics, and risk of psoriasis. J Clin Psychopharmacol 29(2):134–140, 2009 19512974

Brown CS, Bachmann GA, Wan J, et al: Gabapentin for the treatment of vulvodynia: a randomized controlled trial. Obstet Gynecol 131(6):1000–1007, 2018 29742655

Camfferman D, Kennedy JD, Gold M, et al: Eczema and sleep and its relationship to daytime functioning in children. Sleep Med Rev 14(6):359–369, 2010 20392655

Carmichael AJ, Paul CJ: Idiosyncratic dapsone induced manic depression. BMJ 298(6686):1524, 1989 2503107

Catalano G, Catalano MC, Alberts VA: Famotidine-associated delirium: a series of six cases. Psychosomatics 37(4):349–355, 1996 8701013

Chan S, Reddy V, Myers B, et al: High-dose doxepin for the treatment of chronic intractable scalp psoriasis. JAAD Case Rep 24(8):71–73, 2020 33521215

Charleston LIV: Burning mouth syndrome: a review of recent literature. Curr Pain Headache Rep 17(6):336, 2013 23645183

Chaudhry IB, Hallak J, Husain N, et al: Minocycline benefits negative symptoms in early schizophrenia: a randomised double-blind placebo-controlled clinical trial in patients on standard treatment. J Psychopharmacol 26(9):1185–1193, 2012 22526685

Check JH, Chan S: Complete eradication of chronic long standing eczema and keratosis pilaris following treatment with dextroamphetamine sulfate. Clin Exp Obstet Gynecol 41(2):202–204, 2014 24779252

Cheng CY, Su SC, Chen CH, et al: HLA associations and clinical implications in T-cell mediated drug hypersensitivity reactions: an updated review. J Immunol Res 2014:565320, 2014 24901010

Choi EH, Brown BE, Crumrine D, et al: Mechanisms by which psychologic stress alters cutaneous permeability barrier homeostasis and stratum corneum integrity. J Invest Dermatol 124(3):587–595, 2005 15737200

Cipriani R, Perini GI, Rampinelli S: Paroxetine in alopecia areata. Int J Dermatol 40(9):600–601, 2001 11737460

Clegg A, Young JB: Which medications to avoid in people at risk of delirium: a systematic review. Age Ageing 40(1):23–29, 2011 21068014

Cox NH, Gordon PM, Dodd H: Generalized pustular and erythrodermic psoriasis associated with bupropion treatment. Br J Dermatol 146(6):1061–1063, 2002 12072078

Craven JL: Cyclosporine-associated organic mental disorders in liver transplant recipients. Psychosomatics 32(1):94–102, 1991 2003144

Dalgard FJ, Gieler U, Tomas-Aragones L, et al: The psychological burden of skin diseases: a cross-sectional multicenter study among dermatological out-patients in 13 European countries. J Invest Dermatol 135(4):984–991, 2015 25521458

DelRosso L, Hoque R: Eczema: a diagnostic consideration for persistent nocturnal arousals. J Clin Sleep Med 8(4):459–460, 2012 22893779

Demitsu T, Yoneda K, Kakurai M, et al: Clinical efficacy of reserpine as "add-on therapy" to antihistamines in patients with recalcitrant chronic idiopathic urticaria and urticarial vasculitis. J Dermatol 37(9):827–829, 2010 20883370

D'Erme AM, Zanieri F, Campolmi E, et al: Therapeutic implications of adding the psychotropic drug escitalopram in the treatment of patients suffering from moderate-severe psoriasis and psychiatric comorbidity: a retrospective study. J Eur Acad Dermatol Venereol 28(2):246–249, 2014 22963277

Di Prima T, De Pasquale R: Use of an MAO inhibitor in the treatment of psoriasis vulgaris [in Italian]. G Ital Dermatol Venereol 124(9):419–420, 1989 2699608

Dodd S, Maes M, Anderson G, et al: Putative neuroprotective agents in neuropsychiatric disorders. Prog Neuropsychopharmacol Biol Psychiatry 42:135–145, 2013 23178231

Dodiuk-Gad RP, Laws PM, Shear NH: Epidemiology of severe drug hypersensitivity. Semin Cutan Med Surg 33(1):2–9, 2014 25037253

Dos Santos-Ribeiro S, de Salles Andrade JB, Quintas JN, et al: A systematic review of the utility of electroconvulsive therapy in broadly defined obsessive-compulsive-related disorders. Prim Care Companion CNS Disord 20(5):18r02342, 2018 30407758

Dowlatshahi EA, Wakkee M, Herings RM, et al: Increased antidepressant drug exposure in psoriasis patients: a longitudinal population-based cohort study. Acta Derm Venereol 93(5):544–550, 2013 23529077

Dowlatshahi EA, Wakkee M, Arends LR, et al: The prevalence and odds of depressive symptoms and clinical depression in psoriasis patients: a systematic review and meta-analysis. J Invest Dermatol 134(6):1542–1551, 2014 24284419

Drake LA, Millikan LE; Doxepin Study Group: The antipruritic effect of 5% doxepin cream in patients with eczematous dermatitis. Arch Dermatol 131(12):1403–1408, 1995 7492129

Droitcourt C, Nowak E, Rault C, et al: Risk of suicide attempt associated with isotretinoin: a nationwide cohort and nested case-time-control study. Int J Epidemiol 48(5):1623–1635, 2019 31098637

Droitcourt C, Poizeau F, Kerbrat S, et al: Isotretinoin and risk factors for suicide attempt: a population-based comprehensive case series and nested case-control study using 2010–2014 French Health Insurance data. J Eur Acad Dermatol Venereol 34(6):1293–1301, 2020 31587374

Ebata T, Izumi H, Aizawa H, et al: Effects of nitrazepam on nocturnal scratching in adults with atopic dermatitis: a double-blind placebo-controlled crossover study. Br J Dermatol 138(4):631–634, 1998 9640368

Eichenfield DZ, Sprague J, Eichenfield LF: Management of acne vulgaris: a review. JAMA 326(20):2055–2067, 2021 34812859

Eskeland S, Halvorsen JA, Tanum L: Antidepressants have anti-inflammatory effects that may be relevant to dermatology: a systematic review. Acta Derm Venereol 97(8):897–905, 2017 28512664

Farhat LC, Olfson E, Nasir M, et al: Pharmacological and behavioral treatment for trichotillomania: an updated systematic review with meta-analysis. Depress Anxiety 37(8):715–727, 2020 32390221

Fleuret C, Le Toux G, Morvan J, et al: Use of selective serotonin reuptake inhibitors in the treatment of burning mouth syndrome. Dermatology 228(2):172–176, 2014 24557331

Freudenmann RW, Lepping P: Second-generation antipsychotics in primary and secondary delusional parasitosis: outcome and efficacy. J Clin Psychopharmacol 28(5):500–508, 2008 18794644

Gerdes S, Zahl VA, Knopf H, et al: Comedication related to comorbidities: a study in 1203 hospitalized patients with severe psoriasis. Br J Dermatol 159(5):1116–1123, 2008 18717681

Goldburg SR, Strober BE, Payette MJ: Hidradenitis suppurativa: epidemiology, clinical presentation, and pathogenesis. J Am Acad Dermatol 82(5):1045–1058, 2020 31604104

Goldsmith LA, Bolognia JL, Callen JP, et al: American Academy of Dermatology Consensus Conference on the safe and optimal use of isotretinoin: summary and recommendations. J Am Acad Dermatol 50(6):900–906, 2004 15153892

Goldsobel AB, Rohr AS, Siegel SC, et al: Efficacy of doxepin in the treatment of chronic idiopathic urticaria. J Allergy Clin Immunol 78(5 Pt 1):867–873, 1986 3782654

González E, Sanguino RM, Franco MA: Bupropion in atopic dermatitis (letter). Pharmacopsychiatry 39(6):229, 2006 17124645

Gottlieb AB, Chao C, Dann F: Psoriasis comorbidities. J Dermatolog Treat 19(1):5–21, 2008 18273720

Grant JE, Odlaug BL, Kim SW: Lamotrigine treatment of pathologic skin picking: an open-label study. J Clin Psychiatry 68(9):1384–1391, 2007 17915977

Grant JE, Odlaug BL, Kim SW: N-acetylcysteine, a glutamate modulator, in the treatment of trichotillomania: a double-blind, placebo-controlled study. Arch Gen Psychiatry 66(7):756–763, 2009 19581567

Grant JE, Odlaug BL, Chamberlain SR, et al: A double-blind, placebo-controlled trial of lamotrigine for pathological skin picking: treatment efficacy and neurocognitive predictors of response. J Clin Psychopharmacol 30(4):396–403, 2010 20531220

Grant JE, Odlaug BL, Chamberlain SR, et al: Skin picking disorder. Am J Psychiatry 169(11):1143–1149, 2012 23128921

Greene SL, Reed CE, Schroeter AL: Double-blind crossover study comparing doxepin with diphenhydramine for the treatment of chronic urticaria. J Am Acad Dermatol 12(4):669–675, 1985 3886724

Grover S, Kukreti R: HLA alleles and hypersensitivity to carbamazepine: an updated systematic review with meta-analysis. Pharmacogenet Genomics 24(2):94–112, 2014 24336023

Gupta AK, Knowles SR, Gupta MA, et al: Lithium therapy associated with hidradenitis suppurativa: case report and a review of the dermatologic side effects of lithium. J Am Acad Dermatol 32(2 Pt 2):382–386, 1995 7829746

Gupta MA: Review of somatic symptoms in post-traumatic stress disorder. Int Rev Psychiatry 25(1):86–99, 2013a 23383670

Gupta MA: Emotional regulation, dissociation, and the self-induced dermatoses: clinical features and implications for treatment with mood stabilizers. Clin Dermatol 31(1):110–117, 2013b 23245982

Gupta MA, Gupta AK: Chronic idiopathic urticaria associated with panic disorder: a syndrome responsive to selective serotonin reuptake inhibitor antidepressants? Cutis 56(1):53–54, 1995 7555104

Gupta MA, Gupta AK: Psychodermatology: an update. J Am Acad Dermatol 34(6):1030–1046, 1996 8647969

Gupta MA, Gupta AK: Depression and suicidal ideation in dermatology patients with acne, alopecia areata, atopic dermatitis and psoriasis. Br J Dermatol 139(5):846–850, 1998 9892952

Gupta MA, Gupta AK: Olanzapine is effective in the management of some self-induced dermatoses: three case reports. Cutis 66(2):143–146, 2000 10955197

Gupta MA, Gupta AK: Chronic idiopathic urticaria and post-traumatic stress disorder (PTSD): an under-recognized comorbidity. Clin Dermatol 30(3):351–354, 2012 22507051

Gupta MA, Gupta AK: Cutaneous sensory disorder. Semin Cutan Med Surg 32(2):110–118, 2013a 24049969

Gupta MA, Gupta AK: Sleep-wake disorders and dermatology. Clin Dermatol 31(1):118–126, 2013b 23245983

Gupta MA, Gupta AK: Current concepts in psychodermatology. Curr Psychiatry Rep 16(6):449, 2014 24740235

Gupta MA, Gupta AK: Self-induced dermatoses: a great imitator. Clin Dermatol 37(3):268–277, 2019 31178108

Gupta MA, Gupta AK: An elevated leg movement index during sleep in atopic dermatitis and periodic leg movement disorder may be an indication of sympathetic activation common to both (letter). J Clin Sleep Med 16(3):463, 2020 31992432

Gupta MA, Gupta AK, Haberman HF: The self-inflicted dermatoses: a critical review. Gen Hosp Psychiatry 9(1):45–52, 1987 3817460

Gupta MA, Gupta AK, Kirkby S, et al: A psychocutaneous profile of psoriasis patients who are stress reactors: a study of 127 patients. Gen Hosp Psychiatry 11(3):166–173, 1989 2721939

Gupta MA, Gupta AK, Schork NJ, et al: Depression modulates pruritus perception: a study of pruritus in psoriasis, atopic dermatitis, and chronic idiopathic urticaria. Psychosom Med 56(1):36–40, 1994 8197313

Gupta MA, Simpson FC, Gupta AK: Psoriasis and sleep disorders: a systematic review. Sleep Med Rev 29:63–75, 2016 26624228

Gupta MA, Jarosz P, Gupta AK: Posttraumatic stress disorder (PTSD) and the dermatology patient. Clin Dermatol 35(3):260–266, 2017a 28511822

Gupta MA, Simpson FC, Vujcic B, et al: Obstructive sleep apnea and dermatologic disorders. Clin Dermatol 35(3):319–327, 2017b 28511831

Gupta MA, Vujcic B, Gupta AK: Dissociation and conversion symptoms in dermatology. Clin Dermatol 35(3):267–272, 2017c 28511823

Gupta MA, Pur DR, Vujcic B, et al: Use of antiepileptic mood stabilizers in dermatology. Clin Dermatol 36(6):756–764, 2018a 30446200

Gupta MA, Vujcic B, Pur DR, et al: Use of antipsychotic drugs in dermatology. Clin Dermatol 36(6):765–773, 2018b 30446201

Haefner HK, Collins ME, Davis GD, et al: The vulvodynia guideline. J Low Genit Tract Dis 9(1):40–51, 2005 15870521

Hall SD, Wang Z, Huang SM, et al: The interaction between St John's wort and an oral contraceptive. Clin Pharmacol Ther 74(6):525–535, 2003 14663455

Heckmann SM, Kirchner E, Grushka M, et al: A double-blind study on clonazepam in patients with burning mouth syndrome. Laryngoscope 122(4):813–816, 2012 22344742

Heller MM, Wong JW, Lee ES, et al: Delusional infestations: clinical presentation, diagnosis and treatment. Int J Dermatol 52(7):775–783, 2013 23789596

Henderson CA, Highet AS: Depression induced by etretinate. BMJ 298(6678):964, 1989 2497882

Hoffman J, Williams T, Rothbart R, et al: Pharmacotherapy for trichotillomania. Cochrane Database Syst Rev 9(9):CD007662, 2021 34582562

Hoss D, Segal S: Scalp dysesthesia. Arch Dermatol 134(3):327–330, 1998 9521031

Huang YC, Cheng YC: Isotretinoin treatment for acne and risk of depression: a systematic review and meta-analysis. J Am Acad Dermatol 76(6):1068.e9–1076.e9, 2017 28291553

Huber M, Lepping P, Pycha R, et al: Delusional infestation: treatment outcome with antipsychotics in 17 consecutive patients (using standardized reporting criteria). Gen Hosp Psychiatry 33(6):604–611, 2011 21762999

Hughes JE, Barraclough BM, Hamblin LG, et al: Psychiatric symptoms in dermatology patients. Br J Psychiatry 143:51–54, 1983 6882992

Hundley JL, Yosipovitch G: Mirtazapine for reducing nocturnal itch in patients with chronic pruritus: a pilot study. J Am Acad Dermatol 50(6):889–891, 2004 15153889

Hung SI, Chung WH, Liu ZS, et al: Common risk allele in aromatic antiepileptic-drug induced Stevens-Johnson syndrome and toxic epidermal necrolysis in Han Chinese. Pharmacogenomics 11(3):349–356, 2010 20235791

Husain Z, Reddy BY, Schwartz RA: DRESS syndrome, part I: clinical perspectives. J Am Acad Dermatol 68(5):693.e1–693.e14, quiz 706–708, 2013 23602182

Jafferany M, Osuagwu FC: Use of topiramate in skin-picking disorder: a pilot study. Prim Care Companion CNS Disord 19(1), 2017 28129492

Jick SS, Kremers HM, Vasilakis-Scaramozza C: Isotretinoin use and risk of depression, psychotic symptoms, suicide, and attempted suicide. Arch Dermatol 136(10):1231–1236, 2000 11030769

Jones J, Dougherty J, Cannon L: Diphenhydramine-induced toxic psychosis. Am J Emerg Med 4(4):369–371, 1986 3718632

Keller WR, Kum LM, Wehring HJ, et al: A review of anti-inflammatory agents for symptoms of schizophrenia. J Psychopharmacol 27(4):337–342, 2013 23151612

Kelsay K: Management of sleep disturbance associated with atopic dermatitis. J Allergy Clin Immunol 118(1):198–201, 2006 16815155

Keshtkarjahromi M, Mariscal J, Dempsey K, et al: Treatment of severe excoriation disorder with mirtazapine: a case report. Clin Neuropharmacol 44(5):189–190, 2021 34326284

Kimsey LS: Delusional infestation and chronic pruritus: a review. Acta Derm Venereol 96(3):298–302, 2016 26337109

Kimyai-Asadi A, Harris JC, Nousari HC: Critical overview: adverse cutaneous reactions to psychotropic medications. J Clin Psychiatry 60(10):714–725, quiz 726, 1999 10549695

Kinoshita-Ise M, Shear NH: Diagnostic and therapeutic approach to scalp dysesthesia: a case series and published work review. J Dermatol 46(6):526–530, 2019 31106878

Konstantinou GN, Konstantinou GN: Psychiatric comorbidity in chronic urticaria patients: a systematic review and meta-analysis. Clin Transl Allergy 9:42, 2019 31462988

Kontaxakis VP, Ferentinos PP, Havaki-Kontaxaki BJ, et al: Genetic vulnerability and isotretinoin-induced psychiatric adverse events. World J Biol Psychiatry 11(2):158–159, 2010 20109108

Kuhn H, Mennella C, Magid M, et al: Psychocutaneous disease: pharmacotherapy and psychotherapy. J Am Acad Dermatol 76(5):795–808, 2017 28411772

Latini A, Carducci M: Psoriasis during therapy with olanzapine. Eur J Dermatol 13(4):404–405, 2003 12948926

Lepping P, Freudenmann RW: Delusional parasitosis: a new pathway for diagnosis and treatment. Clin Exp Dermatol 33(2):113–117, 2008 18205853

Levenson JL: Psychiatric issues in dermatology, part 1: atopic dermatitis and psoriasis. Prim Psychiatry 15:31–34, 2008a

Levenson JL: Psychiatric issues in dermatology, part 2: alopecia areata, urticaria, and angioedema. Prim Psychiatry 15:31–34, 2008b

Levenson JL, Sharma AA, Ortega-Loayza AG: Somatic symptom disorder in dermatology. Clin Dermatol 35(3):246–251, 2017 28511820

Litt JZ: Litt's Drug Eruptions & Reactions Manual: D.E.R.M. Boca Raton, FL, CRC Press, 2013

Lochner C, Seedat S, Niehaus DJ, et al: Topiramate in the treatment of trichotillomania: an open-label pilot study. Int Clin Psychopharmacol 21(5):255–259, 2006 16877895

Lochner C, Roos A, Stein DJ: Excoriation (skin-picking) disorder: a systematic review of treatment options. Neuropsychiatr Dis Treat 13:1867–1872, 2017 28761349

Luis Blay S: Depression and psoriasis comorbidity: treatment with paroxetine: two case reports. Ann Clin Psychiatry 18(4):271–272, 2006 17162628

Mahtani R, Parekh N, Mangat I, et al: Alleviating the itch-scratch cycle in atopic dermatitis. Psychosomatics 46(4):373–374, 2005 16000683

Marqueling AL, Zane LT: Depression and suicidal behavior in acne patients treated with isotretinoin: a systematic review. Semin Cutan Med Surg 26(4):210–220, 2007 18395669

Marron SE, Tomas-Aragones L, Boira S: Anxiety, depression, quality of life and patient satisfaction in acne patients treated with oral isotretinoin. Acta Derm Venereol 93(6):701–706, 2013 23727704

McGrath EJ, Lovell CR, Gillison F, et al: A prospective trial of the effects of isotretinoin on quality of life and depressive symptoms. Br J Dermatol 163(6):1323–1329, 2010 21137117

McMillan R, Forssell H, Buchanan JA, et al: Interventions for treating burning mouth syndrome. Cochrane Database Syst Rev 11(11):CD002779, 2016 27855478

Medansky RS, Handler RM: Dermatopsychosomatics: classification, physiology, and therapeutic approaches. J Am Acad Dermatol 5(2):125–136, 1981 7021610

Messenger AG, McKillop J, Farrant P, et al: British Association of Dermatologists' guidelines for the management of alopecia areata 2012. Br J Dermatol 166(5):916–926, 2012 22524397

Miranda Varella Pereira G, Soriano Marcolino M, Silveira Nogueira Reis Z, et al: A systematic review of drug treatment of vulvodynia: evidence of a strong placebo effect. BJOG 125(10):1216–1224, 2018 29569822

Miyaoka T, Wake R, Furuya M, et al: Minocycline as adjunctive therapy for patients with unipolar psychotic depression: an open-label study. Prog Neuropsychopharmacol Biol Psychiatry 37(2):222–226, 2012 22349578

Modell JG, Boyce S, Taylor E, et al: Treatment of atopic dermatitis and psoriasis vulgaris with bupropion-SR: a pilot study. Psychosom Med 64(5):835–840, 2002 12271115

Myers B, Reddy V, Chan S, et al: Optimizing doxepin therapy in dermatology: introducing blood level monitoring and genotype testing. J Dermatolog Treat 33(1):87–93, 2022 32347140

Nevoralová Z, Dvořáková D: Mood changes, depression and suicide risk during isotretinoin treatment: a prospective study. Int J Dermatol 52(2):163–168, 2013 23347302

Nguyen DD, Marchese M, Cone EB, et al: Investigation of suicidality and psychological adverse events in patients treated with finasteride. JAMA Dermatol 157(1):35–42, 2021 33175100

Odlaug BL, Grant JE: Pathological skin picking, in Trichotillomania, Skin Picking, and Other Body-Focused Repetitive Behaviors. Edited by Grant JE, Stein DJ, Woods DW, et al. Washington, DC, American Psychiatric Publishing, 2012, pp 21–41

Oliver G, Dean O, Camfield D, et al: N-acetyl cysteine in the treatment of obsessive compulsive and related disorders: a systematic review. Clin Psychopharmacol Neurosci 13(1):12–24, 2015 25912534

Ollaik F, Dagher M, Bachour K, et al: Adrenergic urticaria: a rare underdiagnosed subtype. Int J Dermatol 59(5):615–616, 2020 31736049

Özkaya E, Babuna Kobaner G, Yılmaz Z, et al: Doxepin in difficult-to-treat chronic urticaria: a retrospective, cross-sectional study from Turkey. Dermatol Ther 32(4):e12993, 2019 31175673

Patel KR, Immaneni S, Singam V, et al: Association between atopic dermatitis, depression, and suicidal ideation: a systematic review and meta-analysis. J Am Acad Dermatol 80(2):402–410, 2019 30365995

Patel KR, Lee HH, Rastogi S, et al: Association between hidradenitis suppurativa, depression, anxiety, and suicidality: a systematic review and meta-analysis. J Am Acad Dermatol 83(3):737–744, 2020 31862404

Patel T, Ishiuji Y, Yosipovitch G: Nocturnal itch: why do we itch at night? Acta Derm Venereol 87(4):295–298, 2007 17598030

Perini G, Zara M, Cipriani R, et al: Imipramine in alopecia areata: a double-blind, placebo-controlled study. Psychother Psychosom 61(3–4):195–198, 1994 8066157

Physicians' Desk Reference: Physicians' Desk Reference, 63rd Edition. Montvale, NJ, Physicians' Desk Reference, 2009

Qureshi AA, Abate LE, Yosipovitch G, et al: A systematic review of evidence-based treatments for prurigo nodularis. J Am Acad Dermatol 80(3):756–764, 2019 30261199

Rademaker M: Adverse effects of isotretinoin: a retrospective review of 1743 patients started on isotretinoin. Australas J Dermatol 51(4):248–253, 2010 21198520

Ramirez FD, Chen S, Langan SM, et al: Association of atopic dermatitis with sleep quality in children. JAMA Pediatr 173(5):e190025, 2019 30830151

Rao KS, Menon PK, Hilman BC, et al: Duration of the suppressive effect of tricyclic antidepressants on histamine-induced wheal-and-flare reactions in human skin. J Allergy Clin Immunol 82(5 Pt 1):752–757, 1988 2903876

Rehn LM, Meririnne E, Höök-Nikanne J, et al: Depressive symptoms and suicidal ideation during isotretinoin treatment: a 12-week follow-up study of male Finnish military conscripts. J Eur Acad Dermatol Venereol 23(11):1294–1297, 2009 19522777

Rieder E, Tausk F: Psoriasis, a model of dermatologic psychosomatic disease: psychiatric implications and treatments. Int J Dermatol 51(1):12–26, 2012 22182372

Rodríguez-Cerdeira C, Sánchez-Blanco E, Sánchez-Blanco B, et al: Delusional infestation. Am J Emerg Med 35(2):357–360, 2017 27823940

Rudzki E, Borkowski W, Czubalski K: The suggestive effect of placebo on the intensity of chronic urticaria. Acta Allergol 25(1):70–73, 1970 5468243

Ryback R: Topiramate in the treatment of psoriasis: a pilot study. Br J Dermatol 147(1):130–133, 2002 12100195

Sampogna F, Tabolli S, Abeni D: The impact of changes in clinical severity on psychiatric morbidity in patients with psoriasis: a follow-up study. Br J Dermatol 157(3):508–513, 2007 17627789

Samuels DV, Rosenthal R, Lin R, et al: Acne vulgaris and risk of depression and anxiety: a meta-analytic review. J Am Acad Dermatol 83(2):532–541, 2020 32088269

Sandhu JK, Wu KK, Bui TL, et al: Association between atopic dermatitis and suicidality: a systematic review and meta-analysis. JAMA Dermatol 155(2):178–187, 2019 30540348

Sarifakioglu E, Onur O: Women with scalp dysesthesia treated with pregabalin. Int J Dermatol 52(11):1417–1418, 2013 23557491

Saunte DML, Jemec GBE: Hidradenitis suppurativa: advances in diagnosis and treatment. JAMA 318(20):2019–2032, 2017 29183082

Savage KT, Singh V, Patel ZS, et al: Pain management in hidradenitis suppurativa and a proposed treatment algorithm. J Am Acad Dermatol 85(1):187–199, 2021 32950543

Selles RR, McGuire JF, Small BJ, et al: A systematic review and meta-analysis of psychiatric treatments for excoriation (skin-picking) disorder. Gen Hosp Psychiatry 41:29–37, 2016 27143352

Semiz UB, Inanc L, Bezgin CH: Are trauma and dissociation related to treatment resistance in patients with obsessive-compulsive disorder? Soc Psychiatry Psychiatr Epidemiol 49(8):1287–1296, 2014 24213522

Senra MS, Wollenberg A: Psychodermatological aspects of atopic dermatitis. Br J Dermatol 170(Suppl 1):38–43, 2014 24930567

Shah B, Levenson JL: Use of psychotropic drugs in the dermatology patient: when to start and stop? Clin Dermatol 36(6):748–755, 2018 30446199

Sidbury R, Tom WL, Bergman JN, et al: Guidelines of care for the management of atopic dermatitis, section 4: prevention of disease flares and use of adjunctive therapies and approaches. J Am Acad Dermatol 71(6):1218–1233, 2014 25264237

Soczynska JK, Mansur RB, Brietzke E, et al: Novel therapeutic targets in depression: minocycline as a candidate treatment. Behav Brain Res 235(2):302–317, 2012 22963995

Stockdale CK, Lawson HW: 2013 Vulvodynia Guideline update. J Low Genit Tract Dis 18(2):93–100, 2014 24633161

Strober B, Gooderham M, de Jong EMGJ, et al: Depressive symptoms, depression, and the effect of biologic therapy among patients in Psoriasis Longitudinal Assessment and Registry (PSOLAR). J Am Acad Dermatol 78(1):70–80, 2018 29102053

Sundström A, Alfredsson L, Sjölin-Forsberg G, et al: Association of suicide attempts with acne and treatment with isotretinoin: retrospective Swedish cohort study. BMJ 341:c5812, 2010 21071484

Taghavi Ardakani A, Farrehi M, Sharif MR, et al: The effects of melatonin administration on disease severity and sleep quality in children with atopic dermatitis: a randomized, double-blinded, placebo-controlled trial. Pediatr Allergy Immunol 29(8):834–840, 2018 30160043

Thomas KH, Martin RM, Potokar J, et al: Reporting of drug induced depression and fatal and non-fatal suicidal behaviour in the UK from 1998 to 2011. BMC Pharmacol Toxicol 15:54, 2014 25266008

Thorlacius L, Cohen AD, Gislason GH, et al: Increased suicide risk in patients with hidradenitis suppurativa. J Invest Dermatol 138(1):52–57, 2018 28942360

Thorslund K, Svensson T, Nordlind K, et al: Use of serotonin reuptake inhibitors in patients with psoriasis is associated with a decreased need for systemic psoriasis treatment: a population-based cohort study. J Intern Med 274(3):281–287, 2013 23711088

Turecki G, Brent DA: Suicide and suicidal behaviour. Lancet 387(10024):1227–1239, 2016 26385066

U.S. Food and Drug Administration: Information for healthcare professionals: dangerous or even fatal skin reactions—carbamazepine (marketed as Carbatrol, Equetro, Tegretol and generics). U.S. Food and Drug Administration, 2007. Available at: www.fda.gov/Drugs/DrugSafety/PostmarketDrugSafetyInformationforPatientsandProviders/ucm124718.htm. Accessed July 15, 2015.

U.S. Food and Drug Administration: Risk Evaluation and Mitigation Strategy (REMS). The iPLEDGE Program: single shared system for isotretinoin. U.S. Food and Drug Administration, 2012. Available at: www.fda.gov/downloads/Drugs/DrugSafety/PostmarketDrugSafetyInformationforPatientsandProviders/UCM234639.pdf. Accessed July 30, 2015.

Vallerand IA, Lewinson RT, Parsons LM, et al: Assessment of a bidirectional association between major depressive disorder and alopecia areata. JAMA Dermatol 155(4):475–479, 2019 30649133

Varoni EM, Lo Faro AF, Lodi G, et al: Melatonin treatment in patients with burning mouth syndrome: a triple-blind, placebo-controlled, crossover randomized clinical trial. J Oral Facial Pain Headache 32(2):178–188, 2018 29694465

von Einsiedel RW, Roesch-Ely D, Diebold K, et al: H(2)-histamine antagonist (famotidine) induced adverse CNS reactions with long-standing secondary mania and epileptic seizures. Pharmacopsychiatry 35(4):152–154, 2002 12163986

Warnock JK, Morris DW: Adverse cutaneous reactions to antidepressants. Am J Clin Dermatol 3(5):329–339, 2002a 12069639

Warnock JK, Morris DW: Adverse cutaneous reactions to antipsychotics. Am J Clin Dermatol 3(9):629–636, 2002b 12444805

Warnock JK, Morris DW: Adverse cutaneous reactions to mood stabilizers. Am J Clin Dermatol 4(1):21–30, 2003 12477370

Weisshaar E, Szepietowski JC, Dalgard FJ, et al: European S2k guideline on chronic pruritus. Acta Derm Venereol 99(5):469–506, 2019 30931482

Wong S, Bewley A: Patients with delusional infestation (delusional parasitosis) often require prolonged treatment as recurrence of symptoms after cessation of treatment is common: an observational study. Br J Dermatol 165(4):893–896, 2011 21605110

Woosley RL, Romero KA: QT Drugs List, 2015. Available at: https://www.crediblemeds.org. Accessed May 19, 2015.

Wysowski DK, Pitts M, Beitz J: An analysis of reports of depression and suicide in patients treated with isotretinoin. J Am Acad Dermatol 45(4):515–519, 2001 11568740

Yang CC, Liang CS, Chu CW: Combination of quetiapine immediate release and XR for H1-antihistamine-refractory chronic spontaneous urticaria comorbid with depressive disorder: a case report. Am J Ther 26(6):e727–e728, 2019 30418225

Yang EJ, Beck KM, Koo J: Folie à famille: a systematic review of shared delusional infestation. J Am Acad Dermatol 81(5):1211–1215, 2019 31002848

Yosipovitch G, Xiong GL, Haus E, et al: Time-dependent variations of the skin barrier function in humans: transepidermal water loss, stratum corneum hydration, skin surface pH, and skin temperature. J Invest Dermatol 110(1):20–23, 1998 9424081

Yosipovitch G, Ansari N, Goon A, et al: Clinical characteristics of pruritus in chronic idiopathic urticaria. Br J Dermatol 147(1):32–36, 2002 12100181

Yosipovitch G, Sackett-Lundeen L, Goon A, et al: Circadian and ultradian (12 h) variations of skin blood flow and barrier function in non-irritated and irritated skin—effect of topical corticosteroids. J Invest Dermatol 122(3):824–829, 2004 15086571

Zonios D, Yamazaki H, Murayama N, et al: Voriconazole metabolism, toxicity, and the effect of cytochrome P450 2C19 genotype. J Infect Dis 209(12):1941–1948, 2014 24403552

14

Rheumatological Disorders

James L. Levenson, M.D.
Stephen J. Ferrando, M.D.

Neuropsychiatric disorders are common in patients with rheumatological disorders. On the basis of standardized research interviews, nearly one-fifth of patients with rheumatoid arthritis (RA) are estimated to have a psychiatric disorder, most often a depressive disorder (Levenson and Irwin 2019). Depressed patients with RA are more likely to report pain, are less likely to comply with medications, and have poorer quality of life than other patients with RA. However, physicians underrecognize depression in their patients with RA (Rathbun et al. 2014). A nationwide Japanese study of people with RA found that although only 5% of the participants had been officially diagnosed with depression, 35% had Patient Health Questionnaire–9 scores indicating current depression (Sruamsiri et al. 2017). A large Swedish population-based study found no significant differences in how often antidepressants were prescribed in patients with RA versus matched healthy control subjects despite the higher prevalence of depression in RA (Pedersen et al. 2022). Research on depression in osteoarthritis (OA) has shown similar findings, with high rates of depression associated with increased pain and poorer quality of life (Joshi et al. 2015). Studies of patients with systemic lupus erythematosus found that 30%–50% of the patients had depression, 13%–24% had anxiety, 3%–4% had mania or mixed episodes, and 2%–5% had psychosis (Abrol et al. 2021; Levenson and Irwin 2019). The differential diagnosis of psychiatric disorders in patients with rheumatological disorders includes primary psychiatric disorders, secondary syndromes (e.g., psychosis due to CNS lupus), and side effects of rheumatological medications.

Treatment of Psychiatric Disorders

For the most part, treatment of depression, anxiety, mania, psychosis, delirium, and pain in patients with rheumatological disorders is similar to their treatment in patients with other medical diseases, following the principles covered in other chapters in this book. Treating depression is important because it is a major determinant of outcome and functional capacity in RA (Isnardi et al. 2021). There have been no clinical trials of antidepressants for depression in patients with RA since the second edition of this book, and the evidence base remains very limited (Fiest et al. 2017). Earlier trials in RA have been with selective serotonin reuptake inhibitors (SSRIs) and tricyclic antidepressants (TCAs) but not serotonin-norepinephrine reuptake inhibitors (SNRIs).

There have been 33 clinical trials of antidepressants for back or other pain or OA (Ferreira et al. 2021), with some evidence for benefit. However, despite the wide prevalence of depression in OA, there have been very few trials of antidepressants for depression in OA, none recent. The studies that have been performed suggest that antidepressants are beneficial in the treatment of depression in patients with OA and that improvement in depression is associated with reduced pain and disability (Lin et al. 2003). When pharmacotherapy of depression is part of a collaborative care approach, outcomes are improved over usual care (Lin et al. 2006).

Although current evidence indicates that all antidepressants have about equal efficacy in the treatment of depression, they differ in their analgesic efficacy, tolerability, and potential drug interactions. TCAs have long been recognized as having analgesic benefits, even at low doses (e.g., amitriptyline, 25 mg) and independent of the presence of depression (see also Chapter 17, "Pain Management"). At higher doses, the tolerability and safety of TCAs are poor. Nevertheless, amitriptyline appears to be the antidepressant most often prescribed for patients with OA (van den Driest et al. 2021). SSRIs have comparable antidepressant efficacy but less analgesic efficacy. SNRIs possess more analgesic potential than SSRIs. Most randomized controlled trials (RCTs) showing analgesic efficacy of antidepressants in rheumatological disorders have been of TCAs (e.g., Ash et al. 1999; Grace et al. 1985; both in RA). Subsequently, duloxetine (60–120 mg/day) has been shown to be efficacious in several randomized placebo-controlled trials in OA (e.g., Chappell et al. 2009; Frakes et al. 2011; Micca et al. 2013). A meta-analysis of seven RCTs found duloxetine to have statistically significant, moderate benefits for pain, function, and quality of life for patients with knee OA, but with frequent gastrointestinal side effects (Osani and Bannuru 2019). Drug interactions may occur, although this is generally not a problem with first- and second-line treatments for RA.

Psychopharmacological treatment of neuropsychiatric symptoms (particularly psychosis and mania) in patients with CNS lupus is a challenge, with no guidance from RCTs (Tincani et al. 1996). Most reports have been in children and adolescents (e.g., Lim et al. 2013; Zuniga Zambrano et al. 2014). High-dose corticosteroids are considered a first-line treatment to suppress CNS inflammation; however, they may exacerbate neuropsychiatric symptoms. Second-line agents include azathioprine and cyclophosphamide, and combination therapy is common (Fanouriakis et al. 2016). Antipsychotic drugs are frequently used for symptomatic treatment concurrent with corticosteroids. Clinically, agents with high potency at dopamine D_2 receptors generally appear the most effective, especially in severe cases. Patients with CNS lupus must be monitored closely for extrapyramidal symptoms and seizures. Anticonvulsant mood stabilizers are often used for prophylaxis or treatment of seizures as well as for their mood-stabilizing properties. Benzodiazepines should be used with caution because of the risk of confusion and behavioral disinhibition. However, benzodiazepines have been effective, sometimes combined with electroconvulsive therapy, in catatonia caused by lupus (Boeke et al. 2018).

Psychiatric Side Effects of Rheumatological Medications

The differential diagnosis of psychiatric disorders in patients with rheumatological disorders includes side effects of rheumatological medications. Table

Table 14–1.   Psychiatric side effects of medications used in treating rheumatological disorders

Medication	Psychiatric side effects
Abatacept	None reported
Adalimumab	None reported
Anakinra	Headache
Azathioprine	Delirium
Baricitinib	None reported
Belimumab	None reported
Certolizumab	Headache
Corticosteroids	Mood lability, euphoria, irritability, anxiety, insomnia, mania, depression, psychosis, delirium, cognitive disturbance
Cyclophosphamide	Delirium (at high doses) (rare)
Cyclosporine	Anxiety, delirium, visual hallucinations
Etanercept	None reported
Golimumab	None reported
Hydroxychloroquine	Confusion, psychosis, mania, depression, nightmares, anxiety, aggression, delirium
Immunoglobulin (intravenous)	Delirium, agitation
Infliximab	None reported
Leflunomide	Anxiety
Methotrexate	Delirium (at high doses) (rare)
Mycophenolate mofetil	Anxiety, depression, sedation (all rare)
Nonsteroidal anti-inflammatory drugs (high dose)	Depression, anxiety, paranoia, hallucinations, impaired concentration, hostility, confusion, delirium
Rituximab	None reported

Table 14–1.   Psychiatric side effects of medications used in treating
rheumatological disorders *(continued)*

Medication	Psychiatric side effects
Sulfasalazine	Insomnia, depression, hallucinations
Tacrolimus	Anxiety, delirium, insomnia, restlessness
Tocilizumab	None reported
Tofacitinib	None reported
Upadacitinib	None reported
Voclosporin	Fatigue, tremor, dizziness, hypoesthesia, paresthesia, seizures, headaches, posterior reversible encephalopathy syndrome

14–1 lists the reported psychiatric side effects of rheumatological medications. Most of these come from case reports, and they are not all substantiated. For example, a large prospective cohort study of hydroxychloroquine versus sulfasalazine as an active comparator in patients with RA found no increase in the risk of depression, suicide or suicidal ideation, or psychosis with hydroxychloroquine (Lane et al. 2021). Corticosteroid-induced psychiatric symptoms are reviewed in Chapter 10, "Endocrine and Metabolic Disorders."

Rheumatological Side Effects of Psychotropic Medications: Psychotropic Drug–Induced Lupus

Patients who are taking antipsychotic medications, particularly chlorpromazine, may have positive antinuclear and antiphospholipid antibodies, but most do not develop signs of an autoantibody-associated disease. Compared with other (nonpsychiatric) drugs known to cause a symptomatic lupuslike syndrome, chlorpromazine and carbamazepine carry low risk (0.1%–1%), and several other psychotropics (oxcarbazepine, valproic acid, lamotrigine, phenelzine, prazosin, and lithium) carry very low risk (≤0.1%) (Arnaud et al. 2019). There are isolated case reports of lupus with several antidepressants and donepezil. Drug-induced lupus is actually more commonly caused by rheumatological drugs (most commonly with infliximab and adalimumab) than by psychotropics. CNS involvement is usually absent in drug-induced lupus. Laboratory findings may include mild cytopenia, elevated erythrocyte sedimentation rate, and elevated antinuclear antibody titers. Antihistone antibodies are positive in up to 95% of patients but are not pathognomonic of drug-induced lupus. After discontinuation of the drug, symptoms and antibody titers decline, usually over a period of weeks; however, the recovery can take more than a year (Vedove et al. 2009). Rechallenge is sometimes possible without recurrence, as reported in a case of clozapine-induced lupus (Pathak et al. 2019).

Drug-Drug Interactions

Few important drug interactions occur between rheumatological and psychopharmacological agents. These are summarized in Table 14–2, with the exception of most chemotherapeutic agents (discussed in Chapter 8, "Oncology") and corticosteroids (discussed in Chapter 10). The most important possible interactions involve potential for increased gastrointestinal bleeding when nonsteroidal anti-inflammatory drugs are combined with serotonergic agents, particularly SSRIs, SNRIs, and tertiary-amine TCAs. The potential for synergistic myelosuppressive effects exists with the combination of immunosuppressive agents (sulfasalazine, azathioprine, chemotherapeutic agents) and psychotropics with this effect (e.g., clozapine, carbamazepine). Hydroxychloroquine has been reported to sometimes increase the QTc interval, but this interaction has not been affected by co-prescription with antidepressants (Park et al. 2021) or antipsychotics (Renaldi et al. 2021). Leflunomide is relatively free of interactions.

Key Points

- Depression is highly prevalent among patients with rheumatological disorders.

- Randomized controlled trials have shown antidepressants to be effective for the treatment of depression in patients with rheumatoid arthritis.

Table 14–2. Rheumatological medication–psychotropic medication interactions[a]

Medication	Interaction mechanism	Effects on psychotropic medications and management
Azathioprine	Synergistic myelosuppression	Potential increased risk for blood dyscrasias with some psychotropics (e.g., clozapine, carbamazepine, valproate, mirtazapine)
Hydroxychloroquine		? Increased risk of cardiac arrhythmias with other QT-prolonging agents
Nonsteroidal anti-inflammatory drugs	Additive anticoagulant effect	Increased risk of bleeding with SSRIs, SNRIs, and tertiary-amine TCAs
Sulfasalazine	Additive nausea	Increased nausea with some psychotropics (e.g., SSRIs, SNRIs, cholinesterase inhibitors, anticonvulsants, lithium)
	Synergistic myelosuppression	Potential increased risk for blood dyscrasias with some psychotropics (e.g., clozapine, carbamazepine, valproate, mirtazapine)
Tacrolimus	QT prolongation	Increased risk of cardiac arrhythmias with other QT-prolonging agents, including TCAs, typical antipsychotics, pimozide, risperidone, paliperidone, iloperidone, quetiapine, ziprasidone, and lithium
Upadacitinib, voclosporin	Substrate of CYP3A4	Strong CYP3A4 inducers (carbamazepine, modafinil, armodafinil) should be avoided

Note. CYP = cytochrome P450; SNRIs = serotonin-norepinephrine reuptake inhibitors; SSRIs = selective serotonin reuptake inhibitors; TCAs = tricyclic antidepressants.
[a]Drug interactions between chemotherapeutic agents used in rheumatology (e.g., cyclophosphamide, methotrexate, cyclosporine, tacrolimus) and psychotropic drugs are covered in Chapter 8, "Oncology."

- Tricyclic antidepressants and serotonin-norepinephrine re-uptake inhibitors possess more analgesic potential than do se-lective serotonin reuptake inhibitors.

- Psychiatric drugs are uncommon causes of drug-induced lu-pus, with chlorpromazine and carbamazepine most common among those that cause lupus.

- Among the drugs used to treat rheumatological disorders, cor-ticosteroids are the most likely to cause psychiatric side effects.

References

Abrol E, Coutinho E, Chou M, et al: Psychosis in systemic lupus erythematosus (SLE): 40-year experience of a specialist centre. Rheumatology (Oxford) 60(12):5620–5629, 2021 33629101

Arnaud L, Mertz P, Gavand PE, et al: Drug-induced systemic lupus: revisiting the ever-changing spectrum of the disease using the WHO pharmacovigilance data-base. Ann Rheum Dis 78(4):504–508, 2019 30793701

Ash G, Dickens CM, Creed FH, et al: The effects of dothiepin on subjects with rheu-matoid arthritis and depression. Rheumatology (Oxford) 38(10):959–967, 1999 10534546

Boeke A, Pullen B, Coppes L, et al: Catatonia associated with systemic lupus erythe-matosus (SLE): a report of two cases and a review of the literature. Psychosomat-ics 59(6):523–530, 2018 30270156

Chappell AS, Ossanna MJ, Liu-Seifert H, et al: Duloxetine, a centrally acting analge-sic, in the treatment of patients with osteoarthritis knee pain: a 13-week, random-ized, placebo-controlled trial. Pain 146(3):253–260, 2009 19625125

Fanouriakis A, Pamfil C, Sidiropoulos P, et al: Cyclophosphamide in combination with glucocorticoids for severe neuropsychiatric systemic lupus erythematosus: a retrospective, observational two-centre study. Lupus 25(6):627–636, 2016 26692040

Ferreira GE, McLachlan AJ, Lin CC, et al: Efficacy and safety of antidepressants for the treatment of back pain and osteoarthritis: systematic review and meta-analysis. BMJ 372:m4825, 2021 33472813

Fiest KM, Hitchon CA, Bernstein CN, et al: Systematic review and meta-analysis of interventions for depression and anxiety in persons with rheumatoid arthritis. J Clin Rheumatol 23(8):425–434, 2017 28221313

Frakes EP, Risser RC, Ball TD, et al: Duloxetine added to oral nonsteroidal anti-inflammatory drugs for treatment of knee pain due to osteoarthritis: results of a randomized, double-blind, placebo-controlled trial. Curr Med Res Opin 27(12):2361–2372, 2011 22017192

Grace EM, Bellamy N, Kassam Y, et al: Controlled, double-blind, randomized trial of amitriptyline in relieving articular pain and tenderness in patients with rheumatoid arthritis. Curr Med Res Opin 9(6):426–429, 1985 3886308

Isnardi CA, Capelusnik D, Schneeberger EE, et al: Depression is a major determinant of functional capacity in rheumatoid arthritis. J Clin Rheumatol 27(6S):S180–S185, 2021 32732521

Joshi N, Khanna R, Shah RM: Relationship between depression and physical activity, disability, burden, and health-related quality of life among patients with arthritis. Popul Health Manag 18(2):104–114, 2015 25247246

Lane JCE, Weaver J, Kostka K, et al: Risk of depression, suicide and psychosis with hydroxychloroquine treatment for rheumatoid arthritis: a multinational network cohort study. Rheumatology (Oxford) 60(7):3222–3234, 2021 33367863

Levenson JL, Irwin MR: Rheumatology, in American Psychiatric Publishing Textbook of Psychosomatic Medicine and Consultation-Liaison Psychiatry, 3rd Edition. Edited by Levenson JL. Washington, DC, American Psychiatric Publishing, 2019, pp 683–708

Lim LS, Lefebvre A, Benseler S, et al: Longterm outcomes and damage accrual in patients with childhood systemic lupus erythematosus with psychosis and severe cognitive dysfunction. J Rheumatol 40(4):513–519, 2013 23457384

Lin EH, Katon W, Von Korff M, et al: Effect of improving depression care on pain and functional outcomes among older adults with arthritis: a randomized controlled trial. JAMA 290(18):2428–2429, 2003 14612479

Lin EH, Tang L, Katon W, et al: Arthritis pain and disability: response to collaborative depression care. Gen Hosp Psychiatry 28(6):482–486, 2006 17088163

Micca JL, Ruff D, Ahl J, et al: Safety and efficacy of duloxetine treatment in older and younger patients with osteoarthritis knee pain: a post hoc, subgroup analysis of two randomized, placebo-controlled trials. BMC Musculoskelet Disord 14:137, 2013 23590727

Osani MC, Bannuru RR: Efficacy and safety of duloxetine in osteoarthritis: a systematic review and meta-analysis. Korean J Intern Med 34(5):966–973, 2019 30871298

Park E, Giles JT, Perez-Recio T, et al: Hydroxychloroquine use is not associated with QTc length in a large cohort of SLE and RA patients. Arthritis Res Ther 23(1):271, 2021 34715924

Pathak S, Cherry S, Samad S, et al: Successful clozapine rechallenge in a patient with suspected drug induced lupus. BMJ Case Rep 12(4):e228574, 2019 30948402

Pedersen JK, Andersen K, Svendsen AJ, et al: No difference in antidepressant prescription in rheumatoid arthritis and controls: results from a population-based, matched inception cohort. Scand J Rheumatol 51(3):173–179, 2022 34182890

Rathbun AM, Harrold LR, Reed GW: A description of patient- and rheumatologist-reported depression symptoms in an American rheumatoid arthritis registry population. Clin Exp Rheumatol 32(4):523–532, 2014 24984165

Renaldi J, Koumpouras F, Dong X: Evaluating the risk of QTc prolongation associated with hydroxychloroquine use with antidepressants in lupus patients with fibromyalgia. Lupus 30(11):1844–1848, 2021 34353174

Sruamsiri R, Kaneko Y, Mahlich J: The underrated prevalence of depression in Japanese patients with rheumatoid arthritis: evidence from a nationwide survey in Japan. BMC Rheumatol 1:5, 2017 30886949

Tincani A, Brey R, Balestrieri G, et al: International survey on the management of patients with SLE, II: the results of a questionnaire regarding neuropsychiatric manifestations. Clin Exp Rheumatol 14(Suppl 16):S23–S29, 1996 9049450

van den Driest JJ, Schiphof D, de Wilde M, et al: Antidepressant and anticonvulsant prescription rates in patients with osteoarthritis: a population-based cohort study. Rheumatology (Oxford) 60(5):2206–2216, 2021 33175150

Vedove CD, Del Giglio M, Schena D, et al: Drug-induced lupus erythematosus. Arch Dermatol Res 301(1):99–105, 2009 18797892

Zuniga Zambrano YC, Guevara Ramos JD, Penagos Vargas NE, et al: Risk factors for neuropsychiatric manifestations in children with systemic lupus erythematosus: case-control study. Pediatr Neurol 51(3):403–409, 2014 25160546

15

Critical Care and Surgery

Melissa P. Bui, M.D.

Elisabeth A. Dietrich, M.D.

James L. Levenson, M.D.

Stephen J. Ferrando, M.D.

Psychopharmacological treatment in the critical care setting and perioperative period can be particularly challenging because of severe multiorgan system disease, rapid shifts in clinical status, and the introduction of multiple medications such as anesthetics, analgesics, and antibiotics that may directly influence cognitive functioning and interact with psychotropic drugs. In this chapter, we address the prevention and treatment of delirium; highlight other relevant states of altered mental status commonly encountered among critically ill patients; explore the psychopharmacological treatment of presurgical anxiety and acute and posttraumatic stress syndromes that are often seen in the wake of prolonged critical illness, such as post-ICU syndrome (PICS); review drug-drug interactions that may be encountered in the ICU and surgical

631

settings; and address the management of psychotropic drugs in the perioperative period, including treatment of preoperative anxiety. The reader is referred to relevant chapters in this volume that address psychopharmacological treatment within specific organ system disease states.

Delirium

Delirium, characterized by a rapid-onset disturbance in consciousness, attention and arousal, and cognition, is common in hospitalized patients who are medically ill and is associated with worsened short- and long-term clinical, functional, and neuropsychological outcomes (Desai et al. 2011). It causes lasting distress to patients and families and is an independent predictor of morbidity and mortality, particularly when persisting at hospital discharge (Salluh et al. 2015). On admission to the general hospital, 14%–24% of patients have delirium, and during hospital admission 6%–56% develop delirium, including as many as 87% of the patients in ICUs (Ely et al. 2004). Clinically, delirium has three psychomotor behavior subtypes: hypoactive, hyperactive, and mixed (Thom et al. 2019). The hypoactive form often may be mistaken for depression or missed entirely if patients are not regularly screened for delirium with a validated assessment, highlighting the importance of universal screening for delirium (Pun et al. 2019). The hyperactive and mixed forms are associated with waxing and waning agitation, increased motor activity, hallucinations, and delusions. Although management of behavioral disturbances of delirium accounts for approximately one-third of psychiatric consultation requests (Schellhorn et al. 2009), it is often underdiagnosed and remains challenging to manage, particularly given the limited evidence supporting clear pharmacological prevention or management strategies.

The optimal management of delirium entails systematic delirium screening, particularly among patient populations considered to be at especially high risk (ICU patients, geriatric patients, patients with multimorbidity). Treatment includes identification and treatment of underlying causes (e.g., organ failure, infection, exposure to deliriogenic medications or interventions, metabolic derangements), environmental interventions (i.e., early and progressive mobilization, sleep-wake optimization, frequent orientation), and psychopharmacology to address specific targets of intervention (e.g., agitation, sleep cycle disturbances, withdrawal from substances). It is important to review medications that may cause or exacerbate delirium, including benzodiazepines, opioid analgesics, corticosteroids, anticholinergics, and deliriogenic antibiotics such as cefepime (Payne et al. 2017).

Pharmacological approaches are but one component of delirium management. Numerous studies using multimodal (i.e., combining delirium screening with nonpharmacological and pharmacological intervention) approaches to delirium prevention have documented reduced incidence and duration of delirium, as well as reductions in other important outcomes related to morbidity and care costs (Collinsworth et al. 2016; Hshieh et al. 2015; Pun et al. 2019), which stresses the need for combined nonpharmacological and pharmacological interventions.

Psychopharmacological interventions for the treatment of delirium are aimed at correcting disturbances in one or more neurotransmitter systems (i.e., cholinergic, dopaminergic, noradrenergic, and serotonergic) in order to target emergent or perpetuating symptoms of delirium (e.g., sleep-wake disturbances, agitation leading to disruption of care, perceptual disturbances). Correction of sleep-wake cycle disruptions that are characteristic of delirium is targeted via melatonin (MT1 and MT2), anti-α_1-adrenergic, antihistaminic, and GABA agonist properties. Psychopharmacology clinical trials in the published literature have been aimed at the prevention of delirium in surgical and critically ill patients and the treatment of delirium once diagnosed. Medications studied in randomized controlled trials (RCTs) include haloperidol, ziprasidone, olanzapine, risperidone, aripiprazole, midazolam, propofol, dexmedetomidine, donepezil, and rivastigmine. The treatment of anticholinergic delirium requires specific psychopharmacological intervention and is covered separately later in this chapter (see subsection "Anticholinergic Delirium"). Delirium associated with the coronavirus SARS-CoV-2 disease (COVID-19) is also reviewed. Delirium from alcohol withdrawal is covered in Chapter 18, "Substance Use Disorders."

Delirium Prevention Trials

The high morbidity, mortality, and cost associated with delirium have made it an attractive target for pharmacological intervention, with the aim of identifying a prophylactic intervention capable of reducing the incidence, duration, or severity of the condition. Numerous studies have centered on antipsychotics as a primary point of intervention given their frequent use in managing behavioral symptoms of delirium once it arises. α_2 Agonists, donepezil, and cholinesterase inhibitors also have been explored as potential delirium prevention agents, with mixed success.

Several double-blind RCTs have examined the role for prophylactic use of the typical antipsychotic haloperidol in the prevention of delirium among critically ill patients. Wang et al. (2012) randomly assigned 457 patients age 65 or older who were admitted to the ICU after noncardiac surgery to receive haloperidol (0.5 mg IV bolus injection followed by continuous infusion at a rate of 0.1 mg/hour for 12 hours) or placebo. The primary end point was delirium in the first 7 days, which was less common in the haloperidol group (15.3% vs. 23.2%; RR=0.66; 95% CI=0.45–0.97). Secondary outcomes were better in the haloperidol group as well, including longer mean time to onset of delirium, more delirium-free days, and shorter length of ICU stay. There was no significant difference in all-cause 28-day mortality, and no drug-related side effects were documented. Notably, average Acute Physiology and Chronic Health Evaluation II scores among patients in this study were less than half those of patients in other comparable delirium prevention studies. This may limit findings to patients with less severe illness. In an RCT comparing haloperidol with placebo in preventing delirium in older adults with hip fractures, haloperidol, 0.5 mg, or placebo was administered orally three times daily for 1–3 days before hip replacement surgery and was continued for 3 days postoperatively (Kalisvaart et al. 2005). The incidence of delirium did not differ between the haloperidol and the placebo groups (15.1% vs. 16.5%). However, those taking haloperidol had lower severity of delirium (mean 4 points lower on the Delirium Rating Scale—Revised-98; $P<0.001$), shorter duration of delirium (mean 6.4 days shorter; $P<0.001$), and shorter length of hospital stay (mean 5.5 days shorter; $P<0.001$). Importantly, no drug-related side effects, including extrapyramidal side effects (EPS), were encountered.

Al-Qadheeb et al. (2016) reported lower severity of agitation among patients who developed delirium in a study examining the role of low-dose haloperidol in preventing patients with subsyndromal delirium from becoming fully delirious, as measured by the Intensive Care Delirium Screening Checklist. Although patients in the haloperidol group spent fewer hours per day agitated (Sedation Agitation Scale ≥5; $P=0.008$), there were no significant differences in days alive without delirium or coma, time to first incidence of delirium, delirium duration, days of mechanical ventilation, or mortality. QT prolongation and EPS were also noted to be comparable between the two groups.

The Modifying the INcidence of Delirium (MIND) Trial was a multisite double-blind, placebo-controlled feasibility study comparing the efficacy of haloperidol or ziprasidone and placebo among critically ill patients at high risk for developing delirium (Girard et al. 2010). There were no differences between groups for either the primary end point (delirium-free and coma-free days: haloperidol median [interquartile range] = 14.0 [6.0–18.0] days; ziprasidone = 15.0 [9.1–18.0] days; and placebo = 12.5 [1.2–17.2] days; P = 0.66) or the secondary outcomes (ventilator-free days, P = 0.25; hospital length of stay, P = 0.68; or mortality, P = 0.81). Again, the development of EPS was similar between treatment groups (P = 0.46).

Trials examining atypical antipsychotics as a component of delirium prevention strategies have yielded similar results. A study examining the role of 1 mg of risperidone given sublingually on recovery from anesthesia after elective cardiac surgery found lower incidence of delirium (7 of 63 patients) when compared with placebo (20 of 63 patients) (RR = 0.35; 95% CI = 0.16–0.77) (Prakanrattana and Prapaitrakool 2007). However, the study was not blinded, and the length of ICU stay was not different between groups.

A single prospective randomized placebo-controlled trial randomly assigned 53 neurosurgical patients to receive enteric aripiprazole (15 mg) or placebo for up to 7 days (Mokhtari et al. 2020). Delirium incidence was significantly lower in the aripiprazole group compared with placebo (20% vs. 55%; P = 0.22), with no adverse reactions observed in the treatment group of the study.

Olanzapine, 5 mg, given orally preoperatively and immediately postoperatively was compared with placebo in a large RCT aimed at reducing the incidence of delirium in high-risk patients having joint replacement surgery (Larsen et al. 2010). The incidence of delirium was 15% in the olanzapine group compared with 41% in the placebo group (P < 0.001). In addition, the olanzapine-treated group had lower Delirium Rating Scale—Revised-98 scores during the first 5 postoperative days, needed lower dosages of narcotics, and were more likely to be discharged to home (vs. a rehabilitation facility) compared with the placebo group.

An important trial among palliative care patients showed that prophylactic administration of either haloperidol or risperidone resulted in worse outcomes when compared with placebo (Agar et al. 2017). This multicenter, double-blind, parallel-arm, dose-titrated randomized clinical trial found that patients in the haloperidol and risperidone groups had delirium symptom scores that were significantly higher than in the placebo group (haloperidol average of 0.24 U higher; 95% CI = 0.06–0.42; $P = 0.009$; and risperidone 0.48 U higher; 95% CI = 0.09–0.86; $P = 0.02$) and had more EPS (haloperidol = 0.79; 95% CI = 0.17–1.41; $P = 0.01$; risperidone = 0.73; 95% CI = 0.09–1.37; $P = 0.03$), and patients in the haloperidol group had lower survival (hazard ratio = 1.73; 95% CI = 1.20–2.50; $P = 0.003$). In contrast to the above studies, this trial suggests a higher predisposition to adverse effects from antipsychotics among hospice and palliative care patients.

Given the cholinergic deficit hypothesis of delirium, cholinesterase inhibitors were hypothesized to have potential benefit in delirium prophylaxis among critically ill patients. Three small RCTs comparing donepezil with placebo did not yield significant differences between groups in the incidence of delirium (Liptzin et al. 2005; Marcantonio et al. 2011; Sampson et al. 2007). A placebo-controlled, multicenter, double-blind RCT compared an escalating, twice-a-day dosing strategy of rivastigmine with placebo among critically ill patients with delirium, with a primary outcome of duration of delirium (van Eijk et al. 2010). However, the trial had to be halted early by its data safety review board after there was a disproportionate increase in mortality among the rivastigmine group. Cholinesterase inhibitors are not recommended for use in the prevention of delirium.

Dexmedetomidine, an intravenously administered α_2-receptor agonist sedative that decreases norepinephrine release centrally, has shown significant promise in the prevention of delirium among postoperative patients and in the ICU setting. A meta-analysis by Flükiger et al. (2018) showed that dexmedetomidine was associated with significantly lower overall incidence of delirium when compared with placebo (RR = 0.52; 95% CI = 0.39–0.70; $I^2 = 37\%$), standard sedatives (RR = 0.63; 95% CI = 0.46–0.86; $I^2 = 69\%$), and opioids (RR = 0.61; 95% CI = 0.44–0.83; $I^2 = 0\%$). However, exposure to dexmedetomidine significantly increased the risk of bradycardia and hypotension. Separate meta-analyses by Shen and Zeng had similarly positive findings among noncardiac surgical patients. Shen et al. (2020) found that the overall incidence of postoperative delirium was significantly lower in the dexmedetomidine group than in the control group (RR = 0.51; 95% CI = 0.43–0.61; $P < 0.01$), and Zeng and colleagues (2019) reported that exposure to dexmedetomidine significantly reduced the prevalence of postoperative delirium when compared with placebo (RR = 0.61; 95% CI = 0.34–0.76; P = 0.001; I^2 = 66%). Each meta-analysis identified associations between dexmedetomidine exposure and both bradycardia and hypotension.

Dexmedetomidine also has shown promise in the prevention of delirium when administered nocturnally to ICU patients (Skrobik et al. 2018). When compared with placebo, nocturnal dexmedetomidine was associated with a greater proportion of patients who remained delirium free (dexmedetomidine = 40 of 50 patients [80%] vs. placebo = 27 of 50 patients [54%]; RR = 0.44; 95% CI = 0.23–0.82; P = 0.006).

In the absence of a single pharmacological agent capable of decreasing the incidence of delirium, pioneers in critical care began to evaluate the role for "bundles" of care, deploying multiple evidence-based interventions simultaneously with the goal of improving outcomes among critically ill patients. The ABCDEF bundle (Table 15–1), which was evaluated across 68 sites and led to recruitment of more than 15,000 patients with at least 1 ICU day, resulted in reductions in mortality, ICU and hospital length of stay, days on mechanical ventilation, and incidence of delirium (Marra et al. 2017; Pun et al. 2019). A dose-response relationship was seen between higher bundle compliance and improvements in each of those areas. Complete ABCDEF bundle compliance was associated with reduced incidence of delirium (adjusted OR = 0.60; 95% CI = 0.49–0.72), and partial ABCDEF bundle compliance showed a dose-dependent relationship, with improved adherence to the bundle reflecting lower rates of delirium among study patients.

The ABCDEF bundle reflects the Society of Critical Care Medicine's Pain, Agitation/Sedation, Delirium, Immobility, and Sleep Disruption Guidelines, which do not advocate for the use of either haloperidol or atypical antipsychotics for the prevention or treatment of delirium (Devlin et al. 2018). However, the use of antipsychotics is permitted for the treatment of either psychosis or agitation that threatens the safety of the patient or those caring for them.

In summary, there is limited evidence in critically ill and surgical patients for pharmacological prophylaxis with antipsychotics or dexmedetomidine (Serafim et al. 2015). Adverse events, particularly EPS and torsades de pointes with antipsychotics, have been minimal in prevention trials, and antipsychotics appear to be generally well tolerated within this patient population, with the exception of palliative care and hospice patients. The gold standard for delirium prevention and treatment is the bundled-care approach, which pri-

Table 15–1. ABCDEF bundle to improve outcomes among critically ill patients

Bundle component	Description
A	Assess, prevent, and manage pain
B	Both spontaneous awakening trials and spontaneous breathing trials
C	Choice of analgesia and sedation
D	Delirium: assess, prevent, and manage
E	Early mobility and exercise
F	Family engagement and empowerment

Source. Adapted from Marra et al. 2017.

oritizes delirium monitoring and intervention as one of its core principles. Although many ICUs may not yet have sufficient resources or collaboration to implement the full ABCDEF bundle, partial compliance has also shown significant benefit, and multimodal interventions for delirium remain critical for the practicing psychiatrist to be aware of and advocate for when providing psychiatric consultations to critically ill patients (Collinsworth et al. 2016; Pun et al. 2019).

Delirium Treatment Studies

The first pharmacological RCT in delirium compared haloperidol, chlorpromazine, and lorazepam (mean dosage = 1.4 mg, 36 mg, and 4.6 mg orally per day, respectively) in patients with AIDS (Breitbart et al. 1996). Haloperidol and chlorpromazine were equally effective for both hyperactive and hypoactive variants, but lorazepam was ineffective and even worsened delirium in some patients, necessitating discontinuation. Notably, these patients had mild to moderate delirium symptoms, thus requiring only low dosages of medication, and the incidence of EPS was low.

Subsequent trials have produced mixed results, not surprising given the protean nature of delirium, the range of etiologies, and different treatment settings. The HOPE-ICU study, a double-blind, placebo-controlled RCT in ICU patients, found that haloperidol did not change the duration of delirium

(Page et al. 2013). A prospective interventional cohort study in patients undergoing cardiac surgery found that protocolized treatment with haloperidol did not differ from usual care with regard to delirium incidence or duration, length of stay, or complication rate (Schrøder Pedersen et al. 2014). Only about a third of the delirious palliative care patients from 14 centers across four countries appeared to benefit from haloperidol (Crawford et al. 2013).

Small RCTs comparing haloperidol with atypical antipsychotics generally have not found significant differences in effectiveness and safety in treating delirium. Examples include a single-blind trial comparing haloperidol with risperidone (Han and Kim 2004); a study comparing haloperidol, risperidone, olanzapine, and quetiapine (Yoon et al. 2013); two RCTs comparing haloperidol and olanzapine (Maneeton et al. 2013; Skrobik et al. 2004); and a single-blind trial comparing haloperidol, olanzapine, and risperidone (Grover et al. 2011). None of these studies was placebo controlled.

Hu et al. (2004) compared olanzapine, parenteral haloperidol, and placebo in a heterogeneous group of delirious hospitalized patients. Improvement was greater with both drugs compared with placebo, with no end point difference between the two drugs (Hu et al. 2004).

There are a few placebo-controlled RCTs of atypical antipsychotics. Risperidone reduced the incidence of delirium in elderly patients who were experiencing subsyndromal delirium after on-pump cardiac surgery (Hakim et al. 2012). Two small studies found that delirium resolved more quickly with quetiapine (Devlin et al. 2010; Tahir et al. 2010). The Devlin study was a prospective, randomized, double-blind, placebo-controlled study across three sites that randomly assigned delirious patients to receive quetiapine, 50 mg every 12 hours, or placebo, with open-label as-needed haloperidol available to both groups. The dose of quetiapine was increased in 50-mg increments every 24 hours (maximum of 200 mg every 12 hours) if more than one dose of haloperidol was given in the previous 24 hours. Quetiapine was associated with a shorter time to first resolution of delirium, reduced duration of delirium, less agitation, fewer days of as-needed haloperidol, and increased likelihood of discharge to home. Patients in the quetiapine group had greater levels of sedation, although EPS and QTc interval prolongation were similar across groups.

The largest placebo-controlled RCT of antipsychotics for the treatment of delirium to date is the MIND-USA study, a randomized, double-blind, placebo-controlled trial that assigned critically ill, delirious patients to receive intravenous boluses of haloperidol (maximum dose=20 mg daily), ziprasidone (maximum dose=40 mg daily), or placebo (Girard et al. 2018). No significant differences were found between placebo and treatment arms for either the primary end point (days alive without delirium or coma) or the secondary end points (30- and 90-day survival, time to extubation, and time to ICU and hospital discharge), leading to the conclusion that standing doses of haloperidol or ziprasidone did not significantly alter the duration of delirium. Of note, 89% of delirious patients included in this study had the hypoactive subtype of delirium, for which the use of antipsychotics is not clearly indicated.

As noted earlier in the subsection "Delirium Prevention Trials," some evidence indicates that perioperative sedation with dexmedetomidine reduces the incidence of delirium compared with other sedatives. RCTs of its efficacy in treating delirium found it superior to intravenous haloperidol (Reade et al. 2009) and successful in treating delirium when added to usual care among critically ill patients with delirium receiving mechanical ventilation (Reade et al. 2016). The latter trial, known as the Dexmedetomidine to Lessen ICU Agitation study, documented an increase in ventilator-free hours at 7 days (median difference=17.0 hours; P=0.01) as well as faster resolution of delirium (median difference=16 hours; P=0.01) when compared with placebo (Reade et al. 2016).

In summary, although antipsychotics are widely used in the management of delirium, the evidence base supporting their use remains very modest. A few small RCTs suggested similar efficacy of haloperidol (oral or parenteral), quetiapine, olanzapine, and risperidone for the treatment of delirium; however, the limited number of trials and the limitations and variability of the trial designs prevent firm conclusions about comparative efficacy or adverse effects. Patients taking higher dosages of haloperidol (>4.5 mg/day by injection or >7.5–15 mg/day orally) may have a higher incidence of EPS compared with patients taking olanzapine or risperidone administered orally at more modest equivalent dosages. Dexmedetomidine may be a promising agent for the prevention and treatment of delirium, and larger randomized double-blind comparison trials are indicated.

The Society of Critical Care Medicine's Pain, Agitation/Sedation, Delirium, Immobility, and Sleep Disruption Guidelines do not recommend the use of haloperidol, atypical antipsychotics, or dexmedetomidine for either the prevention or the treatment of delirium. However, haloperidol or atypical antipsychotics may be used to treat symptoms or psychosis or agitation that threatens the safety or well-being of patients or those caring for them. Ideally, the practitioner would select an agent best suited to the symptomatic needs of the individual patient, would use as-needed dosing prior to implementation of a standing regimen, and would discontinue the medication as early as it was safe to do so. Titrating the medication to a particular clinical measurement also may be helpful in minimizing unnecessary exposures; for example, if an as-needed antipsychotic is being used in the management of agitation, the consulting psychiatrist might recommend that a dose be given if the Richmond Agitation Sedation Scale score is +2 or higher. Patients receiving antipsychotic medications should also be closely monitored for the emergence of EPS, QTc interval prolongation, and other potential dangerous sequelae of antipsychotic medications, especially if the patients have underlying cardiac conditions, or comorbid hepatic or renal impairment that may negatively affect drug clearance. Care also should be taken to ensure that patients are fully weaned off antipsychotics prior to hospital discharge, because these medications may be erroneously continued and expose patients to unnecessary risks and side effects from continued use (Fontaine et al. 2018).

QTc Interval Prolongation

Use of antipsychotics among critically ill and postoperative patients must take into account the risk of prolongation of the QTc interval and the potential for development of torsades de pointes (Beach et al. 2013; see also Chapter 2, "Severe Drug Reactions," and Chapter 6, "Cardiovascular Disorders"). Normal QTc interval is less than 430 ms for men and less than 450 ms for women, and a prolonged QTc interval is considered more than 450 ms for men and more than 470 ms for women. In a review of 223 consecutive ICU patients receiving intravenous haloperidol, Sharma et al. (1998) found that 8 patients (3.6%) developed torsades de pointes, which was associated with high dosages (>35 mg), rapid infusion, and preexisting prolonged QTc interval (>500 ms in 84% of patients with torsades de pointes). A U.S. FDA alert warned against the off-label use of intravenous haloperidol, particularly at higher than recommended dosages, citing "at least 28 case reports of QTc prolongation and [torsades de pointes] in the medical literature, some with fatal outcome in the context of off-label intravenous use of haloperidol" (U.S. Food and Drug Administration 2007). Higher dosages and intravenous administration of haloperidol appear to be associated with a higher risk of QT prolongation and torsades de pointes. The warning emphasizes the particular need for caution when using any formulation of haloperidol to treat patients who 1) have other QT-prolonging conditions, including electrolyte imbalance (particularly hypokalemia and hypomagnesemia); 2) have underlying cardiac abnormalities, hypothyroidism, or familial long QT syndrome; or 3) are taking drugs known to prolong the QT interval, including other antipsychotics, tricyclic antidepressants (TCAs), and lithium (Funk et al. 2020). Continuous electrocardiographic monitoring is recommended if patients need high dosages of haloperidol or other antipsychotics, need intravenous administration of haloperidol, or have underlying cardiac conditions that predispose them to either QT prolongation or cardiac arrhythmias. Care also should be taken to ensure that the QTc interval is being accurately measured. Bazett's formula is typically applied in most routine electrocardiograms to automatically calculate the QTc interval, but it has been criticized for being inaccurate, overestimating it in tachycardia and underestimating it in bradycardia. Fridericia's correction and the Framingham approach both provide reasonable alternatives, but there is no consensus on the comparative effectiveness of these approaches with regard to predicting risk for torsades (Funk et al. 2020). It is recommended that patients receiving QT-prolonging drugs who are at risk for QT prolongation have the QT interval measured during peak plasma concentration of the QT-prolonging medication (Al-Khatib et al. 2003).

In critically ill patients with significant agitation and either with prolonged QTc interval or at high risk for the development of cardiac arrhythmias, alternatives to antipsychotics (e.g., dexmedetomidine, valproic acid, very low dosages of benzodiazepines, or physical restraints) should be considered first, with frequent electrocardiographic monitoring to serially reexamine the risk-benefit ratio of antipsychotic exposures. In summary, although there is no absolute QTc interval at which a psychotropic drug is unconditionally contraindicated, the risk-benefit ratio in patients with pretreatment QTc intervals longer than 500 ms must be assessed comprehensively, with careful attention to risk mitigation strategies (Funk et al. 2020).

Dexmedetomidine Pharmacology

Dexmedetomidine, an α_2-receptor agonist that decreases sympathetic tone both centrally and peripherally, was approved by the FDA in 1999 for use in humans as a short-term medication (<24 hours) for analgesia and sedation in the ICU (Gertler et al. 2001). It has also been found to attenuate neuroendo-crine and hemodynamic responses to anesthesia and surgery and to reduce an-esthetic and opioid requirements. Furthermore, it has been shown to reduce neurocognitive impairment in the ICU and perioperatively when compared with both placebo and comparator drugs (Li et al. 2015). Dexmedetomidine must be administered intravenously. It is rapidly and extensively distributed to tissues and rapidly eliminated almost entirely via cytochrome P450 2D6 (CYP2D6), with a half-life of 2–2.5 hours (Karol and Maze 2000). This pat-tern of immediate distribution and fast elimination allows rapid titration and observation of effects. Dexmedetomidine does not require dosage adjustment in renal insufficiency; dosage reduction in hepatic impairment is recommended by the manufacturer without specific dosing guidance. Infusion ranges of 0.2–0.7 µg/kg/hour have been reported in critically ill ICU patients, includ-ing those on ventilatory support and with organ failure (Maldonado et al. 2009; Reade et al. 2009). The most common side effects are hypotension, bra-dycardia, and respiratory suppression. It is a major substrate and inhibitor of CYP2D6 (see "Drug-Drug Interactions" later in this chapter).

COVID-19 Delirium

With the arrival of COVID-19, patients hospitalized with COVID-19 often needed very intensive medical care, including ICU admission, mechanical ventilation, extracorporeal membrane oxygenation, and continuous renal re-placement therapy. The strict isolation precautions needed to minimize the spread of the virus often translated into long periods of social isolation, early and deep sedation among intubated patients, and use of physical restraints. This combination resulted in a high incidence of severe, prolonged delirium that has been associated with increased mortality and elevated rates of post-admission cognitive dysfunction (Ragheb et al. 2021). It has been postulated that in addition to these synergistic environmental contributions to delirium, COVID-19 is thought to cause prolonged symptoms of delirium through its activation of inflammatory and thrombotic pathways, as well as a direct effect on CNS endothelium and parenchyma (Bodro et al. 2020). Preliminary stud-ies have found that delirium is often present among patients with positive test results for COVID-19, even without associated respiratory symptoms, and that rates of agitation, myoclonus, abulia, and alogia are also disproportion-ately elevated among patients with COVID-19 (Baller et al. 2020). Treatment recommendations have focused primarily on the use of prevention management strategies, low-potency antipsychotics, and α_2 agonists, although RCTs and formalized trials have not yet been available to guide the optimal approach to management (Baller et al. 2020).

Anticholinergic Delirium

Acetylcholine deficit is one of the critical pathogenetic mechanisms of delirium (Trzepacz 2000). Medications with antimuscarinic effects (e.g., benztropine, trihexyphenidyl, scopolamine, diphenhydramine, TCAs [especially tertiary-amine compounds]) cause delirium, and patients with impaired cholinergic neurotransmission (i.e., Alzheimer's disease) and other CNS insults (e.g., trauma, hypoxia, stroke) are highly susceptible to their effects. Anticholinergic delirium is addressed by removal of the offending agent, supportive measures, and, in severe refractory cases, treatment with physostigmine (adults 0.5–2 mg, children 0.01–0.03 mg/kg, given intravenously at ≤1 mg/min every 20–30 minutes until symptoms resolve) (Moore et al. 2015).

Catatonia

The high incidence of catatonia among critically ill patients is increasingly being recognized as a significant target for screening and intervention, particularly given the phenotypic overlap between catatonia and delirium. Studies examining the incidence of catatonia in critically ill patients suggest that the condition is more prevalent than was previously realized. A prospective cohort investigation conducted by Wilson et al. (2017) evaluated critically ill patients with the Bush Francis Catatonia Rating Scale, which mapped to DSM-5 Criterion A for catatonia (American Psychiatric Association 2013), as well as the Confusion Assessment Method for the ICU. Of the 136 patients enrolled, 58 (43%) had delirium, 4 (3%) had catatonia, 42 (31%) had both delirium and catatonia, and 32 (24%) had neither. Such high rates of catatonia have not previously been appreciated, with the overlap in clinical symptoms probably confounding a clear distinction between the two syndromes. Nevertheless, these findings challenge current DSM diagnostic criteria, which preclude the diagnosis of medical catatonia in patients with delirium. They also highlight the importance of increasing practitioners' index of suspicion for catatonia among critically ill patients. The management of patients with both catatonia and delirium poses particular challenges given the delicate psychopharmacological balance that must be achieved to treat the patient's catatonia while minimizing the risk of exacerbating the patient's delirium with benzodiazepines and the catatonia with antipsychotics. A thorough medical workup for underlying causes of catatonia remains critically important in this population, as does caution in prescribing antipsychotics and formulating an appropriate treatment plan that includes benzodiazepines or electroconvulsive therapy (Oldham and Lee 2015).

Acute and Posttraumatic Stress in the Critical Care Setting

Posttraumatic stress symptoms and disorders can occur as a result of traumatic physical injury, intensive care, and major surgery (Bienvenu et al. 2013; Jackson et al. 2014). Although much less studied, acute stress disorder symptoms or early-onset PTSD in the critical care setting is prevalent and appears to predict ongoing or later-onset PTSD and cognitive dysfunction (Davydow et al. 2013). Preexisting anxiety disorders, need for sedation with benzodiazepines, and so-called delusional memories (recalled experiences that occurred during a state of delirium and are not based in reality) have all been shown to be associated with increased risk of PTSD among ICU survivors (Burki 2019). Hospitalized patients who experienced blunt physical trauma were screened with the National Stressful Events Survey Acute Stress Disorder Scale, and the tool was found to be predictive for both the development and the severity of PTSD (Rahmat et al. 2021).

PTSD and other psychological, cognitive, and functional deficits have been recognized as having a high prevalence in post-ICU patients and have been considered within a framework of PICS (Rawal et al. 2017). Family members of critically ill patients often experience similar psychological sequelae, a condition called PICS-F (Smith and Rahman 2022). Rawal et al. (2017) recommended that patients experiencing PICS be referred to interdisciplinary PICS clinics consisting of a critical care physician, psychiatrist or neuropsychologist, physiotherapist, and respiratory therapist, but such clinics are uncommon. A Cochrane review investigating the effect of ICU follow-up services found limited effectiveness in terms of improving health-related quality of life (Schofield-Robinson et al. 2018). More studies are needed to guide the optimal management of this patient population. Psychopharmacological treatment of PTSD in the months after a severe injury or ICU stay would be expected to follow usual treatment guidelines, with selective serotonin reuptake inhibitors (SSRIs) being first-line treatment. However, no RCTs have been reported to guide treatment of patients with postsurgical or post-ICU PTSD.

Retrospective studies of PTSD prevention among soldiers who had sustained burns in combat and had at least one surgery found that intraoperative ketamine versus no ketamine (McGhee et al. 2008) was associated with a significant reduction in incident PTSD, but preoperative and intraoperative midazolam (McGhee et al. 2009b) and propranolol (McGhee et al. 2009a) had no significant relationship to PTSD. In an RCT, intravenous ketamine produced rapid improvement in PTSD 24 hours later (Feder et al. 2014); however, a multicenter placebo-controlled RCT examining the effect of low- versus standard-dose ketamine for symptoms of PTSD failed to find a significant dose-related effect of ketamine on PTSD symptoms (Abdallah et al. 2022). Administration of ketamine immediately after a motor vehicle accident also has been found to *increase* PTSD incidence (Schönenberg et al. 2008), so further study is warranted. In a retrospective analysis of traumatic injury victims admitted to the hospital, higher morphine dosages in the week after injury were predictive of lower incidence of PTSD but not of major depression or other anxiety disorder, suggesting a beneficial effect of morphine on fear conditioning (Bryant et al. 2009). A pilot RCT investigating a 14-day prevention strategy for PTSD among hospitalized surgical trauma victims found no differences between propranolol, gabapentin, and placebo (Stein et al. 2007). A Cochrane review of pharmacological intervention to prevent PTSD, including studies in a variety of traumas that included surgery and septic shock, concluded that there was moderate-quality evidence for the efficacy of hydrocortisone but no evidence to support the efficacy of propranolol, escitalopram, temazepam, or gabapentin (Amos et al. 2014). In an RCT of acute adult trauma inpatients, fewer PTSD symptoms were observed in patients undergoing a collaborative care intervention that included psychiatric medication when indicated than in patients receiving usual care (Zatzick et al. 2004).

In summary, data on PTSD prevention are sparse, with studies limited by small sample size and retrospective data. Findings that intraoperative ketamine, higher posttrauma morphine dosages, and stress corticosteroids after trauma and surgery are associated with lower rates of PTSD must be corroborated by further prospective study with these agents, in addition to antidepressants, which are virtually unstudied. One nonpharmacological approach showing great promise is the advent of ICU diaries or a written journal kept by family members and medical staff to document the day-to-day experience of the patient. However, although early studies found lower incidence of PTSD among ICU patients with the aid of an ICU diary, the number of patients with substantial PTSD symptoms at 3 months was not significantly reduced in a larger double-blind RCT (Garrouste-Orgeas et al. 2019).

Psychotropic Drugs in the Perioperative Period

The question of whether to discontinue a psychiatric drug before surgery with general anesthesia is a common and complex one. In one survey of adults before elective surgery, 43% admitted to taking one or more psychotropic medications (Scher and Anwar 1999). Of these, 35% were taking antidepressants, 34% were taking benzodiazepines, 19% were taking combinations, and 11% were taking antipsychotics, lithium, or over-the-counter psychotropics such as melatonin (Scher and Anwar 1999). Another study reported that 16.7% of the American adult population receives prescriptions for psychotropic medications, with 12.0% taking antidepressants; 8.3% taking anxiolytics, sedatives, or hypnotics; and 1.6% taking antipsychotics (Moore and Mattison 2017). The potential risks of continuing a psychotropic drug before surgery include adverse interactions with anesthetic agents, interference with hemodynamic management (e.g., causing hypotension or hypertension), and postoperative complications (e.g., excessive sedation, ileus). Risks of discontinuing the drug include, at best, loss of therapeutic effect and, at worst, rebound exacerbation of the mental disorder or a withdrawal syndrome, particularly if the patient was prescribed opiates or benzodiazepines preoperatively. The evidence base regarding these relative risks is scanty, composed mostly of case reports. Practical and ethical limitations make controlled trials unlikely.

Individual psychotropic medications must be reviewed before surgery to determine the risks and benefits of continuing each medication through the perioperative period, to evaluate any potential drug-drug interactions that the patient may be exposed to during the procedure, and to account for other possible risks to the patient, such as increased risk of bleeding. Additionally, the decision to discontinue a psychotropic medication before surgery should be individualized, taking into account the extent of surgery, the patient's condition (diagnosis, comorbidities, stability), the choice of anesthetic agents, the length of preoperative fasting, and the risks of discontinuation (withdrawal, relapse) (Huyse et al. 2006). Some experts recommend that lithium, monoamine oxidase inhibitors (MAOIs), TCAs, and clozapine be discontinued before surgery; that SSRIs be continued for patients who are mentally and physically stable; and that for all other psychotropics, an individualized decision is needed. One consensus of experts noted that for major procedures, lithium should be held for 72 hours before surgery, whereas for minor procedures lithium can be continued during the perioperative period, including on the day of surgery (Oprea et al. 2022). In the 2021 Consensus Statement on Preoperative Management of Medications for Psychiatric Diseases, the Society for Perioperative Assessment and Quality Improvement also advised that for patients with ADHD undergoing surgery, stimulant medications and atomoxetine should be held on the day of surgery (Oprea et al. 2022). Other experts caution against discontinuation, advising that the safest course of action for most drug therapy is to continue the drug until the time of surgery, particularly for drugs that can cause a withdrawal syndrome (Noble and Kehlet 2000; Smith et al. 1996). Discontinuing psychiatric medications before surgery risks acute psychiatric relapse, complicating postoperative management and recovery from surgery. If a psychiatric medication must be held during the perioperative window, a plan should also be made for when it may be safely restarted postoperatively to avoid any unnecessary withdrawal or risk of psychiatric relapse. Abrupt discontinuation risks withdrawal reactions from anticonvulsants, opiates, benzodiazepines and other hypnotics, serotonergic antidepressants, and TCAs. Of note, abruptly discontinuing TCAs before surgery can increase the likelihood of cholinergic rebound (Henssler et al. 2019).

Seemingly contradictory literature about perioperative management of psychotropics makes establishing clear guidelines difficult. For example, lithium and carbamazepine are reported both to cause resistance to neuromuscular blocking agents (Ostergaard et al. 1989) and to prolong their effects (Melton et al. 1993). Another difficulty in balancing risks is that some psychotropics may actually provide side benefits; for example, antipsychotics may enhance intraoperative hypothermia (Kudoh et al. 2004). In our opinion, the risks of discontinuation usually exceed the risks of continuing most psychotropic drugs. However, one possible exception is serotonergic antidepressants, which in many studies have been associated with an increase in perioperative bleeding. A systematic review of 13 studies concluded that serotonergic antidepressants increased that risk, with ORs of 1.21–4.14 (Mahdanian et al. 2014). A meta-analysis of 42 observational studies found that patients using SSRIs had a 36% higher risk of bleeding (Laporte et al. 2017). However, the absolute increase in risk and the magnitude of blood loss appear to be small, except in patients at high risk for bleeding (e.g., coagulopathy, thrombocytopenia). Another exception to continuing medications through the perioperative period is the cholinesterase inhibitors, which synergistically increase the effects of succinylcholine and similar neuromuscular blocking agents (Russell 2009) and may run the risk of causing or exacerbating postoperative delirium. Given the low risks of temporary cessation of therapy, cholinesterase inhibitors should be stopped before surgery.

Some drugs commonly used in anesthesia have potential interactions with psychotropic medications. For example, because valproic acid is a highly protein-bound drug, patients taking valproic acid may have increased free concentrations of propofol, which is also highly plasma protein bound, thereby reducing the necessary dose of propofol (Hızlı Sayar et al. 2014).

Even MAOIs can be continued with relative safety before surgery, by use of specific "MAOI-safe" anesthetic techniques or substitution of reversible MAOIs (Smith et al. 1996). A consensus of experts recommended continuing MAOIs during the perioperative period with use of an MAOI-safe anesthetic or discontinuing MAOIs for 10–14 days before surgery with guidance from a psychiatrist (Oprea et al. 2022). In some cases, interruption of psychopharmacological therapy may be unavoidable, such as when a patient is unable to take oral medication postoperatively for a long period. General strategies to cope with this possibility include 1) allowing patients to continue their usual drugs until the day of surgery when possible; 2) using alternatives to oral administration if available (see Chapter 3, "Alternative Routes of Drug Administration"); 3) when alternative routes are not available, substituting an alternative drug of the same or a different class, one that can be administered by a non-oral route; and 4) returning gastrointestinal transit times to normal as soon as possible to restore reliable drug absorption from the gut (e.g., avoiding unnecessary gastrointestinal tubes and restrictions on oral intake and using non-opioid or opioid-reduced analgesia combined with early oral nutrition) (Noble and Kehlet 2000).

Special considerations for patients receiving medication-assisted treatment for opioid use disorder should be noted as well. Although buprenorphine's pharmacodynamic profile suggests that it should be discontinued before surgery out of concern that it would competitively inhibit opioid agonists at the μ receptor and reduce analgesic efficacy, multiple studies have demonstrated that standard opioids given to buprenorphine-maintained patients are effective and additive to the baseline analgesia associated with buprenorphine (Harrison et al. 2018). For most patients, maintenance doses of buprenorphine and methadone can be continued through the perioperative period (Harrison et al. 2018). Given oral naltrexone's half-life of 10 hours, current perioperative management recommendations are to discontinue naltrexone 2–3 days before surgery and to restart after abstinence from opioids for 7–10 days (Harrison et al. 2018).

Perioperative testing for patients prescribed psychotropic medications should also be considered. A preoperative electrocardiogram may be helpful, especially for patients taking TCAs, typical or atypical antipsychotics, or lithium (Harbell et al. 2021). Given the risk of QTc interval prolongation associated with hypokalemia and hypomagnesemia, electrolyte levels should be monitored in the perioperative period. Hepatic function should be considered, especially for patients taking psychotropic medications associated with hepatic impairment, such as valproic acid, clozapine, and olanzapine. Serum drug level monitoring during the perioperative period should be considered when clinically appropriate. For patients who continue taking lithium in the perioperative period, urine output, renal function, electrolytes, and lithium levels should be closely monitored.

Treatment of Preoperative Anxiety

Preoperative anxiety is common in adults and children and has been treated with antianxiety medications, particularly benzodiazepines. Concerns have been expressed about whether preoperative sedating medication might delay discharge, especially because an increasing percentage of surgical procedures are being carried out on an outpatient basis. A Cochrane review of 17 studies found no evidence of a difference in time to discharge from the hospital in adult patients who had received anxiolytic premedication (Walker and Smith 2009).

Adults and Preoperative Anxiety

Randomized trials in adults have had mixed results regarding use of preoperative benzodiazepines. Furthermore, studies vary in type of surgery, patient demographics, medication choice, dosage, and timing of medication. Compared with placebo, both oral diazepam (10 mg) in the evening before surgery and midazolam (1.5 mg) at least 15 minutes before surgery resulted in lower preoperative anxiety and a reduction in the usual postoperative increase in cortisol levels (Pekcan et al. 2005). Among women undergoing abdominal hysterectomy, diazepam-treated patients showed lower postoperative anxiety and lower incidence of surgical wound infection up to 30 days after surgery compared with those given placebo (Levandovski et al. 2008). In one trial, premedication with alprazolam, 0.5 mg, decreased preoperative anxiety, with no effect on postoperative pain and morphine consumption when compared with placebo (Joseph et al. 2014). Another trial found that 50 mg of clorazepate the evening before surgery prevented increases in anxiety and sympathoadrenal activity (Meybohm et al. 2007). However, a large placebo-controlled trial found that premedication with lorazepam did not improve the self-reported patient experience the day after surgery but was associated with a modest delay in extubation and a lower rate of early cognitive recovery (Maurice-Szamburski et al. 2015). Another trial showed that premedication with midazolam improved hemodynamic stability and analgesia during anesthesia induction, but it was not effective in reducing preoperative anxiety (Jeon et al. 2018).

Alternative medications also have been found to be beneficial in randomized trials, with similar limitations in study setting and design. A recent systematic review concluded that melatonin was superior to placebo and may have effects similar to those of benzodiazepines in lowering preoperative and postoperative anxiety (Madsen et al. 2020). Premedication with 1,200 mg of gabapentin improved preoperative anxiety, postoperative analgesia, and early knee mobilization after arthroscopic knee surgery compared with placebo (Ménigaux et al. 2005); a subsequent study showed that this dose of gabapentin was effective for preoperative anxiolysis without resulting in sedation or preoperative memory impairment (Adam et al. 2012). Preoperative gabapentin may have other benefits, including attenuation of the hemodynamic response to laryngoscopy and intubation and prevention of chronic postsurgical pain, postoperative nausea and vomiting, and delirium (Kong and Irwin 2007). Although another randomized trial found that the similar drug pregabalin (75–300 mg administered orally) increased perioperative sedation, it failed to reduce preoperative state anxiety or postoperative pain or to improve the recovery process after minor elective surgery procedures (White et al. 2009). However, a subsequent trial showed that premedication with pregabalin, 75 mg, significantly reduced preoperative anxiety in adults scheduled for plastic surgery (Cortés-Martínez et al. 2020), and a systematic review concluded that pregabalin, 150 mg, was effective in decreasing anxiety, stabilizing intraoperative hemodynamics, and managing postoperative pain (Torres-González et al. 2020). Finally, in a trial of moderate- and high-risk gynecological surgery patients, Chen et al. (2008) reported that premedication with mirtazapine (30 mg) reduced the level of preoperative anxiety and the risk of postoperative nausea and vomiting.

In summary, benzodiazepines and other agents, including gabapentin, pregabalin, and mirtazapine, have been documented to be beneficial in reducing preoperative anxiety in many but not all trials. Some studies have highlighted potential benefits of managing postoperative anxiety and pain as well. Given the lack of comparative studies, it is difficult to make a definitive recommendation. Therefore, pharmacological treatment should be individualized and combined with behavioral interventions. One systematic review demonstrated the effect of nonpharmacological strategies, as psychological preparation reduced postoperative pain, negative affect, and hospital length of stay by approximately half a day (Powell et al. 2016).

Children and Preoperative Anxiety

Anxiety about impending surgery occurs in up to 60% of children. Preoperative anxiety in children has been associated with several problematic behaviors, both preoperatively (e.g., agitation, crying, enuresis, the need for physical restraint during anesthetic induction) and postoperatively (e.g., pain, sleeping disturbances, parent-child conflict, separation anxiety) (Wright et al. 2007). Various pharmacological interventions have been studied, including benzodiazepines, α_2-receptor agonists, and hydroxyzine, as well as nonpharmacological strategies, including web-based preparation, parental presence during anesthesia induction, and other forms of distraction (Chaudhary et al. 2014; Kumari et al. 2017; Manyande et al. 2015).

As in adults, many medication trials in children have focused on benzodiazepines. In one trial, oral midazolam as premedication for pediatric surgical patients provided faster onset of sedation, more effective anxiolysis, and easier separation from parents and mask acceptance, when compared with oral α_2 agonists dexmedetomidine and clonidine (Kumari et al. 2017). Another study that compared oral midazolam, 0.5 mg/kg, with oral clonidine, 4 μg/kg, and intranasal dexmedetomidine, 2 μg/kg, found that midazolam was more effective in reducing preoperative anxiety in children scheduled for elective surgery (Bromfalk et al. 2021). Of note, alternative routes of administration are more often needed for young children than for older patients (see also Chapter 3). Sublingual midazolam, 0.2 mg/kg, was found to be as efficacious as oral midazolam, 0.5 mg/kg (Kattoh et al. 2008).

With benzodiazepines' potential for causing respiratory depression and confusion in the postoperative period, several trials have explored alternative anxiolytics in children. For example, intranasal dexmedetomidine was found to be more effective than intranasal midazolam (Diwan et al. 2020) and oral midazolam (Linares Segovia et al. 2014) for managing preoperative anxiety in children. The benefits of premedication with dexmedetomidine include significantly decreased heart rate before anesthesia induction, more effective sedation at separation from parents, and decreased postoperative pain in the pediatric population (Peng et al. 2014). Another study highlighted the benefits of intranasal fentanyl versus intranasal midazolam and dexmedetomidine as premedication in preschool children, including easier separation from parents, earlier onset of sedation and anxiolysis, and shorter duration of action (Chatrath et al. 2018).

Additional anxiolytic benefit from dexmedetomidine can be observed in the postoperative period: children who received premedication with intravenous dexmedetomidine had significantly lower levels of anxiety 2 and 4 hours after surgery, compared with their preoperative anxiety levels; in contrast, children who received intravenous midazolam had no statistically significant differences between their preoperative and postoperative anxiety levels (Du et al. 2019). Perioperative gabapentin also has been shown to decrease postoperative anxiety in pediatric surgical patients (Tomaszek et al. 2020).

Although melatonin has shown promise for preoperative anxiety in adults, studies in children have yielded mixed results. In one trial, melatonin was as effective as midazolam in alleviating preoperative anxiety in children and was associated with a tendency toward faster recovery and a lower incidence of agitation and sleep disturbance postoperatively (Samarkandi et al. 2005). Although two subsequent studies found midazolam to be more effective than melatonin (Isik et al. 2008; Kain et al. 2009), use of melatonin alongside nonpharmacological strategies as part of a multimodal approach significantly decreased the incidence of emergence delirium in children compared with those receiving midazolam (Singla et al. 2021).

Although studies have explored the use of benzodiazepines, α_2 agonists, and other agents for pediatric preoperative anxiolysis, there is no definitive conclusion on the most effective agent based on the current literature. Consequently, pharmacological intervention should be tailored to each patient and used along with nonpharmacological strategies such as web-based preparation, parental presence during anesthesia induction, and other forms of distraction.

Adverse Neuropsychiatric Effects of Critical Care and Surgical Drugs

Drugs used in critical care and surgery may have adverse neuropsychiatric effects. These drugs are summarized in Table 15–2 and discussed below.

Nitrous Oxide

Nitrous oxide anesthesia has been associated with reversible and irreversible cognitive impairment and psychotic symptoms; however, the causal nature of these symptoms remains controversial because studies fail to account for multiple concurrent causal factors (Sanders et al. 2008). Potential mechanisms proposed include antagonism of the N-methyl-D-aspartate receptor and disruption of cortical methionine synthase, which may lead to B_{12} and folate deficiency. Women, young patients, and older adults with B_{12} deficiency appear to be most susceptible.

Inhalational Anesthetics and Succinylcholine

Inhalational anesthetics and succinylcholine may cause malignant hyperthermia, which is similar to neuroleptic malignant syndrome (see Chapter 2) in that it is characterized by delirium, autonomic instability, rigidity, and tremor. Antipsychotic medications have not been reported to predispose to this effect. Malignant hyperthermia is treated with dantrolene and supportive care.

Table 15–2.   Psychiatric adverse effects of medications used in critical care and surgery

Medication	Psychiatric adverse effects
Inhalational anesthetics	
Desflurane, enflurane, halothane, isoflurane, methoxyflurane, and sevoflurane	Malignant hyperthermia syndrome: delirium, autonomic instability, muscular rigidity, tremor
Neuromuscular blockers	
Succinylcholine	Malignant hyperthermia syndrome: delirium, autonomic instability, muscular rigidity, tremor
Nitrous oxide	Psychosis, reversible and irreversible cognitive impairment
Sympathomimetic agents	
Dobutamine, dopamine, epinephrine, isoproterenol, and norepinephrine	Fear, anxiety, restlessness, tremor, insomnia, confusion, irritability, mania, psychosis
Vasodilators	
Amrinone, isosorbide, milrinone, nesiritide, nitroglycerin, and nitroprusside	Increased intracranial pressure, syncope
Intravenous sedative and anesthesia induction agents	
Etomidate, midazolam, and propofol	Excessive sedation, respiratory suppression, delirium (especially in combination with sedative-hypnotics and opioid analgesics)
Ketamine	Dissociation, psychosis, blunted affect, emotional withdrawal

Sympathomimetic Amines

Sympathomimetic amines include dopamine, dobutamine, and other drugs. Central effects of these medications include fear, anxiety, restlessness, tremor, insomnia, confusion, irritability, weakness, psychotic states, appetite reduction, nausea, and vomiting.

Vasodilator Hypotensive Agents

Vasodilator hypotensive agents include nitroglycerin and nitroprusside. Increases in intracranial pressure can occur with central vasodilation. In patients whose intracranial pressure is already elevated, sodium nitroprusside should be used only with extreme caution.

Drug-Drug Interactions

Multiple drug-drug interactions are possible because of the use of psychopharmacological agents in the critical care and perisurgical arena (Table 15–3). Most of these potential interactions (e.g., for antibiotics, corticosteroids, analgesics, and cardiovascular medications) are covered in the relevant organ system disease chapters and in Chapter 1, "Pharmacokinetics, Pharmacodynamics, and Principles of Drug-Drug Interactions." The focus in this chapter is on anesthetic agents and intravenously administered agents used in the critical care setting.

Inhalational Anesthetics

Pharmacodynamic effects of inhalational anesthetics (e.g., enflurane, halothane, isoflurane, methoxyflurane, desflurane, sevoflurane) include excessive sedation and respiratory suppression with sedating psychotropic drugs (sedative-hypnotics, barbiturates, drugs with antihistaminergic properties) and hypotensive effects with α_1-blocking psychotropics (e.g., TCAs, MAOIs, antipsychotics). Halothane in combination with sympathomimetic psychotropic drugs (e.g., norepinephrine reuptake inhibitors [NRIs], serotonin-norepinephrine reuptake inhibitors [SNRIs], TCAs, psychostimulants) may cause arrhythmias secondary to halothane-induced myocardial sensitization to these agents. The mechanisms of neuroleptic malignant syndrome (see Chapter 2) and malignant hyperthermia are thought to be divergent, and there are no reports of antipsychotic treatment increasing the risk of malignant hyperthermia postoperatively.

Table 15–3. Critical care and perioperative medication–psychotropic medication interactions

Medication	Interaction mechanism	Effects on psychotropic medications and management
Inhalational anesthetics		
Desflurane, enflurane, halothane, isoflurane, methoxyflurane, and sevoflurane	Additive sedation	Increased sedation with sedative-hypnotics and antihistaminic psychotropics (TCAs, antipsychotics)
	Additive hypotensive effect	Increased risk of hypotension with drugs that block α_1-adrenergic receptors (e.g., TCAs, MAOIs, typical and atypical antipsychotics)
	Halothane: sensitization of myocardium	Arrhythmias with sympathomimetic psychotropics (NRIs, SNRIs, TCAs, psychostimulants)
Nitrous oxide	Activation of supraspinal $GABA_A$ receptors	Sedative-hypnotics and propofol may block anesthetic activity of nitrous oxide.
	Potentiation of noradrenergic mechanisms	Additive analgesia with noradrenergic agents (SNRIs, NRIs, TCAs)
Nondepolarizing neuromuscular blocking agents		
Pancuronium and tubocurarine	Reversal of antinicotinic neuromuscular blockade	Cholinesterase inhibitors antagonize anesthesia because of these agents and should be stopped 2 weeks before surgery.
	Unknown mechanism	Lithium and carbamazepine have been found to both potentiate and inhibit neuromuscular blockade.

Table 15–3. Critical care and perioperative medication–psychotropic medication interactions (continued)

Medication	Interaction mechanism	Effects on psychotropic medications and management
Depolarizing neuromuscular blocking agents		
Suxamethonium (succinylcholine)	Increasing acetylcholine-mediated neuromuscular depolarization	Cholinesterase inhibitors may increase the duration of action of these agents.
	Blockade of depolarization	Psychotropics with anticholinergic properties (trihexyphenidyl, benztropine, TCAs, antipsychotics) may antagonize depolarization and reduce effectiveness.
Sedative-hypnotic induction agents		
Etomidate, midazolam, and propofol	Additive sedation	Increased sedation with sedative-hypnotics and antihistaminic psychotropics (TCAs, antipsychotics).
α_2-Adrenergic sedatives		
Dexmedetomidine	Additive sedation	Increased sedation with sedative-hypnotics and antihistaminic psychotropics (TCAs, antipsychotics)
	Inhibition of CYP2D6	May inhibit the metabolism of psychotropics metabolized by this isozyme (e.g., TCAs, mirtazapine, venlafaxine, risperidone, opioids, atomoxetine) if given chronically (see Chapter 1), but there are no apparent interactions with short-term use.

Table 15–3. Critical care and perioperative medication–psychotropic medication interactions *(continued)*

Medication	Interaction mechanism	Effects on psychotropic medications and management
α_2-Adrenergic sedatives *(continued)*		
Ketamine	Substrate of CYP2B6 (major), CYP2C9 (minor), CYP3A4 (major)	May increase the effect of CNS depressants. CYP3A4 inhibitors may increase the serum concentration of ketamine.
Sympathomimetic inotropic and pressor agents		
Dopamine, epinephrine, isoproterenol, and norepinephrine	Monoamine oxidase inhibition	Treatment with MAOIs 2–3 weeks before initiation of these agents may augment hypertensive effects and cause hypertensive crisis.
	Reversal of pressor effect	Risk of severe hypotension with coadministration of agents with β_2 agonist activity (epinephrine, isoproterenol) and drugs that block α_1-adrenergic receptors (e.g., TCAs, typical and atypical antipsychotics). Norepinephrine should be used as a pressor agent in this situation.
	Additive noradrenergic effects	With dopaminergic and noradrenergic psychotropics (e.g., bupropion, atomoxetine, duloxetine, TCAs), augmentation of hypertensive effects and CNS activation.
Dobutamine	Hypokalemia	Increased risk of cardiac arrhythmias with QT-prolonging agents, including TCAs, typical antipsychotics, pimozide, risperidone, paliperidone, iloperidone, quetiapine, ziprasidone, and lithium.

Table 15–3. Critical care and perioperative medication–psychotropic medication interactions *(continued)*

Medication	Interaction mechanism	Effects on psychotropic medications and management
Vasodilators		
Amrinone, isosorbide, milrinone, nesiritide, nitroglycerin, and nitroprusside	Additive hypotensive effects	Augmentation of hypotensive effects when combined with drugs that block α_1-adrenergic receptors (e.g., TCAs, MAOIs, typical and atypical antipsychotics) or with phosphodiesterase type 5 inhibitors.

Note. CYP=cytochrome P450; MAOIs=monoamine oxidase inhibitors; NRIs=norepinephrine reuptake inhibitors; SNRIs=serotonin-norepinephrine reuptake inhibitors; TCAs=tricyclic antidepressants.

Nitrous Oxide

The analgesic action of nitrous oxide is partially dependent on both the inhibition of supraspinal $GABA_A$ receptors and the activation of spinal $GABA_A$ receptors. Agents that activate the supraspinal $GABA_A$ receptor, such as midazolam and propofol, may interfere with nitrous oxide analgesia by inhibiting the activation of the descending inhibitory neurons (Sanders et al. 2008). Noradrenergic agents (e.g., TCAs, SNRIs, NRIs) and opioids may potentiate analgesia due to nitrous oxide via its activation of locus coeruleus and opioidergic neurons.

Nondepolarizing Neuromuscular Blocking Agents

Nondepolarizing neuromuscular blocking agents (e.g., tubocurarine, pancuronium) act by competitive inhibition at nicotinic cholinergic receptors, producing paralysis. Cholinesterase inhibitors may antagonize this type of neuromuscular blockade and, in fact, are used to reverse it. Cholinesterase inhibitors should be discontinued several weeks before surgery involving neuromuscular blocking agents (Russell 2009). Lithium and carbamazepine may both potentiate and inhibit neuromuscular blockade by these agents (Melton et al. 1993; Ostergaard et al. 1989).

Depolarizing Neuromuscular Blocking Agents

In contrast to the nondepolarizing agents, succinylcholine (suxamethonium) has acetylcholine-like actions; cholinesterase inhibitors prolong the duration of action of succinylcholine by inhibiting its plasma cholinesterase-mediated metabolism and increasing acetylcholine-mediated neuromuscular depolarization. Anticholinergic drugs may antagonize succinylcholine effects.

Sedative-Hypnotic Induction and Continuous Sedation Agents

Coadministration of sedative-hypnotic induction and continuous sedation agents (propofol, midazolam, etomidate) with CNS depressant psychotropics, including benzodiazepines, nonbenzodiazepine hypnotics, and antihistaminic drugs, may synergistically result in excessive sedation and respiratory suppression.

Dexmedetomidine

Because dexmedetomidine is a substrate and inhibitor of CYP2D6, pharmacokinetic interactions with some psychotropics might be expected, especially with prolonged infusion of this agent (see Chapter 1 for a listing of CYP2D6-interacting psychotropic drugs) (Karol and Maze 2000). With short-term use, dexmedetomidine does not appear to have pharmacokinetic interactions. Dosage modifications of some concomitant medications (e.g., some anesthetics, sedatives, hypnotics, antihistaminic medications, opioids) may be needed primarily because of common pharmacodynamic actions of the two drugs.

Sympathomimetic Agents

Sympathomimetic agents (e.g., dopamine, dobutamine, epinephrine, norepinephrine, isoproterenol) are often used for vasoconstriction, bronchodilation, combination with local anesthetics, and treatment of hypersensitizing reactions. Concurrent use of MAOIs (including tranylcypromine, phenelzine, moclobemide, and selegiline) with sympathomimetic agents may prolong and intensify cardiac stimulation and vasopressor effects because of increased release of catecholamines, which accumulate in intraneuronal storage sites during MAOI therapy. This interaction may result in headache, cardiac arrhythmias, vomiting, or sudden and severe hypertensive or hyperpyretic crises. For patients who have been receiving MAOIs within 3 weeks before administration of sympathomimetic agents, the initial dosage of dopamine should be reduced to no more than one-tenth of the usual dosage. It should also be noted that linezolid, a commonly used antibiotic in the ICU setting, is also an MAOI, and the patient's medication regimen should be considered accordingly to minimize exposure to sympathetic amines (Quinn and Stern 2009) (see also Chapter 12, "Infectious Diseases").

Dopamine may interact pharmacodynamically with noradrenergic agents, such as TCAs, NRIs, SNRIs, and psychostimulants, to cause a marked increase in heart rate and/or blood pressure. Patients with preexisting hypertension may have increased risk of an exaggerated pressor response with these drugs. Dobutamine may cause hypokalemia, so administration of this drug with QTc-prolonging psychotropic drugs requires close cardiac and serum potassium monitoring. Unlike dopamine, dobutamine does not appear to be an MAO substrate (Yan et al. 2002); however, absent substantial clinical data, caution is warranted when combining dobutamine with irreversible MAOIs.

Vasodilators

The principal pharmacological action of vasodilators (isosorbide dinitrate and mononitrate, nitroglycerin, nitroprusside, milrinone, amrinone, nesiritide) is relaxation of vascular smooth muscle and consequent dilation of peripheral arteries and veins. Excessive hypotension may result through additive effects when vasodilators are used with psychotropics with α_1-antagonist properties, such as TCAs, MAOIs, and phenothiazines; atypical antipsychotics; and phosphodiesterase type 5 inhibitors, such as sildenafil, vardenafil, and tadalafil.

Key Points

- Delirium prevention and treatment require early assessment of patients at risk, identification and treatment of underlying causes, implementation of environmental interventions, and use of psychopharmacology to target agitation, hallucinations, and sleep-wake disruptions.

- For the prevention of delirium, a few randomized controlled trials (RCTs) in select patient populations undergoing surgery support the efficacy of olanzapine and dexmedetomidine in reducing the incidence of delirium and haloperidol in reducing the severity and duration of delirium.

- For the treatment of delirium not due to sedative or alcohol withdrawal, large double-blind RCTs have not shown significant benefit from antipsychotics, donepezil, or cholinesterase inhibitors. The Society of Critical Care Medicine does not support the use of antipsychotics in the treatment of delirium.

- If antipsychotics are needed to treat specific symptoms of delirium that threaten the safety of the patient or others, the minimum necessary dosage should be used, and the medication should be discontinued at the earliest feasible time. Generally, patients should not continue antipsychotics after hospital discharge unless targeting specific residual psychotic symptoms.

- Currently, the multimodal behavioral ABCDEF bundle is the gold standard for prevention and treatment of delirium among critically ill patients. Those providing psychiatric consultation to critically ill patients may advocate for adoption of the ABCDEF bundle and may highlight elements of the bundle that can be adopted in a piecemeal fashion (e.g., early and progressive mobilization, minimization of sedation, family involvement).

- The decision to continue or stop a psychotropic drug in the perioperative period should be individualized, with consideration of the extent of surgery, the patient's medical condition, the choice of anesthetic agents, the length of preoperative fasting, and the risks of drug discontinuation.

- The greatest perioperative risk exists with lithium, monoamine oxidase inhibitors, tricyclic antidepressants, and clozapine.

- For preoperative anxiety in adults and children, benzodiazepines are the most widely used agents; however, other agents such as gabapentin and α-adrenergic antagonists such as clonidine and dexmedetomidine may be viable alternatives.

- For PTSD secondary to illness or injury, evidence from small RCTs suggests efficacy of stress doses of hydrocortisone in reducing PTSD symptoms after cardiac surgery and septic shock. Evidence for other agents, such as propranolol, intraoperative ketamine, and opioid analgesics, is scant and inconclusive.

- In the critical care setting, psychotropic drugs should be prescribed with caution given the significant potential for pharmacodynamic and pharmacokinetic interactions with anesthetics and other agents.

References

Abdallah CG, Roache JD, Gueorguieva R, et al: Dose-related effects of ketamine for antidepressant-resistant symptoms of posttraumatic stress disorder in veterans and active duty military: a double-blind, randomized, placebo-controlled multicenter clinical trial. Neuropsychopharmacology 47(8):1574–1581, 2022 35046508

Adam F, Bordenave L, Sessler DI, et al: Effects of a single 1200-mg preoperative dose of gabapentin on anxiety and memory. Ann Fr Anesth Reanim 31(10):e223–e227, 2012 22770920

Agar MR, Lawlor PG, Quinn S, et al: Efficacy of oral risperidone, haloperidol, or placebo for symptoms of delirium among patients in palliative care: a randomized clinical trial. JAMA Intern Med 177(1):34–42, 2017 27918778

Al-Khatib SM, LaPointe NM, Kramer JM, et al: What clinicians should know about the QT interval [Erratum in: JAMA 290(10):1318, 2003]. JAMA 289(16):2120–2127, 2003 12709470

Al-Qadheeb NS, Skrobik Y, Schumaker G, et al: Preventing ICU subsyndromal delirium conversion to delirium with low-dose IV haloperidol: a double-blind, placebo-controlled pilot study. Crit Care Med 44(3):583–591, 2016 26540397

American Psychiatric Association: Diagnostic and Statistical Manual of Mental Disorders, 5th Edition. Arlington, VA, American Psychiatric Association, 2013

Amos T, Stein DJ, Ipser JC: Pharmacological interventions for preventing posttraumatic stress disorder (PTSD). Cochrane Database Syst Rev (7):CD006239, 2014 25001071

Baller EB, Hogan CS, Fusunyan MA, et al: Neurocovid: pharmacological recommendations for delirium associated with COVID-19. Psychosomatics 61(6):585–596, 2020 32828569

Beach SR, Celano CM, Noseworthy PA, et al: QTc prolongation, torsades de pointes, and psychotropic medications. Psychosomatics 54(1):1–13, 2013 23295003

Bienvenu OJ, Gellar J, Althouse BM, et al: Post-traumatic stress disorder symptoms after acute lung injury: a 2-year prospective longitudinal study. Psychol Med 43(12):2657–2671, 2013 23438256

Bodro M, Compta Y, Sánchez-Valle R: Presentations and mechanisms of CNS disorders related to COVID-19. Neurol Neuroimmunol Neuroinflamm 8(1):e923, 2020 33310765

Breitbart W, Marotta R, Platt MM, et al: A double-blind trial of haloperidol, chlorpromazine, and lorazepam in the treatment of delirium in hospitalized AIDS patients. Am J Psychiatry 153(2):231–237, 1996 8561204

Bromfalk Å, Myrberg T, Walldén J, et al: Preoperative anxiety in preschool children: a randomized clinical trial comparing midazolam, clonidine, and dexmedetomidine. Paediatr Anaesth 31(11):1225–1233, 2021 34403548

Bryant RA, Creamer M, O'Donnell M, et al: A study of the protective function of acute morphine administration on subsequent posttraumatic stress disorder. Biol Psychiatry 65(5):438–440, 2009 19058787

Burki TK: Post-traumatic stress in the intensive care unit. Lancet Respir Med 7(10):843–844, 2019 31204253

Chatrath V, Kumar R, Sachdeva U, et al: Intranasal fentanyl, midazolam and dexmedetomidine as premedication in pediatric patients. Anesth Essays Res 12(3):748–753, 2018 30283188

Chaudhary S, Jindal R, Girotra G, et al: Is midazolam superior to triclofos and hydroxyzine as premedicant in children? J Anaesthesiol Clin Pharmacol 30(1):53–58, 2014 24574594

Chen CC, Lin CS, Ko YP, et al: Premedication with mirtazapine reduces preoperative anxiety and postoperative nausea and vomiting. Anesth Analg 106(1):109–113, 2008 18165563

Collinsworth AW, Priest EL, Campbell CR, et al: A review of multifaceted care approaches for the prevention and mitigation of delirium in intensive care units. J Intensive Care Med 31(2):127–141, 2016 25348864

Cortés-Martínez LA, Cardoso-García LE, Galván-Talamantes Y, et al: Pregabalin as a premedication for anxiety in patients undergoing plastic surgery: randomized double-blind, placebo-controlled study. Cir Cir 88(5):548–553, 2020 33064711

Crawford GB, Agar MM, Quinn SJ, et al: Pharmacovigilance in hospice/palliative care: net effect of haloperidol for delirium. J Palliat Med 16(11):1335–1341, 2013 24138282

Davydow DS, Zatzick D, Hough CL, et al: In-hospital acute stress symptoms are associated with impairment in cognition 1 year after intensive care unit admission. Ann Am Thorac Soc 10(5):450–457, 2013 23987665

Desai SV, Law TJ, Needham DM: Long-term complications of critical care. Crit Care Med 39(2):371–379, 2011 20959786

Devlin JW, Roberts RJ, Fong JJ, et al: Efficacy and safety of quetiapine in critically ill patients with delirium: a prospective, multicenter, randomized, double-blind, placebo-controlled pilot study. Crit Care Med 38(2):419–427, 2010 19915454

Devlin JW, Skrobik Y, Gélinas C, et al: Executive summary: clinical practice guidelines for the prevention and management of pain, agitation/sedation, delirium, immobility, and sleep disruption in adult patients in the ICU. Crit Care Med 46(9):1532–1548, 2018 30113371

Diwan G, Bharti AK, Rastogi K, et al: Comparison of intranasal dexmedetomidine and midazolam as premedication in pediatric surgical patients: a prospective, randomized double-blind study. Anesth Essays Res 14(3):384–389, 2020 34092846

Du Z, Zhang XY, Qu SQ, et al: The comparison of dexmedetomidine and midazolam premedication on postoperative anxiety in children for hernia repair surgery: a randomized controlled trial. Paediatr Anaesth 29(8):843–849, 2019 31125470

Ely EW, Shintani A, Truman B, et al: Delirium as a predictor of mortality in mechanically ventilated patients in the intensive care unit. JAMA 291(14):1753–1762, 2004 15082703

Feder A, Parides MK, Murrough JW, et al: Efficacy of intravenous ketamine for treatment of chronic posttraumatic stress disorder: a randomized clinical trial. JAMA Psychiatry 71(6):681–688, 2014 24740528

Flükiger J, Hollinger A, Speich B, et al: Dexmedetomidine in prevention and treatment of postoperative and intensive care unit delirium: a systematic review and meta-analysis. Ann Intensive Care 8(1):92, 2018 30238227

Fontaine GV, Mortensen W, Guinto KM, et al: Newly initiated in-hospital antipsychotics continued at discharge in non-psychiatric patients. Hosp Pharm 53(5):308–315, 2018 30210148

Funk MC, Beach SR, Bostwick JR, et al: QTc prolongation and psychotropic medications. Am J Psychiatry 177(3):273–274, 2020 32114782

Garrouste-Orgeas M, Flahault C, Vinatier I, et al: Effect of an ICU diary on posttraumatic stress disorder symptoms among patients receiving mechanical ventilation: a randomized clinical trial. JAMA 322(3):229–239, 2019 31310299

Gertler R, Brown HC, Mitchell DH, et al: Dexmedetomidine: a novel sedative-analgesic agent. Proc (Bayl Univ Med Cent) 14(1):13–21, 2001 16369581

Girard TD, Pandharipande PP, Carson SS, et al: Feasibility, efficacy, and safety of antipsychotics for intensive care unit delirium: the MIND randomized, placebo-controlled trial. Crit Care Med 38(2):428–437, 2010 20095068

Girard TD, Exline MC, Carson SS, et al: Haloperidol and ziprasidone for treatment of delirium in critical illness. N Engl J Med 379(26):2506–2516, 2018 30346242

Grover S, Kumar V, Chakrabarti S: Comparative efficacy study of haloperidol, olanzapine and risperidone in delirium. J Psychosom Res 71(4):277–281, 2011 21911107

Hakim SM, Othman AI, Naoum DO: Early treatment with risperidone for subsyndromal delirium after on-pump cardiac surgery in the elderly: a randomized trial. Anesthesiology 116(5):987–997, 2012 22436797

Han CS, Kim YK: A double-blind trial of risperidone and haloperidol for the treatment of delirium. Psychosomatics 45(4):297–301, 2004 15232043

Harbell MW, Dumitrascu C, Bettini L, et al: Anesthetic considerations for patients on psychotropic drug therapies. Neurol Int 13(4):640–658, 2021 34940748

Harrison TK, Kornfeld H, Aggarwal AK, et al: Perioperative considerations for the patient with opioid use disorder on buprenorphine, methadone, or naltrexone maintenance therapy. Anesthesiol Clin 36(3):345–359, 2018 30092933

Henssler J, Heinz A, Brandt L, et al: Antidepressant withdrawal and rebound phenomena. Dtsch Arztebl Int 116(20):355–361, 2019 31288917

Hızlı Sayar G, Eryılmaz G, Semieoğlu S, et al: Influence of valproate on the required dose of propofol for anesthesia during electroconvulsive therapy of bipolar affective disorder patients. Neuropsychiatr Dis Treat 10:433–438, 2014 24623978

Hshieh TT, Yue J, Oh E, et al: Effectiveness of multicomponent nonpharmacological delirium interventions: a meta-analysis. JAMA Intern Med 175(4):512–520, 2015 25643002

Hu H, Deng W, Yang H, et al: A prospective random control study: comparison of olanzapine and haloperidol in senile delirium. Chongqing Medical Journal 8:1234–1237, 2004

Huyse FJ, Touw DJ, van Schijndel RS, et al: Psychotropic drugs and the perioperative period: a proposal for a guideline in elective surgery. Psychosomatics 47(1):8–22, 2006 16384803

Isik B, Baygin O, Bodur H: Premedication with melatonin vs midazolam in anxious children. Paediatr Anaesth 18(7):635–641, 2008 18616492

Jackson JC, Pandharipande PP, Girard TD, et al: Depression, post-traumatic stress disorder, and functional disability in survivors of critical illness in the BRAIN-ICU study: a longitudinal cohort study. Lancet Respir Med 2(5):369–379, 2014 24815803

Jeon S, Lee HJ, Do W, et al: Randomized controlled trial assessing the effectiveness of midazolam premedication as an anxiolytic, analgesic, sedative, and hemodynamic stabilizer. Medicine (Baltimore) 97(35):e12187, 2018 30170468

Joseph TT, Krishna HM, Kamath S: Premedication with gabapentin, alprazolam or a placebo for abdominal hysterectomy: effect on pre-operative anxiety, post-operative pain and morphine consumption. Indian J Anaesth 58(6):693–699, 2014 25624531

Kain ZN, MacLaren JE, Herrmann L, et al: Preoperative melatonin and its effects on induction and emergence in children undergoing anesthesia and surgery. Anesthesiology 111(1):44–49, 2009 19546692

Kalisvaart KJ, de Jonghe JF, Bogaards MJ, et al: Haloperidol prophylaxis for elderly hip-surgery patients at risk for delirium: a randomized placebo-controlled study. J Am Geriatr Soc 53(10):1658–1666, 2005 16181163

Karol MD, Maze M: Pharmacokinetics and interaction pharmacodynamics of dexmedetomidine in humans. Baillieres Clin Anaesthesiol 14:261–269, 2000

Kattoh T, Katome K, Makino S, et al: Comparative study of sublingual midazolam with oral midazolam for premedication in pediatric anesthesia [in Japanese]. Masui 57(10):1227–1232, 2008 18975537

Kong VK, Irwin MG: Gabapentin: a multimodal perioperative drug? Br J Anaesth 99(6):775–786, 2007 18006529

Kudoh A, Takase H, Takazawa T: Chronic treatment with antipsychotics enhances intraoperative core hypothermia. Anesth Analg 98(1):111–115, 2004 14693598

Kumari S, Agrawal N, Usha G, et al: Comparison of oral clonidine, oral dexmedetomidine, and oral midazolam for premedication in pediatric patients undergoing elective surgery. Anesth Essays Res 11(1):185–191, 2017 28298782

Laporte S, Chapelle C, Caillet P, et al: Bleeding risk under selective serotonin reuptake inhibitor (SSRI) antidepressants: a meta-analysis of observational studies. Pharmacol Res 118:19–32, 2017 27521835

Larsen KA, Kelly SE, Stern TA, et al: Administration of olanzapine to prevent postoperative delirium in elderly joint-replacement patients: a randomized, controlled trial. Psychosomatics 51(5):409–418, 2010 20833940

Levandovski R, Ferreira MB, Hidalgo MP, et al: Impact of preoperative anxiolytic on surgical site infection in patients undergoing abdominal hysterectomy. Am J Infect Control 36(10):718–726, 2008 18834731

Li B, Wang H, Wu H, Gao C: Neurocognitive dysfunction risk alleviation with the use of dexmedetomidine in perioperative conditions or as ICU sedation: a meta-analysis. Medicine (Baltimore) 94(14):e597, 2015 25860207

Linares Segovia B, García Cuevas MA, Ramírez Casillas IL, et al: Pre-anesthetic medication with intranasal dexmedetomidine and oral midazolam as an anxiolytic: a clinical trial [in Spanish]. An Pediatr (Barc) 81(4):226–231, 2014 24472331

Liptzin B, Laki A, Garb JL, et al: Donepezil in the prevention and treatment of postsurgical delirium. Am J Geriatr Psychiatry 13(12):1100–1106, 2005 16319303

Madsen BK, Zetner D, Møller AM, et al: Melatonin for preoperative and postoperative anxiety in adults. Cochrane Database Syst Rev 12(12):CD009861, 2020 33319916

Mahdanian AA, Rej S, Bacon SL, et al: Serotonergic antidepressants and perioperative bleeding risk: a systematic review. Expert Opin Drug Saf 13(6):695–704, 2014 24717049

Maldonado JR, Wysong A, van der Starre PJ, et al: Dexmedetomidine and the reduction of postoperative delirium after cardiac surgery. Psychosomatics 50(3):206–217, 2009 19567759

Maneeton B, Maneeton N, Srisurapanont M, et al: Quetiapine versus haloperidol in the treatment of delirium: a double-blind, randomized, controlled trial. Drug Des Devel Ther 7(7):657–667, 2013 23926422

Manyande A, Cyna AM, Yip P, et al: Non-pharmacological interventions for assisting the induction of anaesthesia in children. Cochrane Database Syst Rev 2015(7):CD006447, 2015 26171895

Marcantonio ER, Palihnich K, Appleton P, et al: Pilot randomized trial of donepezil hydrochloride for delirium after hip fracture. J Am Geriatr Soc 59(Suppl 2):S282–S288, 2011 22091574

Marra A, Ely EW, Pandharipande PP, et al: The ABCDEF bundle in critical care. Crit Care Clin 33(2):225–243, 2017 28284292

Maurice-Szamburski A, Auquier P, Viarre-Oreal V, et al: Effect of sedative premedication on patient experience after general anesthesia: a randomized clinical trial. JAMA 313(9):916–925, 2015 25734733

McGhee LL, Maani CV, Garza TH, et al: The correlation between ketamine and posttraumatic stress disorder in burned service members. J Trauma 64(2 Suppl):S195–S198, discussion S197–S198, 2008 18376165

McGhee LL, Maani CV, Garza TH, et al: The effect of propranolol on posttraumatic stress disorder in burned service members. J Burn Care Res 30(1):92–97, 2009a 19060728

McGhee LL, Maani CV, Garza TH, et al: The relationship of intravenous midazolam and posttraumatic stress disorder development in burned soldiers. J Trauma 66(4 Suppl):S186–S190, 2009b 19359964

Melton AT, Antognini JF, Gronert GA: Prolonged duration of succinylcholine in patients receiving anticonvulsants: evidence for mild up-regulation of acetylcholine receptors? Can J Anaesth 40(10):939–942, 1993 8222033

Ménigaux C, Adam F, Guignard B, et al: Preoperative gabapentin decreases anxiety and improves early functional recovery from knee surgery. Anesth Analg 100(5):1394–1399, 2005 15845693

Meybohm P, Hanss R, Bein B, et al: Comparison of premedication regimes: a randomized, controlled trial [in German]. Anaesthesist 56(9):890–892, 2007 17551699

Mokhtari M, Farasatinasab M, Jafarpour Machian M, et al: Aripiprazole for prevention of delirium in the neurosurgical intensive care unit: a double-blind, randomized, placebo-controlled study. Eur J Clin Pharmacol 76(4):491–499, 2020 31900543

Moore PW, Rasimas JJ, Donovan JW: Physostigmine is the antidote for anticholinergic syndrome. J Med Toxicol 11(1):159–160, 2015 25339374

Moore TJ, Mattison DR: Adult utilization of psychiatric drugs and differences by sex, age, and race. JAMA Intern Med 177(2):274–275, 2017 27942726

Noble DW, Kehlet H: Risks of interrupting drug treatment before surgery. BMJ 321(7263):719–720, 2000 10999886

Oldham MA, Lee HB: Catatonia vis-à-vis delirium: the significance of recognizing catatonia in altered mental status. Gen Hosp Psychiatry 37(6):554–559, 2015 26162545

Oprea AD, Keshock MC, O'Glasser AY, et al: Preoperative management of medications for psychiatric diseases: Society for Perioperative Assessment and Quality Improvement consensus statement. Mayo Clin Proc 97(2):397–416, 2022 35120702

Ostergaard D, Engbaek J, Viby-Mogensen J: Adverse reactions and interactions of the neuromuscular blocking drugs. Med Toxicol 4(5):351–368, 1989 2682131

Page VJ, Ely EW, Gates S, et al: Effect of intravenous haloperidol on the duration of delirium and coma in critically ill patients (Hope-ICU): a randomised, double-blind, placebo-controlled trial. Lancet Respir Med 1(7):515–523, 2013 24461612

Payne LE, Gagnon DJ, Riker RR, et al: Cefepime-induced neurotoxicity: a systematic review. Crit Care 21(1):276, 2017 29137682

Pekcan M, Celebioglu B, Demir B, et al: The effect of premedication on preoperative anxiety. Middle East J Anaesthesiol 18(2):421–433, 2005 16438017

Peng K, Wu SR, Ji FH, Li J: Premedication with dexmedetomidine in pediatric patients: a systematic review and meta-analysis. Clinics (Sao Paulo) 69(11):777–786, 2014 25518037

Powell R, Scott NW, Manyande A, et al: Psychological preparation and postoperative outcomes for adults undergoing surgery under general anaesthesia. Cochrane Database Syst Rev 2016(5):CD008646, 2016 27228096

Prakanrattana U, Prapaitrakool S: Efficacy of risperidone for prevention of postoperative delirium in cardiac surgery. Anaesth Intensive Care 35(5):714–719, 2007 17933157

Pun BT, Balas MC, Barnes-Daly MA, et al: Caring for critically ill patients with the ABCDEF bundle: results of the ICU Liberation Collaborative in over 15,000 adults. Crit Care Med 47(1):3–14, 2019 30339549

Quinn DK, Stern TA: Linezolid and serotonin syndrome. Prim Care Companion J Clin Psychiatry 11(6):353–356, 2009 20098528

Ragheb J, McKinney A, Zierau M, et al: Delirium and neuropsychological outcomes in critically ill patients with COVID-19: a cohort study. BMJ Open 11(9):e050045, 2021 34535480

Rahmat S, Velez J, Farooqi M, et al: Post-traumatic stress disorder can be predicted in hospitalized blunt trauma patients using a simple screening tool. Trauma Surg Acute Care Open 6(1):e000623, 2021 33880413

Rawal G, Yadav S, Kumar R: Post-intensive care syndrome: an overview. J Transl Int Med 5(2):90–92, 2017 28721340

Reade MC, O'Sullivan K, Bates S, et al: Dexmedetomidine vs. haloperidol in delirious, agitated, intubated patients: a randomised open-label trial. Crit Care 13(3):R75, 2009 19454032

Reade MC, Eastwood GM, Bellomo R, et al: Effect of dexmedetomidine added to standard care on ventilator-free time in patients with agitated delirium: a randomized clinical trial. JAMA 315(14):1460–1468, 2016 26975647

Russell WJ: The impact of Alzheimer's disease medication on muscle relaxants. Anaesth Intensive Care 37(1):134–135, 2009 19160552

Salluh JI, Wang H, Schneider EB, et al: Outcome of delirium in critically ill patients: systematic review and meta-analysis. BMJ 350:h2538, 2015 26041151

Samarkandi A, Naguib M, Riad W, et al: Melatonin vs. midazolam premedication in children: a double-blind, placebo-controlled study. Eur J Anaesthesiol 22(3):189–196, 2005 15852991

Sampson EL, Raven PR, Ndhlovu PN, et al: A randomized, double-blind, placebo-controlled trial of donepezil hydrochloride (Aricept) for reducing the incidence of postoperative delirium after elective total hip replacement. Int J Geriatr Psychiatry 22(4):343–349, 2007 17006875

Sanders RD, Weimann J, Maze M: Biologic effects of nitrous oxide: a mechanistic and toxicologic review. Anesthesiology 109(4):707–722, 2008 18813051

Schellhorn SE, Barnhill JW, Raiteri V, et al: A comparison of psychiatric consultation between geriatric and non-geriatric medical inpatients. Int J Geriatr Psychiatry 24(10):1054–1061, 2009 19326400

Scher CS, Anwar M: The self-reporting of psychiatric medications in patients scheduled for elective surgery. J Clin Anesth 11(8):619–621, 1999 10680101

Schofield-Robinson OJ, Lewis SR, Smith AF, et al: Follow-up services for improving long-term outcomes in intensive care unit (ICU) survivors. Cochrane Database Syst Rev 11(11):CD012701, 2018 30388297

Schönenberg M, Reichwald U, Domes G, et al: Ketamine aggravates symptoms of acute stress disorder in a naturalistic sample of accident victims. J Psychopharmacol 22(5):493–497, 2008 18208917

Schröder Pedersen S, Kirkegaard T, Balslev Jørgensen M, et al: Effects of a screening and treatment protocol with haloperidol on post-cardiotomy delirium: a prospective cohort study. Interact Cardiovasc Thorac Surg 18(4):438–445, 2014 24357472

Serafim RB, Bozza FA, Soares M, et al: Pharmacologic prevention and treatment of delirium in intensive care patients: a systematic review. J Crit Care 30(4):799–807, 2015 25957498

Sharma ND, Rosman HS, Padhi ID, et al: Torsades de pointes associated with intravenous haloperidol in critically ill patients. Am J Cardiol 81(2):238–240, 1998 9591913

Shen QH, Li HF, Zhou XY, et al: Dexmedetomidine in the prevention of postoperative delirium in elderly patients following non-cardiac surgery: a systematic review and meta-analysis. Clin Exp Pharmacol Physiol 47(8):1333–1341, 2020 32215933

Singla L, Mathew PJ, Jain A, et al: Oral melatonin as part of multimodal anxiolysis decreases emergence delirium in children whereas midazolam does not: a randomised, double-blind, placebo-controlled study. Eur J Anaesthesiol 38(11):1130–1137, 2021 34175857

Skrobik YK, Bergeron N, Dumont M, et al: Olanzapine vs haloperidol: treating delirium in a critical care setting. Intensive Care Med 30(3):444–449, 2004 14685663

Skrobik Y, Duprey MS, Hill NS, et al: Low-dose nocturnal dexmedetomidine prevents ICU delirium: a randomized, placebo-controlled trial. Am J Respir Crit Care Med 197(9):1147–1156, 2018 29498534

Smith MS, Muir H, Hall R: Perioperative management of drug therapy, clinical considerations. Drugs 51(2):238–259, 1996 8808166

Smith S, Rahman O: Post intensive care syndrome. StatPearls, 2022. Available at: http://www.ncbi.nlm.nih.gov/books/NBK558964. Accessed October 5, 2022.

Stein MB, Kerridge C, Dimsdale JE, et al: Pharmacotherapy to prevent PTSD: results from a randomized controlled proof-of-concept trial in physically injured patients. J Trauma Stress 20(6):923–932, 2007 18157888

Tahir TA, Eeles E, Karapareddy V, et al: A randomized controlled trial of quetiapine versus placebo in the treatment of delirium. J Psychosom Res 69(5):485–490, 2010 20955868

Thom RP, Levy-Carrick NC, Bui M, et al: Delirium. Am J Psychiatry 176(10):785–793, 2019 31569986

Tomaszek L, Fenikowski D, Maciejewski P, et al: Perioperative gabapentin in pediatric thoracic surgery patients—randomized, placebo-controlled, phase 4 trial. Pain Med 21(8):1562–1571, 2020 31596461

Torres-González MI, Manzano-Moreno FJ, Vallecillo-Capilla MF, et al: Preoperative oral pregabalin for anxiety control: a systematic review. Clin Oral Investig 24(7):2219–2228, 2020 32468485

Trzepacz PT: Is there a final common neural pathway in delirium? Focus on acetylcholine and dopamine. Semin Clin Neuropsychiatry 5(2):132–148, 2000 10837102

U.S. Food and Drug Administration: Information for healthcare professionals: haloperidol (marketed as Haldol, Haldol Decanoate, and Haldol Lactate). 2007. Available at: https://www.fda.gov/drugs/postmarket-drug-safety-information-patients-and-providers/haloperidol-marketed-haldol-haldol-decanoate-and-haldol-lactate-information. Accessed April 28, 2016.

van Eijk MM, Roes KC, Honing ML, et al: Effect of rivastigmine as an adjunct to usual care with haloperidol on duration of delirium and mortality in critically ill patients: a multicentre, double-blind, placebo-controlled randomised trial. Lancet 376(9755):1829–1837, 2010 21056464

Walker KJ, Smith AF: Premedication for anxiety in adult day surgery. Cochrane Database Syst Rev (4):CD002192, 2009 19821294

Wang W, Li HL, Wang DX, et al: Haloperidol prophylaxis decreases delirium incidence in elderly patients after noncardiac surgery: a randomized controlled trial. Crit Care Med 40(3):731–739, 2012 22067628

White PF, Tufanogullari B, Taylor J, et al: The effect of pregabalin on preoperative anxiety and sedation levels: a dose-ranging study. Anesth Analg 108(4):1140–1145, 2009 19299776

Wilson JE, Carlson R, Duggan MC, et al: Delirium and catatonia in critically ill patients: the delirium and catatonia prospective cohort investigation. Crit Care Med 45(11):1837–1844, 2017 28841632

Wright KD, Stewart SH, Finley GA, et al: Prevention and intervention strategies to alleviate preoperative anxiety in children: a critical review. Behav Modif 31(1):52–79, 2007 17179531

Yan M, Webster LT Jr, Blumer JL: Kinetic interactions of dopamine and dobutamine with human catechol-O-methyltransferase and monoamine oxidase in vitro. J Pharmacol Exp Ther 301(1):315–321, 2002 11907189

Yoon HJ, Park KM, Choi WJ, et al: Efficacy and safety of haloperidol versus atypical antipsychotic medications in the treatment of delirium. BMC Psychiatry 13(13):240, 2013 24074357

Zatzick D, Roy-Byrne P, Russo J, et al: A randomized effectiveness trial of stepped collaborative care for acutely injured trauma survivors. Arch Gen Psychiatry 61(5):498–506, 2004 15123495

Zeng H, Li Z, He J, et al: Dexmedetomidine for the prevention of postoperative delirium in elderly patients undergoing noncardiac surgery: a meta-analysis of randomized controlled trials. PLoS One 14(8):e0218088, 2019 31419229

16

Organ Transplantation

Marian Fireman, M.D.
Andrea F. DiMartini, M.D.
Catherine C. Crone, M.D.

Transplantation engenders many biopsychosocial stressors, resulting in rates of anxiety and mood symptoms, delirium, and cognitive disorders in transplant cohorts that are similar to or higher than rates in other medically ill populations. Untreated psychiatric disorders can have effects on psychiatric and transplant medical outcomes and adherence to necessary posttransplant routines. Pharmacotherapy is an essential component of the psychiatric care of many transplant recipients.

Organ disease alters many aspects of drug pharmacokinetics, changing the bioavailability and disposition of medications and both the intended therapeutic action and side effects. For a full review of pharmacokinetics of psychotropic drugs in general and in hepatic, renal, bowel, heart, and lung diseases in particular, the reader is referred to Chapter 1, "Pharmacokinetics,

Pharmacodynamics, and Principles of Drug-Drug Interactions," and the respective chapters on these organ systems. Our primary focus for this chapter is on key points in the management of psychopathology in adult transplant recipients. Topics include the physiological properties of the newly transplanted organ in relation to drug pharmacokinetics, the psychopharmacological treatment of psychiatric illness that arises pretransplant to posttransplant, and the neuropsychiatric adverse effects and drug-drug interactions related to immunosuppressant medications. Considering these pharmacological issues and the wide interpatient variability, we provide guidelines for drug choice and dosing.

Posttransplant Pharmacological Considerations

Posttransplant Organ Functioning

For most recipients, a newly transplanted organ functions immediately, such that normal physiological parameters are quickly restored and pharmacokinetic abnormalities resolve. For patients with stable liver or kidney functioning within the first month after transplant, the clearance and steady-state volume of distribution of drugs have been shown to be similar to those of healthy volunteers (Hebert et al. 2003). Thus, most transplant recipients can be treated with standard therapeutic drug dosing, assuming that they have recovered from the immediate postoperative complications (e.g., sedation, delirium, ileus) and are able to take oral medications.

For some recipients, however, the transplanted organ does not assume autonomous normal physiological functioning immediately, or the organ may assume normal functioning slowly over time. Posttransplant pharmacokinetic studies addressing these issues have been conducted mostly in liver and kidney recipients because of the importance of these organs in drug pharmacokinetics. Such studies have investigated only immunosuppressive medications because of the need to achieve and maintain stable immunosuppressant levels to prevent organ rejection, the ability to monitor serum levels, and the narrow therapeutic range of these drugs. These data can provide general guidance on psychotropic medication prescribing in specific types of posttransplant organ dysfunction.

Primary nonfunction, occurring in 3%–4% of liver and renal transplant recipients (Kemmer et al. 2007; U.S. Renal Data System 2008), is primary graft failure that results in death or retransplantation within 30 days of the transplant. For liver recipients with primary nonfunction, survival beyond the fifth postoperative day is uncommon, and life support until another organ becomes available is the focus of therapy. The ICU team will often use intravenous benzodiazepines, propofol, dexmedetomidine, or opioids for rapid sedation and pain management.

The most common allograft complication affecting pharmacokinetics in the immediate posttransplant period is delayed graft function (DGF). DGF occurs in 10%–50% of liver recipients (Angelico 2005). Such patients were shown to need half the immunosuppressant dosage needed by those without DGF, and these dosing requirements did not correlate with body weight. This finding suggests that in the early posttransplant period, metabolic capacity rather than volume of distribution is the critical factor in pharmacokinetics (Hebert et al. 2003).

DGF occurs in 25%–50% of renal transplant recipients and is defined as the need for dialysis within the first week after transplant (Shoskes and Cecka 1998; U.S. Renal Data System 2008). Immunosuppressant pharmacokinetic studies show that DGF alters pharmacokinetics by mechanisms that increase the free fraction of parent drugs and renally excreted metabolites (Shaw et al. 1998). Delayed renal elimination of immunosuppressants for patients in severe or acute renal impairment after transplant can result in levels three to six times higher than those in nonimpaired recipients for both renally excreted drugs and their metabolites (Shaw et al. 1998). DGF also affects the binding of drugs to plasma proteins, even in the absence of hypoalbuminemia (Shaw et al. 1998).

Posttransplant Organ Rejection

Acute cellular rejection occurs in 20%–70% of liver transplant recipients, most often within the first 3 weeks after transplant, and results in transient graft dysfunction. Delirium may be a clinical manifestation. Acute rejection is most commonly treated with high-dose steroids, effective in 65%–80% of cases. Alternative therapies include antibody treatments, such as monoclonal therapy and antithymocyte globulin (Cooper 2020; Lake 2003). These agents, particularly high-dose steroids, can cause serious neuropsychiatric side effects (see the subsection "Neuropsychiatric Effects of Immunosuppressant Medications and Their Treatment" later in this chapter).

Chronic graft rejection, manifested by gradual obliteration of small bile ducts and microvascular changes, occurs in about 5%–10% of liver recipients and responds poorly to changes in immunosuppression. Patients may have jaundice or difficult-to-manage pruritus. Loss of liver synthetic function may not be evident until very late in the course (Lake 2003).

An estimated 20%–60% of kidney recipients experience an episode of acute rejection, most often within the first 6 months after transplant. However, up to 30% of recipients with stable or improving renal function will actually be in an undetected rejection episode (Rush et al. 1998; Shapiro et al. 2001). With treatment, acute rejection typically resolves quickly, with restoration of prerejection renal function, whereas undetected subclinical rejection can result in gradually worsening renal function over time, with eventual graft loss (Rush et al. 1998).

Nearly 50% of heart transplant recipients experience an episode of acute rejection (either humoral or cellular) within the first posttransplant year. Most episodes are treated with the addition of steroids to the baseline immunosuppressive regimen. Ischemic injury usually occurs in the early posttransplant period and can also cause allograft dysfunction (Michaels et al. 2003). Sinus node dysfunction or atrioventricular block necessitating permanent pacing occurs in 5%–19% of heart transplant recipients and may be associated with rejection (Collins et al. 2003). Psychotropics, particularly those with the potential to prolong the QTc interval or cause conduction delay by other mechanisms, should be used with caution in these patients (see also Chapter 6, "Cardiovascular Disorders").

General Posttransplant Issues

In addition to overt DGF or rejection, some recipients have transient physiological abnormalities in the weeks after transplant that could also affect pharmacokinetics (e.g., liver congestion or renal hypoperfusion in heart recipients, fluid overload in kidney recipients, liver hypoperfusion and fluid overload in liver recipients). Liver transplant recipients often develop pretransplant altered hemodynamics with fluid retention (i.e., ascites, peripheral edema, and pleural effusions) or hepatorenal syndrome. Generally, once normal hemodynamics are restored after transplant, hepatorenal syndrome resolves. Nonetheless, up to 20% of patients may develop persisting fluid retention in the form of moderate to large pleural and peritoneal fluid collections, resulting in fluctuating drug volume of distribution. In addition, nearly 20% of liver recipients need postoperative dialysis in the days to weeks after transplant, mostly to treat resolving hepatorenal syndrome and volume overload (Contreras et al. 2002). Principles of psychotropic management during hemodialysis should be applied (see Chapter 5, "Renal and Urological Disorders").

In addition, underlying disease processes or other comorbid organ insufficiencies that are not corrected by organ transplant may have an effect on drug pharmacokinetics. For example, patients with cystic fibrosis who receive a lung transplant may continue to have delayed gastric emptying, pancreatic insufficiency with malabsorption, and altered liver metabolism and renal clearance that impair normal cyclosporine kinetics (Reynaud-Gaubert et al. 1997).

Chronic graft rejection is potentially reversible in the early stages but not once chronic dysfunction has set in, after which progressive graft failure may occur. Thus, for transplant recipients, adherence to lifelong immunosuppressants is critical. Unfortunately, for all organ types, immunosuppressant nonadherence is a major risk factor for rejection and may be responsible for up to 30% of graft loss and late deaths after the initial recovery period (Bunzel and Laederach-Hofmann 2000). Attempts to identify and alleviate immunosuppressant side effects may increase adherence. Unfortunately, the treatment of most types of graft dysfunction (DGF or acute or chronic rejection) typically requires an increase in the dosage of the primary calcineurin-inhibiting medication or the addition of other immunosuppressants, including monoclonal antibodies, steroids, mycophenolate, and sirolimus, which tend to create or exacerbate neuropsychiatric side effects (see the subsection "Neuropsychiatric Effects of Immunosuppressant Medications and Their Treatment" later in this chapter). Additionally, depression has been implicated in cases of nonadherence, and mood symptoms should be elicited and treated.

Finally, for all organ types, calcineurin-inhibiting immunosuppressants are nephrotoxic, and chronic use results in renal failure for 10%–20% of recipients by 5 years after transplant (Ojo et al. 2003). Thus, the quality of renal function should always be considered, especially for long-term transplant recipients.

With the resumption of normal graft function, psychotropic medications that may have been prescribed at lower dosages before transplant to account for diminished metabolism or elimination may need to be adjusted to higher dosages after transplant. Another important consideration is pain management for patients taking chronic opioids before transplant; higher than average dosages of narcotic analgesics may be needed perioperatively. In one specific example, patients undergoing methadone maintenance therapy, for whom methadone was also used as their postoperative pain medication, needed an average methadone dosage increase of 60% after transplant, presumably to adjust for chronic downregulation of μ opiate pain receptors from chronic methadone exposure (Weinrieb et al. 2004) and improvement in metabolism after transplant.

Living Organ Donation Issues: Recipients and Donors

Living donor liver transplant recipients make up only about 4% of liver transplant procedures in the United States (Health Resources and Services Administration Division of Transplantation 2022), but these recipients need special pharmacological consideration. Because living donor liver transplant recipients receive grafts that are 55%–60% of normal liver volume, they initially need smaller doses of medication. Pharmacokinetic studies with immunosuppressants suggest that their medication doses should be 30% lower than doses given to deceased donor liver transplant recipients to achieve similar therapeutic levels in the early postoperative period (Jain et al. 2008). In addition to the fact that a smaller liver clears drugs less readily, animal models suggest that glucuronide conjugation is impaired during the first several weeks of hepatic regeneration (Jain et al. 2008).

Living donor liver transplant recipients can experience an uncommon technical complication called small-for-size syndrome (SFSS). SFSS occurs when a partial liver graft is unable to meet the functional demands of the recipient, resulting in a clinical syndrome characterized by postoperative liver dysfunction. The incidence of SFSS is reported to be 5%–10% after partial liver transplant but may be higher depending on the status of the recipient and the type of graft used (Tucker and Heaton 2005). SFSS is characterized by prolonged cholestasis, elevated liver enzymes, and coagulopathy combined with manifestations of portal hypertension such as ascites. Without any intervention, approximately 50% of recipients with SFSS die of sepsis within 6 weeks after transplant (Dahm et al. 2005). Using psychotropics for these patients requires close attention to liver function, fluid status, and coagulopathy.

For living liver donors, little is known about the rate and extent of the restoration of hepatic function, especially after right lobe hepatectomy, a procedure involving more extensive removal of hepatic tissue (50%–60% of the liver mass). Existing literature suggests that the liver mass of donors can return to approximately 80%–100% of baseline by several weeks to months after donation, despite biochemical abnormalities persisting beyond 2 months (Nadalin et al. 2004). One preliminary study of donor liver function showed that hepatic galactose elimination capacity, a measure of liver function, was only 50% by 10 days after hepatic resection despite rapid return of liver volume (Jochum et al. 2006). By 3 months, complete function was restored (Jochum et al. 2006).

Psychotropic considerations for live liver donors must take into account the time since donation and the potential for incomplete restoration of metabolic capacity. Long-term hepatic function in liver donors is unknown but is assumed to return to normal. Several studies of liver donors' psychological outcomes evaluated via specific psychiatric assessments found that substantial percentages of liver donors, 10%–14%, have symptoms that meet criteria for depressive and/or anxiety disorders within the first year after donation (Erim et al. 2006, 2007; Fukunishi et al. 2001).

Kidney donors lose half of their functional nephron mass with donor nephrectomy. In the year after nephrectomy, donor creatinine clearance can decrease by 30% compared with preoperative levels but still be within normal limits (Bieniasz et al. 2009). With long-term follow-up, kidney donors continue to have 72%–77% of predonation creatinine clearance and an incidence of proteinuria as high as 31% (Najarian et al. 1992; Zafar et al. 2002). Although most donors experience a decrease in glomerular filtration rate immediately after donation, the risk of end-stage renal failure is low, approximately 0.2%–0.5% (Azar et al. 2007). In one study, after 1-year follow-up, 9.3% of donors were prescribed antidepressants for severe depression, suggesting a substantial need for psychotropics in donors (Azar et al. 2007).

Psychotropic Medications in Transplant Recipients

Although no psychotropic medication is absolutely contraindicated for use in transplant recipients, specific precautions and careful selection are necessary. Patients in end-stage organ failure are typically more sensitive to medication side effects. For example, patients with psychomotor retardation or cognitive impairment due to uremia, hypoxia, or hepatic encephalopathy often cannot tolerate psychotropics with significant sedating side effects (e.g., benzodiazepines, mirtazapine, paroxetine). Pharmacokinetic changes (e.g., delayed absorption, altered volume of distribution, impaired metabolism, reduced excretion) caused by organ failure will also necessitate dosing adjustments. After transplant, drug-drug interactions become a greater concern because patients are maintained on a broad array of medications (e.g., immunosuppressants, antihypertensives, antibiotics, lipid-lowering agents, hypoglycemic drugs).

QTc interval prolongation is an important issue for patients prescribed psychotropic medications. Many psychotropics are known to prolong the QTc interval, and some have been associated with torsades de pointes, a malignant ventricular arrhythmia. Many pretransplant patients may be taking other medications with known potential to cause QTc interval prolongation or torsades de pointes. After transplant, the immunosuppressant medications (e.g., cyclosporine, tacrolimus) are known to prolong the QTc interval. Furthermore, posttransplant patients are often prescribed other medications with potential to prolong the QTc interval. Care must be taken when prescribing multiple medications known to prolong the QTc interval; frequent electrocardiographic monitoring or cardiology consultation may be necessary (Funk et al. 2020).

In the following subsections, we provide guidance by drug class regarding the selection of psychotropics with respect to specific side effects and organ disease. These guidelines apply both to pretransplant patients with organ failure and to posttransplant patients without complete restoration of organ function. Because few data are available specifically on transplant recipients, information on non–transplant recipients with advanced organ disease is included.

Antidepressants

The prevalence of depressive and anxiety disorders among transplant recipients is high and contributes to increased morbidity and mortality if the depression or anxiety is left untreated. Patients often do well with antidepressant therapy, and appropriate medication treatment should not be avoided because of concerns about organ disease. Antidepressants may provide additional benefits to the management of organ failure symptoms, such as nausea, anorexia, insomnia, pruritus, pain, and intradialytic hypotension. After transplant, antidepressants can be helpful not only for primary psychiatric disorders but also for disorders that are secondary to immunosuppressants.

Selective Serotonin Reuptake Inhibitors

Selective serotonin reuptake inhibitors (SSRIs) are the primary choice for transplant recipients because of their relative safety. Although relatively unstudied in posttransplant patients, citalopram, sertraline, paroxetine, and fluoxetine have been studied to various degrees in patients with end-stage organ disease (Gottlieb et al. 2007; Kalender et al. 2007; Lacasse et al. 2004), with generally positive results; however, caution must be exercised because of the very limited number of randomized controlled trials.

SSRIs inhibit platelet activation and may prolong bleeding time. Although possibly beneficial for patients with congestive heart failure who are prone to thromboembolism, SSRIs carry some risk for patients with cirrhosis, who are prone to bleeding as a result of varices, coagulopathy, and thrombocytopenia (Serebruany et al. 2003; Weinrieb et al. 2003). SSRIs should be used with caution in patients already taking drugs that increase bleeding risk (e.g., acetylsalicylic acid [aspirin] and other nonsteroidal anti-inflammatory drugs, antiplatelet agents) (Weinrieb et al. 2005). All of the SSRIs may cause some degree of QTc interval prolongation, although citalopram is the only agent that carries recommendations for dose limitation (Funk et al. 2020).

Among the SSRIs, citalopram and escitalopram have the fewest drug-drug interactions. U.S. FDA recommendations call for limiting citalopram dosage to 40 mg/day; dosages not greater than 20 mg/day for patients with hepatic impairment or older than 60 are suggested (Beach et al. 2013). Citalopram was effective for mild to moderate depression in depressed lung transplant recipients (Silvertooth et al. 2004).

Sertraline has the second fewest drug interactions of the SSRIs and is often the SSRI of choice because of issues of cost and decreased likelihood of QT prolongation as compared with citalopram. It significantly reduced itch scores in patients with cholestatic jaundice, independent of effects on depression (Mayo et al. 2007). In patients on dialysis, it lessened intradialytic hypotension, a common hemodialysis complication (Yalcin et al. 2002).

Paroxetine is generally associated with greater weight gain than other SSRIs, which may be beneficial for poor nutritional status, a common problem among patients with end-stage organ disease. In depressed patients with end-stage renal disease, paroxetine combined with psychotherapy reduced depression and improved nutritional status (e.g., serum albumin, predialysis serum urea nitrogen) (Koo et al. 2005). Tolerability is a concern because of paroxetine's anticholinergic side effects and discontinuation syndrome.

Fluvoxamine is generally avoided in transplant recipients because it is a strong inhibitor of multiple cytochrome P450 (CYP) isozymes. Use of this agent may result in adverse drug-drug interactions.

Vilazodone, approved by the FDA in 2011 for treatment of major depression, is both an SSRI and a partial serotonin type 1A (5-HT$_{1A}$) agonist. It does not appear to cause electrocardiographic changes. The metabolism of vilazodone may be inhibited by strong CYP3A4 inhibitors (Wang et al. 2015). Vortioxetine is an SSRI with additional agonist activity at 5-HT$_{1A}$ and 5-HT$_{1B}$ receptors and inhibitory activity at 5-HT$_3$, 5-HT$_7$, and 5-HT$_{1D}$ receptors. Levels of vortioxetine may be affected by CYP2D6 inhibitors (Garnock-Jones 2014). Vilazodone and vortioxetine are expensive compared with other antidepressants, and there is little experience with use of these medications for patients with end-organ disease or organ transplants.

Mirtazapine

Mirtazapine is a unique agent that preferentially blocks presynaptic α_2, histamine, and 5-HT$_2$ and 5-HT$_3$ receptors. By blocking 5-HT$_3$ receptors, mirtazapine provides antiemetic effects, a valuable feature for transplant recipients with nausea from medications and organ failure (Kim et al. 2004). Mirtazapine may relieve persistent pruritus caused by uremia or cholestasis by blockade of histamine, 5-HT$_2$, and 5-HT$_3$ receptors (Davis et al. 2003). It may increase appetite and promote weight gain, which can be advantageous for some patients, but after transplant, mirtazapine may accentuate immunosuppressant-induced weight gain and hyperlipidemia (Kim et al. 2004; McIntyre et al. 2006). It may cause agranulocytosis, neutropenia, and other reductions in hematological parameters and should be used cautiously in patients taking drugs that can cause blood dyscrasias (e.g., immunosuppressants, interferon). Although rare, these events can be especially serious in immunocompromised patients. Because mirtazapine lacks inhibitory effects on CYP isozymes, there is little risk of drug-drug interactions (Crone and Gabriel 2004). Mirtazapine should not be combined with clonidine because these agents act in opposition at central α_2 receptors. Combination of these agents may result in loss of effectiveness of clonidine for treatment of hypertension (Abo-Zena et al. 2000).

Bupropion

Although the activating side effects associated with bupropion can be difficult for some patients to tolerate, activation and lack of sedation can be useful for transplant recipients with persistent fatigue. Bupropion also may be useful for smoking cessation, an important issue in transplant recipients because of long-term risk for malignancy (Wagena et al. 2005). It can elevate blood pressure and should be used with caution in end-stage organ disease and post-transplant patients with preexisting and persistent hypertension associated with immunosuppressants. Although the risk of seizures is low at therapeutic doses, cautious use is needed for patients at risk for seizures from other causes (e.g., hepatic encephalopathy, high-dose immunosuppression). Bupropion is a strong inhibitor of CYP2D6, so care must be exercised when it is combined with medications metabolized by this isozyme. Although most immunosuppressants are not metabolized by CYP2D6, other medications frequently prescribed to transplant recipients (e.g., other psychotropics and β-blockers) are CYP2D6 substrates. In addition, use of lower doses is recommended in end-stage liver disease.

Serotonin-Norepinephrine Reuptake Inhibitors

Venlafaxine, desvenlafaxine, and duloxetine can elevate blood pressure, and caution should be exercised as with bupropion. Duloxetine has been reported to cause severe liver toxicity in rare cases (Billioti de Gage et al. 2018; see also Chapter 4, "Gastrointestinal Disorders"). Levomilnacipran, the most recently approved medication in this class, is a more potent inhibitor of norepinephrine reuptake. This action may improve cognition but may also cause elevations in heart rate and blood pressure. Levels of levomilnacipran are affected by renal function, and doses must be decreased in moderate to severe renal impairment. Levels of levomilnacipran may be increased by strong CYP3A4 inhibitors (Scott 2014). As with other new agents, little is known about the use of this drug in transplant recipients.

Nefazodone

The risk of serious hepatotoxicity and CYP3A4 inhibition makes nefazodone an undesirable choice for transplant recipients. There have been several cases of immunosuppressant toxicity resulting from nefazodone's inhibition of CYP3A4 (see the subsection "Drug-Drug Interactions" later in this chapter).

Trazodone

Trazodone is similar in action to nefazodone but lacks significant hepatotoxicity. The sedating side effects are helpful for persistent insomnia but may be intolerable for patients with psychomotor slowing or cognitive impairment, common among patients with end-stage organ disease and neuropsychiatric side effects from immunosuppressants. Care is needed for patients with heart disease who are more prone to its orthostatic and arrhythmogenic effects. Trazodone does not appear to have effects on the CYP isozymes.

Tricyclic Antidepressants

Tricyclic antidepressants (TCAs) are a secondary choice in the transplant population because of safety and tolerability issues. TCAs have significant effects on the cardiovascular system, producing quinidine-like (type 1A) antiarrhythmic activity, orthostatic hypotension, intraventricular conduction delay, QTc interval prolongation, and increased heart rate (Fusar-Poli et al. 2006). Weight gain, changes in lipid levels, and anticholinergic side effects may be undesirable for transplant recipients (McIntyre et al. 2008). Secondary-amine TCAs (desipramine, nortriptyline) are preferred over tertiary-amine TCAs because of a less severe adverse-effect profile. Nortriptyline offers the advantage of established therapeutic drug levels and reports of safe use by some transplant recipients (Kay et al. 1991).

Monoamine Oxidase Inhibitors

In general, monoamine oxidase inhibitors pose excessive safety and tolerability risks (e.g., drug-drug interactions, potential hypertensive crises) in transplant recipients. Transdermal selegiline may be an option for treatment-resistant patients who are unable to take oral medications or who lack adequate bowel absorption (Pae et al. 2007; see also Chapter 3, "Alternative Routes of Drug Administration").

Ketamine and Esketamine

Ketamine and esketamine are pharmacologically novel treatments for adult patients with treatment-resistant depression. There are concerns about the use of these treatments in the general population, including safety, efficacy, tolerability, patient selection, and risk for precipitation of substance use disorders.

Esketamine is the *S*-enantiomer of ketamine, and both agents are dissociative hallucinogens used as general anesthetics. Both have a high affinity for the phencyclidine site of the *N*-methyl-D-aspartate receptor. Ketamine is generally used intravenously, and esketamine is used intranasally. There are no published studies or case reports to date on the use of these agents in patients with end-organ disease or organ transplants, and several potential adverse effects seen in medically healthy patients suggest caution in these populations. Dissociative reactions are commonly reported, but these generally resolve in several hours. These agents may induce psychosis in vulnerable patients, although the absolute risk is unclear. The most common neurological side effects are dizziness, drowsiness, and light-headedness; no persistent cognitive deficits have been reported. Hemodynamic adverse effects are common, particularly with ketamine. Patients receiving these treatments must be monitored closely for increases in heart rate and blood pressure and treated as appropriate.

Ketamine and esketamine are metabolized by CYP3A4 and CYP2B6. Inhibitors and inducers of these isoenzymes may have effects on the metabolism of ketamine and esketamine, but clinical significance is unclear. Neither agent appears to have clinically meaningful induction or inhibition of the CYP isoenzymes (McIntyre et al. 2021). Cyclosporine has been noted to increase ketamine toxicity in animal models (Robinson et al. 2017).

Brexanolone

Brexanolone, a modulator of $GABA_A$ receptors and an analogue of the neurosteroid allopregnanolone, is approved for the treatment of postpartum depression. Brexanolone should be avoided in patients with end-stage renal disease. Brexanolone can inhibit CYP2C9, so caution should be exercised when brexanolone is administered with medications metabolized by this isoenzyme (Edinoff et al. 2021b). Currently no studies or case reports have been done on the use of this medication in the transplant population (see also Chapter 11, "Obstetrics and Gynecology").

Psychostimulants

Methylphenidate and dextroamphetamine are effective for short-term treatment of depressive symptoms in medically ill patients. Both offer the advantage of rapid onset of action and are useful in reducing apathy, fatigue, and cognitive dulling. Methylphenidate was markedly effective for at least four of eight liver transplant recipients experiencing depression, apathy, and cognitive impairment (Plutchik et al. 1998). Although supraventricular tachycardia has been reported in a heart recipient treated with methylphenidate, stimulants have been used safely for patients with significant cardiac disease without marked changes in blood pressure or heart rate (Come and Shapiro 2005; Masand et al. 1991). Nevertheless, close monitoring for elevations in blood pressure or heart rate or for worsening congestive heart failure is necessary.

Several new formulations of psychostimulants have been released since 2015, including an amphetamine extended-release oral suspension, amphetamine extended-release oral dissolving tablet, mixed amphetamine salts, amphetamine extended-release oral solution, and amphetamine immediate-release oral dissolving tablet. Newer formulations of methylphenidate also have been released. It is unclear whether any of these will offer an advantage over previous formulations for organ transplant recipients or for patients with end-organ disease, and no current reviews or case studies are available in the literature.

Modafinil has been used clinically in transplant recipients; however, particularly at dosages of 400 mg/day or more, modafinil inhibits CYP2C9 and CYP2C19 and weakly induces CYP1A2 and CYP2B6. At higher dosages, modafinil is a moderate to strong inducer of CYP3A4, which may be problematic in combination with immunosuppressants (see the subsection "Drug-Drug Interactions" later in this chapter). Armodafinil has metabolic interactions similar to those of modafinil.

Atomoxetine is a selective norepinephrine reuptake inhibitor used for the treatment of ADHD. It is not classified as a stimulant. No reports of atomoxetine use in transplant recipients have been published. However, because of CYP2D6 inhibition and warnings about potential hepatotoxicity, other medications are preferred.

Viloxazine, a serotonin-norepinephrine modulating agent, is approved for the treatment of ADHD in children ages 6–17 years. There are no published studies regarding its use in organ transplant recipients. Viloxazine is a potent CYP1A2 inhibitor, and dose reductions may be necessary for patients taking agents metabolized by CYP1A2. Viloxazine is contraindicated for patients with severe hepatic impairment, and dose reductions are needed for patients with moderate to severe renal insufficiency (Edinoff et al. 2021a).

Benzodiazepines

Benzodiazepines are effective in providing anxiolysis to transplant recipients but may worsen sedation, respiratory suppression, preexisting cognitive impairment, or encephalopathy in patients with end-stage organ disease. Lorazepam, oxazepam, and temazepam require only glucuronidation and may be a safer choice for patients with cirrhosis (Crone and Gabriel 2004) or impaired posttransplant hepatic function. Clonazepam has been successfully used to manage steroid-induced mania in transplant recipients.

Buspirone

Buspirone, a serotonin partial agonist, is marketed for the treatment of generalized anxiety disorder. It is often ineffective for patients who have previously received benzodiazepines. It may be helpful in transplant recipients with anxiety because it does not cause respiratory depression, but its metabolism may be affected by inhibitors of CYP3A4 and P-glycoprotein.

Antipsychotic Agents

Antipsychotics are commonly used for transplant recipients to manage agitation and psychosis associated with acute delirium, mood disorders secondary to immunosuppressants (e.g., mania), and comorbid primary psychiatric disorders (e.g., bipolar disorder, schizophrenia). They can also be used for anxiolysis (e.g., for patients with advanced pulmonary disease or patients being weaned off ventilators). A concern is their risk of QTc interval prolongation, torsades de pointes, and sudden death (Funk et al. 2020; Pacher and Kecskemeti 2004; see also Chapter 6). Transplant recipients often have other risk factors for cardiac arrhythmia (e.g., electrolyte imbalance, renal or hepatic disease, heart failure, ventricular hypertrophy, other QTc-prolonging drugs).

Haloperidol

Haloperidol is the primary typical antipsychotic used for transplant recipients because of its varied routes of administration, therapeutic efficacy, overall tolerability, and few side effects. It is an excellent choice for managing agitation or psychosis in delirious transplant recipients (see also Chapter 15, "Critical Care and Surgery"). In rare cases, extremely high dosages of intravenous haloperidol (>1,000 mg/day) have been safely used to control severe agitation (Levenson 1995). Haloperidol can also treat psychosis from immunosuppressant neurotoxicity (see the subsection "Neuropsychiatric Effects of Immunosuppressant Medications and Their Treatment" later in this chapter) (Tripathi and Panzer 1993). Extrapyramidal side effects should be monitored in transplant recipients with encephalopathy. QTc interval prolongation should be monitored closely in patients taking haloperidol, particularly intravenous haloperidol (Beach et al. 2013; Funk et al. 2020).

Atypical Antipsychotics

Atypical antipsychotics may be used for agitation, insomnia, anxiety, mania, and delirium associated with end-stage organ disease or posttransplant immunosuppressant reactions; however, no literature specific to transplant patients has been published. Atypical antipsychotics may cause weight gain, hyperlipidemia, and glucose intolerance, exacerbating the similar effects of immunosuppressant drugs. Olanzapine and quetiapine are often used in these patients for their sedating side effects and lower risk of QTc interval prolongation. Aripiprazole may be a useful choice if sedation is not desired; it also has the lowest risk of QTc interval prolongation (Beach et al. 2013; Funk et al. 2020).

Several newer agents have been approved in recent years, but to date there are no studies or case reports regarding the use of these agents in the transplant population. Olanzapine/samidorphan may cause less weight gain than some of the other atypical antipsychotics, but samidorphan is an opioid antagonist with action at μ, κ, and δ opioid receptors, so it cannot be used with opioid agonist agents for pain (Potkin et al. 2020). Asenapine is now available in transdermal form, which may be useful for patients unable to take oral medications and for whom parenteral medications are less desirable. Other new antipsychotic agents include amisulpride (not available in the United States in oral form; approved in the United States only as an antiemetic), lumateperone, brexpiprazole, and cariprazine, as well as newer formulations of paliperidone (intramuscular, available for dosing every 3 months and every 6 months) and aripiprazole. As previously noted, little is known about the use of these agents in the organ transplant population. If these agents are used, attention should be paid to whether dosing adjustments are needed in renal or hepatic impairment, whether the agents cause significant QTc interval prolongation, and the pharmacokinetic properties of these agents.

Mood Stabilizers

Lithium is complicated to use for patients awaiting transplant and those who are recent recipients because of problems with fluid imbalance. Other mood stabilizers pose more of a challenge after transplant because they interact with immunosuppressants, altering immunosuppressant drug levels. The choice of mood stabilizer for a transplant recipient depends on the patient's history of symptoms, prior treatment, and type of organ disease.

Lithium

Maintaining lithium levels within a narrow therapeutic window is complicated in transplant recipients. For patients with dehydration, congestive heart failure, cirrhosis, nephrotic syndrome, or cystic fibrosis, sodium retention mechanisms are activated and lithium clearance is reduced (Thomsen and Schou 1999). Fluctuating fluid status from dehydration (due to fever, sweating, or decreased intake) or fluid overload (e.g., edema, ascites) can also make maintenance of stable nontoxic lithium levels difficult (Thomsen and Schou 1999). Cyclosporine, a common immunosuppressant, increases lithium levels by altering proximal tubular reabsorption (Vincent et al. 1987). Other drugs used before or after transplant (e.g., angiotensin converting enzyme inhibitors, spironolactone, calcium channel blockers) can alter lithium levels. Lithium can cause renal tubular damage with loss of urine-concentrating ability (see Chapter 5). After transplant, these potential adverse effects of lithium must be carefully considered, especially when lithium is combined with nephrotoxic immunosuppressant therapy. Lithium can cause weight gain, cognitive slowing, and tremor, potentially aggravating common posttransplant problems (DasGupta and Jefferson 1990).

Valproic Acid

Valproic acid is a less desirable choice for patients with preexisting hepatic impairment, and its use for treatment of short-term immunosuppressant mood instability is not advisable given its potentially serious side effects (e.g., hepatotoxicity, thrombocytopenia, platelet dysfunction). Reduced serum albumin concentrations due to cirrhosis, renal disease, cachexia, other catabolic states, as well as elevated free fatty acid concentrations in the setting of diabetes, hemodialysis, and hypertriglyceridemia, can raise free valproic acid levels, resulting in an increased risk of sedation, cognitive slowing, and lethargy (Haroldson et al. 2000).

Carbamazepine and Oxcarbazepine

Carbamazepine may cause leukopenia and poses a rare risk of serious blood dyscrasias, including aplastic anemia and agranulocytosis, which are especially concerning for patients taking immunosuppressants or those who are immunocompromised because of end-stage organ disease (Schatzberg and DeBattista 2015). It may alter vitamin D levels and bone turnover, potentially increasing the risk for osteoporosis from immunosuppressant therapy (Mintzer et al. 2006). For patients with renal failure or cirrhosis, levels of carbamazepine and its pharmacologically active metabolite 10,11-epoxide should be closely monitored (Tutor-Crespo et al. 2008). Carbamazepine may induce CYP3A4, lowering tacrolimus and cyclosporine levels (see the subsection "Drug-Drug Interactions" later in this chapter). Oxcarbazepine, although not associated with blood dyscrasias, is a weak inducer of CYP3A4 and can reduce immunosuppressant levels (Rösche et al. 2001; Wang and Ketter 2002). Hyponatremia has been observed in up to 50% of patients taking oxcarbazepine, and oxcarbazepine use also has been associated with lower vitamin D levels and increased bone turnover (Asconapé 2002; Mintzer et al. 2006).

Gabapentin

Gabapentin can be used to treat anxiety disorders, neuropathic pain (e.g., immunosuppressant-induced neuropathy, postherpetic neuralgia), restless legs syndrome, and uremic pruritus (Colman and Stadel 1999; Molnar et al. 2006; Naini et al. 2007). These conditions are common in transplant recipients, particularly those with renal failure. Because gabapentin is renally excreted rather than hepatically metabolized, the dosage must be reduced in proportion to the decline in creatinine clearance (Wong et al. 1995).

Topiramate

Topiramate is generally undesirable for transplant recipients because of its tendency to cause cognitive impairment and possible metabolic acidosis (Schatzberg and DeBattista 2015). Cognitive side effects are especially problematic for patients with cognitive dysfunction due to end-stage organ disease or high-dose immunosuppressants.

Lamotrigine

Lamotrigine, originally developed as an antiepileptic, appears to inhibit uptake of serotonin, norepinephrine, and dopamine. It has been approved for maintenance therapy for adults with bipolar disorder. Lamotrigine carries the risk of serious side effects, including Stevens-Johnson syndrome, hepatotoxicity, and hemophagocytic lymphohistiocytosis, a rare and potentially devastating immune system disorder (Mufson 2018). Given these risks, experience with lamotrigine in the organ transplant population is limited, and this agent should be used with great caution, if at all.

Medications Used to Treat Sleep Disorders

Several medications for the treatment of sleep disorders have been approved in recent years. These include the melatonin agonists, such as tasimelteon, and the orexin agonists, such as lemborexant and suvorexant. No information was found in the literature regarding the use of these agents in organ transplant recipients. Practitioners prescribing these agents should be aware of any toxicities, dosing adjustments needed in organ failure, and pharmacokinetics and potential drug-drug interactions. Suvorexant may be useful for delirium prophylaxis (Xu et al. 2020).

Other Medications

The vesicular monoamine transporter 2 inhibitors used to treat tardive dyskinesia and pimavanserin for psychosis in Parkinson's disease have been approved in recent years. Little is known about the use of these agents in the organ transplant population.

Medications Used to Treat Substance Use Disorders

Medications to reduce cravings or block the effect of substances and potentially diminish relapse risk for alcohol, opioids, and tobacco have not been systematically studied in transplant recipients. Nevertheless, the known pharmacodynamics of these drugs can provide guidance for their use (see Chapter 18, "Substance Use Disorders"). These medications may be particularly useful in reducing complications from recurrent tobacco, alcohol, and other substance use in transplant recipients. Immunosuppressed patients are at higher risk for malignancy, recurrence of liver disease, and infectious diseases associated with use of tobacco, alcohol, and other substances. Tobacco use after transplant places patients at high risk for malignancy, particularly lung cancer, and patients receiving transplants for acute alcoholic hepatitis may be at higher risk for posttransplant alcohol use. These medications can modify these risks.

For treating alcohol use disorder, disulfiram is not advised for transplant recipients because of possible serious side effects and significant interactions with medications requiring CYP metabolism (e.g., posttransplant immunosuppressants) (Chick 1999; DiMartini et al. 2005; Krahn and DiMartini 2005). Acamprosate should be used cautiously because rare cases of cardiomyopathy, heart failure, and renal failure have occurred. In renal impairment (creatinine clearance = 30–50 mL/min), a half dose should be given; acamprosate is contraindicated for creatinine clearance of 30 mL/min or less (Overman et al. 2003; Saivin et al. 1998). Naltrexone, an opioid antagonist, is contraindicated in severe hepatic disease and may cause hepatotoxicity, particularly at dosages of 300 mg/day or more (Krahn and DiMartini 2005). Naltrexone may be helpful for short-term treatment of pruritus in severe liver disease (Parés 2014). Postoperative use is contraindicated because of antagonism of opioid analgesia. Patients surveyed after liver transplant were reluctant to use naltrexone because of potential hepatotoxicity (Weinrieb et al. 2001).

For tobacco use disorder, nicotine replacement therapies are generally contraindicated for patients with serious heart disease because of the potential for increasing angina and heart rate and possibly exacerbating arrhythmias. Caution is advised, especially in heart transplant recipients. Varenicline is renally excreted, and dose reductions are recommended for patients who have renal insufficiency or those undergoing dialysis. Side effects (e.g., nausea, vomiting) may be problematic for transplant recipients.

Transplant recipients undergoing methadone maintenance therapy for opioid use disorder can be successfully managed, including through the provision of adequate postoperative analgesia. For patients with renal or hepatic failure, dosage adjustment may be needed to minimize side effects and prevent worsening uremic or hepatic encephalopathy; however, higher dosages may be needed after transplant because of resumption of normal metabolic capacity. Perioperatively, patients undergoing methadone maintenance therapy need careful attention to pain control. The dosage can be increased for pain control or continued at a maintenance level with a different opioid added for acute postoperative pain. Sedation, respiratory depression, and other symptoms of opioid toxicity should be monitored (Jiao et al. 2010). Drug-drug interactions are common, particularly those mediated through CYP3A4 interactions. It is of note that methadone metabolism is not thought to be affected by cyclosporine (Indiana University Division of Clinical Pharmacology 2022; Meissner et al. 2014). A few cases of buprenorphine-induced hepatotoxicity in patients with known hepatitis C have been reported. Buprenorphine is metabolized by CYP3A4, and drug-drug interactions must be considered (Zuin et al. 2009), although these are less common than drug-drug interactions with methadone. Buprenorphine is not recommended perioperatively because it may precipitate withdrawal in patients taking opioids. Methadone has significant potential for QTc interval prolongation, whereas QTc interval prolongation with buprenorphine is minimal. If use of buprenorphine instead of methadone is possible, it may be a better choice for patients with end-organ disease and posttransplant patients.

Drug-Specific Issues

Neuropsychiatric Effects of Immunosuppressant Medications and Their Treatment

Immunosuppressants commonly cause medical side effects (e.g., hyperglycemia, hypertension, nephrotoxicity, infections, increased risk for cancer), as well as neuropsychiatric side effects (Table 16–1). Patients with neuropsychiatric symptoms often take combinations of immunosuppressants, making the contribution of any specific drug to the symptoms sometimes difficult to establish.

The mainstays of transplant immunosuppression are the calcineurin-inhibiting immunosuppressants cyclosporine and tacrolimus. Both drugs have similar neuropsychiatric side effects. Up to 40%–60% of transplant recipients experience mild symptoms, including tremulousness, headache, restlessness, insomnia, vivid dreams, photophobia, hyperesthesias or dysesthesias, anxiety, and agitation (Magee 2006; Tombazzi et al. 2006). Moderate to severe side effects—cognitive impairment, coma, seizures, focal neurological deficits, dysarthria, cortical blindness, and delirium—occur less often but can affect 21%–32% of patients during the early postoperative period (Bechstein 2000).

Table 16–1.   Neuropsychiatric side effects of immunosuppressants

Medication	Neuropsychiatric side effects
Calcineurin inhibitors (cyclosporine/tacrolimus)	Fatigue, insomnia, anxiety, agitation, confusion, depression, hallucinations, cognitive impairment, seizures, neuropathy
Corticosteroids (e.g., prednisone)	Euphoria, depression, anxiety, agitation, insomnia, hallucinations, delusions, delirium, personality changes, cognitive impairment
Sirolimus	Pain, tremor, insomnia, headache
Everolimus	Pain, fatigue, nervousness, insomnia
Azathioprine	Neuropsychiatric side effects rare
Mycophenolate/ mycophenolic acid	Anxiety, depression, seizures, agitation, weakness, headache, insomnia, tremor
Belatacept	Pain, headache, dizziness, tremor, insomnia, anxiety; associated with CNS posttransplant lymphoproliferative disorder
Monoclonal antibodies[a]	
Basiliximab	Insomnia, fatigue, pain, headache, tremor
Alemtuzumab	Insomnia, anxiety
Rituximab	Anxiety, depression, delirium, hallucinations

[a]Daclizumab, another monoclonal antibody, was removed from the market in 2018 because of reports of inflammatory encephalitis and meningoencephalitis.
Source. Alloway et al. 1998; Bajjoka and Anandan 2002; Bartynski and Boardman 2007; Bechstein 2000; Di Maira et al. 2020; DiMartini et al. 2008; Kershner and Wang-Cheng 1989; Magee 2006; National Library of Medicine 2015; Tombazzi et al. 2006.

Neuropsychiatric effects are more common with parenteral administration and early posttransplant, perhaps because of higher serum levels during this period.

Calcineurin-inhibiting immunosuppressants have been associated with posterior reversible leukoencephalopathy syndrome, which produces a variety of symptoms depending on the location of the lesions. Symptoms may include headache, visual disturbances, seizures, focal neurological symptoms, decreased consciousness, and coma. Patients with moderate to severe symptoms should have a CT scan or MRI of the brain to evaluate for characteristic cortical and subcortical white matter changes, typically involving the parietal or occipital lobes (Bartynski and Boardman 2007). Cases have been reported involving the anterior brain, cerebellum, and brain stem (Bartynski and Boardman 2007). Specific findings on fluid-attenuated inversion recovery MRI sequences and apparent diffusion coefficient mapping (sensitive to water diffusion) are especially useful in identifying the characteristic vasogenic edema seen in posterior reversible leukoencephalopathy syndrome (Ahn et al. 2003).

Neuropsychiatric adverse effects of high-dose corticosteroid treatment are reviewed in Chapter 10, "Endocrine and Metabolic Disorders."

Sirolimus, a non–calcineurin-inhibiting immunosuppressant, appears to have mild neuropsychiatric side effects, including pain, tremor, insomnia, and headache. Azathioprine rarely causes neuropsychiatric side effects. Neuropsychiatric side effects with mycophenolate appear to be milder than those described with calcineurin-inhibiting immunosuppressants, but up to 20% of patients may complain of symptoms such as anxiety, depression, seizures, agitation, weakness, headache, insomnia, and tremor (Alloway et al. 1998; DiMartini et al. 2005). Everolimus also appears to have mild neuropsychiatric side effects, including pain, fatigue, nervousness, and insomnia.

Belatacept, a T-cell costimulation blocker used primarily for renal transplant recipients, may cause headache. Belatacept and other immunosuppressants have been associated with CNS posttransplant lymphoproliferative disorder (Castellano-Sanchez et al. 2004; National Library of Medicine 2015).

Monoclonal antibodies, used for induction immunosuppression or adjunctive therapy, have generally mild and uncommon neuropsychiatric side effects. Muromonab-CD3 is an exception but is no longer used or available in the United States. Rituximab is associated with progressive multifocal leukoencephalopathy (Kranick et al. 2007).

Evaluation of posttransplant neuropsychiatric symptoms must include careful consideration of all possible etiologies, such as metabolic disturbances, infections, organ insufficiency, medication effects, and drug interactions. If side effects are believed to be secondary to calcineurin-inhibiting immunosuppressants, it may be necessary, if medically possible, to decrease the dose or switch to a different agent if symptoms are severe or life-threatening. In general, symptoms resolve with reduction or discontinuation of the calcineurin-inhibiting immunosuppressant. Anticonvulsants can successfully treat calcineurin-inhibiting immunosuppressant–induced seizures and are not needed in the long term. Seizures may also cease if calcineurin-inhibiting immunosuppressant dosage reduction or discontinuation is possible. Corticosteroid-induced symptoms generally improve dramatically as the medication is tapered after transplant.

If treatment of neuropsychiatric symptoms is needed, it is important to choose medications with the fewest side effects, fewest active metabolites, and least toxicity. Benzodiazepines may be used safely in the short term for sleep disturbances, anxiety, and agitation; long-term treatment with these agents is usually not advisable. SSRIs are generally considered first-line treatment for depressive and anxiety disorders (see subsection "Selective Serotonin Reuptake Inhibitors" earlier in this chapter). Haloperidol and other antipsychotics can be used for symptoms of delirium, hallucinations, delusions, mania, mood lability, irritability, and agitation.

Drug-Drug Interactions

Drug interactions commonly occur with immunosuppressants and other drugs frequently needed by transplant recipients (e.g., antihypertensives, antimicrobials, lipid-modifying agents, antiulcer drugs, analgesics, psychotropics). Most immunosuppressants have significant toxicities and narrow therapeutic indexes. Glucocorticoids, calcineurin-inhibiting immunosuppressants, sirolimus, everolimus, and corticosteroids are all CYP3A4 substrates (Table 16–2). Inhibitors and inducers of CYP3A4 may cause clinically significant drug level changes, resulting in toxicity or inadequate immunosuppression. Glucocorticoids induce CYP3A4 and may decrease levels of drugs metabolized by CYP3A4 (e.g., quetiapine) (Indiana University Division of Clinical Pharmacology 2022; Pascussi et al. 2003).

Several drug interactions are particularly relevant to psychiatrists (Tables 16–3 and 16–4). Among SSRIs, paroxetine is the most potent inhibitor of CYP2D6, which may increase the risk for drug-drug interactions. Fluoxetine has been well tolerated and successfully used in patients with cardiac disease and renal failure (Gottlieb et al. 2007; Kalender et al. 2007); however, its long half-life and its potential for drug-drug interactions make it less desirable for the medically ill (Crone and Gabriel 2004). Both fluoxetine and its active metabolite, norfluoxetine, are inhibitors of CYP1A2, CYP2D6, CYP2C19, and CYP3A4. Because of its ability to inhibit CYP3A4, fluoxetine theoretically could prolong the metabolism of cyclosporine, tacrolimus, and sirolimus.

Table 16–2. Immunosuppressant metabolism and effects on metabolic systems

Immunosuppressant medication	Metabolized by	Inhibits	Induces
Corticosteroids	CYP3A4	CYP3A4 (high dose)	CYP3A4 (low dose)
Cyclosporine	CYP3A4 P-glycoprotein	CYP3A4 P-glycoprotein	—
Sirolimus	CYP3A4 P-glycoprotein	—	—
Everolimus	CYP3A4 P-glycoprotein	CYP3A4 P-glycoprotein	—
Tacrolimus	CYP3A4 P-glycoprotein UGT	UGT	—

Note. CYP=cytochrome P450; UGT=uridine 5′-diphosphate glucuronosyltransferase.
Source. Augustine et al. 2007; Fireman et al. 2004; National Library of Medicine 2015; Warrington et al. 2004.

However, a small study failed to detect significant changes in cyclosporine levels when fluoxetine was used (Strouse et al. 1996). No change in cyclosporine levels occurred in a small group of transplant recipients treated with citalopram (Liston et al. 2001). Sertraline inhibits CYP2D6 at dosages greater than 200 mg/day and is a weak inhibitor of CYP3A4. One study reported that cyclosporine clearance was inhibited by sertraline (Lill et al. 2000), but another study failed to show any significant changes in cyclosporine levels for patients taking sertraline, paroxetine, or fluoxetine (Markowitz et al. 1998). Although there are no reports of elevated immunosuppressant levels with fluvoxamine, it is the least desirable choice among SSRIs because of its risk of drug-drug interactions (Crone and Gabriel 2004). It is a strong inhibitor of CYP1A2 and inhibits CYP2C9, CYP2C19, and CYP3A4. Nefazodone, a CYP3A4 inhibitor, has been implicated in a number of case reports as causing toxic calcineurin-inhibiting immunosuppressant levels, leading in two cases to acute renal insufficiency and delirium and in two cases to elevated liver enzymes (Campo et al. 1998; Garton 2002; Helms-Smith et al. 1996; Wright et al. 1999). St.

Table 16–3.   Immunosuppressant medication–psychotropic
medication interactions

Medication	Metabolic effect	Effects on psychotropic medications and management
Corticosteroids	Induce CYP3A4	Reduced levels and possibly subtherapeutic effect for pimozide, quetiapine, ziprasidone, iloperidone, fentanyl, meperidine, tramadol, buspirone, buprenorphine, benzodiazepines (except oxazepam, lorazepam, temazepam)
Cyclosporine	Inhibits CYP3A4	Increased levels and toxicities for pimozide, quetiapine, ziprasidone, iloperidone, fentanyl, meperidine, tramadol, buspirone, buprenorphine, vilazodone, levomilnacipran, benzodiazepines (except oxazepam, lorazepam, temazepam)
	Inhibits P-glycoprotein	Possible increase in bioavailability and toxicity for P-glycoprotein substrates, including carbamazepine, lamotrigine, phenytoin, paroxetine, venlafaxine, olanzapine, quetiapine, risperidone
	Unknown mechanism	Ketamine toxicity possible
Tacrolimus	QT prolongation	Increased QT prolongation in combination with other QT-prolonging drugs such as tricyclic antidepressants, methadone, typical antipsychotics, pimozide, risperidone, paliperidone, iloperidone, quetiapine, ziprasidone, other atypical antipsychotics, lithium

Note.   CYP = cytochrome P450.

John's wort, a popular herbal remedy for depression, is an inducer of CYP3A4 and P-glycoprotein. Use of St. John's wort can result in reduced levels of calcineurin-inhibiting immunosuppressants and has resulted in transplant rejection (Fireman et al. 2004). In summary, it appears that only antidepressants that strongly inhibit or induce CYP3A4 may have clinically meaningful in-

Table 16–4. Psychotropic medication–immunosuppressant medication and other important drug interactions

Medication	Pharmacokinetic effect	Effects on immunosuppressant medications and management
Carbamazepine, oxcarbazepine, and phenytoin	Induce CYP3A4	Increased metabolism and reduced exposure and therapeutic effect of CYP3A4 substrates, including corticosteroids, cyclosporine, tacrolimus, sirolimus
Armodafinil and modafinil	Inhibit CYP2C9, CYP2C19	Caution with medications metabolized by CYP2C9, CYP2C19
St. John's wort	Induces CYP3A4 and P-glycoprotein	Reduced bioavailability and increased metabolism leading to reduced exposure and therapeutic effect of CYP3A4 or P-glycoprotein substrates, including corticosteroids, cyclosporine, tacrolimus, sirolimus
Fluvoxamine and nefazodone	Inhibits CYP3A4	Reduced metabolism and increased exposure and toxicities of CYP3A4 substrates, including corticosteroids, cyclosporine, tacrolimus, sirolimus
Bupropion and atomoxetine	Inhibit CYP2D6	May affect levels of medications metabolized by CYP2D6
Viloxazine	Inhibits CYP1A2	May need dose reductions of medications metabolized by CYP1A2

Note. CYP=cytochrome P450.

teractions with immunosuppressants (i.e., inhibitors nefazodone and perhaps fluvoxamine and inducer St. John's wort). In turn, calcineurin-inhibiting immunosuppressants may increase levels of psychotropics metabolized by CYP3A4, whereas glucocorticoids may decrease levels (Indiana University Division of Clinical Pharmacology 2022; Madhusoodanan et al. 2014). Information about pharmacokinetics is continuously evolving, and practitioners are encouraged to review the pharmacokinetics of the agents they prescribe and check immunosuppressant levels as needed if the potential for drug-drug interactions exists.

In one case, a transplant recipient's cyclosporine level declined 50% because of CYP3A4 induction by modafinil, 200 mg/day (Cephalon 1998). Carbamazepine may lower drug levels of tacrolimus and cyclosporine by causing CYP3A4 induction (Baciewicz and Baciewicz 1989; Campana et al. 1996; Chabolla and Wszolek 2006), which can increase the risk of organ rejection due to inadequate immunosuppression.

The immunosuppressant drugs have important pharmacodynamic interactions. Calcineurin-inhibiting immunosuppressants are nephrotoxic, and nephrotoxicity may increase when calcineurin-inhibiting immunosuppressants are combined with aminoglycosides, amphotericin B, nonsteroidal anti-inflammatory drugs, vancomycin, and probably lithium (Alloway et al. 1998). Lithium should be used only when necessary for patients with end-organ failure and in posttransplant patients because side effects, drug-drug interactions, and changes in fluid status combined with the narrow therapeutic index of lithium make management quite complex. Frequent assessment of renal function, creatinine clearance, and lithium levels is necessary. In addition, immunosuppressants, psychotropics, and many other medications may prolong the QT interval and have the potential to cause torsades de pointes; care must be taken when prescribing combinations of these medications.

Gastrointestinal symptoms (e.g., nausea, vomiting, diarrhea) are common adverse effects of immunosuppressant medications in more than 60% of patients undergoing combination therapy (Pescovitz and Navarro 2001). Gastrointestinal symptoms should always be evaluated, especially before administering psychotropic medications with similar adverse effects (e.g., SSRIs, venlafaxine).

Immunosuppressants have significant metabolic side effects (e.g., weight gain, glucose intolerance, hyperlipidemia) (Alloway et al. 1998; Augustine et al. 2007; Bajjoka and Anandan 2002). These side effects must be considered when psychotropic medications with similar effects, such as some of the atypical antipsychotics, are to be used. Psychotropic medications with minimal metabolic side effects should be considered (see drug choices in the earlier section "Psychotropic Medications in Transplant Recipients").

Conclusion

Transplantation is a challenging process for patients and medical professionals alike. Patients undergo acute and chronic pathophysiological changes and will be subjected to powerful medications with potentially serious side effects. In addition, psychiatric disorders are common in these patients, and the identification and prompt treatment of these disorders are important aspects of transplant care. We have reviewed the essential aspects of the transplant process relevant to pharmacotherapy. This chapter should provide the information necessary to deal with the psychotropic needs of this unique and complex patient population.

Key Points

- Psychiatric consultation can aid in the correct diagnosis and the correct choice of proper medication.

- No psychotropic medications are absolutely contraindicated for use in transplant recipients, but clinicians should carefully consider the type of organ disease, stage in the transplantation process, drug, dosage, potential for side effects, and possible drug-drug interactions.

- Patients should begin taking a psychotropic medication at a low dosage, and the dosage should be slowly titrated upward.

- Patients with organ disease often have some degree of cognitive impairment or encephalopathy and tend to be more sensitive to sedative and cognitive side effects of psychotropic medications.

- Selection of psychotropic medications should take into consideration other potential benefits a drug might provide to aid symptoms of organ disease (e.g., additionally treating pruritus, restless legs syndrome, nausea, anorexia, fatigue).

- Encephalopathy can be mistaken for depression, psychosis, mania, and anxiety disorders. Careful diagnosis is necessary to avoid use of psychotropic medications that may aggravate a patient's symptoms (e.g., worsen agitation or confusion).

- After transplantation, medications that inhibit or induce cyto-chrome P450 (CYP) 3A4 should be avoided if possible because most immunosuppressants are CYP3A4 substrates.

- Immunosuppressants and many psychotropics may cause QTc interval prolongation, and care must be taken when prescribing these medications in combination.

- Although neuropsychiatric symptoms or changes in mental status may have many possible etiologies in the early post-transplant period, the possibility that symptoms reflect im-munosuppressive medication side effects should always be entertained. Symptoms may diminish with a decrease in immu-nosuppressive medications.

- Drug-drug interactions should be carefully considered because patients may be taking a wide variety of medications in addition to immunosuppressants that may pose a risk of significant inter-actions with psychotropics.

References

Abo-Zena RA, Bobek MB, Dweik RA: Hypertensive urgency induced by an interac-tion of mirtazapine and clonidine. Pharmacotherapy 20(4):476–478, 2000 10772378

Ahn KJ, Lee JW, Hahn ST, et al: Diffusion-weighted MRI and ADC mapping in FK506 neurotoxicity. Br J Radiol 76(912):916–919, 2003 14711782

Alloway RR, Holt C, Somerville KT: Solid organ transplant, in Pharmacotherapy Self-Assessment Program, 3rd Edition. Kansas City, KS, American College of Clinical Pharmacy, 1998, pp 219–272

Angelico M: Donor liver steatosis and graft selection for liver transplantation: a short review. Eur Rev Med Pharmacol Sci 9(5):295–297, 2005 16231593

Asconapé JJ: Some common issues in the use of antiepileptic drugs. Semin Neurol 22(1):27–39, 2002 12170391

Augustine JJ, Bodziak KA, Hricik DE: Use of sirolimus in solid organ transplantation. Drugs 67(3):369–391, 2007 17335296

Azar SA, Nakhjavani MR, Tarzamni MK, et al: Is living kidney donation really safe? Transplant Proc 39(4):822–823, 2007 17524822

Baciewicz AM, Baciewicz FA Jr: Cyclosporine pharmacokinetic drug interactions. Am J Surg 157(2):264–271, 1989 2644865

Bajjoka IE, Anandan JV: Liver transplantation, in Pharmacotherapy Self-Assessment Program, 4th Edition. Kansas City, KS, American College of Clinical Pharmacy, 2002, pp 169–202

Bartynski WS, Boardman JF: Distinct imaging patterns and lesion distribution in posterior reversible encephalopathy syndrome. AJNR Am J Neuroradiol 28(7):1320–1327, 2007 17698535

Beach SR, Celano CM, Noseworthy PA, et al: QTc prolongation, torsades de pointes, and psychotropic medications. Psychosomatics 54(1):1–13, 2013 23295003

Bechstein WO: Neurotoxicity of calcineurin inhibitors: impact and clinical management. Transpl Int 13(5):313–326, 2000 11052266

Bieniasz M, Domagala P, Kwiatkowski A, et al: The assessment of residual kidney function after living donor nephrectomy. Transplant Proc 41(1):91–92, 2009 19249485

Billioti de Gage S, Collin C, Le-Tri T, et al: Antidepressants and hepatotoxicity: a cohort study among 5 million individuals registered in the French National Health Insurance database. CNS Drugs 32(7):673–684, 2018 29959758

Bunzel B, Laederach-Hofmann K: Solid organ transplantation: are there predictors for posttransplant noncompliance? A literature overview. Transplantation 70(5):711–716, 2000 11003346

Campana C, Regazzi MB, Buggia I, et al: Clinically significant drug interactions with cyclosporin: an update. Clin Pharmacokinet 30(2):141–179, 1996 8906896

Campo JV, Smith C, Perel JM: Tacrolimus toxic reaction associated with the use of nefazodone: paroxetine as an alternative agent. Arch Gen Psychiatry 55(11):1050–1052, 1998 9819077

Castellano-Sanchez AA, Li S, Qian J, et al: Primary central nervous system posttransplant lymphoproliferative disorders. Am J Clin Pathol 121(2):246–253, 2004 14983939

Cephalon: Provigil (modafinil) product information. 1998. Available at: www.accessdata.fda.gov/drugsatfda_docs/label/2015/020717s037s038lbl.pdf. Accessed October 5, 2022.

Chabolla DR, Wszolek ZK: Pharmacologic management of seizures in organ transplant. Neurology 67(12 Suppl 4):S34–S38, 2006 17190920

Chick J: Safety issues concerning the use of disulfiram in treating alcohol dependence. Drug Saf 20(5):427–435, 1999 10348093

Collins KK, Thiagarajan RR, Chin C, et al: Atrial tachyarrhythmias and permanent pacing after pediatric heart transplantation. J Heart Lung Transplant 22(10):1126–1133, 2003 14550822

Colman E, Stadel BV: Gabapentin for postherpetic neuralgia. JAMA 282(2):134–135, 1999 10411191

Come CE, Shapiro PA: Supraventricular tachycardia associated with methylphenidate treatment in a heart transplant recipient. Psychosomatics 46(5):461–463, 2005 16145192

Contreras G, Garces G, Quartin AA, et al: An epidemiologic study of early renal replacement therapy after orthotopic liver transplantation. J Am Soc Nephrol 13(1):228–233, 2002 11752042

Cooper JE: Evaluation and treatment of acute rejection in kidney allografts. Clin J Am Soc Nephrol 15(3):430–438, 2020 32066593

Crone CC, Gabriel GM: Treatment of anxiety and depression in transplant patients: pharmacokinetic considerations. Clin Pharmacokinet 43(6):361–394, 2004 15086275

Dahm F, Georgiev P, Clavien PA: Small-for-size syndrome after partial liver transplantation: definition, mechanisms of disease and clinical implications. Am J Transplant 5(11):2605–2610, 2005 16212618

DasGupta K, Jefferson JW: The use of lithium in the medically ill. Gen Hosp Psychiatry 12(2):83–97, 1990 2407615

Davis MP, Frandsen JL, Walsh D, et al: Mirtazapine for pruritus. J Pain Symptom Manage 25(3):288–291, 2003 12614964

Di Maira T, Little EC, Berenguer M: Immunosuppression in liver transplant. Best Pract Res Clin Gastroenterol 46–47:101681, 2020 33158467

DiMartini AF, Dew MA, Trzepacz PT: Organ transplantation, in The American Psychiatric Publishing Textbook of Psychosomatic Medicine. Edited by Levenson J. Washington, DC, American Psychiatric Publishing, 2005, pp 675–700

DiMartini A, Crone C, Fireman M, et al: Psychiatric aspects of organ transplantation in critical care. Crit Care Clin 24(4):949–981, x, 2008 18929948

Edinoff AN, Akuly HA, Wagner JH, et al: Viloxazine in the treatment of attention deficit hyperactivity disorder. Front Psychiatry 12:789982, 2021a 34975586

Edinoff AN, Odisho AS, Lewis K, et al: Brexanolone, a GABA-A modulator in the treatment of post-partum depression in adults: a comprehensive review. Front Psychiatry 12:789982, 2021b 34594247

Erim Y, Beckmann M, Valentin-Gamazo C, et al: Quality of life and psychiatric complications after adult living donor liver transplantation. Liver Transpl 12(12):1782–1790, 2006 17133566

Erim Y, Beckmann M, Kroencke S, et al: Psychological strain in urgent indications for living donor liver transplantation. Liver Transpl 13(6):886–895, 2007 17539009

Fireman M, DiMartini AF, Armstrong SC, et al: Immunosuppressants. Psychosomatics 45(4):354–360, 2004 15232051

Fukunishi I, Sugawara Y, Takayama T, et al: Psychiatric disorders before and after living-related transplantation. Psychosomatics 42(4):337–343, 2001 11496023

Funk MC, Beach SR, Bostwick JR, et al: QTc prolongation and psychotropic medications. Am J Psychiatry 177(3):273–274, 2020 32114782

Fusar-Poli P, Picchioni M, Martinelli V, et al: Anti-depressive therapies after heart transplantation. J Heart Lung Transplant 25(7):785–793, 2006 16818121

Garnock-Jones KP: Vortioxetine: a review of its use in major depressive disorder. CNS Drugs 28(9):855–874, 2014 25145538

Garton T: Nefazodone and cyp450 3a4 interactions with cyclosporine and tacrolimus1 (letter). Transplantation 74(5):745, 2002 12352898

Gottlieb SS, Kop WJ, Thomas SA, et al: A double-blind placebo-controlled pilot study of controlled-release paroxetine on depression and quality of life in chronic heart failure. Am Heart J 153(5):868–873, 2007 17452166

Haroldson JA, Kramer LE, Wolff DL, et al: Elevated free fractions of valproic acid in a heart transplant patient with hypoalbuminemia. Ann Pharmacother 34(2):183–187, 2000 10676827

Health Resources and Services Administration Division of Transplantation: Organ Donation and Transplantation Dashboard. Health Resources and Services Administration, Healthcare Systems Bureau, Division of Transplantation, 2022. Available at: https://data.hrsa.gov/topics/health-systems/organ-donation. Accessed January 15, 2022.

Hebert MF, Wacher VJ, Roberts JP, et al: Pharmacokinetics of cyclosporine pre- and post-liver transplantation. J Clin Pharmacol 43(1):38–42, 2003 12520626

Helms-Smith KM, Curtis SL, Hatton RC: Apparent interaction between nefazodone and cyclosporine (letter). Ann Intern Med 125(5):424, 1996 8702104

Indiana University Division of Clinical Pharmacology: Drug Interactions Flockhart Table. 2022. Available at: https://drug-interactions.medicine.iu.edu/MainTable.aspx. Accessed February 10, 2022.

Jain A, Venkataramanan R, Sharma R, et al: Pharmacokinetics of mycophenolic acid in live donor liver transplant patients vs deceased donor liver transplant patients. J Clin Pharmacol 48(5):547–552, 2008 18440919

Jiao M, Greanya ED, Haque M, et al: Methadone maintenance therapy in liver transplantation. Prog Transplant 20(3):209–214, quiz 215, 2010 20929104

Jochum C, Beste M, Penndorf V, et al: Quantitative liver function tests in donors and recipients of living donor liver transplantation. Liver Transpl 12(4):544–549, 2006 16482561

Kalender B, Ozdemir AC, Yalug I, et al: Antidepressant treatment increases quality of life in patients with chronic renal failure. Ren Fail 29(7):817–822, 2007 17994449

Kay J, Bienenfeld D, Slomowitz M, et al: Use of tricyclic antidepressants in recipients of heart transplants. Psychosomatics 32(2):165–170, 1991 2027938

Kemmer N, Secic M, Zacharias V, et al: Long-term analysis of primary nonfunction in liver transplant recipients. Transplant Proc 39(5):1477–1480, 2007 17580166

Kershner P, Wang-Cheng R: Psychiatric side effects of steroid therapy. Psychosomatics 30(2):135–139, 1989 2652177

Kim J, Phongsamran P, Park S: Use of antidepressant drugs in transplant recipients. Prog Transplant 14(2):98–104, 2004 15264454

Koo JR, Yoon JY, Joo MH, et al: Treatment of depression and effect of antidepression treatment on nutritional status in chronic hemodialysis patients. Am J Med Sci 329(1):1–5, 2005 15654172

Krahn LE, DiMartini A: Psychiatric and psychosocial aspects of liver transplantation. Liver Transpl 11(10):1157–1168, 2005 16184540

Kranick SM, Mowry EM, Rosenfeld MR: Progressive multifocal leukoencephalopathy after rituximab in a case of non-Hodgkin lymphoma. Neurology 69(7):704–706, 2007 17698796

Lacasse Y, Beaudoin L, Rousseau L, et al: Randomized trial of paroxetine in end-stage COPD. Monaldi Arch Chest Dis 61(3):140–147, 2004 15679006

Lake JR: Liver transplantation, in Current Diagnosis and Treatment in Gastroenterology, 2nd Edition. Edited by Friedman S. New York, McGraw Hill, 2003, pp 813–834

Levenson JL: High-dose intravenous haloperidol for agitated delirium following lung transplantation. Psychosomatics 36(1):66–68, 1995 7871137

Lill J, Bauer LA, Horn JR, et al: Cyclosporine-drug interactions and the influence of patient age. Am J Health Syst Pharm 57(17):1579–1584, 2000 10984808

Liston HL, Markowitz JS, Hunt N, et al: Lack of citalopram effect on the pharmacokinetics of cyclosporine. Psychosomatics 42(4):370–372, 2001 11496034

Madhusoodanan S, Velama U, Parmar J, et al: A current review of cytochrome P450 interactions of psychotropic drugs. Ann Clin Psychiatry 26(2):120–138, 2014 24812650

Magee CC: Pharmacology and side effects of cyclosporine and tacrolimus. UpToDate, March 29, 2006. Available at: www.uptodate.com/contents/pharmacology-and-side-effects-of-cyclosporine-and-tacrolimus?source=search_result&search=pharmacology+of+cyclosporine+and+tacrolimus&selectedTitle=1%7E150. Accessed April 29, 2016.

Markowitz JS, Gill HS, Hunt NM, et al: Lack of antidepressant-cyclosporine pharmacokinetic interactions. J Clin Psychopharmacol 18(1):91–93, 1998 9472853

Masand P, Pickett P, Murray GB: Psychostimulants for secondary depression in medical illness. Psychosomatics 32(2):203–208, 1991 2027944

Mayo MJ, Handem I, Saldana S, et al: Sertraline as a first-line treatment for cholestatic pruritus. Hepatology 45(3):666–674, 2007 17326161

McIntyre RS, Soczynska JK, Konarski JZ, et al: The effect of antidepressants on lipid homeostasis: a cardiac safety concern? Expert Opin Drug Saf 5(4):523–537, 2006 16774491

McIntyre RS, Panjwani ZD, Nguyen HT, et al: The hepatic safety profile of duloxetine: a review. Expert Opin Drug Metab Toxicol 4(3):281–285, 2008 18363543

McIntyre RS, Rosenblat JD, Nemeroff CB, et al: Synthesizing the evidence for ketamine and esketamine in treatment-resistant depression: an international expert opinion on available evidence and implementation. Am J Psychiatry 178(5):383–399, 2021 33726522

Meissner K, Blood J, Francis AM, et al: Cyclosporine-inhibitable cerebral drug transport does not influence clinical methadone pharmacodynamics. Anesthesiology 121(6):1281–1291, 2014 25072223

Michaels PJ, Espejo ML, Kobashigawa J, et al: Humoral rejection in cardiac transplantation: risk factors, hemodynamic consequences and relationship to transplant coronary artery disease. J Heart Lung Transplant 22(1):58–69, 2003 12531414

Mintzer S, Boppana P, Toguri J, et al: Vitamin D levels and bone turnover in epilepsy patients taking carbamazepine or oxcarbazepine. Epilepsia 47(3):510–515, 2006 16529614

Molnar MZ, Novak M, Mucsi I: Management of restless legs syndrome in patients on dialysis. Drugs 66(5):607–624, 2006 16620140

Mufson JM: Lamotrigine: pharmacology, clinical utility and new safety concerns. Am J Psychiatry Resid J 13(12):2–4, 2018

Nadalin S, Testa G, Malagó M, et al: Volumetric and functional recovery of the liver after right hepatectomy for living donation. Liver Transpl 10(8):1024–1029, 2004 15390329

Naini AE, Harandi AA, Khanbabapour S, et al: Gabapentin: a promising drug for the treatment of uremic pruritus. Saudi J Kidney Dis Transpl 18(3):378–381, 2007 17679749

Najarian JS, Chavers BM, McHugh LE, et al: 20 years or more of follow-up of living kidney donors. Lancet 340(8823):807–810, 1992 1357243

National Library of Medicine: DailyMed. 2015. Available at: https://dailymed.nlm.nih.gov/dailymed. Accessed July 4, 2016.

Ojo AO, Held PJ, Port FK, et al: Chronic renal failure after transplantation of a non-renal organ. N Engl J Med 349(10):931–940, 2003 12954741

Overman GP, Teter CJ, Guthrie SK: Acamprosate for the adjunctive treatment of alcohol dependence. Ann Pharmacother 37(7–8):1090–1099, 2003 12841823

Pacher P, Kecskemeti V: Cardiovascular side effects of new antidepressants and antipsychotics: new drugs, old concerns? Curr Pharm Des 10(20):2463–2475, 2004 15320756

Pae CU, Lim HK, Han C, et al: Selegiline transdermal system: current awareness and promise. Prog Neuropsychopharmacol Biol Psychiatry 31(6):1153–1163, 2007 17614182

Parés A: Old and novel therapies for primary biliary cirrhosis. Semin Liver Dis 34(3):341–351, 2014 25057957

Pascussi JM, Gerbal-Chaloin S, Drocourt L, et al: The expression of CYP2B6, CYP2C9 and CYP3A4 genes: a tangle of networks of nuclear and steroid receptors. Biochim Biophys Acta 1619(3):243–253, 2003 12573484

Pescovitz MD, Navarro MT: Immunosuppressive therapy and post-transplantation diarrhea. Clin Transplant 15(Suppl 4):23–28, 2001 11778784

Plutchik L, Snyder S, Drooker M, et al: Methylphenidate in post liver transplant patients. Psychosomatics 39(2):118–123, 1998 9584537

Potkin SG, Kunovac J, Silverman BL, et al: Efficacy and safety of a combination of olanzapine and samidorphan in adult patients with an acute exacerbation of schizophrenia: outcomes from the randomized phase 3 ENLIGHTEN-1 study. J Clin Psychiatry 81(2):e1–e9, 2020 32141723

Reynaud-Gaubert M, Viard L, Girault D, et al: Improved absorption and bioavailability of cyclosporine A from a microemulsion formulation in lung transplant recipients affected with cystic fibrosis. Transplant Proc 29(5):2450–2453, 1997 9270807

Robinson BL, Dumas M, Ali SF, et al: Cyclosporine exacerbates ketamine toxicity in zebrafish: mechanistic studies on drug-drug interaction. J Appl Toxicol 37(12):1438–1447, 2017 28569378

Rösche J, Fröscher W, Abendroth D, et al: Possible oxcarbazepine interaction with cyclosporine serum levels: a single case study. Clin Neuropharmacol 24(2):113–116, 2001 11307049

Rush D, Nickerson P, Gough J, et al: Beneficial effects of treatment of early subclinical rejection: a randomized study. J Am Soc Nephrol 9(11):2129–2134, 1998 9808101

Saivin S, Hulot T, Chabac S, et al: Clinical pharmacokinetics of acamprosate. Clin Pharmacokinet 35(5):331–345, 1998 9839087

Schatzberg AF, DeBattista C: Manual of Clinical Psychopharmacology, 8th Edition. Washington, DC, American Psychiatric Publishing, 2015

Scott LJ: Levomilnacipran extended-release: a review of its use in adult patients with major depressive disorder. CNS Drugs 28(11):1071–1082, 2014 25270036

Serebruany VL, Glassman AH, Malinin AI, et al: Selective serotonin reuptake inhibitors yield additional antiplatelet protection in patients with congestive heart failure treated with antecedent aspirin. Eur J Heart Fail 5(4):517–521, 2003 12921813

Shapiro R, Randhawa P, Jordan ML, et al: An analysis of early renal transplant protocol biopsies—the high incidence of subclinical tubulitis. Am J Transplant 1(1):47–50, 2001 12095037

Shaw LM, Mick R, Nowak I, et al: Pharmacokinetics of mycophenolic acid in renal transplant patients with delayed graft function. J Clin Pharmacol 38(3):268–275, 1998 9549665

Shoskes DA, Cecka JM: Deleterious effects of delayed graft function in cadaveric renal transplant recipients independent of acute rejection. Transplantation 66(12):1697–1701, 1998 9884262

Silvertooth EJ, Doraiswamy PM, Clary GL, et al: Citalopram and quality of life in lung transplant recipients. Psychosomatics 45(3):271–272, 2004 15123855

Strouse TB, Fairbanks LA, Skotzko CE, et al: Fluoxetine and cyclosporine in organ transplantation: failure to detect significant drug interactions or adverse clinical events in depressed organ recipients. Psychosomatics 37(1):23–30, 1996 8600490

Thomsen K, Schou M: Avoidance of lithium intoxication: advice based on knowledge about the renal lithium clearance under various circumstances. Pharmacopsychiatry 32(3):83–86, 1999 10463373

Tombazzi CR, Waters B, Shokouh-Amiri MH, et al: Neuropsychiatric complications after liver transplantation: role of immunosuppression and hepatitis C. Dig Dis Sci 51(6):1079–1081, 2006 16865574

Tripathi A, Panzer MJ: Cyclosporine psychosis. Psychosomatics 34(1):101–102, 1993 8426884

Tucker ON, Heaton N: The "small for size" liver syndrome. Curr Opin Crit Care 11(2):150–155, 2005 15758596

Tutor-Crespo MJ, Hermida J, Tutor JC: Relative proportions of serum carbamazepine and its pharmacologically active 10,11-epoxy derivative: effect of polytherapy and renal insufficiency. Ups J Med Sci 113(2):171–180, 2008 18509811

U.S. Renal Data System: USRDS 2008 annual data report: atlas of chronic kidney disease and end-stage renal disease in the United States. National Institutes of Health, National Institute of Diabetes and Digestive and Kidney Diseases, 2008. Available at: www.usrds.org/atlas08.aspx. Accessed July 14, 2016.

Vincent HH, Wenting GJ, Schalekamp MA, et al: Impaired fractional excretion of lithium: a very early marker of cyclosporine nephrotoxicity. Transplant Proc 19(5):4147–4148, 1987 3314004

Wagena EJ, Knipschild PG, Huibers MJ, et al: Efficacy of bupropion and nortriptyline for smoking cessation among people at risk for or with chronic obstructive pulmonary disease. Arch Intern Med 165(19):2286–2292, 2005 16246996

Wang PW, Ketter TA: Pharmacokinetics of mood stabilizers and new anticonvulsants. Psychopharmacol Bull 36(1):44–66, 2002 12397847

Wang SM, Han C, Lee SJ, et al: Vilazodone for the treatment of major depressive disorder: focusing on its clinical studies and mechanism of action. Psychiatry Investig 12(2):155–163, 2015 25866514

Warrington JS, Greenblatt DJ, Von Moltke LL: Role of CYP3A enzymes in the biotransformation of triazolam in rat liver. Xenobiotica 34(5):463–471, 2004 15370962

Weinrieb RM, Van Horn DH, McLellan AT, et al: Alcoholism treatment after liver transplantation: lessons learned from a clinical trial that failed. Psychosomatics 42(2):110–116, 2001 11239123

Weinrieb RM, Auriacombe M, Lynch KG, et al: A critical review of selective serotonin reuptake inhibitor-associated bleeding: balancing the risk of treating hepatitis C-infected patients. J Clin Psychiatry 64(12):1502–1510, 2003 14728113

Weinrieb RM, Barnett R, Lynch KG, et al: A matched comparison study of medical and psychiatric complications and anesthesia and analgesia requirements in methadone-maintained liver transplant recipients. Liver Transpl 10(1):97–106, 2004 14755785

Weinrieb RM, Auriacombe M, Lynch KG, et al: Selective serotonin re-uptake inhibitors and the risk of bleeding. Expert Opin Drug Saf 4(2):337–344, 2005 15794724

Wong MO, Eldon MA, Keane WF, et al: Disposition of gabapentin in anuric subjects on hemodialysis. J Clin Pharmacol 35(6):622–626, 1995 7665723

Wright DH, Lake KD, Bruhn PS, et al: Nefazodone and cyclosporine drug-drug interaction. J Heart Lung Transplant 18(9):913–915, 1999 10528754

Xu S, Cui Y, Shen J, et al: Suvorexant for the prevention of delirium: a meta-analysis. Medicine (Baltimore) 99(30):e21043, 2020 32791676

Yalcin AU, Sahin G, Erol M, et al: Sertraline hydrochloride treatment for patients with hemodialysis hypotension. Blood Purif 20(2):150–153, 2002 11818677

Zafar MN, Jawad F, Aziz T, et al: Donor follow-up in living-related renal transplantation. Transplant Proc 34(6):2443–2444, 2002 12270473

Zuin M, Giorgini A, Selmi C, et al: Acute liver and renal failure during treatment with buprenorphine at therapeutic dose. Dig Liver Dis 41(7):e8–e10, 2009 18294936

17

Pain Management

Christina M. van der Feltz-Cornelis, M.D., Ph.D.

James L. Levenson, M.D.

According to the Global Burden of Disease Study, pain is globally the most commonly reported symptom, with low back pain and migraine as the leading causes of years lost to disabilities in 2016, contributing 57.6 million (7.2%) and 45.1 million (5.6%) of total years lost, respectively (GBD 2016 Disease and Injury Incidence and Prevalence Collaborators 2017). This is more than the total affected by cancer, heart disease, and diabetes combined in the United States (Institute of Medicine 2011). Both acute and chronic pain are associated with depression and anxiety (de Heer et al. 2014, 2018), and based on clinical experience, up to 40% of psychiatric patients use over-the-counter painkillers without their psychiatrist's knowledge. Impairments in multiple quality-of-life and functional domains lead to sickness absence from work and are highly costly, making the treatment of pain a major personal and public health concern (Coggon et al. 2012). Nevertheless, evidence indicates that undertreatment occurs (Bonnewyn et al. 2009).

Clinically, pain can be divided into neuropathic, nociceptive, and mixed pain. Examples of neuropathic pain include painful polyneuropathies and postherpetic neuralgia (Johnson and Rice 2014), trigeminal neuralgia, and complex regional pain syndrome (CRPS), for which tricyclic and other antidepressants as well as anticonvulsants have been studied extensively. Nociceptive pain can be musculoskeletal (e.g., low back pain) or visceral in nature (e.g., irritable bowel syndrome). Fibromyalgia is an example of mixed pain.

Opioids have been prescribed for chronic noncancer pain management (Department of Veterans Affairs and Department of Defense 2010) based on adoption of the World Health Organization pain ladder, which was originally developed for treatment of cancer pain in 1986 (Ventafridda et al. 1985). However, this emphasis on prescription of opioids has been a major factor in the development of an epidemic of opioid addiction and drug overdose deaths (Volkow and McLellan 2016). New guidelines advise monitoring opioid addiction risk from the start of treatment and using nonopioid medications, such as antidepressants and anticonvulsants, that were originally considered optional adjuvant medication in the World Health Organization guideline (Miller 2004), if possible. They also recommend focusing on physical exercise and psychological treatment, such as cognitive-behavioral therapy (Dowell et al. 2016).

Psychiatric Comorbidity

Somatic Symptom Disorder With Pain

In DSM-5's somatic symptom disorder, basing diagnosis on the absence of a medical explanation of somatic symptoms was abandoned in favor of the presence of significant distress in relation to the somatic symptom, whether it exists in the context of a known medical condition or not (American Psychiatric Association 2013). One subclassification is somatic symptom disorder with pain, which occurs in approximately 15% of somatic symptom disorder cases and is associated with elevated biomarkers such as interleukin-6 and high-sensitivity C-reactive protein (Van der Feltz-Cornelis et al. 2020). Loneliness, social isolation, and childhood abuse are associated with acute and chronic pain (Allen et al. 2020; Blyth et al. 2007). It is well known that social rejection is associated with emotional pain. Brain regions that show a significant change in activation following a rejection stimulus include cortical regions such as the cingulate, insular, orbitofrontal, and prefrontal cortex and subcortical regions such as the angular gyrus, hippocampus, striatum, tegmental area, and temporal pole. These regions correspond to pain, distress, and memory retrieval; reward, romantic love, and dopaminergic circuits; and emotion regulation and behavioral adaptation (van der Watt et al. 2021). Physical injury and social rejection activate similar brain centers. Many patients who use opioid medications long term for the treatment of chronic pain have both physical and social pain, and these medications may produce a state of persistent opioid dependence that suppresses the endogenous opioid system that is essential for human socialization and reward processing (Sullivan and Ballantyne 2021). Psychological and physical domains interrelate and can cause significant decreases in quality of life regardless of the etiology of the pain (Rief and Martin 2014).

Substance Use

The prevalence of substance dependence or addiction in patients with chronic pain ranges from 3% to 48% depending on the population sampled, and 60% of patients admitted taking more than prescribed (Setnik et al. 2017). The core criteria for a substance use disorder in patients with chronic pain include the loss of control in the use of the medication, excessive preoccupation with the medication despite adequate analgesia, and adverse consequences associated with its use. Persistent pain can lead to increased focus on opioid medications and measures to ensure an adequate medication supply. Patients understandably fear the reemergence of pain and withdrawal symptoms if they run out of medication. Drug-seeking behavior may be the result of an anxious patient trying to maintain a previous level of pain control. However, opiate prescriptions have increased dramatically in recent decades, and unlike in cancer treatment, it has emerged that opioid use disorder can occur in patients who began taking opioids for treatment of chronic pain. Therefore, serious efforts should be made to avoid or reduce opiate prescription in chronic noncancer pain.

Integrating care for chronic pain with innovative stepped-care models of substance abuse treatment would probably improve outcomes by tailoring the intensity of treatment to the individual patient's needs (Haibach et al. 2014).

Depression and Suicidality

Pain is a risk factor for the development of common mental disorders. Moderate to very severe pain more than doubles the risk of developing mood or anxiety disorders (de Heer et al. 2018). Chronic pain is commonly comorbid with a depressive or anxiety disorder, with pain severity and associated disability strongly associated with severity of depressive and anxiety symptoms. Even after remission of depressive or anxiety disorders, disabling and severely limiting pain occurs more than three times more often than in people who never had a depressive or anxiety disorder. This difference was greatest in chest pain rather than in gastrointestinal or musculoskeletal pain, but the chest pain was not related to cardiorespiratory illness (de Heer et al. 2014). Pain and the disability that comes with it increase the risk for suicidal ideation, and this occurs in the context of depressive comorbidity but also independently. Therefore, exploration of suicidality in relation to pain should be part of the clinical examination of patients with pain (de Heer et al. 2018; Lerman et al. 2015).

Among the vegetative and somatic symptoms of depression, pain is second only to insomnia (Bras et al. 2010). Depression with comorbid pain is more resistant to treatment, but pain often subsides with improvement in depressive symptoms (Kroenke et al. 2008). In addition to having greater efficacy for the treatment of neuropathic pain, serotonin-norepinephrine reuptake inhibitors (SNRIs) and tricyclic antidepressants (TCAs) are associated with higher rates of improvement and lower rates of relapse than selective serotonin reuptake inhibitors (SSRIs) (Cohen and Mao 2014).

Anxiety, Fear, Catastrophizing, Anger, and Sleep

Patients with chronic pain syndromes have higher rates of both anxiety symptoms and anxiety disorders, such as generalized anxiety disorder, panic disorder, agoraphobia, and PTSD (Outcalt et al. 2015). Fear of pain, movement, reinjury, and other negative consequences that result in the avoidance of activities promotes the transition to and sustaining of chronic pain and its associated disabilities, such as muscular reactivity, deconditioning, and guarded movement. This restriction of activities can result in physiological changes, such as weight gain and muscle atrophy, that can lead to functional deterioration. In fibromyalgia, patients who think treatment of their illness will not be effective are at increased risk for more anxiety symptoms. Strengthening beliefs that treatment can help and reducing catastrophic thinking therefore seem crucial in the treatment of fibromyalgia (de Heer et al. 2017).

Addressing anxiety is also of paramount importance in pain due to known medical conditions. Anxiety plays a prominent role in patients with coronary heart disease and chest pain, with chest pain inducing anxiety more than depression. Treatment of patients with coronary heart disease and chest pain should aim to deconstruct potentially catastrophic cognitions and strengthen emotional coping (de Heer et al. 2020).

Ample evidence also indicates that pain and poor sleep commonly occur together, although the direction of causality in their association remains unclear (Wong and Fielding 2012). Sleep impairments have been shown to reliably predict exacerbations of chronic pain better than pain predicts sleep disturbances, however. It is likely that sleep disturbances adversely affect key processes in the development and maintenance of chronic pain, but further research is needed to elucidate the underlying mechanisms (Finan et al. 2013). Treating the sleep disturbance may improve pain control (Alföldi et al. 2014).

Pain Description and Management

The painDETECT questionnaire can be used to prepare medication treatment by classifying the pain as nociceptive, neuropathic, or mixed pain. It was specifically validated for this purpose in patients with low back pain and showed good sensitivity and specificity (Freynhagen et al. 2006). A summative score for nine items can range from 1 to 38. A score of 19 or higher indicates that a neuropathic pain component is likely. In the case of a score of 12 or less, nociceptive pain is more likely. A score of 13–18 is classified as mixed pain.

Pain Plus Depression

Acute Pain

Acute pain is usually the result of trauma from surgery, injury, or exacerbation of chronic disease, especially musculoskeletal conditions. Acute pain management is usually successful with straightforward strategies such as relaxation; immobilization; analgesics such as nonsteroidal anti-inflammatory drugs (NSAIDs), acetaminophen, and opioids; and massage. Acute pain management initiated as early as possible and focused on preventing the occurrence and reemergence of pain may allow for lower total dosages of analgesics. The absence of signs consistent with acute pain, such as elevated heart rate, elevated blood pressure, and diaphoresis, does not rule out the presence of pain.

Analgesics, especially opioids, should be prescribed only for pain relief. Although analgesia may produce other benefits, symptoms commonly coinciding with acute pain, such as insomnia or anxiety, should be managed separately from pain. Sleep deprivation and anxiety may intensify the sensation of pain and increase requests for more medication. Reducing anxiety and insomnia often reduces analgesic needs. In acute pain management, psychiatric consultation is requested when a patient needs more analgesia than expected or has a history of substance abuse. Patients with an active or recent history of opioid addiction and those receiving methadone maintenance therapy have increased tolerance to opioids and may need opioid doses up to 50% higher. Adequate treatment of acute pain is a priority, and opioids may be needed for that; however, opioid use should be carefully monitored, preferably provided only for the expected duration of the acute pain episode, and followed by guided tapering and replacement with other pain medication if some pain relief is still needed. Inadequate dosing is significantly more common than abuse or diversion. Dosage should be carefully individualized rather than based on preconceived expectations.

Selected Chronic Pain Conditions

Neuropathic Pain

Postherpetic neuralgia.   Postherpetic neuralgia is pain, often described as burning, stabbing, or throbbing, that persists or recurs at the site of shingles at least 3 months after an acute varicella zoster rash. Postherpetic neuralgia occurs in about 10% of patients with acute herpes zoster; occurs in more than 50% of patients older than 65 who have shingles; and is more likely in people with cancer, diabetes, or immunosuppression. It occurs in less than 6% of immunocompetent people, however (Johnson and Rice 2014). Approximately 8.2% of hospital admissions are for the treatment of postherpetic neuralgia (Cocchio et al. 2019).

TCAs, anticonvulsants (e.g., carbamazepine, valproic acid, pregabalin, gabapentin), and opioids are the most common effective treatments for postherpetic neuralgia and may have potential for its prevention. Amitriptyline, gabapentin, and pregabalin provide pain relief in 50%–60% of patients with postherpetic neuralgia (Panickar and Serpell 2015), and a 5% lidocaine patch is approved for postherpetic neuralgia (Derry et al. 2014). Unless otherwise contraindicated, TCAs should be the first choice for treating postherpetic neuralgia, followed by gabapentin or pregabalin (Moore et al. 2014). There are no clinical trials of SNRIs for postherpetic neuralgia. Unfortunately, opioids continue to be prescribed more often than other agents (Gudin et al. 2019). Gabapentin was not effective in prevention of neuralgia in acute shingles (Bulilete et al. 2019).

Diabetic peripheral neuropathy pain.   Up to 90% of patients with diabetes mellitus experience painful diabetic neuropathy, with duration of illness and poor glycemic control as contributing risk factors (Schreiber et al. 2015). This pain is described as constant burning to episodic, paroxysmal, and lancinating in quality and results from axonal degeneration and segmental demyelination. First-line pharmacological treatments for diabetic peripheral neuropathy pain include TCAs, SNRIs, and calcium channel modulating anticonvulsants (Sloan et al. 2021), which appear to be of comparable efficacy (Snedecor et al. 2014). Other anticonvulsants have been shown to be effective in smaller studies. Experimental and clinical evidence have shown that opioids can be helpful in pain control as well if used as an adjuvant to first-line treatments (Schreiber et al. 2015).

Central poststroke pain and spinal cord injury.   Pain is common following stroke (8% of patients) or spinal cord trauma (60%–70% of patients). Symptoms of spinal cord injury pain or central poststroke pain are often poorly localized, vary over time, and include allodynia (>50% of patients with central poststroke pain), hyperalgesia, dysesthesias, and muscle and visceral pain regardless of sensory deficits. Pain is described as burning, aching, lancinating, or pricking.

Central poststroke pain is difficult to treat; conventional analgesics and opioids have been shown to be ineffective (Scuteri et al. 2020). Based on current evidence, amitriptyline, lamotrigine, and gabapentinoids should be used as first-line pharmacotherapy for central poststroke pain. Other agents, such as fluvoxamine, steroids, and intravenous infusions of lidocaine, ketamine, or propofol, can be considered in severe treatment-resistant cases (Choi et al. 2021). One small open-label trial showed some potential benefit from duloxetine (Kim et al. 2019). Intravenous lidocaine may be the most efficacious agent, but the need for intravenous administration limits its use. Topical lidocaine may be beneficial for some patients (Hans et al. 2008). Magnetic stimulation and invasive electrical stimulation also have been shown to be effective for carefully selected patients (Flaster et al. 2013).

Trigeminal neuralgia.   Trigeminal neuralgia (tic douloureux) is a chronic pain syndrome with a prevalence of about 0.015% (Montano et al. 2015). It is characterized by severe, paroxysmal, recurrent, lancinating pain with a unilateral distribution of cranial nerve V, most commonly the mandibular division. Sensory or motor deficits are not usually present. Less commonly, the facial or glossopharyngeal nerve is involved, with pain distribution to the ear, posterior pharynx, tongue, or larynx. Episodes of pain can be spontaneous or evoked by nonpainful stimuli to trigger zones, activities such as talking or chewing, or environmental conditions. Between episodes, patients are typically pain free. Uncontrolled pain with frequent or severe prolonged attacks increases the risk of insomnia, weight loss, social withdrawal, anxiety, panic attacks, and depression, including suicide.

Carbamazepine is the first-line agent for pharmacotherapy for trigeminal neuralgia and the only medication whose use is supported by multiple controlled trials. Oxcarbazepine is a reasonable first-line alternative with comparable efficacy. For nonresponders, lamotrigine, gabapentin, pregabalin, botulinum toxin type A, baclofen, and phenytoin may be used as monotherapy or as adjuncts, but the evidence for these is weak (Bendtsen et al. 2019). Given the pathophysiological similarities of trigeminal neuralgia with postherpetic neuralgia and painful peripheral neuropathies, other medications such as the TCAs and SNRIs seem appropriate to consider, but no clinical trials have been reported. For refractory cases, microvascular surgical decompression, ablation, and neuromodulation therapies are options (Bendtsen et al. 2019).

Complex regional pain syndrome.   *CRPS* is a broad term describing excess and prolonged pain and inflammation that follows an injury to an arm or leg or cause of immobilization, often with hyperalgesia or allodynia to cutaneous stimuli. CRPS has acute (recent, short-term) and chronic (lasting more than 6 months) forms. CRPS used to be known as reflex sympathetic dystrophy or causalgia. Other symptoms include changes in skin color or temperature and swelling on the arm or leg below the site of injury. CRPS is more common in women but can occur in anyone at any age, with a peak around age 40. It is rare in older adults, who have less inflammation after injury, and in young children. Although CRPS improves over time, eventually going away in most people, the rare severe or prolonged cases are profoundly disabling. The prognosis also depends on any underlying pathology that affects general nerve health, such as diabetes or conditions affecting circulation. Smoking affects the outcome adversely (National Institute of Neurological Disorders and Stroke 2021). Most CRPS illnesses are caused by improper function of the peripheral C-fiber nerve fibers that carry pain messages to the brain. Their excess firing triggers inflammation designed to promote healing and rest after injury. In some people, the nerve injury is obvious, but for others a specialist may be needed to locate and treat the injury. Poor circulation can impede nerve and tissue healing. Blood vessels in the affected limb can dilate to leak fluid into the surrounding tissue, causing red, swollen skin. This can deprive underlying muscles and deeper tissues of oxygen and nutrients, which can cause muscle weakness and joint pain. When skin blood vessels overconstrict, the skin becomes cold and white, gray, or bluish. CRPS develops in the limbs because circulation is constrained there. Breaking the cycle by reducing limb swelling and restoring circulation is often the key that permits recovery to begin. The affected limb should be kept elevated when resting or sleeping in order to help excess fluid to return to the heart; the patient should exercise every day (these do not have to be long exercise sessions) to improve circulation and oxygenation and use compression stockings and sleeves (National Institute of Neurological Disorders and Stroke 2021). Motor neglect is a common complication in CRPS. It is a potentially reversible condition that includes a loss of function without a loss of strength, reflexes, or sensation, with a presumed mechanism of learned nonuse and resulting cortical remapping of motor areas.

Regarding treatment, intensive rehabilitation is the current gold standard and includes mirror therapy, motor imagery, desensitization, and graded return to activities to improve function and reverse cortical changes (Zangrandi et al. 2021). A new development is to provide such training by gait training and virtual imagery (De Keersmaecker et al. 2019). This is a form of virtual mirror therapy where the patient walks on a treadmill and sees a full-body graphic rendering of themselves walking in real time in a virtual environment in front of them on a large patient-facing screen (de Villiers et al. 2021).

Treatment also includes psychotherapy, to address any psychological sequelae, and pharmacotherapy. Symptoms often improve with NSAIDs or corticosteroids in the acute, or inflammatory, stage of the disease. Evidence suggests efficacy for gabapentin, carbamazepine, TCAs, and opioids. Increased risk for substance use disorders limits the use of opioids to prescribing contingent on functional improvement; currently, extensive research to find alternative treatments to opioids for pain reduction is ongoing (National Institutes of Health 2019). Randomized controlled trials (RCTs) of calcitonin and bisphosphonates for CRPS found reduced pain and improved joint mobility (National Institute of Neurological Disorders and Stroke 2021). As a last step, invasive procedures should be limited to selected cases and considered only after psychosomatic assessment.

Phantom limb pain.   Feeling pain in a body part that has actually been removed is a common occurrence and can occur in limbs or after mastectomy (Björkman et al. 2017). It can gradually fade away; however, it can also become a lifelong debilitating chronic pain syndrome, leading to sleep deprivation, depression, and suicidality, and can be unresponsive to traditional combinations of strong opioids, adjuvant pain medications, antidepressants, local anesthetics, nerve stimulators, hypnotics, and psychotropics. Drug treatment is seldom more effective than placebo (Srejic and Banimahd 2021). However, morphine, tramadol, gabapentin, calcitonin, intramuscular botulinum toxin, and ketamine have been shown to reduce phantom pain in controlled studies (McCormick et al. 2014). A recent case description of a successful treatment of a difficult 2-year-long treatment-resistant case with sublingual buprenorphine/naloxone suggests that although traditional escalating pure μ opioid receptor agonists and adjuvant neuropathic pain combinations often have disappointing efficacy in the treatment of resistant phantom limb pain, the combination of buprenorphine and naloxone has a potent combination of mechanisms of action: potent long-acting μ agonist/antagonist, κ-receptor antagonist, δ-receptor antagonist, and novel opioid receptor-like 1 agonist effects (Srejic and Banimahd 2021). This anecdotal finding warrants further research; however, nonpharmacological interventions may be more promising.

A systematic review of 10 RCTs evaluating treatments found that repetitive transcranial magnetic stimulation and transcranial direct current stimulation were effective therapies to reduce pain perception, anxiety, and depression symptoms in patients with phantom limb pain (Garcia-Pallero et al. 2022). However, the value of deep brain stimulation and motor cortex stimulation remains controversial. Another systematic review of 142 RCTs found only strong evidence for imagery-based therapies as well (Hyung and Wiseman-Hakes 2022).

Headache

Migraine.   Approximately 90% of the U.S. population will develop a headache within their lifetime, and headache disorders account for more disability-adjusted life-years than all other neurological disorders combined. Among primary headache disorders, the two most common are migraine and tension-type headache, with migraine identified as the most disabling (Goetz et al. 2022).

About 18% of women and 6% of men have migraines, with peak incidence between ages 30 and 40. Common migraine is a unilateral pulsatile headache, which may be associated with other symptoms such as nausea, vomiting, photophobia, and phonophobia. The classic form of migraine adds visual prodromal symptoms (National Institute for Health and Care Excellence 2021a). A systematic review showed that fixed-dose combinations of aspirin, paracetamol (acetaminophen), and caffeine were more than twice as effective as placebo in alleviating pain within 2 hours (Diener et al. 2022).

Placebo-controlled clinical trials suggest the use of NSAIDs and triptans for acute treatment of migraine attacks and propranolol, metoprolol, flunarizine, valproate, topiramate, and TCAs as prophylactic agents (National Institute for Health and Care Excellence 2021c). For chronic migraine (headache occurring on 15 or more days per month for more than 3 months), topiramate, amitriptyline, onabotulinumtoxinA, and cognitive-behavioral therapy have been shown to be effective (Carod-Artal 2014).

In chronic migraine, a new development is the use of the neuropeptide calcitonin gene-related peptide (CGRP) injectables for prevention. CGRP is known to play a central role in the underlying pathophysiology of migraine. In comparison to the effective triptan class of antimigraine treatments, the CGRP antagonists possess comparable efficacy but a superior cardiovascular safety profile (Srinivasan et al. 2022). For example, eptinezumab reduced monthly migraine days by approximately 8 days compared with placebo. More patients who received eptinezumab experienced at least 75% reduction in monthly migraine days compared with placebo, resulting in a number needed to treat (NNT) as low as six, depending on the study population and the dose. The preventive effect was noticed on postinfusion day 1. The most common treatment-emergent adverse events were nausea and fatigue, and the incidence of hypersensitivity or study withdrawal was low (Morgan and Joyner 2021). Discontinuation of the drug because of high costs led to relapse in patients with chronic migraine, suggesting that ongoing administration is needed for prevention (Vernieri et al. 2021).

Chronic daily headache.   Chronic daily headache affects about 5% of the population and includes constant (transformed) migraine, medication overuse headache, chronic tension-type headaches, new-onset daily persistent headache, cluster headache, and hemicrania continua (National Institute for Health and Care Excellence 2021c). Patients with chronic daily headache are more likely to overuse medication, leading to rebound headache; experience psychiatric comorbidity such as depression and anxiety; report functional disability; and experience stress-related headache exacerbations. According to the National Institute for Health and Care Excellence (2021c) guideline, combination aspirin, paracetamol, and caffeine can be a first treatment. Preventive treatment is seldom needed for tension headache, but if prophylaxis is considered necessary, amitriptyline can be effective, initially 10 mg at night, increased if necessary to a maintenance dosage of 50–75 mg at night if no comorbid depressive disorder is present and a maximum of 150 mg at night in the case of comorbid depressive disorder (National Institute for Health and Care Excellence 2021b). Medication overuse headache may be considered if the patient has been taking simple analgesics on 15 or more days a month, or codeine-containing analgesics, ergotamines, or triptans on 10 or more days a month. If so, these drugs should be stopped (abruptly, not gradually) and the headache reassessed 4 weeks later; the patient may need to be warned about temporarily exacerbating headache. Psychological treatments such as cognitive-behavioral therapy and mindfulness-based treatment are effective as well in reduction of primary headache attacks (Lee et al. 2019).

Fibromyalgia

Fibromyalgia is a chronic pain syndrome characterized by widespread musculoskeletal pain in all four limbs and trunk, stiffness, and tender points. These symptoms are usually accompanied by poor sleep, fatigue, and cognitive and gastrointestinal symptoms. Research into the causes of fibromyalgia is ongoing. Current research suggests that fibromyalgia may be a syndrome of dysfunctional central pain processing influenced by a variety of processes, including infection, physical trauma, psychological traits, and psychopathology (Cheng et al. 2022). Several possible causes have been explored, such as diet, inflammation, damage to thinly myelinated and unmyelinated nerve fibers causing small fiber pathology (Karl et al. 2021), physical trauma, menopause (Ozcivit et al. 2021), genetic polymorphism associated with mitochondrial metabolism (Janssen et al. 2021; Martínez-Lara et al. 2020), and psychosocial factors. Placebo-controlled trials suggest pain reduction with gabapentin (Moore et al. 2014), and both amitriptyline and duloxetine are effective in treating pain, fatigue, and sleep problems in patients with fibromyalgia, especially in the case of comorbid depression (de Farias et al. 2020). Exercise (da Silva et al. 2022), aquatic exercise, and infrared light treatment also improve pain (Salm et al. 2019).

Pain in Sickle Cell Disease

Pain is the hallmark of sickle cell disease: more than 50% of the patients report chronic pain (Knisely et al. 2022). Sickle cell pain is mainly nociceptive, resulting from tissue ischemia and microcirculatory vaso-occlusion by sickled or less malleable red blood cells. It may be acute or chronic, with acute painful episodes most often affecting long bones and joints and the lower back. A recent review concluded that continuous administration of intravenous morphine accompanied by oral analgesics, including NSAIDs and acetaminophen, is the most commonly used practice for treating sickle cell disease in patients presenting with a vaso-occlusive pain crisis. Possible effectiveness of tinzaparin, isoxsuprine, and pethidine as therapeutic options may be considered. However, there is no recommendation for a certain agent to be prescribed (Hejazi et al. 2021). Although TCAs and SNRIs are frequently prescribed, no clinical trials have been done in sickle cell disease. The benefits of long-term opioids must be balanced against the risks of addiction (Mo et al. 2021).

Nociceptive Pain

Tissue injury and inflammation trigger the release of local mediators of pain and inflammation, including prostaglandins, serotonin, bradykinin, adenosine, and cytokines. These substances sensitize tissue nociceptors and produce the sensation of pain. Somatic (musculoskeletal) and visceral pain are generally nociceptive in origin but may also have neuropathic elements. Somatic pain is a localized stabbing or sharp pain, whereas visceral pain is diffuse, with aching, pressure, colicky, or sharp qualities. Musculoskeletal pain includes soft tissue injuries, intra-articular disorders, bone pain, muscle pain syndromes, and neck and low-back conditions. Mild to moderate nociceptive pain generally responds to NSAIDs, but severe pain may require opioids. Expert consensus guidelines recommend arthritis education, exercise (particularly aquatic) and dietary management, topical NSAIDs, cyclooxygenase isoenzyme 2 (COX-2) inhibitors, and NSAIDs with proton pump inhibitors for patients without cardiovascular comorbidities and intra-articular corticosteroids or hyaluronic acid for osteoarthritis pain of the knee but not the hip. Acetaminophen/paracetamol and oral and transdermal opioids were not recommended (Bannuru et al. 2019). In addition, duloxetine has been shown to be well tolerated and effective in treating osteoarthritis knee pain in both younger and older adults (Risser et al. 2013). As a new development, a recent meta-analysis of nine RCTs found that tanezumab reduces pain and improves function in patients with knee and hip osteoarthritis (Zhang et al. 2021).

Malignant Pain

One-third of newly diagnosed oncology patients and 65%–85% of those with advanced disease report significant pain (National Cancer Institute 2021). Management of malignancy-related pain is often suboptimal; many patients receive subtherapeutic doses of analgesics despite published guidelines for cancer pain management (National Cancer Institute 2021). Cancer pain may have both nociceptive and neuropathic components. Neuropathic pain is often managed with anticonvulsants, TCAs, SNRIs, or opioids. Mild nociceptive pain can be managed with acetaminophen or NSAIDs, but most patients with malignancies experience moderate to severe pain, generally treated with opioids. Short-acting opioids are used for initiation of therapy, for pain that is highly variable, or in medically unstable patients. Once analgesic needs become stable, patients should be switched to long-half-life or sustained-release forms. Inadequate opioid dosing often results because of fear of addiction or respiratory depression. Patients become opioid tolerant with long-term dosing and may need dose increases to maintain pain control (Fielding et al. 2013).

Pharmacological Treatment

Opioids

Opioids are a group of drugs comprising a range of substances, including opiates and their synthetic analogues. Opiates are the naturally occurring alkaloids found in the opium poppy and include morphine, codeine, and thebaine. Their semisynthetic derivatives include heroin, hydrocodone, oxycodone, and buprenorphine. Opioids also include a range of synthetic or pharmaceutical opioids, such as methadone, pethidine, tramadol, and fentanyl (World Health Organization 1994). In this chapter, we use the term *opioids*.

Opioids reduce the sensory and affective components of pain by interacting with μ, δ, and κ opioid receptors located on the peripheral nerves in the CNS modulating pain transmission. Opioids are potent analgesics for all types of neuropathic and nociceptive pain. Controversy surrounds the long-term use of opioids for chronic nonmalignant pain. Studies are generally less than 18 months in duration and are complicated by high rates of discontinuation because of adverse events or insufficient pain relief. Opioids should be slowly tapered and discontinued if the burdens (side effects, toxicities, aberrant drug-related behaviors) outweigh the objective benefits (analgesia, functional improvement).

Successful treatment with opioids requires the assessment and documentation of improvements in function and analgesia without accompanying adverse side effects and aberrant behaviors. Suitable patients are those with moderate or severe pain persisting for more than 3 months and adversely affecting function or quality of life.

As stated previously, in view of the opioid addiction crisis that resulted from excessive opioid prescription for chronic pain, other treatments should be considered for chronic pain, and opioid prescription should be a last resort.

Before opioid treatment is initiated, additional factors, such as the patient's specific pain syndrome, response to other therapies, and potential for aberrant drug-related behaviors (misuse, abuse, addiction, diversion), should be considered. See also Chapter 18, "Substance Use Disorders." A patient's suitability for chronic opioid therapy can be assessed with standardized questionnaires. Commonly used instruments include the following:

- Opioid Risk Tool: www.drugabuse.gov/sites/default/files/opioidrisktool.pdf
- Diagnosis, Intractability, Risk, Efficacy risk assessment tool: https://advancedhealth.com/wp-content/uploads/2018/03/DIRE-Risk-Assessment-Tool.pdf
- Screener and Opioid Assessment for Patients With Pain: www.mcstap.com/docs/SOAPP-5.pdf

Instruments to measure treatment outcomes, including analgesia, activities of daily living, adverse events, and potential aberrant drug-related behaviors, are as follows:

- The Pain Assessment and Documentation Tool (https://nida.nih.gov/sites/default/files/PainAssessmentDocumentationTool.pdf). The presence of aberrant drug-related behaviors should always be evaluated.
- The Current Opioid Misuse Measure (available for download at http://womenshealthcouncil.org/current-opioid-misuse-measure-comm-tool) is used to evaluate patients who are taking opioids for concurrent signs or symptoms of intoxication, emotional volatility, poor response to medication, addiction, health care use patterns, and problematic medication behaviors. A nine-item electronic version was developed and validated (McCaffrey et al. 2019).

Clinically available opioids include naturally occurring compounds such as morphine and codeine; semisynthetic derivatives such as hydromorphone, oxymorphone, hydrocodone, oxycodone, dihydrocodeine, and buprenorphine; and synthetic opioid analgesics such as fentanyl, meperidine/pethidine, methadone, tramadol, pentazocine, and propoxyphene.

Because of its hydrophilicity, morphine has poor oral bioavailability (22%–48%) and delayed CNS access and onset of action. This delay prolongs the analgesic effect of morphine relative to its plasma half-life, which decreases the potential for accumulation and toxicity. Morphine is a more effective epidural or spinal analgesic than oxycodone.

Codeine is a prodrug that is active only when it is metabolized to morphine.

Oxycodone is an opioid analgesic with high oral bioavailability (>60%), a faster onset of action, and more predictable plasma levels than morphine. This makes it more likely to result in addiction than slower-working opioids. In comparison with morphine, oxycodone has similar analgesic efficacy, releases less histamine, and causes fewer hallucinations (Cavalcanti et al. 2014).

Hydrocodone is similar to oxycodone in terms of rapid oral absorption and onset of analgesia and the likelihood of developing addiction. Hydrocodone is metabolized by N-demethylation to hydromorphone, which has properties similar to those of morphine but lower rates of side effects.

Fentanyl is a synthetic pharmaceutical drug, 50–100 times stronger than morphine, making it far more dangerous than other opioids. It is used to relieve severe pain, such as after surgery or during cancer treatment, and breakthrough pain (i.e., flare-ups of intense pain despite round-the-clock narcotic treatment). It can be provided as a lozenge on a plastic stick administered under the tongue like a lollipop, as a sublingual spray or tablet that dissolves quickly under the tongue, as a nasal spray, or as an injectable. It is highly lipophilic, with affinity for neuronal tissues and the potential for transdermal or transmucosal delivery. The duration of action of transdermal preparations is up to 72 hours, with considerable interindividual variability. Fentanyl works by blocking pain receptors in the brain and increasing production of dopamine. Like other potent opioid receptor drugs, fentanyl carries massive risk for addiction and abuse regardless of its prescription form. The National Institute on Drug Abuse has warned that fentanyl does not show up on routine urine toxicology screens and pointed out the substance's immense potency and addictive potential (Addiction Center 2021; Skolnick 2022).

Meperidine is known as pethidine in Europe. It can cause seizures and an agitated delirium, believed to be caused by accumulation of the active metabolite normeperidine, which has anticholinergic properties. This is particularly a concern for patients with renal insufficiency, because normeperidine is eliminated by the kidneys. It is not being prescribed in the United States and in Europe currently, except for small quantities in Eastern Europe. It is still used in Central America, the Caribbean, and Africa (United Nations 2021).

Tramadol is a "semi-opioid" that weakly binds to μ opioid receptors and weakly inhibits the reuptake of serotonin and norepinephrine. Tramadol should be preferred over fast- and short-half-life opioids such as oxycodone to lower addiction risk. Also, tramadol has the extra benefit of a positive effect on mood (Bumpus 2020). There is a risk for serotonin syndrome when tramadol is used in conjunction with other agents that inhibit the reuptake of serotonin. Also, tramadol abuse is rising as physicians in the United States become more reluctant to prescribe other opioids and may think that tramadol is not addictive; however, it is.

Methadone warrants special consideration in the treatment of chronic pain because of its low cost, high bioavailability, rapid onset of action, slow hepatic clearance, multiple receptor affinities, lack of neurotoxic metabolites, and incomplete cross-tolerance with other opioids. However, compared with other opioids, methadone has significantly greater risk of inadvertent overdose because of the longer time for adaptation with oral use and greater variation in plasma half-life (15–120 hours) (Sandoval et al. 2005). Extensive tissue distribution and prolonged half-life prevent withdrawal symptoms when methadone is dosed once a day. However, elimination is biphasic, and the more rapid elimination phase equates with analgesia that is limited to approximately 6 hours. Repeated dosing, with accumulation in tissue, may increase analgesia duration to 8–12 hours. Therefore, it should usually be given twice daily. Methadone was shown to be effective for chronic pain in a study of 100 patients, with a mean duration of treatment of 11 months (Peng et al. 2008). Methadone is also associated with QTc interval prolongation and torsades de pointes, especially when given intravenously or at high doses, and increased rates of all-cause mortality at all doses (Ray et al. 2015).

Buprenorphine is a strong agonist and partial antagonist of opioid receptors. It is available as parenteral, sublingual, and transdermal formulations. Unlike full μ opioid agonists, buprenorphine shows a ceiling effect on receptors not directly involved in pain transmission, such as at the rewarding areas, which may limit the abuse potential and result in a wider safety margin. Buprenorphine is an effective analgesic with similar or even better tolerability compared with other opioids; at low doses, its effectiveness and tolerability can play an important role in the treatment of chronic pain as the preferential first-line opioid in clinical practice. This makes it a valid therapeutic option for the management of chronic pain (Fishman and Kim 2018). As a long-acting agonist, buprenorphine prevents withdrawal and craving and stabilizes opioid receptors. As a high-affinity agonist, buprenorphine blocks other opioids from binding, preventing misuse of other opioids (United Nations 2021). According to an Italian expert consensus study, buprenorphine would be preferred over other opioids in most cases if used for chronic pain (Mattia et al. 2021). More information can be found in Chapter 18.

The most common side effect of chronic opioid therapy is decreased gastrointestinal motility, causing constipation, vomiting, and abdominal pain. Oral opioids differ in their propensity to cause symptoms of gastrointestinal dysmotility. An often unrecognized side effect of opioids is a paradoxical development of chronic abdominal pain called *narcotic bowel syndrome*. It can cause worsening pain despite increasing doses of opioid used to treat the pain (Farmer et al. 2017). Transdermal opioids (fentanyl, buprenorphine) have fewer gastrointestinal side effects than oral opioids.

Long-term opioid administration may result in analgesic tolerance or opioid-induced hyperalgesia, which may be due to alterations in psychophysiological pathways (Arout et al. 2015; Wachholtz et al. 2015). When tolerance develops, coadministration of other analgesics, opioid rotation to a more potent agonist, or intermittent cessation of certain agents may restore analgesic effect (Vorobeychik et al. 2008). Opioid rotation from morphine or hydromorphone may be beneficial because the 3-glucuronide metabolites of either drug can accumulate within the cerebrospinal fluid and produce neuroexcitatory effects, such as allodynia, myoclonus, delirium, and seizures (Smith 2000). Rotation to mixed agonist-antagonist opioids (buprenorphine, pentazocine) may precipitate withdrawal symptoms in patients undergoing chronic opioid therapy.

As the supply of opioids has increased over the past two decades in an effort to better treat pain, the number of deaths associated with prescription opioids has increased dramatically. Several factors have been associated with this increase, including too high doses for naive patients, too rapid titration of doses, insufficient patient monitoring, and insufficient knowledge of drug metabolism and drug interactions (Agarin et al. 2015).

Antidepressants

Pain in combination with depressive disorder can be treated with an algorithm that was developed as an alternative to the World Health Organization pain ladder (de Heer et al. 2013).

At the beginning of treatment, depending on assessment with the pain-DETECT questionnaire that the pain is mostly nociceptive or neuropathic, the patient will receive medication accordingly. In case of nociceptive pain, the first step is acetaminophen up to 1,000 mg three times daily. The second step is a COX inhibitor, given their efficacy for nociceptive pain, provided that the patient is younger than 70 and does not have cardiac conditions. In the case of neuropathic pain, gabapentin is given as the second step. However, in some countries, addiction problems with gabapentin are common, so this should be closely monitored or avoided altogether if the patient is known to be prone to addiction. If an opioid is provided, that is only done as a last step. Tramadol may be preferred over other opioids because it has the extra benefit of a serotonergic positive effect on mood, but that also carries a risk for serotonin syndrome, and it is as addictive as the other opioids.

The analgesic properties of antidepressants are underappreciated. The neurobiology of pain suggests that all antidepressants might be effective for treatment of chronic pain. TCAs and SNRIs, in particular, are prescribed for many chronic pain syndromes, including diabetic neuropathy, postherpetic neuralgia, central pain, poststroke pain, tension-type headache, migraine, and oral-facial pain (Riediger et al. 2017). The analgesic effect of antidepressants is independent of their antidepressant effect and is thought to be mediated primarily by the blockade of reuptake of norepinephrine and serotonin, increasing their levels and enhancing the activation of descending inhibitory neurons in the dorsal horn of the spinal cord. Antidepressants may also produce antinociceptive effects by other mechanisms. For example, TCAs block a subtype of sodium channel implicated in neuropathic pain (Patel and Dickenson 2022).

TCAs have been shown in controlled trials to effectively treat central poststroke pain, postherpetic neuralgia, painful diabetic and nondiabetic polyneuropathy, and postmastectomy pain syndrome, but not spinal cord injury pain, phantom limb pain, or pain in HIV neuropathy. A systematic review of 67 RCTs showed evidence that SNRIs are 1.5 times more likely to achieve clinically meaningful pain improvement, with an NNT of seven inpatients with neuropathic pain. There was some evidence for a clinically meaningful benefit for rubefacients such as capsaicin (NNT=7) and opioids (NNT=8) and very low certainty of evidence for TCAs. Acupuncture was ineffective. All drug classes, except TCAs, had a greater likelihood of deriving a clinically meaningful benefit than having withdrawals due to adverse events (Falk et al. 2021).

Duloxetine, venlafaxine, desvenlafaxine, and milnacipran are SNRIs that inhibit the presynaptic reuptake of serotonin, norepinephrine, and, to a lesser extent, dopamine. They are associated with fewer side effects than TCAs and can be titrated more quickly, but titration cannot be monitored by serum levels. Guidelines for the treatment of neuropathic pain recommend duloxetine at adequate doses as an effective treatment (Lunn et al. 2014).

In clinical trials, the efficacy of SSRIs in chronic pain syndromes has been inconsistent and disappointing, especially in the treatment of neuropathic pain. In a Cochrane review, Banzi et al. (2015) found SSRIs to be no more efficacious than placebo for migraine and less efficacious than TCAs for tension-type headache.

Anticonvulsants

Anticonvulsants are effective for treating a variety of neuropathic pain syndromes, including trigeminal neuralgia, diabetic neuropathy, and postherpetic neuralgia, and for migraine prophylaxis (Falk et al. 2021; Seidel et al. 2013). They reduce pain by inhibiting excessive neuronal activity.

First-Generation Anticonvulsants
Carbamazepine is the most widely studied first-generation anticonvulsant effective for neuropathic pain (Wiffen et al. 2014).

Second-Generation Anticonvulsants
Newer anticonvulsants were developed to target novel pharmacological mechanisms for the suppression of nociceptive processes. Gabapentin and pregabalin show significant effects against neuropathic pain, but oxcarbazepine does not (Falk et al. 2021). Gabapentin demonstrated analgesic efficacy in placebo-controlled trials of diabetic peripheral neuropathy pain, postherpetic neuralgia, fibromyalgia, and postamputation phantom limb pain (Moore et al. 2014). Pregabalin, a gabapentin analogue with rapid onset of action and better bioavailability, is effective for the treatment of painful diabetic neuropathy, postherpetic neuralgia, and central neuropathic pain associated with spinal cord injury. Its most common side effects include sedation, peripheral edema, dizziness, and dry mouth (Toth 2014). Pregabalin has been shown to reduce postoperative pain but causes increased sedation and visual disturbances (Mishriky et al. 2015). Gabapentin and pregabalin are entirely renally excreted, so the dosage must be lowered for patients with impaired renal function. For patients undergoing chronic hemodialysis, a single dose of the drug is given three times a week after dialysis (Atalay et al. 2013).

A Cochrane review showed that large high-quality, long-duration studies reporting clinically useful levels of pain relief for individual participants provided no convincing evidence that lamotrigine is effective in treating neuropathic pain and fibromyalgia at dosages of 200–400 mg/day. Given the availability of more effective treatments, including other anticonvulsants and antidepressants, lamotrigine does not have a significant place in therapy based on the available evidence. The adverse-effect profile of lamotrigine is also of concern (Wiffen et al. 2013a, 2013b, 2013c).

Third-Generation Anticonvulsants
Topiramate offers the advantages of minimal hepatic metabolism and unchanged renal excretion, few drug interactions, a long half-life, and the unusual side effect of weight loss. Topiramate is effective for migraine prophylaxis

(National Institute for Health and Care Excellence 2021c) and reduction of neuropathic pain (Falk et al. 2021), but the not-uncommon side effect of cognitive impairment can limit its utility.

When prescribing anticonvulsants, one should remember that they may induce serotonin syndrome because of their serotonergic properties, especially for patients who are taking multiple other serotonergic agents (Prakash et al. 2021).

Benzodiazepines

Benzodiazepines are commonly prescribed for insomnia, anxiety, and occasionally spasticity for patients with chronic pain, but they usually work only in the short term against sleep problems and anxiety and mostly not at all for pain. Also, dependency may occur within 6 weeks of use. Clonazepam may provide long-term relief for cancer-related neuropathic pain (Howard et al. 2014).

Antipsychotics

Antipsychotics have been studied in a variety of chronic pain conditions, including diabetic neuropathy, postherpetic neuralgia, headache, facial pain, pain associated with AIDS and cancer, and musculoskeletal pain. Compared with typical antipsychotics, atypical antipsychotics offer a broader therapeutic spectrum and have lower rates of extrapyramidal side effects.

A meta-analysis of 11 controlled trials suggested that some antipsychotics have analgesic efficacy in headache (haloperidol) and trigeminal neuralgia (pimozide), but antipsychotics' role in chronic pain is mainly as add-on therapy to other agents (Seidel et al. 2013). Another systematic review found that atypical antipsychotics may reduce pain in fibromyalgia and headache/migraine (Jimenez et al. 2018). However, they are associated with metabolic disruptions, such as weight gain and new-onset diabetes, which somewhat offset their benefits.

Results are difficult to interpret because comorbid depressive, anxiety, and sleep disorders in patients with fibromyalgia might respond to treatment with atypical antipsychotics.

Calcium Channel Blockers

The most frequently prescribed calcium channel modulators for neuropathic pain are the gabapentinoids gabapentin and pregabalin (Patel et al. 2018). If gabapentin is or is not effective in treating a condition, then the same is very likely to be true for pregabalin for that condition.

Capsaicin

Topically applied capsaicin has moderate to poor efficacy in the treatment of chronic musculoskeletal or neuropathic pain but is clearly more effective at high doses if tolerated (Falk et al. 2021).

Drug-Drug Interactions

In this section, we review only drug interactions between psychotropic drugs and opioids, triptans, NSAIDs, and local anesthetics. (Selected interactions are listed in Table 17–1.) Most pharmacokinetic interactions between pain drugs and psychotropic drugs result from psychotropic drug–mediated inhibition or induction of cytochrome P450 (CYP)–mediated drug metabolism. Many opioids are metabolized by CYP2D6, an enzyme significantly inhibited by fluoxetine, paroxetine, moclobemide, and bupropion. The triptan antimigraine medications rizatriptan, sumatriptan, and zolmitriptan undergo metabolism by monoamine oxidase A. Monoamine oxidase inhibitors (MAOIs) increase the levels of these drugs and possibly their toxicity. Mexiletine, a CYP1A2 inhibitor, may inhibit metabolism of olanzapine and clozapine. NSAIDs, including COX-2 inhibitors but not acetylsalicylic acid (aspirin), may precipitate lithium toxicity by reducing its excretion (Hersh et al. 2007). Valproate inhibition of glucuronidation increases lamotrigine levels severalfold and may cause toxicity unless lamotrigine dosage is reduced by at least 50% (Gidal et al. 2003). See Chapter 1, "Pharmacokinetics, Pharmacodynamics, and Principles of Drug-Drug Interactions," for a general discussion of drug interactions.

Pharmacodynamic interactions also occur between pain medications and psychotropic agents. The increased risk of gastrointestinal bleeding with NSAIDs and serotonergic antidepressants is covered in Chapter 4, "Gastrointestinal Disorders." The phenylpiperidine series opioids, meperidine (pethidine), fentanyl, tramadol, methadone, dextromethorphan, and propoxyphene are weak serotonin reuptake inhibitors and may precipitate serotonin syndrome in combination with MAOIs (including some fatalities), TCAs, SSRIs,

Table 17–1. Pain medication–psychotropic medication interactions

Pain medication	Interaction mechanism	Clinical effect(s) and management
Opioids		
Dextromethorphan, fentanyl, meperidine (pethidine), methadone, propoxyphene, tramadol	Increased serotonin activity (have serotonin reuptake inhibitor activity)	Possible serotonin syndrome or hyperpyrexia when combined with SSRIs, SNRIs, MAOIs, or TCAs. Avoid concurrent use; discontinue offending opioid. Consider morphine for pain management.
Methadone	Prolonged QT interval	Potentiates QT prolongation induced by TCAs or antipsychotics (typical and atypical). May lead to cardiac arrhythmias or torsades de pointes. Avoid concurrent use. Consider other opioid analgesic.
Nonsteroidal anti-inflammatory drugs		
Celecoxib (and other cyclooxygenase isoenzyme 2 inhibitors), ibuprofen, naproxen	Reduced renal blood flow	Reduced lithium elimination, leading to lithium toxicity. Monitor lithium levels; reduce lithium dosage. Consider acetylsalicylic acid (aspirin).
Antimigraine agents		
Almotriptan, eletriptan, frovatriptan, naratriptan, rizatriptan, sumatriptan, zolmitriptan	Serotonin agonist activity	Possible serotonin syndrome in combination with SSRIs, SNRIs, MAOIs, or TCAs. Use with caution. Instruct patient about symptoms.

Table 17–1. Pain medication–psychotropic medication interactions *(continued)*

Pain medication	Interaction mechanism	Clinical effect(s) and management
Local anesthetic		
Mexiletine	Inhibition of cytochrome P450 1A2	Increased levels of olanzapine or clozapine, possibly increasing toxicity. Avoid concurrent use. Reduce antipsychotic dose.

Note.   MAOIs = monoamine oxidase inhibitors; SNRIs = serotonin-norepinephrine reuptake inhibitors; SSRIs = selective serotonin reuptake inhibitors; TCAs = tricyclic antidepressants.

SNRIs, and other serotonergic drugs. Morphine, codeine, oxycodone, and buprenorphine are less likely to precipitate serotonin toxicity. The constipating effects of opioids are additive in combination with drugs possessing anticholinergic activity, including TCAs and anticholinergic agents used to treat extrapyramidal symptoms (e.g., trihexyphenidyl, benztropine). Methadone is associated with prolonged QTc interval (Ehret et al. 2007), which is exacerbated in the presence of CYP3A4 inhibitors (e.g., fluvoxamine, fluoxetine, nefazodone) and other QT-prolonging agents (e.g., TCAs, typical and atypical antipsychotics). In 2006, the U.S. FDA issued an alert warning of possible serotonin syndrome precipitated by the combined use of SSRIs or SNRIs and triptan antimigraine medications, but subsequent experience has shown that this rarely occurs, and co-prescription is not contraindicated (Orlova et al. 2018). For a full discussion of serotonin syndrome, see Chapter 2, "Severe Drug Reactions."

Key Points

- In opioid prescription, functional outcomes should be determined before therapy is initiated.

- Choice of medication depends on classification of pain as neuropathic, nociceptive, or mixed, depending on the painDETECT questionnaire.

- Opioids should be avoided as much as possible in nonmalignant chronic pain.

- The alternative pain medication ladder described in this chapter builds on earlier steps so as to achieve optimal analgesic effect while avoiding opioids as long as possible.

- Major depressive disorder is underdiagnosed and undertreated, so patients should be treated aggressively if disabling pain persists.

- Opioids should be avoided in the presence of major depressive disorder.

- Gabapentin, pregabalin, and topiramate are primarily renally excreted.

- Caution is needed when combining valproate and lamotrigine; the lamotrigine dosage should be reduced by 50%.

- Cytochrome P450 2D6 inhibitors, including several antidepressants, inhibit opioid metabolism.

References

Addiction Center: Fentanyl addiction, abuse, and treatment. 2021. Available at: https://www.addictioncenter.com/opiates/fentanyl. Accessed November 7, 2021.

Agarin T, Trescot AM, Agarin A, et al: Reducing opioid analgesic deaths in America: what health providers can do. Pain Physician 18(3):E307–E322, 2015 26000678

Alföldi P, Wiklund T, Gerdle B: Comorbid insomnia in patients with chronic pain: a study based on the Swedish Quality Registry for Pain Rehabilitation (SQRP). Disabil Rehabil 36(20):1661–1669, 2014 24320022

Allen SF, Gilbody S, Atkin K, et al: The associations between loneliness, social exclusion and pain in the general population: a N=502,528 cross-sectional UK Biobank study. J Psychiatr Res 130:68–74, 2020 32791383

American Psychiatric Association: Diagnostic and Statistical Manual of Mental Disorders, 5th Edition. Arlington, VA, American Psychiatric Publishing, 2013

Arout CA, Edens E, Petrakis IL, et al: Targeting opioid-induced hyperalgesia in clinical treatment: neurobiological considerations. CNS Drugs 29(6):465–486, 2015 26142224

Atalay H, Solak Y, Biyik Z, et al: Cross-over, open-label trial of the effects of gabapentin versus pregabalin on painful peripheral neuropathy and health-related quality of life in haemodialysis patients. Clin Drug Investig 33(6):401–408, 2013 23572323

Bannuru RR, Osani MC, Vaysbrot EE, et al: OARSI guidelines for the non-surgical management of knee, hip, and polyarticular osteoarthritis. Osteoarthritis Cartilage 27(11):1578–1589, 2019 31278997

Banzi R, Cusi C, Randazzo C, et al: Selective serotonin reuptake inhibitors (SSRIs) and serotonin-norepinephrine reuptake inhibitors (SNRIs) for the prevention of tension-type headache in adults. Cochrane Database Syst Rev 5(5):CD011681, 2015 25931277

Bendtsen L, Zakrzewska JM, Abbott J, et al: European Academy of Neurology guideline on trigeminal neuralgia. Eur J Neurol 26(6):831–849, 2019 30860637

Björkman B, Lund I, Arnér S, et al: The meaning and consequences of amputation and mastectomy from the perspective of pain and suffering. Scand J Pain 14:100–107, 2017 28850422

Blyth FM, Macfarlane GJ, Nicholas MK: The contribution of psychosocial factors to the development of chronic pain: the key to better outcomes for patients? Pain 129(1–2):8–11, 2007 17398007

Bonnewyn A, Katona C, Bruffaerts R, et al: Pain and depression in older people: comorbidity and patterns of help seeking. J Affect Disord 117(3):193–196, 2009 19217167

Bras M, Dordević V, Gregurek R, et al: Neurobiological and clinical relationship between psychiatric disorders and chronic pain. Psychiatr Danub 22(2):221–226, 2010 20562750

Bulilete O, Leiva A, Rullán M, et al: Efficacy of gabapentin for the prevention of postherpetic neuralgia in patients with acute herpes zoster: a double blind, randomized controlled trial. PLoS One 14(6):e0217335, 2019 31166976

Bumpus JA: Low-dose tramadol as an off-label antidepressant: a data mining analysis from the patients' perspective. ACS Pharmacol Transl Sci 3(6):1293–1303, 2020 33344902

Carod-Artal FJ: Tackling chronic migraine: current perspectives. J Pain Res 7:185–194, 2014 24748814

Cavalcanti IL, Carvalho AC, Musauer MG, et al: Safety and tolerability of controlled-release oxycodone on postoperative pain in patients submitted to the oncologic head and neck surgery. Rev Col Bras Cir 41(6):393–399, 2014 25742404

Cheng JC, Anzolin A, Berry M, et al: Dynamic functional brain connectivity underlying temporal summation of pain in fibromyalgia. Arthritis Rheumatol 74(4):700–710, 2022 34725971

Choi HR, Aktas A, Bottros MM: Pharmacotherapy to manage central post-stroke pain. CNS Drugs 35(2):151–160, 2021 33550430

Cocchio S, Baldovin T, Furlan P, et al: Cross-sectional study on hospitalizations related to herpes zoster in an Italian region, 2008–2016. Aging Clin Exp Res 31(1):145–150, 2019 29766448

Coggon D, Ntani G, Palmer KT, et al: The CUPID (Cultural and Psychosocial Influences on Disability) study: methods of data collection and characteristics of study sample. PLoS One 7(7):e39820, 2012 22792189

Cohen SP, Mao J: Neuropathic pain: mechanisms and their clinical implications. BMJ 348:f7656, 2014 24500412

da Silva JM, de Barros BS, Almeida GJ, et al: Dosage of resistance exercises in fibromyalgia: evidence synthesis for a systematic literature review up-date and meta-analysis. Rheumatol Int 42(3):413–429, 2022 34652480

de Farias ÁD, Eberle L, Amador TA, et al: Comparing the efficacy and safety of duloxetine and amitriptyline in the treatment of fibromyalgia: overview of systematic reviews. Adv Rheumatol 60(1):35, 2020 32641165

de Heer EW, Dekker J, van Eck van der Sluijs JF, et al: Effectiveness and cost-effectiveness of transmural collaborative care with consultation letter (TCCCL) and duloxetine for major depressive disorder (MDD) and (sub)chronic pain in collaboration with primary care: design of a randomized placebo-controlled multi-centre trial: TCC:PAINDIP. BMC Psychiatry 13:147, 2013 23705849

de Heer EW, Gerrits MM, Beekman AT, et al: The association of depression and anxiety with pain: a study from NESDA. PLoS One 9(10):e106907, 2014 25330004

de Heer EW, Vriezekolk JE, van der Feltz-Cornelis CM: Poor illness perceptions are a risk factor for depressive and anxious symptomatology in fibromyalgia syndrome: a longitudinal cohort study. Front Psychiatry 8:217, 2017 29163236

de Heer EW, Ten Have M, van Marwijk HWJ, et al: Pain as a risk factor for common mental disorders: results from the Netherlands Mental Health Survey and Incidence Study-2: a longitudinal, population-based study. Pain 159(4):712–718, 2018 29252911

de Heer EW, Palacios JE, Adèr HJ, et al: Chest pain, depression and anxiety in coronary heart disease: consequence or cause? A prospective clinical study in primary care. J Psychosom Res 129:109891, 2020 31865173

De Keersmaecker E, Lefeber N, Geys M, et al: Virtual reality during gait training: does it improve gait function in persons with central nervous system movement disorders? A systematic review and meta-analysis. NeuroRehabilitation 44(1):43–66, 2019 30814368

Department of Veterans Affairs; Department of Defense: Clinical practice guideline: management of opioid therapy for chronic pain. 2010. Available at: https://www.va.gov/painmanagement/docs/cpg_opioidtherapy_summary.pdf. Accessed October 6, 2022.

Derry S, Wiffen PJ, Moore RA, et al: Topical lidocaine for neuropathic pain in adults. Cochrane Database Syst Rev 7(7):CD010958, 2014 25058164

de Villiers E, Stone T, Wang N-W, et al: Virtual Environment Rehabilitation for Patients with Motor Neglect Trial (VERMONT): a single-center randomized controlled feasibility trial. Brain Sci 11(4):464, 2021 33917497

Diener HC, Gaul C, Lehmacher W, et al: Aspirin, paracetamol (acetaminophen) and caffeine for the treatment of acute migraine attacks: a systemic review and meta-analysis of randomized placebo-controlled trials. Eur J Neurol 29(1):350–357, 2022 34519136

Dowell D, Haegerich TM, Chou R: CDC guideline for prescribing opioids for chronic pain. MMWR Recomm Rep 65(1)(RR-1):1–49, 2016 26987082

Ehret GB, Desmeules JA, Broers B: Methadone-associated long QT syndrome: improving pharmacotherapy for dependence on illegal opioids and lessons learned for pharmacology. Expert Opin Drug Saf 6(3):289–303, 2007 17480178

Falk J, Thomas B, Kirkwood J, et al: PEER systematic review of randomized controlled trials: management of chronic neuropathic pain in primary care. Can Fam Physician 67(5):e130–e140, 2021 33980642

Farmer AD, Gallagher J, Bruckner-Holt C, et al: Narcotic bowel syndrome. Lancet Gastroenterol Hepatol 2(5):361–368, 2017 28397700

Fielding F, Sanford TM, Davis MP: Achieving effective control in cancer pain: a review of current guidelines. Int J Palliat Nurs 19(12):584–591, 2013 24356502

Finan PH, Goodin BR, Smith MT: The association of sleep and pain: an update and a path forward. J Pain 14(12):1539–1552, 2013 24290442

Fishman MA, Kim PS: Buprenorphine for chronic pain: a systemic review. Curr Pain Headache Rep 22(12):83, 2018 30291571

Flaster M, Meresh E, Rao M, et al: Central poststroke pain: current diagnosis and treatment. Top Stroke Rehabil 20(2):116–123, 2013 23611852

Freynhagen R, Baron R, Gockel U, et al: painDETECT: a new screening questionnaire to identify neuropathic components in patients with back pain. Curr Med Res Opin 22(10):1911–1920, 2006 17022849

Garcia-Pallero MÁ, Cardona D, Rueda-Ruzafa L, et al: Central nervous system stimulation therapies in phantom limb pain: a systematic review of clinical trials. Neural Regen Res 17(1):59–64, 2022 34100428

GBD 2016 Disease and Injury Incidence and Prevalence Collaborators: Global, regional, and national incidence, prevalence, and years lived with disability for 328 diseases and injuries for 195 countries, 1990–2016: a systematic analysis for the Global Burden of Disease Study 2016. Lancet 390(10100):1211–1259, 2017 28919117

Gidal BE, Sheth R, Parnell J, et al: Evaluation of VPA dose and concentration effects on lamotrigine pharmacokinetics: implications for conversion to lamotrigine monotherapy. Epilepsy Res 57(2–3):85–93, 2003 15013050

Goetz A, McCormick S, Phillips R, et al: CE: diagnosing and managing migraine. Am J Nurs 122(1):32–43, 2022 34882585

Gudin J, Fudin J, Wang E, et al: Treatment patterns and medication use in patients with postherpetic neuralgia. J Manag Care Spec Pharm 25(12):1387–1396, 2019 31589557

Haibach JP, Beehler GP, Dollar KM, et al: Moving toward integrated behavioral intervention for treating multimorbidity among chronic pain, depression, and substance-use disorders in primary care. Med Care 52(4):322–327, 2014 24556895

Hans GH, Robert DN, Van Maldeghem KN: Treatment of an acute severe central neuropathic pain syndrome by topical application of lidocaine 5% patch: a case report. Spinal Cord 46(4):311–313, 2008 17607309

Hejazi RA, Mandourah NA, Alsulami AS, et al: Commonly used agent for acute pain management of sickle cell anemia in Saudi emergency department: a narrative review. Saudi Pharm J 29(6):487–496, 2021 34194255

Hersh EV, Pinto A, Moore PA: Adverse drug interactions involving common prescription and over-the-counter analgesic agents. Clin Ther 29(Suppl):2477–2497, 2007 18164916

Howard P, Twycross R, Shuster J, et al: Benzodiazepines. J Pain Symptom Manage 47(5):955–964, 2014 24681184

Hyung B, Wiseman-Hakes C: A scoping review of current non-pharmacological treatment modalities for phantom limb pain in limb amputees. Disabil Rehabil 44(19):5719–5740, 2022 34293999

Institute of Medicine: Relieving Pain in America: A Blueprint for Transforming Prevention, Care, Education, and Research. Committee on Advancing Pain Research, Care, and Education. Washington, DC, National Academies Press, 2011. Available at: https://books.nap.edu/openbook.php?record_id=13172. Accessed October 6, 2022.

Janssen LP, Medeiros LF, Souza A, et al: Fibromyalgia: a review of related polymorphisms and clinical relevance. An Acad Bras Cienc 93(Suppl 4):e20210618, 2021 34730627

Jimenez XF, Sundararajan T, Covington EC: A systematic review of atypical antipsychotics in chronic pain management: olanzapine demonstrates potential in central sensitization, fibromyalgia, and headache/migraine. Clin J Pain 34(6):585–591, 2018 29077621

Johnson RW, Rice AS: Clinical practice: postherpetic neuralgia. N Engl J Med 371(16):1526–1533, 2014 25317872

Karl F, Bischler T, Egenolf N, et al: Fibromyalgia vs small fiber neuropathy: diverse keratinocyte transcriptome signature. Pain 162(10):2569–2577, 2021 33675632

Kim NY, Lee SC, Kim YW: Effect of duloxetine for the treatment of chronic central poststroke pain. Clin Neuropharmacol 42(3):73–76, 2019 31085946

Knisely MR, Tanabe PJ, Walker JKL, et al: Severe persistent pain and inflammatory biomarkers in sickle cell disease: an exploratory study. Biol Res Nurs 24(1):24–30, 2022 34189962

Kroenke K, Shen J, Oxman TE, et al: Impact of pain on the outcomes of depression treatment: results from the RESPECT trial. Pain 134(1–2):209–215, 2008 18022319

Lee HJ, Lee JH, Cho EY, et al: Efficacy of psychological treatment for headache disorder: a systematic review and meta-analysis. J Headache Pain 20(1):17, 2019 30764752

Lerman SF, Rudich Z, Brill S, et al: Longitudinal associations between depression, anxiety, pain, and pain-related disability in chronic pain patients. Psychosom Med 77(3):333–341, 2015 25849129

Lunn MP, Hughes RA, Wiffen PJ: Duloxetine for treating painful neuropathy, chronic pain or fibromyalgia. Cochrane Database Syst Rev (1):CD007115, 2014 24385423

Martínez-Lara A, Moreno-Fernández AM, Jiménez-Guerrero M, et al: Mitochondrial imbalance as a new approach to the study of fibromyalgia. Open Access Rheumatol 12:175–185, 2020 32922097

Mattia C, Luongo L, Innamorato M, et al: An Italian expert consensus on the use of opioids for the management of chronic non-oncological pain in clinical practice: focus on buprenorphine. J Pain Res 14:3193–3206, 2021 34675646

McCaffrey SA, Black RA, Villapiano AJ, et al: Development of a brief version of the Current Opioid Misuse Measure (COMM): the COMM-9. Pain Med 20(1):113–118, 2019 29237039

McCormick Z, Chang-Chien G, Marshall B, et al: Phantom limb pain: a systematic neuroanatomical-based review of pharmacologic treatment. Pain Med 15(2):292–305, 2014 24224475

Miller E: The World Health Organization analgesic ladder. J Midwifery Womens Health 49(6):542–545, 2004 15544984

Mishriky BM, Waldron NH, Habib AS: Impact of pregabalin on acute and persistent postoperative pain: a systematic review and meta-analysis. Br J Anaesth 114(1):10–31, 2015 25209095

Mo G, Jang T, Stewart C, et al: Chronic opioid use in patients with sickle cell disease. Hematology 26(1):415–416, 2021 34102090

Montano N, Conforti G, Di Bonaventura R, et al: Advances in diagnosis and treatment of trigeminal neuralgia. Ther Clin Risk Manag 11:289–299, 2015 25750533

Moore RA, Wiffen PJ, Derry S, et al: Gabapentin for chronic neuropathic pain and fibromyalgia in adults. Cochrane Database Syst Rev (4):CD007938, 2014 24771480

Morgan KW, Joyner KR: Eptinezumab: a calcitonin gene-related peptide monoclonal antibody infusion for migraine prevention. SAGE Open Med 9:20503121211050186, 2021 34659764

National Cancer Institute: Cancer Pain (PDQ). PDQ Supportive and Palliative Care Editorial Board, May 7, 2021. Available at: www.cancer.gov/about-cancer/treatment/side-effects/pain/pain-pdq. Accessed December 20, 2021.

National Institute for Health and Care Excellence: Headaches in over 12s: diagnosis and management. Clinical Guideline [CG150], December 17, 2021a. Available at: www.nice.org.uk/guidance/cg150. Accessed December 20, 2021.

National Institute for Health and Care Excellence: NICE guideline: chronic tension headache CF150. 2021b. Available at: https://southwest.devonformularyguidance.nhs.uk/formulary/chapters/4.-central-nervous-system/tension-headache. Accessed December 20, 2021.

National Institute for Health and Care Excellence: NICE guideline: drugs for acute migraine. May 2021c. Available at: https://cks.nice.org.uk/topics/migraine/prescribing-information/drugs-for-acute-migraine. Accessed December 20, 2021.

National Institute of Neurological Disorders and Stroke: Complex regional pain syndrome fact sheet. 2021. Available at: www.ninds.nih.gov/Disorders/Patient-Caregiver-Education/Fact-Sheets/Complex-Regional-Pain-Syndrome-Fact-Sheet. Accessed December 20, 2021.

National Institutes of Health: NIH Heal Initiative. 2019. Available at: www.heal.nih.gov. Accessed December 20, 2021.

Orlova Y, Rizzoli P, Loder E: Association of coprescription of triptan antimigraine drugs and selective serotonin reuptake inhibitor or selective norepinephrine reuptake inhibitor antidepressants with serotonin syndrome. JAMA Neurol 75(5):566–572, 2018 29482205

Outcalt SD, Kroenke K, Krebs EE, et al: Chronic pain and comorbid mental health conditions: independent associations of posttraumatic stress disorder and depression with pain, disability, and quality of life. J Behav Med 38(3):535–543, 2015 25786741

Ozcivit IB, Erel CT, Durmusoglu F: Can fibromyalgia be considered a characteristic symptom of climacterium? Postgrad Med J Aug 9, 2021:postgradmedj-2021-140336 34373344 Epub ahead of print

Panickar A, Serpell M: Guidelines for general practitioners on treatment of pain in post-herpetic neuralgia. The Shingles Support Society, 2015. Available at: https://www.herpes.org.uk/wp-content/uploads/2015/10/Guidelines-for-PHN-by-Dr-Serpell.pdf. Accessed October 7, 2022.

Patel R, Dickenson AH: Neuropharmacological basis for multimodal analgesia in chronic pain. Postgrad Med 134(3):245–259, 2022 34636261

Patel R, Montagut-Bordas C, Dickenson AH: Calcium channel modulation as a target in chronic pain control. Br J Pharmacol 175(12):2173–2184, 2018 28320042

Peng P, Tumber P, Stafford M, et al: Experience of methadone therapy in 100 consecutive chronic pain patients in a multidisciplinary pain center. Pain Med 9(7):786–794, 2008 18564997

Prakash S, Rathore C, Rana K, et al: Antiepileptic drugs and serotonin syndrome: a systematic review of case series and case reports. Seizure 91:117–131, 2021 34153897

Ray WA, Chung CP, Murray KT, et al: Out-of-hospital mortality among patients receiving methadone for noncancer pain. JAMA Intern Med 175(3):420–427, 2015 25599329

Riediger C, Schuster T, Barlinn K, et al: Adverse effects of antidepressants for chronic pain: a systematic review and meta-analysis. Front Neurol 8:307, 2017 28769859

Rief W, Martin A: How to use the new DSM-5 somatic symptom disorder diagnosis in research and practice: a critical evaluation and a proposal for modifications. Annu Rev Clin Psychol 10:339–367, 2014 24387234

Risser RC, Hochberg MC, Gaynor PJ, et al: Responsiveness of the Intermittent and Constant Osteoarthritis Pain (ICOAP) scale in a trial of duloxetine for treatment of osteoarthritis knee pain. Osteoarthritis Cartilage 21(5):691–694, 2013 23485934

Salm DC, Belmonte LAO, Emer AA, et al: Aquatic exercise and Far Infrared (FIR) modulates pain and blood cytokines in fibromyalgia patients: a double-blind, randomized, placebo-controlled pilot study. J Neuroimmunol 337:577077, 2019 31655422

Sandoval JA, Furlan AD, Mailis-Gagnon A: Oral methadone for chronic noncancer pain: a systematic literature review of reasons for administration, prescription patterns, effectiveness, and side effects. Clin J Pain 21(6):503–512, 2005 16215336

Schreiber AK, Nones CF, Reis RC, et al: Diabetic neuropathic pain: physiopathology and treatment. World J Diabetes 6(3):432–444, 2015 25897354

Scuteri D, Mantovani E, Tamburin S, et al: Opioids in post-stroke pain: a systematic review and meta-analysis. Front Pharmacol 11:587050, 2020 33424596

Seidel S, Aigner M, Ossege M, et al: Antipsychotics for acute and chronic pain in adults. Cochrane Database Syst Rev 8(8):CD004844, 2013 23990266

Setnik B, Roland CL, Pixton GC, et al: Prescription opioid abuse and misuse: gap between primary-care investigator assessment and actual extent of these behaviors among patients with chronic pain. Postgrad Med 129(1):5–11, 2017 27782769

Skolnick P: Treatment of overdose in the synthetic opioid era. Pharmacol Ther 233:108019, 2022 34637841

Sloan G, Selvarajah D, Tesfaye S: Pathogenesis, diagnosis and clinical management of diabetic sensorimotor peripheral neuropathy. Nat Rev Endocrinol 17(7):400–420, 2021 34050323

Smith MT: Neuroexcitatory effects of morphine and hydromorphone: evidence implicating the 3-glucuronide metabolites. Clin Exp Pharmacol Physiol 27(7):524–528, 2000 10874511

Snedecor SJ, Sudhorshan L, Cappelleri JC, et al: Systematic review and meta-analysis of pharmacological therapies for painful diabetic neuropathy. Pain Pract 14(2):167–184, 2014 23534696

Srejic U, Banimahd F: Haunting of the phantom limb pain abolished by buprenorphine/naloxone. BMJ Case Rep 14(2):e237009, 2021 33608331

Srinivasan K, Kozminski K, Zhang Y, et al: Pharmacological, pharmacokinetic, pharmacodynamic and physicochemical characterization of FE 205030: a potent, fast acting, injectable CGRP receptor antagonist for the treatment of acute episodic migraine. J Pharm Sci 111(1):247–261, 2022 34217775

Sullivan MD, Ballantyne JC: When physical and social pain coexist: insights into opioid therapy. Ann Fam Med 19(1):79–82, 2021 33355099

Toth C: Pregabalin: latest safety evidence and clinical implications for the management of neuropathic pain. Ther Adv Drug Saf 5(1):38–56, 2014 25083261

United Nations: World Drug Report 2021 (United Nations publication, sales no. E.21.XI.8). June 2021. Available at: www.unodc.org/res/wdr2021/field/WDR21_Booklet_1.pdf. Accessed October 7, 2022.

Van der Feltz-Cornelis CM, Bakker M, Kaul A, et al: IL-6 and hsCRP in somatic symptom disorders and related disorders. Brain Behav Immun Health 9:100176, 2020 34589907

van der Watt ASJ, Spies G, Roos A, et al: Functional neuroimaging of adult-to-adult romantic attachment separation, rejection, and loss: a systematic review. J Clin Psychol Med Settings 28(3):637–648, 2021 33392890

Ventafridda V, Saita L, Ripamonti C, et al: WHO guidelines for the use of analgesics in cancer pain. Int J Tissue React 7(1):93–96, 1985 2409039

Vernieri F, Brunelli N, Messina R, et al: Discontinuing monoclonal antibodies targeting CGRP pathway after one-year treatment: an observational longitudinal cohort study. J Headache Pain 22(1):154, 2021 34922444

Volkow ND, McLellan AT: Opioid abuse in chronic pain—misconceptions and mitigation strategies. N Engl J Med 374(13):1253–1263, 2016 27028915

Vorobeychik Y, Chen L, Bush MC, et al: Improved opioid analgesic effect following opioid dose reduction. Pain Med 9(6):724–727, 2008 18816332

Wachholtz A, Foster S, Cheatle M: Psychophysiology of pain and opioid use: implications for managing pain in patients with an opioid use disorder. Drug Alcohol Depend 146:1–6, 2015 25468815

Wiffen PJ, Derry S, Lunn MP, et al: Topiramate for neuropathic pain and fibromyalgia in adults. Cochrane Database Syst Rev 8(8):CD008314, 2013a 23996081

Wiffen PJ, Derry S, Moore RA, et al: Antiepileptic drugs for neuropathic pain and fibromyalgia: an overview of Cochrane reviews. Cochrane Database Syst Rev (11):CD010567, 2013b 24217986

Wiffen PJ, Derry S, Moore RA: Lamotrigine for chronic neuropathic pain and fibromyalgia in adults. Cochrane Database Syst Rev (12):CD006044, 2013c 24297457

Wiffen PJ, Derry S, Moore RA, et al: Carbamazepine for chronic neuropathic pain and fibromyalgia in adults. Cochrane Database Syst Rev 4(4):CD005451, 2014 24719027

Wong WS, Fielding R: The co-morbidity of chronic pain, insomnia, and fatigue in the general adult population of Hong Kong: prevalence and associated factors. J Psychosom Res 73(1):28–34, 2012 22691556

World Health Organization: Lexicon of Alcohol and Drug Terms. Geneva, World Health Organization, 1994

Zangrandi A, Demers FA, Schneider C: Complex regional pain syndrome: a comprehensive review on neuroplastic changes supporting the use of non-invasive neurostimulation in clinical settings. Front Pain Res (Lausanne) 2:732343, 2021 35295500

Zhang B, Tian X, Qu Z, et al: Relative efficacy and safety of tanezumab for osteoarthritis: a systematic review and meta-analysis of randomized-controlled trials. Clin J Pain 37(12):914–924, 2021 34608021

18

Substance Use Disorders

Jozef Bledowski, M.D.

Substance use disorders are present in a significant portion of the population, with a disproportionate representation in the medically ill. It is well known that substance use disorders increase the risk for accidental and intentional injury, precipitation of acute and chronic medical illness, both extended hospital stays and incidence of leaving against medical advice, and significant delays in illness recovery. Therefore, it is not surprising that substance use disorders are commonly encountered in both inpatient and outpatient medical settings. With regard to substance use in the United States, the 2020 National Survey on Drug Use and Health (Substance Abuse and Mental Health Services Administration 2021) found that among individuals age 12 years or older, 20.7% used nicotine-containing products (including tobacco and vaping devices) in the past month, with 63.1% of the adolescents ages 12–17 in that group solely vaping nicotine; 22.2% engaged in binge drinking (defined as five or more drinks for males or four or more drinks for females on a single occasion), and 6.4% engaged in heavy alcohol use (defined as binge drinking on at least 5 days out of a month) in the past month, with the highest percentage of alcohol users in both categories being young adults ages 18–25; and 21.4% used illicit drugs (the definition of which included marijuana, cocaine, heroin, hallucinogens, inhalants, methamphetamine, prescription pain relievers, stimulants, tranquilizers, and sedatives) in the past year, with marijuana being the most commonly used, followed by prescription pain relievers, with the highest percentage of use in both groups also being among young adults ages 18–25.

It is estimated that approximately 15%–30% of hospitalized patients and up to 36% of medically hospitalized patients receiving psychiatric consultation have at least one comorbid substance use disorder (Katz et al. 2008; Schellhorn et al. 2009). Adverse effects of substance intoxication, overdose, withdrawal, and chronic use are common among medically ill patients. Although the overwhelming burden of alcohol and tobacco use is well established in a large proportion of medically ill patients, misuse of prescription medications (particularly opioid analgesics and benzodiazepines) has also reached epidemic proportions and is now commonly encountered in both ambulatory and inpatient medical settings. Furthermore, with the decriminalization of marijuana in most states and U.S. territories; the availability of so-called designer drugs (e.g., 3,4-methylenedioxymethamphetamine [MDMA], synthetic cannabinoids [K2, Spice], synthetic cathinones [bath salts]); the ready availability of unregulated psychoactive herbal extracts (e.g., kratom); and the rising incidence of recreational over-the-counter drug use (e.g., dextromethorphan, pseudoephedrine), it is imperative for the treating provider to also be aware of the potential use of these substances during the evaluation of a medically ill patient.

In this chapter, I discuss pharmacological management of select intoxication syndromes and withdrawal syndromes, and management of abstinence and craving in select substance use disorders, with special emphasis on the medically ill and pregnancy. Reference tables are included outlining potential neuropsychiatric adverse effects and drug-drug interactions of these agents.

Substance Intoxication

Severe intoxication can be life-threatening, but few antidotes exist. Thus, intoxication is managed primarily with supportive measures. The major exceptions are opioid and benzodiazepine overdoses. Mortality data from the

National Center for Injury Prevention and Control (Centers for Disease Control and Prevention 2020) indicate that unintentional poisonings, including overdoses, remain the leading cause of unintentional death in adults ages 25–44 in the United States, surpassing all other unintentional causes of death. In addition, the age-adjusted rates of death due to drug overdose continue to rise, with opioids being the most common substances associated with overdose death (Hedegaard et al. 2020). However, among opioids, the rates of overdose death due to heroin have decreased, whereas the rates of overdose death due to fentanyl and similar synthetic opioids have been increasing (Hedegaard et al. 2020).

Naloxone is a competitive opioid receptor antagonist with particularly high affinity for μ opioid receptors, making it the drug of choice in managing acute opioid intoxication and overdose. It was initially approved by the U.S. FDA in 1971. Naloxone is available in a parenteral formulation (administered via intravenous, intramuscular, or subcutaneous route) and has become available in a noninjectable nasal spray. In addition to the parenteral and nasal spray formulations, naloxone can be administered via inhalation, endotracheal, sublingual, and buccal routes (Kim and Nelson 2015). Given its extensive first-pass hepatic metabolism and low bioavailability when given orally, naloxone has much greater bioavailability when the drug is administered via parenteral, intranasal, or inhalation routes. Parenteral routes of naloxone administration are preferred if possible and have been shown to have a quicker onset of action and to be associated with a reduced need for additional rescue doses of naloxone compared with the intranasal route of administration (Dietze et al. 2019). Nonetheless, in some instances, parenteral naloxone administration may not be available or feasible, underscoring the utility of alternative routes of administration such as nasal spray. Although naloxone is rapidly effective in reversing the effects of most opioids, administration in synthetic opioid intoxication or overdose, as is seen with fentanyl or its analogues, can result in reduced effectiveness because of the high lipophilicity resulting in quick uptake but slow and prolonged dissociation from adipose tissue, high μ opioid receptor binding affinity, and much higher potency of fentanyl and similar agents (Armenian et al. 2018). Similarly, given that buprenorphine has a considerably high affinity for and slower rate of association with and dissociation from the μ opioid receptor, buprenorphine intoxication also requires higher or repeated doses of naloxone, which can result in a delay in its effectiveness (Kim and Nelson 2015).

Naloxone is generally safe to use in the medically ill and is without abso-lute contraindications. In addition to acute agitation, the most common and potentially adverse consequence of naloxone administration is the precipita-tion of acute opioid withdrawal. More commonly seen in chronic opioid users (including chronic pain patients), acute opioid withdrawal precipitated by naloxone can cause sympathetic hyperactivity, uncommonly resulting in ma-lignant hypertension, arrhythmias, and seizures (Kim and Nelson 2015). The use of higher doses of naloxone has been associated with an increased risk of pulmonary complications, including aspiration pneumonia, pneumonitis, and pulmonary edema (Farkas et al. 2020). Nevertheless, the benefit of using nal-oxone clearly outweighs any potential risk, particularly when opioid intoxica-tion results in life-threatening respiratory compromise. In fact, recent programs have encouraged ready availability of naloxone in high-risk populations, even going so far as to provide community organizations, as well as family members and friends of opioid-addicted individuals, free access to naloxone (Avetian et al. 2018). For this reason, in 2014 the FDA approved a naloxone autoinjector that can be easily administered (intramuscularly or subcutaneously) by a fam-ily member or caregiver. Similarly, in 2015 the FDA approved the intranasal formulation of naloxone, which is now commonly prescribed and dispensed to opioid users and their families in the outpatient setting and can be used by first responders in the prehospital setting.

The emergence and rise of the use and overuse of synthetic opioids, par-ticularly fentanyl and similar analogues, in the United States have renewed in-terest in alternative and potentially more effective antidotes. Nalmefene, a competitive μ opioid receptor antagonist, was initially approved by the FDA in 1995 for intravenous use in the treatment of acute opioid overdose; how-ever, it was subsequently pulled from the market, primarily because of its high cost. Nalmefene has a longer half-life and higher potency as compared with naloxone, making it an appealing alternative in treating overdoses from syn-thetic and long-acting opioids (Skolnik 2022). Nalmefene has been used in Europe for quite some time and is approved by the European Medicines Agency (EMA) for treatment of alcohol use disorder (see the "Alcohol Abstinence and Craving" subsection later in this chapter).

There is a lack of well-controlled studies assessing the potential fetal risk associated with naloxone use in humans, so such risk cannot be ruled out. Fur-thermore, the use of naloxone in pregnancy can precipitate severe withdrawal in the mother and fetus, which can then result in fetal distress and preterm labor (ACOG Committee on Health Care for Underserved Women and American Society of Addiction Medicine 2012; Zelner et al. 2015). There is also a potential risk of precipitating hypertensive crisis with naloxone use in women during labor (Schoenfeld et al. 1987). Therefore, naloxone should be reserved for cases in which there is clear potential for reduction in morbidity or mortality, such as in opioid overdose.

Benzodiazepine overdoses, either alone or in combination with other substances, are common, although mortality is typically low if the benzodiazepine is ingested alone. Flumazenil, an imidazobenzodiazepine, functions as a competitive antagonist at the benzodiazepine binding site on the GABA$_A$ receptor and is FDA approved as an antidote in the management of benzodiazepine intoxication (both therapeutic or iatrogenic, such as in conscious sedation or anesthesia, and secondary to recreational or suicidal overdose). Flumazenil has a fairly low bioavailability when given by mouth; therefore, it is administered primarily parenterally. However, it can be administered orally and even rectally, albeit at higher doses, when necessary for long-term management and prevention of re-sedation, particularly in comatose patients (Weinbroum et al. 1997). Its rapid onset of action makes it quite effective in managing acute benzodiazepine overdose.

Flumazenil also can be used to reverse general anesthesia and promote quicker recovery and to manage overdose with nonbenzodiazepine sedative-hypnotics (e.g., zolpidem, zaleplon, eszopiclone). Despite its potential utility, flumazenil carries a significant potential for adverse effects. The most common side effects include acute agitation, dizziness, nausea, and vomiting. Serious and potentially life-threatening adverse effects include seizures, bradycardia, hypotension, and ventricular arrhythmias (Longmire and Seger 1993). However, with appropriate administration, flumazenil does not typically produce significant hemodynamic changes (Weinbroum et al. 1997). The risk of seizures with flumazenil use is higher in patients with seizure disorders and head injury, as well as in habitual or chronic sedative-hypnotic users. Of particular concern is the use of flumazenil in combined benzodiazepine and proarrhythmic or proconvulsant drug ingestions (e.g., tricyclic antidepressants, carbamazepine, phenothiazines, isoniazid, theophylline, clozapine), which may significantly increase the risk for treatment-emergent seizures and ventricular arrhythmias (Seger 2004). Such risks are reduced by starting with low-dose flumazenil via slow infusion and titration (Weinbroum et al. 1997). In weighing the above benefits and risks, routine use of flumazenil in benzodiazepine overdose is not recommended at this time (Penninga et al. 2016).

There is a lack of controlled human studies of flumazenil use in pregnancy. The consensus is that its use in pregnancy should be reserved for cases in which there is clear risk of morbidity or mortality in the mother or fetus and supportive measures are either inadequate or impractical (Zelner et al. 2015).

Substance Use Disorders

Several pharmacological options are available for the treatment of withdrawal states, as well as for the maintenance of abstinence, by managing cravings or blocking the central effects of certain substances. Nevertheless, data are limited on the use of these agents in the medically ill. Therefore, discussion of the pharmacological properties and potential adverse effects requires extrapolation to the medically ill. Of particular focus in this chapter are alcohol, sedative-hypnotics, opioids, tobacco, stimulants, and cannabis, along with some additional information on other relevant and more novel substances.

Alcohol Use Disorder

Alcohol use disorder (AUD) is one of the most commonly encountered substance use disorders in the medically ill. It has been estimated that 21%–42% of patients admitted to general medical wards and 30%–40% of those admitted to ICUs have signs and symptoms that meet diagnostic criteria for AUD (de Wit et al. 2010). In fact, close to 50% of all trauma patients have detectable serum alcohol levels at the time of admission (de Wit et al. 2010). Heavy alcohol use can cause hypoglycemia; electrolyte imbalances (hyponatremia, hypokalemia, hypomagnesemia, and hypophosphatemia); deficiency of thiamine, folate, and other B vitamins; bone marrow suppression, leading to thrombocytopenia and even pancytopenia; cardiotoxicity resulting in arrhythmias and left ventricular dysfunction; acute and chronic hepatic failure (cirrhosis); renal insufficiency or failure; pancreatitis; increased risk of bleeding; and increased risk of nosocomial infections and sepsis. These effects result in increased requirement for critical care services, longer hospital length of stay, delayed rehabilitation, and a twofold increase in mortality (de Wit et al. 2010; Moss and Burnham 2006; O'Brien et al. 2007).

Alcohol Withdrawal Syndrome

Alcohol withdrawal syndrome (AWS) is characterized by a constellation of symptoms, including autonomic hyperarousal and neurological dysfunction, that can lead to potentially life-threatening sequelae. AWS typically occurs approximately 6–24 hours after a steep drop in blood alcohol levels or complete cessation of alcohol consumption. Uncomplicated AWS typically peaks in 48–72 hours and subsides in 5–7 days, although residual sequelae, such as anxiety, insomnia, and autonomic hyperarousal, can last much longer. Common symptoms of AWS include anxiety, insomnia, irritability, nausea and vomiting, tremulousness, perceptual disturbances (visual, auditory, tactile), diaphoresis, tachycardia, and hypertension. These symptoms can then progress to delirium tremens with severe autonomic instability, extreme fluctuations in heart rate and blood pressure, hyperthermia, arrhythmias, clouding of sensorium, delirium, psychosis, seizures, coma, and even death.

Although more than 50% of patients with AUD experience some degree of withdrawal, most experience only mild symptoms without further progression (Mirijello et al. 2015). Contrary to long-held beliefs, most people with AUD do not develop severe alcohol withdrawal symptoms. In fact, the prevalence of severe withdrawal leading to delirium tremens in patients admitted for AWS is between 3% and 5% (Schuckit 2014). Delirium tremens carries a mortality risk of between 1% and 4% in otherwise uncomplicated inpatients, and this risk can be as high as 20% in the hospitalized medically ill (Maldonado et al. 2014; Schuckit 2014). Less severe withdrawal symptoms can still be dangerous in more vulnerable patients. For example, less severe increases in heart rate and blood pressure may precipitate myocardial infarction in a patient with marginal coronary reserve.

The risk for added morbidity, extended length of stay, delayed rehabilitation, and potential long-term cognitive sequelae as a direct result of complicated withdrawal underscores the importance of early identification and treatment of medically ill patients at risk for developing severe AWS. The most commonly used instrument for measuring AWS severity, the revised Clinical Institute Withdrawal Assessment for Alcohol (CIWA-Ar), is highly subjective and was standardized primarily in an uncomplicated alcohol-dependent population (Sullivan et al. 1989). More recently, a shorter and more efficient version of CIWA-Ar was developed, the Brief Alcohol Withdrawal Scale, which focuses mostly on the more objective elements of the

CIWA-Ar scale (i.e., tremor, diaphoresis, agitation, confusion or disorientation, and perceptual disturbances). This version has a higher sensitivity in identifying mild to moderate alcohol withdrawal as compared with the CIWA-Ar, takes much less time to administer, and is effective in specialized acute detoxification settings, as well as in medical-surgical and intensive care settings (Lindner et al. 2019; Rastegar et al. 2017, 2021). An alternative alcohol withdrawal measurement instrument, the modified Minnesota Detoxification Scale, does not rely on patient participation, rather emphasizing more objective findings such as vital signs and physical examination findings (e.g., tremors, diaphoresis), as well as other observational findings (e.g., level of agitation, presence or absence of seizures). This instrument is especially useful in patients who cannot communicate effectively, such as those commonly encountered in the critical care setting (Heavner et al. 2018).

Screening instruments for AUD, such as the Alcohol Use Disorders Identification Test (AUDIT), its revised version (AUDIT-PC), and the CAGE (cut down, annoyed, guilty, eye-opener) questionnaire, have been studied in medically ill patients and have been shown to be sensitive indicators of current or past problematic alcohol use (Bohn et al. 1995; Soderstrom et al. 1997). Among these screening tools, the AUDIT-PC has shown potential utility in predicting AWS in medically hospitalized patients (Pecoraro et al. 2014). However, the ability of these screening instruments to specifically identify patients who are at highest risk for developing severe, clinically significant alcohol withdrawal has not been established. To rectify this, Maldonado and colleagues (2014) developed a screening instrument, the Prediction of Alcohol Withdrawal Severity Scale (PAWSS), to identify medically ill patients who are at greatest risk for developing severe alcohol withdrawal. This scale includes factors such as history of alcohol withdrawal, history of withdrawal seizures or delirium tremens, concomitant use of sedative-hypnotics, recent drinking history, blood alcohol level on admission, and physical evidence of autonomic hyperactivity. Although the PAWSS has been validated for use in hospitalized medically ill patients, its generalizability across all inpatient medical settings (e.g., ICUs) warrants further study (Maldonado et al. 2015). Early identification of at-risk medically ill patients before they develop withdrawal symptoms can facilitate decisions to initiate pharmacological prophylactic measures in those at highest risk, mitigating unnecessary administration of benzodiazepines and other GABAergic agents.

The effective management of alcohol withdrawal in the medically ill involves implementation of vigilant monitoring parameters and correction of associated and comorbid physiological insults, including the correction of electrolyte imbalances (particularly sodium, potassium, magnesium, and phosphorus), as well as adequate nutritional supplementation. Of greatest concern is the increased propensity for medically ill patients with AUD to develop thiamine (vitamin B_1) deficiency, which can then lead to the development of Wernicke's encephalopathy and, if left untreated, Korsakoff's amnestic syndrome, collectively referred to as Wernicke-Korsakoff syndrome (WKS). Studies have shown that most cases of WKS occur in patients with AUD (Harper et al. 1995). Patients with chronic AUD are at significant risk for developing WKS because of reduced thiamine absorption in the gastrointestinal tract, reduced thiamine storage in the liver stemming from hepatocyte necrosis, increased metabolic demand due to consumption of simple carbohydrates commonly found in alcoholic beverages, and poor dietary intake of thiamine (Thomson 2000). Importantly, the classic triad of altered mental status, nystagmus, and ataxia, historically used to diagnose Wernicke's encephalopathy, is not present in most patients who are later confirmed to have WKS. For this reason, Caine and colleagues (1997) developed operational criteria that require only two of the following signs to be present for a diagnosis: history of dietary deficiency, oculomotor abnormalities (nystagmus, ophthalmoplegia, or gaze palsy), cerebellar dysfunction (ataxia, unsteady gait, dysdiadochokinesia, past pointing, or impairment in heel-shin testing), and altered mental status (confusion or memory impairment).

Thiamine should be administered parenterally (preferably intravenously, so as to establish an adequate concentration gradient to promote passive diffusion across the blood-brain barrier) and before glucose is administered, so as to prevent depletion of existing neuronal thiamine stores. Although current practice in the United States (Isenberg-Grzeda et al. 2014) has been to supplement with 50–100 mg/day of thiamine, guidelines implemented by the Royal College of Physicians in the United Kingdom (Thomson et al. 2002) call for higher doses of thiamine in patients who may be at risk for or are already developing signs or symptoms of WKS. They recommend parenteral thiamine, 500 mg three times daily, for the first 3 days, followed by 250 mg/day for 5 additional days or longer, depending on clinical response (Isenberg-Grzeda et al. 2014; Thomson et al. 2002). Although no general consensus regarding thiamine dosing strategies exists, evidence suggests that practitioners in the United States have been underdosing thiamine, particularly in the population most at risk for WKS (Isenberg-Grzeda et al. 2014). Furthermore, it is important to remember that thiamine deficiency also occurs in severely medically ill patients without AUD (e.g., hyperemesis gravidarum, anorexia nervosa, AIDS- and cancer-related cachexia, prolonged stays in the ICU). High-dose parenteral thiamine supplementation is especially indicated when AWS occurs alongside one of these other conditions.

Although supportive measures are most often sufficient to manage mild AWS in medically ill patients, more intensive interventions are needed to manage moderate to severe AWS. Pharmacological prophylaxis and management of alcohol withdrawal historically have been accomplished primarily by administration of GABA agonists (typically benzodiazepines and less often barbiturates). Benzodiazepines are the most frequently used and most proven pharmacological agents for effectively managing AWS. They act by binding to the benzodiazepine site on the $GABA_A$ receptor, changing the receptor conformation to facilitate binding of the inhibitory neurotransmitter GABA, which then increases the frequency of chloride ion channel opening. Benzodiazepines can have unintended consequences, such as delirium, respiratory depression, and paradoxical disinhibition, particularly in medically ill or vulnerable patients (e.g., older adults; patients with history of head injury or preexisting neurocognitive disorder, respiratory insufficiency, or sleep apnea). Benzodiazepine use is a major risk factor for the development of delirium in intensive care patients (Pandharipande et al. 2006). Benzodiazepines and other sedative-hypnotics can also contribute to the development of hepatic encephalopathy. Because of the potential life-threatening sequelae of advanced AWS, one must not fail to treat this condition. Thus, clinicians should carefully consider the risks and benefits of benzodiazepine treatment in medically ill patients. Benzodiazepines have historically been considered the most effective agents in halting the progression of AWS, preventing and treating withdrawal-related seizures, and treating delirium tremens (Mirijello et al. 2015). Decisions regarding which benzodiazepine to use in managing AWS should be individualized to each patient. Specifically, factors affecting drug metabolism and clearance, such as the patient's age and the presence of hepatic impairment, should be considered when choosing a benzodiazepine. The most commonly used long-acting benzodiazepines for AWS, chlordiazepoxide and diazepam, initially undergo hepatic oxidation (Phase I hepatic metabolism), thereby producing active metabolites, which allows less frequent dosing and a smoother taper, making them favored agents in fixed-dose and loading-dose strategies. However, these pharmacokinetic properties can result in the accumulation of active metabolites in individuals with reduced hepatic clearance, such as the elderly and those with hepatic congestion due to heart failure or cirrhosis. This can result in respiratory depression and delirium. Hence, in patients with impaired hepatic function, the shorter-acting agents lorazepam and oxazepam are favored for managing AWS. Both lorazepam and oxazepam bypass hepatic oxidation and undergo clearance via glucuronidation (Phase II hepatic metabolism), thereby not producing active metabolites. Even with these agents, caution is warranted in severe hepatic and renal impairment. Of the most commonly used benzodiazepines in the management of AWS, lorazepam, chlordiazepoxide, and diazepam are available in both parenteral and oral formulations; oxazepam is available only in an oral formulation, limiting its use in the critically ill (Mirijello et al. 2015). There is a concern with high-dose lorazepam infusions, particularly for critically ill patients, because they can cause propylene glycol toxicity, resulting in metabolic acidosis, acute tubular necrosis, seizures, and arrhythmias (Horinek et al. 2009).

Benzodiazepines have been associated with congenital malformations (cleft lip or palate, cardiovascular malformations, and duodenal atresia) with their use in the first trimester. However, systematic reviews did not support a link between benzodiazepine exposure in the first trimester and major congenital malformations (Bellantuono et al. 2013; Grigoriadis et al. 2019). Benzodiazepine use in pregnancy also has been associated with preterm labor and fetal distress, as well as increased risk of spontaneous abortion, low birth weight, and low Apgar scores (Grigoriadis et al. 2020). Decisions about the use of benzodiazepines must take into account the potential risks of untreated AWS in pregnancy, such as fetal distress, precipitation of preterm labor, and the inherent risks of AWS to the mother (DeVido et al. 2015).

Both standing (fixed-dose and loading-dose) and symptom-triggered dosing strategies exist for benzodiazepines in the management of AWS. Earlier studies have shown that symptom-triggered benzodiazepine administration in AWS can reduce total benzodiazepine requirements and duration of treatment, but this is contingent on the careful systematic execution of such protocols in well-controlled settings (DeCarolis et al. 2007; Saitz et al. 1994).

More recent studies suggest that although symptom-triggered dosing strategies have their advantages, both loading-dose and fixed-dose strategies appear to be equally efficacious and may be preferred in cases of severe alcohol withdrawal, especially when such strategies are used in the early stages (Maldonado et al. 2012).

Although benzodiazepines are still regarded as the gold standard in the management of AWS, their use carries some well-known risks, especially in the medically ill population. Most notably, benzodiazepine use increases risk for delirium, excessive sedation, respiratory depression, and falls. For this reason, there has been a renewed interest in developing pharmacological strategies that use nonbenzodiazepine alternatives for AWS (Maldonado 2017). Other pharmacological agents have been shown to have potential utility as monotherapies and adjunctive therapies in select patient populations. Alternative agents for the management of AWS include barbiturates (e.g., phenobarbital), propofol, ketamine, baclofen, anticonvulsants (e.g., carbamazepine, oxcarbazepine, gabapentin, pregabalin, valproic acid, topiramate, and lamotrigine), and sympatholytic agents such as α_2 agonists (e.g., clonidine, dexmedetomidine, guanfacine).

Barbiturates, like benzodiazepines, bind to the $GABA_A$ receptor but at different binding sites. In contrast to benzodiazepines, barbiturates facilitate the action of GABA by increasing the duration (rather than frequency) of chloride ion channel opening, as well as directly stimulating the chloride ion channels at higher doses, which contributes to their narrow therapeutic index, toxicity, and potential for lethality. Although no longer as commonly used because of their significant drug-drug interactions and narrow therapeutic index, barbiturates still have potential utility in select patients as monotherapy or adjunctive therapy in managing AWS. Phenobarbital, a long-acting barbiturate, is the most commonly used barbiturate in treating AWS. It has been shown to be an effective adjunct and comparable alternative to benzodiazepines in emergency department, general medical, and intensive care settings (Nejad et al. 2020; Nguyen and Lam 2020; Nisavic et al. 2019; Rosenson et al. 2013). A systematic review of studies examining phenobarbital use in AWS concluded that phenobarbital, used as monotherapy or adjunctively with benzodiazepines, provided similar or better outcomes as compared with benzodiazepine monotherapy, particularly with early and aggressive phenobarbital dosing strategies (Hammond et al. 2017). However, phenobarbital carries higher risk when used in the medically ill, particularly in the elderly and those with hepatic impairment, primarily because of the potential for accumulation of active metabolites, which can then cause oversedation, respiratory depression, and delirium. Phenobarbital is an inducer of cytochrome P450 (CYP) enzymes; therefore, significant drug-drug interactions may preclude its use in patients who are following complex pharmacological regimens. Overall, phenobarbital remains a viable treatment option, particularly for complicated and severe alcohol withdrawal; however, its use should be carefully individualized.

Propofol is a parenteral (intravenous) sedative that is used for induction and maintenance of anesthesia exclusively in the emergency, critical care, and procedural settings. It is a GABA$_A$ agonist as well as an N-methyl-D-aspartate (NMDA) receptor antagonist, has a short half-life, and is highly lipophilic. Propofol has been shown in case series to be effective in managing benzodiazepine-refractory delirium tremens (Hughes et al. 2014; McCowan and Marik 2000). Of note, propofol carries a risk of respiratory depression, hypotension, bradycardia, and, less commonly, hypertriglyceridemia, acute pancreatitis, and propofol infusion syndrome (Asghar et al. 2020; Hemphill et al. 2019; Marik 2004).

Ketamine, a noncompetitive NMDA receptor antagonist and rapid-acting dissociative anesthetic and analgesic agent, has a limited evidence base supporting its use in AWS, primarily as an adjunct to benzodiazepines in severe, treatment-refractory alcohol withdrawal or delirium tremens (Pizon et al. 2018; Shah et al. 2018). Ketamine can cause clinically significant elevations in blood pressure and heart rate, as well as respiratory depression, in addition to "emergence phenomena," which can result in severe anxiety, agitation, paranoia, perceptual disturbances or hallucinations, and delirium (Manasco et al. 2020).

Baclofen, a GABA$_B$ receptor agonist, appeared to be comparable to a benzodiazepine in two small-scale randomized trials (Addolorato et al. 2006; Gulati et al. 2019). Because of the sparsity and very low quality of available evidence, baclofen is not recommended for routine use in managing AWS (Liu and Wang 2019). Furthermore, given that baclofen is available only in oral and intrathecal formulations, its versatility, particularly in severe AWS, is limited. However, because baclofen is primarily renally excreted, with only minimal hepatic metabolism, it can be considered as an alternative or adjunctive option for the management of AWS in patients with severe hepatic impairment and for whom conventional strategies for managing AWS have failed.

Baclofen is generally safe to use in the medically ill; however, it can cause somnolence, lethargy, hypotonia, hyporeflexia, hypothermia, hypotension, bradycardia, respiratory depression, delirium, and seizures (Romito et al. 2022).

In pregnancy, phenobarbital is known to cross the placenta and has been associated with major congenital malformations, cleft lip or palate, and prenatal growth retardation (Veroniki et al. 2017). The risk of major congenital malformations with phenobarbital use in pregnancy appears to be dose dependent, with the greatest risk seen at dosages of 80 mg/day or greater (Tomson et al. 2018). In addition, phenobarbital poses a risk for respiratory and overall CNS depression and therefore should be used with extreme caution in pregnancy and lactation. Propofol is highly lipophilic and readily crosses the placenta. There is a lack of available evidence to fully evaluate the potential risks associated with propofol use in pregnancy and lactation; however, if use is deemed necessary, propofol is recommended only for short-term (<3 hours) use because there is a risk of maternal hypotension and neonatal CNS depression. Ketamine is known to cross the placenta; however, there is a lack of available evidence to fully evaluate risks in pregnancy and lactation at this time. A recent systematic review of hypnotic agents in patients undergoing cesarean delivery found that ketamine use for induction of general anesthesia was associated with lower Apgar scores (Houthoff Khemlani et al. 2018). If ketamine use is deemed to be clinically necessary, it is recommended that use be of short duration (<3 hours) because of the risk of respiratory depression and neonatal CNS depression. Last, there is a lack of available human studies to fully determine the potential risks associated with baclofen use in pregnancy and lactation. Because of a relative lack of available observational data, the extent of baclofen absorption across the placenta has not been fully evaluated. Oral (in contrast to intrathecal) baclofen has been associated with neonatal withdrawal syndrome, especially with prolonged use of baclofen during pregnancy (Romito et al. 2022). Furthermore, a recent pharmacokinetic study suggested that newborn serum baclofen levels at and immediately after birth may be at their highest, at least partially because of the slower elimination half-life of baclofen in newborns (Balakirouchenane et al. 2021). Thus, baclofen should be used with extreme caution in managing AWS in pregnancy.

Anticonvulsants also have been used to manage AWS and are garnering increased attention as alternatives to benzodiazepines (Maldonado 2017). Anticonvulsants exert their effects via myriad mechanisms, including binding to and inhibiting voltage-gated sodium channels (carbamazepine, oxcarbazepine, valproate, topiramate, and lamotrigine) and voltage-gated calcium channels (gabapentin, pregabalin, and valproate), facilitation of GABAergic transmission by promoting presynaptic GABA release and inhibition of GABA catabolism (valproate), inhibition of glutamatergic activity via NMDA receptor blockade (topiramate), and reduction of presynaptic glutamate release (lamotrigine) (Sills and Rogawski 2020). A Cochrane review of 56 studies of anticonvulsants for alcohol withdrawal did not show a statistically significant difference in CIWA-Ar scores or major outcomes (delirium tremens, life-threatening adverse events) between anticonvulsants and placebo or anticonvulsants compared with each other; however, anticonvulsants did show a protective benefit against seizures (Minozzi et al. 2010). In this particular review, carbamazepine was the only anticonvulsant associated with a statistically significant reduction in alcohol withdrawal symptoms when compared with benzodiazepines (Minozzi et al. 2010). Recent systematic reviews and meta-analyses of randomized controlled trials have not supported the use of anticonvulsants as first-line treatment for AWS at any level of severity, citing high dropout rates and poor quality of existing evidence (Lai et al. 2022; Rojo-Mira et al. 2022). Of the anticonvulsants, carbamazepine and oxcarbazepine, valproate, gabapentin and pregabalin, and topiramate have been shown to have some potential utility as adjunctive therapies in treating AWS (Hammond et al. 2015). Overall, when considering anticonvulsants in managing AWS, the evidence is, at most, supportive of adjunctive or second-line use, and such use should be based on individualized, patient-specific circumstances.

Although also covered elsewhere in this book, it is again worth mentioning the more relevant pharmacokinetic properties and potential adverse effects of some of the more commonly used anticonvulsants in patients with AUD and AWS. Carbamazepine is a known CYP inducer (primarily CYP3A4) and also induces its own metabolism and hence requires more frequent monitoring and dosing adjustments. Valproate (including valproic acid and divalproex sodium) is a well-known CYP inhibitor (particularly CYP2C9). Gabapentin and pregabalin do not undergo hepatic metabolism and are excreted via the kidney unchanged. Topiramate is also predominantly renally excreted, without significant hepatic metabolism (Asconape 2014). It is also a carbonic anhydrase inhibitor, thus increasing the risk for development of metabolic acidosis and formation of renal calculi. Furthermore, topiramate often causes cognitive dysfunction and paresthesias. It should also be noted that valproate is highly protein-bound and should be used with caution in patients who are also taking warfarin because it can displace warfarin from protein binding sites, increasing serum levels of the unbound warfarin and thereby increasing bleeding risk. This drug-drug interaction is especially important to recognize in patients with AUD, given their heightened risk of liver impairment and bone marrow suppression, which also increases bleeding risk because of reduced production of coagulation factors and platelets. Valproate is also independently associated with an increased risk for thrombocytopenia, which may further compound bleeding risk in patients with AUD; therefore, valproate should be used with caution (Buoli et al. 2018). Last, given the heightened risk of hyponatremia in heavy alcohol users, it is important to mention that many anticonvulsants have been associated with hyponatremia, with oxcarbazepine and carbamazepine carrying the highest risk (Lu and Wang 2017). These factors underscore the need to carefully consider both acute and chronic medical comorbidities when choosing an anticonvulsant for managing AWS.

Use of most anticonvulsants in pregnancy, especially in the first trimester, should be done with extreme caution. Among the anticonvulsants, valproate carries the highest risk of major congenital malformations (particularly neural tube defects, cleft lip or palate, hypospadias, and clubfoot) and should be avoided in pregnancy (Tomson et al. 2019; Veroniki et al. 2017). Carbamazepine and topiramate also carry a significant risk for major congenital malformations and should be avoided in pregnancy (Veroniki et al. 2017). There is a relative lack of sufficient data to make any firm conclusions about risk associated with gabapentin (and pregabalin) use in pregnancy; however, a recent meta-analysis found that the risk of major congenital malformations with gabapentin use was similar to that in unexposed control subjects (Veroniki et al. 2017). Among the anticonvulsants, lamotrigine and oxcarbazepine have been associated with the lowest risk of adverse fetal outcomes, including major congenital malformations (Tomson et al. 2018, 2019). There appears to be a dose-dependent relationship for risk of developing major congenital malformations with use of valproate, carbamazepine, and lamotrigine (Tomson et al. 2018, 2019). Furthermore, valproate and topiramate have been associated with an increased risk of combined fetal losses, with both (particularly topiramate) also being associated with increased risk for intrauterine growth retardation (Tomson et al. 2019; Veroniki et al. 2017). Last, in utero valproate exposure also has been associated with increased risk for development of cognitive impairment and behavioral abnormalities (i.e., autism spectrum disorders, ADHD, difficulty with socialization and motor function) (Tomson et al. 2019).

The sympatholytic drugs (primarily α_2 agonists) have been shown in some studies to be useful in the management of AWS, particularly as adjunctive agents. Specifically, these agents may assist in tempering the autonomic hyperactivity associated with AWS. The α_2 agonists clonidine and dexmedetomidine have been the most widely studied and have been found to be effective primarily as adjuncts to benzodiazepines in treating AWS (Muzyk et al. 2011). Clonidine is available in oral tablet (both immediate- and extended-release) and transdermal patch formulations, as well as in an injectable solution for epidural or intrathecal use (mainly for adjunctive analgesia in intractable and postoperative pain). The oral tablet can also be administered sublingually and appears to have equivalent pharmacokinetics in the event that a patient is unable to accept medications enterally (Cunningham et al. 1994). Dexmedetomidine is a very highly selective, centrally acting α_2 agonist, administered intravenously and used primarily in the critical care setting. It is an alternative to standard sedation protocols for managing agitation or delirium in mechanically ventilated patients, as well as for facilitating extubation for patients who are having difficulty weaning off mechanical ventilation (Buckley et al. 2021; Pandharipande et al. 2007, 2010). It has garnered attention as a potentially useful agent in managing treatment-refractory and severe AWS in critically ill patients, particularly because of its benzodiazepine-sparing effect (Frazee et al. 2014; Mueller et al. 2014). This benzodiazepine-sparing effect is particularly beneficial for critically ill patients because reduced benzodiazepine burden can help in decreasing the risk of delirium and respiratory depression. A systematic review of studies in adult ICU patients with alcohol withdrawal–related delirium (a known indicator of severe alcohol withdrawal) concluded that the addition of dexmedetomidine to benzodiazepines reduced delirium severity, as measured by associated reduction in CIWA scores (Woods et al. 2015). However, use of adjunctive dexmedetomidine in AWS has been associated with an increased ICU length of stay (Yavarovich et al. 2019). Last, guanfacine, which is also a centrally acting α_2 agonist, can be considered as an alternative to clonidine and dexmedetomidine in managing AWS. Guanfacine is available only in oral tablet (both immediate- and extended-release) formulations. Guanfacine has a much higher affinity for the α_{2A} receptor and a much longer half-life than clonidine. Guanfacine is also a much better anxiolytic than clonidine. Although there have been no formal human studies using guanfacine for AWS, Maldonado (2017) reported successful use of guanfacine in complicated AWS and has incorporated it into a novel benzodiazepine-sparing algorithm for managing AWS. Overall, although monotherapy is not recommended at this time, use of α_2 agonists (particularly dexmedetomidine) as adjuncts in severe or treatment-refractory AWS should be strongly considered, especially in the critically ill population.

Both clonidine and dexmedetomidine have been associated with significant hypotension and bradycardia, whereas guanfacine has much less of an effect on hemodynamics and is much less likely to result in significant hypotension. Furthermore, especially when used long term, clonidine has the potential to cause rebound tachycardia and hypertension with abrupt discontinuation. By virtue of its much longer half-life, guanfacine is less prone to this effect.

There is a lack of human studies to fully evaluate the potential risks associated with clonidine, guanfacine, and dexmedetomidine use in pregnancy and lactation. As with most drugs in this pregnancy risk category, use should be based on careful consideration of potential risks and benefits, with the assumption that there will indeed be some degree of fetal exposure.

Most of the available studies have examined α_2 agonists, and β-blockers have not been as widely studied and seem to have limited utility in AWS. Therefore, use of β-blockers in AWS is not recommended at this time. It should also be noted that these agents can mask sympathetic symptoms associated with AWS, often falsely lowering CIWA-Ar scores. β-Blockers (particularly nonselective ones) are contraindicated in patients with asthma, chronic obstructive pulmonary disease, hypoglycemia, and some cardiac conduction abnormalities (e.g., second- and third-degree heart block).

Antipsychotics are not specifically indicated for managing AWS but can be beneficial as adjunctive therapies for managing associated agitation and delirium. Haloperidol, in particular, has been extensively and safely used in the medically ill. It can be administered via multiple routes (e.g., intramuscular, intravenous, oral, rectal), further adding to its versatility, particularly in critical care settings. Alternatively, sedating atypical antipsychotics (particularly olanzapine and quetiapine) can be used and may be more effective adjuncts in promoting sleep-wake cycle restoration and managing agitation in patients with delirium tremens. Caution should be exercised when using antipsychotics in patients with AWS, particularly because of the drugs' potential for lowering seizure threshold and inducing cardiac arrhythmias. Antipsychotic use in delirium is discussed in more detail elsewhere in this book.

Finally, although intravenous ethanol infusions have historically been used to manage AWS, this practice has fallen out of favor, primarily because of the narrow therapeutic index, inability to safely dose, and potential for multiorgan toxicity. Furthermore, a randomized controlled trial in critically ill patients did not support the use of intravenous ethanol infusion over diazepam in AWS prophylaxis (Weinberg et al. 2008).

Alcohol Abstinence and Craving

The main drugs that are FDA approved for the maintenance of abstinence in AUD are disulfiram, naltrexone (both a daily oral formulation and a monthly intramuscular formulation), and acamprosate.

Disulfiram functions via aversive conditioning, exerting its effects primarily by inhibition of the hepatic enzyme aldehyde dehydrogenase, resulting in the accumulation of toxic acetaldehyde. This precipitates an acute reaction resulting in nausea, vomiting, flushing, hypotension, dizziness, diaphoresis, headache, and anxiety or panic symptoms. Patients who are taking disulfiram and providers who are caring for these patients should be cautioned against using products containing alcohol (e.g., mouthwash, medications such as cough syrup and certain intravenous solutions, foods cooked in alcohol, hand sanitizer, alcohol swabs) because some patients are so sensitive that even slight contact (topical or olfactory) can precipitate this violent reaction. A challenge with using disulfiram, possibly more than with drugs that function by reducing cravings, is the significant potential for noncompliance. The strongest evidence supporting the efficacy of disulfiram in maintaining abstinence and reducing relapse in AUD is based mostly on open-label trials performed in supervised settings (Skinner et al. 2014). Disulfiram is available only in an oral tablet formulation; it relies exclusively on enteral absorption and hepatic metabolism. Disulfiram is potentially hepatotoxic, has precipitated fulminant hepatic failure, and is contraindicated in patients with end-stage liver disease. It is also potentially cardiotoxic and can precipitate arrhythmias and congestive heart failure, particularly in patients with cardiovascular risk factors. Furthermore, severe disulfiram toxicity can precipitate both sensorimotor and cognitive adverse effects (e.g., peripheral neuropathy, visual disturbances, weakness, fatigue, confusion, florid delirium). Disulfiram should not be administered until at least 12 hours after the last use of alcohol, to avoid precipitation of the disulfiram reaction.

Naltrexone functions primarily as a competitive antagonist at the μ opioid receptor and to a lesser extent at the κ and δ opioid receptors. The once-daily oral formulation was approved by the FDA for treating AUD in 1994, and a monthly intramuscular depot formulation was approved in 2006. Naltrexone tablets can also be crushed and made into a liquid formulation for oral administration. Naltrexone promotes abstinence by blocking critical pathways in the reward center of the brain that are responsible for the reinforcing effects of alcohol, as well as by reducing cravings for alcohol. A systematic review and meta-analysis of seven randomized placebo-controlled trials showed that monthly depot naltrexone reduced total drinking days and heavy drinking days per month compared with placebo (Murphy et al. 2022). Administering naltrexone to a patient who is taking or has recently taken opioids can rapidly precipitate opioid withdrawal (Quigley and Boyce 2001). Patients who have recently used opioids (including opioid receptor agonists such as tramadol) should typically wait at least 7–10 days before starting naltrexone, to avoid precipitation of acute withdrawal. It is recommended that patients taking oral naltrexone stop the medication at least 3 days before scheduled procedures that may require the use of centrally acting opioid agonists. Those taking the monthly depot formulation of naltrexone present a greater challenge and should forgo opioid agonist therapy (i.e., scheduled surgeries or procedures) for at least 3 weeks after the administration of depot naltrexone. Although administration of opioids in the fourth week after depot naltrexone administration is possible, it often requires use of much larger doses of opioids to provide adequate analgesia (Curatolo and Trinh 2014). However, because of opioid receptor upregulation and increased receptor sensitivity, patients are at a significantly higher risk for respiratory depression and autonomic instability with administration of opioids during the fourth week after depot naltrexone administration, thereby necessitating close monitoring (Curatolo and Trinh 2014).

Oral naltrexone is heavily hepatically metabolized, whereas the depot formulation bypasses first-pass hepatic oxidation. Both formulations carry the risk of hepatotoxicity and should be used with caution in patients with liver impairment (Garbutt 2010). Guidelines recommend avoiding use of naltrexone when a patient's transaminases are elevated to three times the normal range and in patients with end-stage liver disease (Ross and Peselow 2009). Overall, oral naltrexone is relatively safe and has not been shown to increase risk for serious adverse events when compared with placebo (Bolton et al. 2019).

Acamprosate is the third FDA-approved medication for AUD, having gained formal approval in 2004. It has a fairly complex mechanism of action, exerting influence primarily via modulation of glutamatergic (NMDA) and GABAergic receptors (Plosker 2015). Like naltrexone, acamprosate functions by reducing cravings; in contrast to naltrexone, however, acamprosate functions primarily by inhibiting negative reinforcement (Ross and Peselow 2009). Acamprosate is available only in an oral tablet formulation and is fairly well tolerated, with the most common side effects being mild to moderate gastrointestinal distress (primarily diarrhea; possibly nausea or vomiting and flatulence) and anorexia (Plosker 2015). Although there have been reports of increased anxiety, depression, and suicidality with acamprosate use, these adverse effects are relatively rare (Plosker 2015). In a meta-analysis of 122 randomized clinical trials, both acamprosate and naltrexone were found to reduce propensity for return to drinking, and no statistically significant difference was found between the two (Jonas et al. 2014). A more recent meta-analysis of 64 randomized controlled trials, which included both pharmacological and psychosocial interventions for maintaining abstinence in AUD, showed that acamprosate was the only intervention associated with an increased probability of 12-month abstinence at a moderate degree of certainty in the primary care setting (Cheng et al. 2020). Acamprosate does not undergo hepatic metabolism and is excreted unchanged by the kidney. It does not cause any significant CYP drug-drug interactions and can be used safely in individuals with hepatic impairment. Caution should be exercised in patients with reduced glomerular filtration rate (i.e., older adults and patients with renal insufficiency), and acamprosate should generally be avoided in end-stage renal disease (Plosker 2015).

Nalmefene is a μ and δ opioid receptor antagonist, as well as partial agonist at the κ opioid receptor (Mann et al. 2016). Although not currently used in the United States, oral nalmefene is commonly used in Europe and was approved by the EMA in 2013 for reducing alcohol intake in patients with AUD. Nalmefene has been shown to reduce the degree of alcohol consumption (both heavy drinking days and total daily alcohol consumption) in patients with AUD (Mann et al. 2016). Nalmefene has a longer half-life and less propensity for inducing hepatotoxicity than naltrexone, making it a potential alternative for patients with liver impairment (Ross and Peselow 2009). A recent open-label study of as-needed nalmefene in patients with AUD confirmed that it can indeed be safely used by patients with mild liver impairment (Mueller et al. 2020).

Although human studies of disulfiram, naltrexone, acamprosate, or nalmefene use in pregnancy and lactation are lacking, the available evidence indicates that naltrexone and acamprosate may be the safest options (Kelty et al. 2021). Disulfiram has been associated with an increased risk of congenital malformations (e.g., limb defects), as well as autonomic instability triggered by the alcohol-disulfiram reaction, which may lead to fetal distress; therefore, disulfiram use should be avoided in pregnancy (DeVido et al. 2015; Kelty et al. 2021). Given the current lack of data regarding the safety profile of nalmefene in pregnancy and lactation, its use in this population is cautioned at this time. Nevertheless, especially given the well-known risks of maternal alcohol consumption on fetal development, the use of pharmacological agents in treatment of AUD in pregnancy should be strongly considered.

Other agents that may have abstinence-promoting utility in AUD have also been studied, with the most evidence for anticonvulsants, particularly topiramate and gabapentin (Blodgett et al. 2014; Hammond et al. 2015; Kranzler et al. 2019). Studies have also suggested the potential utility of baclofen, serotonergic agents (e.g., selective serotonin reuptake inhibitors [SSRIs], ondansetron), aripiprazole, and, more recently, varenicline for AUD (Edwards et al. 2011; Gandhi et al. 2020). Although baclofen may hold promise for promoting abstinence in heavy drinkers, results from randomized controlled trials remain mixed, with higher dosages (>60 mg/day) generally being difficult to tolerate (Minozzi et al. 2018; Pierce et al. 2018). Likewise, although varenicline appears to assist in reducing alcohol cravings, a recent systematic review and meta-analysis of the available randomized placebo-controlled trials showed that it does not promote a statistically significant decrease in alcohol consumption in patients with AUD (Gandhi et al. 2020). Although not currently being used for AUD in the United States, sodium oxybate, the sodium salt of γ-hydroxybutyric acid, has been approved in Austria and Italy both for managing AWS and as an abstinence-promoting agent (Keating 2014). Postmarketing surveillance of sodium oxybate has confirmed that it is relatively safe and without serious adverse effects when used properly in patients with

AUD who do not have significant psychiatric comorbidities or history of polysubstance use (Addolorato et al. 2020). The abuse potential associated with sodium oxybate limits its usefulness. Because hepatic impairment is common among patients with AUD, abstinence-promoting medications that do not require hepatic metabolism would be desirable in these instances. Baclofen, gabapentin, and topiramate may be considered if acamprosate is not feasible for such patients. Furthermore, baclofen is the only abstinence-promoting agent that has been evaluated and found safe for use in patients with AUD and advanced liver disease (Mosoni et al. 2018). Overall, the evidence base is still not strong enough to make specific recommendations about first-line use of these agents for AUD at this time.

Sedative-, Hypnotic-, or Anxiolytic-Related Disorders

Sedative, hypnotic, and anxiolytic medications are commonly prescribed and quite readily abused. Benzodiazepines, barbiturates, and GABAergic sleep aids (i.e., zolpidem, eszopiclone, and zaleplon) fall into this category. Benzodiazepines with a short half-life, particularly alprazolam, have the highest potential for abuse and dependence. Although it shares many clinical similarities with AWS, withdrawal from benzodiazepines may, in contrast, have a delayed onset (particularly with benzodiazepines that have a long half-life) and more protracted course.

Sedative, hypnotic, and anxiolytic withdrawal can be more severe than withdrawal from other substances, including alcohol. The management of such withdrawal is similar to that of AWS, which is discussed in the subsection "Alcohol Withdrawal Syndrome" earlier in this chapter. Management typically involves use of a GABAergic agent because most have fairly good cross-reactivity. The exception is alprazolam, which has a novel chemical structure with a triazole ring that seems to have higher binding affinity for a certain subgroup of the benzodiazepine receptor as compared with other benzodiazepines (Ait-Daoud et al. 2018). As a result, alprazolam withdrawal can often be difficult to manage and refractory to treatment with the most common benzodiazepines (i.e., lorazepam, chlordiazepoxide, oxazepam, and diazepam) and barbiturates (i.e., phenobarbital) used in managing AWS. In fact, alprazolam withdrawal often requires the use of alprazolam or clonazepam, which has been shown to be a potentially effective alternative in managing alprazolam withdrawal (Ait-Daoud et al. 2018).

Last, the GABA$_B$ agonist baclofen (discussed in the earlier subsection "Alcohol Use Disorder"), which is commonly used for management of spasticity in patients with spinal cord injury or pathology, has been associated with a potentially life-threatening withdrawal syndrome, similar in presentation to other GABAergic withdrawal syndromes. In comparison with oral baclofen, abrupt cessation or discontinuation of intrathecal baclofen (administered via an intrathecal pump) appears to carry the highest risk of precipitating a severe and potentially life-threatening withdrawal syndrome (Romito et al. 2022). Baclofen withdrawal is most effectively managed by reinstituting baclofen, preferably via the same route of administration as was used before the onset of withdrawal (Romito et al. 2022).

Opioid Use Disorder

Opioid use disorder (OUD) is among the most common substance use disorders in the medically ill. OUD is highly comorbid with chronic pain and blood-borne infectious diseases (particularly hepatitis C and HIV/AIDS). Now having reached epidemic proportions, OUD and resultant withdrawal states are common in general medical wards and ICUs.

Opioid Withdrawal Syndrome

Opioid withdrawal syndrome (OWS) is characterized by autonomic hyperactivity, which results in restlessness, diaphoresis, yawning, rhinorrhea, lacrimation, piloerection, mydriasis, myalgias, and gastrointestinal distress (e.g., cramps, nausea, vomiting, diarrhea). The most commonly administered scale to measure the severity of OWS is the Clinical Opiate Withdrawal Scale. Although OWS is not typically considered life-threatening, fatalities and significant morbidity have been reported with ultrarapid detoxification methods, such as those using naltrexone implants (Hamilton et al. 2002). OWS still has a significant effect on the medically ill, often protracting hospital stays and increasing the risk of complications.

Methadone, a synthetic opioid, was approved by the FDA for the management of OUD in 1972. It functions as a full agonist at the μ opioid receptor. Its long half-life and high receptor binding affinity made it the traditional choice agent for the management of OWS, as well as for maintenance therapy in promoting abstinence and reducing opioid craving (discussed in the next subsection). Methadone can be given orally (as a tablet or solution) and intravenously. It is primarily hepatically metabolized and is a substrate of CYP3A4; therefore, significant drug-drug interactions exist (see Table 18–2 later in this chapter). Of particular importance is the potential for certain antiretrovirals (e.g., efavirenz, darunavir, nevirapine), rifampin, St. John's wort, carbamazepine, phenytoin, and phenobarbital to reduce plasma levels of methadone and effectively precipitate opioid withdrawal (Meemken et al. 2015; Tetrault and Fiellin 2012). Common side effects include sedation, constipation, diaphoresis, urinary retention, and decreased libido. Of greatest concern is the potential for methadone to cause QTc interval prolongation, which ultimately resulted in a black box warning issued by the FDA in 2006. This risk is further increased when methadone is used intravenously, when it is used concomitantly with other QTc-prolonging agents, or when it is combined with drugs that inhibit CYP3A4, such as ritonavir, quetiapine, fluoxetine, fluconazole, and ciprofloxacin (Meemken et al. 2015; Mujtaba et al. 2013; Tetrault and Fiellin 2012). Given the high prevalence of HIV/AIDS infection in intravenous opioid users, potential drug-drug interactions are of significant importance (see also Chapter 12, "Infectious Diseases"). No significant drug-drug interactions exist between methadone and antiretrovirals commonly used to treat hepatitis C infection (Meemken et al. 2015).

Buprenorphine, a semisynthetic opioid, was approved by the FDA for the management of OUD in 2002. It is a partial agonist at the μ opioid receptor and potent antagonist at the κ opioid receptor. Buprenorphine is commonly used to treat OWS and for maintenance therapy in OUD (discussed in the next subsection). A systematic review of randomized controlled trials has shown that buprenorphine is as effective as methadone in managing OWS (Gowing et al. 2017). Buprenorphine has become a preferential alternative to methadone for management of opioid withdrawal, particularly in the medically ill. This is especially because of its lower risk of QTc interval prolongation, as well as its partial agonist and antagonist properties, which impart a ceiling effect that minimizes respiratory depression with dose escalation (Ciraulo et al. 2006; Fareed et al. 2013). Furthermore, buprenorphine, although also a substrate of CYP3A4, has fewer significant drug-drug interactions, particularly with antiretrovirals used to treat HIV, as compared with methadone (Meemken et al. 2015). The exceptions are the antiretroviral drugs atazanavir and ritonavir, which inhibit CYP3A4 and can significantly increase serum levels of buprenorphine and its active metabolite, norbuprenorphine (Meemken et al. 2015).

Much as with methadone, there are no significant drug-drug interactions between buprenorphine and antivirals used in the treatment of hepatitis C infection (Meemken et al. 2015).

Buprenorphine undergoes extensive first-pass metabolism and has low bioavailability when administered orally; therefore, it is typically administered sublingually (in a dissolvable tablet or film) or buccally (in a dissolvable film) either alone or in its combined formulation with naloxone (which is added to deter misuse and diversion) (Ciraulo et al. 2006). Buprenorphine is also available in an extended-release monthly subcutaneous depot formulation and in a 6-month subdermal implant (no longer available in the United States), both having been FDA approved for maintenance treatment of OUD (see the next subsection for additional information). It has also been successfully used intravenously for managing acute opioid withdrawal in medically ill patients (Welsh et al. 2002). A transdermal formulation of buprenorphine is currently approved only for the management of chronic pain, not for OUD or OWS. Caution should be exercised when using buprenorphine in patients with hepatic impairment, particularly those with severe impairment. Buprenorphine, as well as the buprenorphine/naloxone combination, is relatively contraindicated for use in end-stage liver disease. Use in patients undergoing chronic opioid therapy or in those needing acute opioid analgesic therapy, such as in the postoperative setting, can precipitate OWS. The propensity for buprenorphine to occupy μ and κ opioid receptor sites with high binding affinity and slow dissociation blocks the analgesic effects of full opioid agonists and potentially precipitates withdrawal. For this reason, it was previously common practice to hold or avoid using buprenorphine in patients with OUD when use of a full opioid agonist was anticipated, such as in the perioperative setting. However, this practice has now fallen out of favor, largely because of the increased risk for relapse and overdose in this patient population. For this reason, a multisociety expert panel recently developed guidelines that help to demystify and encourage the use of buprenorphine both for analgesia and to mitigate OWS in patients with OUD in the perioperative setting (Kohan et al. 2021). Given its partial agonist properties, buprenorphine can indeed be used as an alternative monotherapy for patients with coexisting OUD and chronic pain or in the acute perioperative setting, reducing the risk of fatal respiratory depression. Along these lines, low-dose or microdose buprenorphine (with initial doses typically ranging from 0.2 to 0.5 mg) cross-titration strategies have successfully been used to transition patients from full opioid agonist therapy to buprenorphine maintenance therapy without precipitating significant OWS (Ahmed et al. 2021). Although such strategies typically necessitate that the buprenorphine sublingual film or tablet be cut into halves or quarters, use of the buccal film formulation, which comes in smaller (microgram) doses, has been shown to be an effective alternative before transitioning to the final, higher dose of the sublingual buprenorphine maintenance formulation (Weimer et al. 2021).

Although buprenorphine has a long half-life, its analgesic effects are more short-lived. Therefore, recommendations for managing acute pain in the perioperative and peripartum setting often involve dosing buprenorphine more frequently throughout the day (e.g., every 6–8 hours) and/or supplementing with nonopioid analgesics (e.g., nonsteroidal anti-inflammatory drugs, acetaminophen), regional blocks, or short-half-life full opioid agonists in either oral or intravenous (including patient-controlled analgesia) formulations (Buresh et al. 2020; Hickey et al. 2022). Furthermore, buprenorphine has dose-dependent μ opioid receptor saturation, which should be kept in mind if also considering concomitant use of a short-acting full opioid agonist for acute pain control, given that higher than usual doses of a short-acting full agonist may be needed (Buresh et al. 2020; Greenwald et al. 2014; Hickey et al. 2022).

α_2 Agonists have long been used as alternatives to opioid agonists in the management of OWS. Two of the most widely used α_2 agonists for OWS are clonidine and lofexidine. In randomized controlled trials, both have been shown to be superior to placebo in ameliorating OWS symptoms (Gowing et al. 2016). Whereas clonidine is used off label, lofexidine was approved by the FDA in 2018 specifically for the management of OWS. The pharmacological properties and use of clonidine were discussed earlier in the subsection "Alcohol Withdrawal Syndrome." Lofexidine is available only in an oral tablet formulation and is approved for use in managing OWS for up to 14 days. Although significantly more expensive, lofexidine appears to have a more favorable safety profile and is less likely to cause hypotension, sedation, and rebound hypertension as compared with clonidine (Fishman et al. 2019; Gowing et al. 2016). α_2 Agonists may be preferred for medically complicated patients with end-stage liver disease or cardiac conduction abnormalities, which may preclude use of buprenorphine and methadone, respectively. Furthermore, these agents may be preferred as adjuncts to opioid agonist therapy in complicated OWS, as well as for use as monotherapy in situations that require a washout or abstinence period from opioid agonists (e.g., starting naltrexone).

Methadone has historically been regarded as the treatment of choice for managing OWS in pregnancy; however, with the introduction of buprenorphine (and the buprenorphine/naloxone combination), evidence suggests that both have comparable efficacy and can be used safely in pregnancy and lactation (Link et al. 2020; Lund et al. 2013; Minozzi et al. 2020). Furthermore, there does not appear to be a heightened risk of teratogenicity with methadone, buprenorphine, or buprenorphine/naloxone use in pregnancy (Klaman et al. 2017). It should be noted that serum levels of methadone and buprenorphine may decrease because of increased clearance, especially in advanced stages of pregnancy, which then necessitates dosage escalation to adequately control or prevent OWS (Klaman et al. 2017). In addition, the decision governing the choice of opioid agonist to use in managing OWS should also take into consideration the complexities associated with peripartum pain management in this patient population. Adverse effects in pregnancy and lactation, which are mostly limited to CNS and respiratory depression and neonatal abstinence syndrome, should be weighed against the potential benefit of reducing the possible risk of maternal-fetal distress associated with opioid withdrawal that can precipitate preterm labor and other complications (Minozzi et al. 2020). After successful detoxification, current guidelines encourage continuation of maintenance therapy in breastfeeding women who are receiving a stable dose of methadone, buprenorphine, or buprenorphine/naloxone, given the obvious relapse prevention benefits to the mother, as well as reduced severity of neonatal abstinence syndrome in the child (Klaman et al. 2017). Compared with methadone, prenatal exposure to buprenorphine alone or in combination with naloxone has the added benefits of decreased frequency and severity of neonatal abstinence syndrome and shorter duration of neonatal hospitalization (Jones et al. 2010; Meyer et al. 2015; Wiegand et al. 2015). Last, lofexidine, like other α_2 agonists (discussed in more detail in the earlier subsection "Alcohol Withdrawal Syndrome"), has not been extensively studied in pregnancy and lactation; therefore, potential risk cannot be ruled out at this time.

Opioid Abstinence and Craving

Methadone and buprenorphine (particularly the formulation with naloxone) are the most commonly used pharmacological agents for reducing craving and promoting abstinence in individuals with OUD. At fixed moderate to high doses, both methadone and buprenorphine have been found to be equally efficacious and have similar side-effect profiles when used as maintenance treatment for OUD (Mattick et al. 2014). However, when compared using fixed low-dose (methadone ≤40 mg; buprenorphine 2–6 mg) and flexible dosing regimens, methadone has been shown to be more effective than buprenorphine in treatment retention (Mattick et al. 2014). Both are discussed in more detail in the previous subsection, "Opioid Withdrawal Syndrome."

In addition to its transmucosal formulations, the FDA approved a buprenorphine 6-month subdermal implant formulation in 2016, targeted toward patients with OUD who were stable on a low to moderate maintenance dose of buprenorphine. Although subsequently approved by the EMA in 2019 and still available in Europe, the buprenorphine implant has been discontinued by its U.S. manufacturer and is no longer available in the United States. Furthermore, the high cost of the buprenorphine implant, as well as the need for surgical insertion and removal, limits its availability to certain patient populations in select clinical settings. Buprenorphine is also available in a monthly extended-release subcutaneous depot formulation that was approved by the FDA in 2017 and has been shown to be safe, generally well tolerated, and effective in promoting abstinence in patients with OUD (Andorn et al. 2020; Haight et al. 2019). In addition, a weekly subcutaneous depot formulation of buprenorphine has been developed and is currently awaiting final FDA approval. The weekly depot formulation has been shown to be a safe, well-tolerated, and effective maintenance treatment option for patients with moderate to severe OUD (Walsh et al. 2017). Although less commonly used, naltrexone (both the oral and the monthly intramuscular depot formulations) has also received FDA approval for reducing cravings and preventing relapse in OUD. Additional information about the pharmacological properties, safety profile, and use of naltrexone in medically ill patients can be found in the earlier subsection "Alcohol Abstinence and Craving." Although generally less favored because of a higher rate of premature discontinuation, the extended-release depot formulation of naltrexone may be a more favorable alternative in certain supervised settings, such as in the criminal justice system, where patients' adherence can be more closely monitored (Jarvis et al. 2018).

Tobacco Use Disorder

Tobacco use, specifically cigarette smoking, is the leading cause of preventable illness and death in the United States (Cornelius et al. 2020; U.S. Department of Health and Human Services 2014). Cigarette smoking has been associated with the development of multiple acute and chronic illnesses, including adenocarcinoma of the lung, hepatocellular carcinoma, colorectal cancer, chronic obstructive pulmonary disease, cardiovascular disease, congenital malformations (cleft lip or palate), ectopic pregnancy, spontaneous abortion, macular degeneration, and diabetes (U.S. Department of Health and Human Services 2014). A comprehensive discussion of the implications of tobacco use in the medically ill is beyond the scope of this chapter. However, it is important to note that smoked tobacco products, because of the polycyclic aromatic hydrocarbons formed during combustion, are inducers of the CYP1A2 enzyme, thereby reducing serum levels of substrates such as warfarin and clozapine. Pharmacological treatment strategies exist to prevent and ameliorate withdrawal symptoms and promote abstinence by reducing cravings associated with nicotine.

Tobacco Withdrawal

Tobacco withdrawal can result in severe anxiety, irritability, restlessness, dysphoria, insomnia, and appetite stimulation. Such symptoms can obviously complicate medical treatment. The psychoactive substance nicotine is primarily responsible for the highly addictive nature of tobacco. Nicotine replacement therapy (NRT) remains the mainstay in the prevention and management of nicotine withdrawal in medical settings (Rigotti et al. 2008). NRT is available as a transdermal patch, a lozenge, gum, a nasal spray, and an inhaler. NRT is safe to use in most medically ill patients, but caution should be exercised in patients with recent coronary events, especially given nicotine's potential for myocardial excitability (e.g., tachycardia, hypertension, increased cardiac work or demand, precipitation of arrhythmias) (Sobieraj et al. 2013). NRT has been proven safe in long-term studies, with no significant adverse outcomes in a study during which it was used for up to 52 weeks (Schnoll et al. 2015). Furthermore, NRT has been shown to increase rates of smoking cessation by 50%–60%, regardless of setting (Hartmann-Boyce et al. 2018).

NRT use in pregnancy is deemed relatively safe, with a recent systematic review finding that there is no significant risk for major congenital malformations; however, this same review determined that there may be a heightened risk of infantile colic and development of ADHD in children born to mothers receiving NRT, warranting further study in this regard (Blanc et al. 2021). Similarly, an earlier study also confirmed the safety of NRT in pregnancy, concluding that there was no significant evidence of system-specific congenital anomalies, apart from a very small number of respiratory anomalies (Dhalwani et al. 2015). It should be noted that nicotine readily crosses the placenta, and maternal nicotine metabolism is increased during pregnancy, which may necessitate higher doses of NRT to stave off withdrawal or reduce nicotine cravings (Blanc et al. 2021). However, because of a concomitant reduction in fetal nicotine clearance, higher NRT doses may increase fetal toxicity, necessitating caution when considering dose escalation (Blanc et al. 2021).

Tobacco Abstinence and Craving

The primary agents used in maintaining tobacco abstinence function by either direct nicotine replacement or reduction of cravings by alternative mechanisms. NRT, bupropion, and varenicline are the mainstays of treatment. NRT is discussed at length in the previous subsection. Bupropion, a norepinephrine-dopamine reuptake inhibitor, is thought to exert its effects on nicotine craving by enhancing the dopaminergic pathways in reward centers of the brain. It is also an antagonist at nicotinic acetylcholine receptors, which further aids in reducing nicotine cravings. Bupropion is FDA approved for smoking cessation and is available in both immediate- and extended-release oral tablet formulations. Evidence suggests that bupropion increases rates of long-term smoking cessation and is as efficacious as NRT but not as well tolerated. It also may be less efficacious than varenicline (Howes et al. 2020). Bupropion can be used safely in medically ill patients, with caution in patients who have a history of seizures and in those whose seizure threshold may be decreased (e.g., because of a recent cerebrovascular accident or traumatic brain injury, withdrawal from alcohol or sedatives, or medications that are known to lower seizure threshold). Seizure risk is significant with bupropion doses greater than 450 mg and with use of the immediate-release formulation. Furthermore, because bupropion is a potent CYP2D6 inhibitor, drug-drug interactions can occur. The most common side effects of bupropion include insomnia, anxiety, dry mouth, and appetite suppression.

Varenicline was approved by the FDA in 2006 for smoking cessation and is administered in an oral tablet formulation for this indication. It is a partial agonist at the $\alpha4\beta2$ nicotinic acetylcholine receptor subtype, which functions to reduce nicotine cravings and promote abstinence. Furthermore, because of its high receptor binding affinity, varenicline prevents nicotine from binding at this receptor, thereby reducing the degree of dopaminergic stimulation in the mesolimbic pathways. Varenicline has been shown to be the most effective pharmacotherapy for smoking cessation when compared with NRT, bupropion, and electronic cigarettes (e-cigarettes) (Thomas et al. 2022). The most common adverse effects associated with varenicline are nausea, headache, and insomnia. Among the most serious, albeit less common, adverse effects are precipitation of mood instability, hostility, severe depression, and suicidality, which prompted the FDA to initially issue a black box warning. The black box warning was subsequently removed after a large multicenter, randomized, placebo-controlled trial in 8,058 participants did not show a statistically significant increase in neuropsychiatric adverse events in patients with and without underlying psychiatric disorders who were taking varenicline, bupropion, or NRT for smoking cessation (Anthenelli et al. 2016). Although the incidence of neuropsychiatric adverse effects was higher in patients with an underlying psychiatric disorder, a secondary analysis of the study confirmed that varenicline and bupropion were not associated with a statistically significant increased risk of neuropsychiatric adverse effects in patients with psychotic, anxiety, or mood disorders when compared with NRT or placebo (Evins et al. 2019). Regardless, it is still recommended to exercise caution when using varenicline in patients with serious psychiatric illness, especially if their illness is not well controlled. Despite some studies raising concerns about potential cardiovascular risk with varenicline, randomized placebo-controlled trials evaluating varenicline use in patients with and without underlying cardiovascular disease have shown that there is no increase in the risk of cardiovascular adverse events with its use (Benowitz et al. 2018; Sterling et al. 2016). Therefore, the use of approved pharmacotherapies, including varenicline, for smoking cessation is strongly encouraged, especially in patients with cardiovascular risk factors. Varenicline is primarily renally excreted and is without significant drug-drug interactions. Caution should be exercised when prescribing varenicline to patients with renal impairment.

The use of NRT in pregnancy is discussed in detail in the previous subsection. Evidence for use of bupropion and varenicline in pregnancy and lactation is lacking; however, no definitive evidence currently indicates that either treatment imparts harm during pregnancy (Turner et al. 2019).

Last, it is important to mention that e-cigarettes are readily available and have been touted as potential agents to help facilitate tobacco or cigarette smoking cessation. At this time, there appears to be evidence of moderate certainty that nicotine-containing e-cigarettes are efficacious in promoting abstinence when compared with NRT (Hartmann-Boyce et al. 2021). However, the evidence is still lacking to make any definitive conclusions about the safety of long-term e-cigarette use. This is especially important to consider given reported cases of e-cigarette or vaping product use–associated acute lung injury (Jonas and Raj 2020).

Cocaine- and Other Stimulant-Related Disorders

Cocaine and methamphetamine are among the stimulants that are the most pervasive and commonly abused by the medically ill. Cocaine use in particular is linked to serious cardiac sequelae, including malignant hypertension, myocardial infarction, arrhythmias, dilated cardiomyopathy, and resultant heart failure (Phillips et al. 2009). Caution should be exercised when using certain medications otherwise commonly administered to cardiac patients. Historically, β-blockers were considered to be contraindicated, primarily because of the theoretical risk for unopposed α_1 receptor agonism, which can cause coronary vasoconstriction in cocaine intoxication. Therefore, use of medications such as labetalol that have mixed α and β receptor antagonist properties may be preferred. In addition, partially as a result of the cardiovascular effects of cocaine (e.g., vasoconstriction, rhabdomyolysis), acute kidney injury is not uncommon (Goel et al. 2014). Both cocaine and other psychostimulants (e.g., methamphetamine) are known to be associated with an increased risk for stroke, with methamphetamines being associated primarily with hemorrhagic strokes and cocaine with both ischemic and hemorrhagic strokes (Lappin and Sara 2019; Westover et al. 2007). In addition, cocaine and psychostimulants are associated with seizures, movement disorders (e.g., dyskinesias, tics, early-onset Parkinson's disease with chronic use), and hypothalamic dysregulation resulting in hyperpyrexia (Lappin and Sara 2019; Sanchez-Ramos 2015). Hypothalamic temperature dysregulation coupled with rhabdomyolysis and relative dopamine depletion (often seen with cocaine toxicity and in chronic use) can increase risk for (or mimic) neuroleptic malignant syndrome (NMS). Therefore, caution should be exercised when using antipsychotics (or other dopamine antagonists) for managing acute agitation associated with psychostimulant intoxication, primarily because of the risk for precipitating NMS. As a result, with the exception of managing stimulant-induced psychosis (in which case antipsychotics are preferred), benzodiazepines are preferred as first-line agents for managing agitation related to psychostimulant intoxication.

Stimulant withdrawal does not typically cause medical instability and results in CNS depression, most often manifesting with fatigue, sluggishness, hypersomnolence, hyperphagia, irritability, and dysphoria. No medications are specifically approved for the management of stimulant withdrawal, which is self-limiting and responsive to supportive interventions. However, several medications have been studied for the management of cravings associated with stimulant use. These include dopaminergic agents (e.g., amphetamines, bupropion, disulfiram by virtue of its function as a dopamine β-hydroxylase inhibitor), GABAergic agents (particularly topiramate), serotonergic agents (e.g., ondansetron, SSRIs), and agents with multimodal, dopaminergic, and glutamatergic mechanisms such as modafinil (Chan et al. 2019; Karila et al. 2008; Ross and Peselow 2009). A Cochrane review did not support the use of psychostimulants (i.e., dexamphetamine, bupropion, methylphenidate, and modafinil) in managing amphetamine use disorder (Pérez-Mañá et al. 2013). A separate Cochrane review examining the use of psychostimulants (i.e., bupropion, dexamphetamine, lisdexamfetamine, methylphenidate, modafinil, mazindol, methamphetamine, mixed amphetamine salts, and selegiline) for the treatment of cocaine use disorder yielded mixed results. Very low-quality evidence suggests that psychostimulants increase cocaine abstinence when compared with placebo but do not reduce cocaine use among those who cannot achieve abstinence (Castells et al. 2016). Therefore, use of psychostimulants for the treatment of stimulant use disorders is not recommended at this time; however, further studies are needed to make firmer conclusions in this regard. Topiramate may have some potential utility in managing cocaine use disorder, specifically in helping to extend periods of abstinence; however, the studies to date remain inconclusive (Singh et al. 2016).

Cannabis- and Synthetic Cannabinoid–Related Disorders

Cannabis use is prevalent among the medically ill, especially now with legislation legalizing both the medicinal and the recreational use of marijuana in various states. A discussion of the safety and efficacy of cannabis in treating various medical conditions (e.g., glaucoma, chronic intractable cancer-related pain, spasticity associated with multiple sclerosis, anorexia or cachexia associated with HIV/AIDS and cancer) is beyond the scope of this chapter and is presented elsewhere (Whiting et al. 2015). Cannabis use is associated with short-term memory deficits, inattention, executive dysfunction, impaired coordination, somnolence, hyperphagia, symptoms of chronic bronchitis, increased anxiety, euphoria, and perceptual disturbances (Hoch et al. 2015; Volkow et al. 2014). In addition, use of cannabis, primarily because of its psychoactive component, Δ-9-tetrahydrocannabinol (THC), has been associated with a dose-dependent risk of precipitating frank psychosis, as well as an earlier onset of psychotic illness, ranging in severity from mild paranoia to schizophrenia spectrum disorders in vulnerable individuals (Hasan et al. 2020). Furthermore, cannabis can cause a condition known as cannabinoid hyperemesis syndrome, which is associated with intractable, cyclic nausea and vomiting in patients who regularly use marijuana (typically seen with heavy use) and is transiently relieved with hot baths, resolving altogether with cessation of cannabis use (Sorensen et al. 2017). Last, it has been reported that most cases of lung injury associated with vaping have been linked to THC-containing e-cigarettes and may be a result of the presence of vitamin E acetate in THC-containing cartridges (Cherian et al. 2020).

Synthetic cannabinoids (e.g., K2, Spice) include a wide array of laboratory-created cannabinoid receptor agonists that have significantly more potent binding affinity at the CB_1 receptor when compared with THC in naturally occurring cannabis (Castaneto et al. 2014). This, in turn, is thought to contribute to the increased toxicity of synthetic cannabinoids (Castaneto et al. 2014). Symptoms associated with synthetic cannabinoid intoxication range from anxiety, blurred vision, diaphoresis, myoclonic jerks, tremors, tachycardia, and hypertension to acute renal failure, frank affective disturbances, aggression or hostility, seizures, psychosis, delirium, and catatonia (Castaneto et al. 2014; Pourmand et al. 2018). Although many synthetic cannabinoids are illegal, the development of analogues with slight variations in chemical structure makes them difficult to regulate (Kesner and Lovinger 2021). These substances often go undetected on standard toxicology screens, and the frequent variations in chemical structure make it challenging to keep up with the development of accurate detection assays; furthermore, the assays that do exist typically require that urine or blood samples be sent to third-party laboratories, which delays turnaround time for results (Pourmand et al. 2018).

Cannabis withdrawal syndrome (CWS) is a distinct clinical entity, typically occurring in patients on abrupt cessation of prolonged or heavy cannabis use and including a combination of at least three of the following symptoms: irritability; anger or aggression; anxiety; sleep disturbances (including insomnia and vivid dreams); decreased appetite; restlessness; depressed mood; and physical symptoms marked by abdominal pain, tremors, diaphoresis, fevers, chills, or headache (American Psychiatric Association 2013). Withdrawal from naturally occurring and synthetic cannabinoids manifests similarly; however, synthetic cannabinoid withdrawal typically occurs more rapidly and is more severe in intensity (Kesner and Lovinger 2021). Management of CWS is typically supportive. At this time, no medications are approved for treating CWS or cannabis use disorder. Studies looking at THC preparations or derivatives (i.e., nabiximols and dronabinol) for mitigation of withdrawal symptoms and cravings have shown some potential benefit; however, further studies are needed to make any specific recommendations in this regard (Nielsen et al. 2019). Further studies are also needed to address the potential utility of gabapentin, oxytocin, and *N*-acetylcysteine for cannabis use disorder or CWS (Nielsen et al. 2019).

Other Substance Use Disorders

Several other recreationally used or abused substances, some with multimodal mechanisms of action, affect monoamine, opioid, GABAergic, cholinergic, and/or glutamatergic pathways. In addition to commonly prescribed and over-the-counter medications, as well as readily available inhalants, these substances include novel agents that seem to have exploded onto the scene within the past decade. Some of these agents are extracted from naturally occurring plants, whereas others are synthetic analogues. An extensive discussion of each of these substances is beyond the scope of this chapter; however, discussion of some common agents, key clinical findings, and specific management recommendations is warranted.

The hallucinogens include both naturally occurring and synthetic compounds. Examples of common hallucinogens include phencyclidine (PCP; angel dust), lysergic acid diethylamide (LSD; acid), dimethyltryptamine, ketamine (special K), dextromethorphan (DXM; skittles, robo), psilocybin (magic mushrooms, shrooms; produced by various species of fungi), mescaline (found mainly in various cactus species, such as peyote), and *Salvia divinorum* (plant containing the psychoactive compound salvinorin A). Hallucinogens commonly precipitate perceptual disturbances and contribute to an altered sense of self, time, and space. There may also be frank dissociation, euphoria, and emotional as well as physical numbing. Some degree of sympathetic activation resulting in tachycardia and hypertension is common.

PCP and ketamine are NMDA receptor antagonists and dissociative agents. PCP intoxication can be quite dramatic, often resulting in significant disinhibition and agitation or hostility, accompanied by prominent sympathomimetic (e.g., tachycardia, hypertension, diaphoresis) and cholinergic (e.g., bronchospasm, sialorrhea, flushing, miosis) signs and symptoms (Passie and Halpern 2014). Vertical and/or horizontal nystagmus is often present, and patients can become floridly delirious or even comatose (Dominici et al. 2015). There is also evidence of increased muscle tone, which can precipitate dystonic reactions and rhabdomyolysis, as well as temperature dysregulation, resulting in hyperthermia (Passie and Halpern 2014; Pourmand et al. 2018). Complications can include cardiac conduction abnormalities, arrhythmias, renal failure (due to rhabdomyolysis), hypertensive crisis, intracranial hemorrhage, and increased risk for NMS. As a result, benzodiazepines are preferred first-line agents in managing agitation due to PCP intoxication, given that antipsychotics can contribute to worsening muscle rigidity and hyperthermia, as well as increased risk for NMS (Pourmand et al. 2018). Intravenous hydration should also be administered to treat or prevent rhabdomyolysis. Ketamine has similar properties to PCP; however, its effects are much less profound in comparison (Passie and Halpern 2014). Ketamine is discussed further in the earlier subsection "Alcohol Withdrawal Syndrome." As with other hallucinogens, management of PCP and ketamine intoxication is primarily supportive.

MDMA ("ecstasy," E, "molly") is an analogue of methamphetamine with some similarities to the hallucinogens. As with LSD, psilocybin, and mescaline, MDMA is also serotonergic, hence contributing to the vivid experiences and "connection" that individuals feel to others and to their environment when they are under its influence. MDMA causes sympathetic activation and can result in an increase in cardiac workload, malignant hypertension that predisposes the individual to stroke and acute myocardial infarction, and disseminated intravascular coagulation (Pourmand et al. 2014). Typical MDMA intoxication often results in feelings of euphoria and increased psychomotor activity, which can further exacerbate hypertension and tachycardia and also contribute to hyperthermia (Passie and Halpern 2014). Tremors and muscle rigidity also can be seen, which may cause rhabdomyolysis and predispose the individual to renal failure. Because of MDMA's serotonergic properties, bruxism, vivid dreams, and gastrointestinal distress also occur. Caution should be taken when using serotonergic agents given the potential for precipitating serotonin syndrome. Like SSRIs, MDMA stimulates release of antidiuretic hormone, which can result in hyponatremia (Pourmand et al. 2014). As with PCP, MDMA intoxication can be managed by supportive measures (hydration, reassurance, redirection, correction of metabolic or electrolyte abnormalities) followed by use of benzodiazepines to manage agitation if necessary.

The synthetic cathinones, more commonly known as bath salts, have properties similar to those of MDMA. They are derivatives of cathinone, the psychoactive alkaloid in the khat plant, which is found in parts of East Africa, the Arabian Peninsula, and Afghanistan (Soares et al. 2021). Khat is typically chewed and produces a stimulant-like effect. Synthetic cathinones cause sympathomimetic effects and also have some hallucinogenic and serotonergic properties. Presenting signs may include tachycardia, hypertension, hyperthermia, diaphoresis, muscle rigidity, rhabdomyolysis resulting in renal failure, adverse cardiovascular effects resulting in stroke or cardiac arrest, disseminated intravascular coagulation, and multiorgan failure; neuropsychiatric adverse effects include profound agitation or aggression, psychosis, florid delirium, and seizures (Soares et al. 2021). Given the prominent serotonergic properties of the cathinone derivatives, individuals using these substances are at risk for serotonin syndrome. Temperature dysregulation, coupled with muscle breakdown or rigidity along with dehydration, can also predispose patients to NMS. Recommended treatment is supportive measures and benzodiazepines for agitation. As with MDMA, antipsychotics and other dopamine antagonists and serotonergic agents should be used with extreme caution.

The opioid receptor agonists kratom (containing the psychoactive plant alkaloid mitragynine) and desomorphine (known as krokodil, a semisynthetic opioid derivative of codeine) have arrived more recently in the United States, coming from Southeast Asia and Eastern Europe (primarily Russia and Ukraine), respectively (Pourmand et al. 2018). Both can cause significant CNS and respiratory depression, but kratom tends to also have some stimulant-like properties at lower doses (Pourmand et al. 2018). Kratom leaves are chewed or typically ingested in a pill or extract form. Krokodil, conversely, is injected and often causes significant local necrosis at the injection site, which can spread and evolve into gangrene (Florez et al. 2017). Furthermore, the homemade synthesis of krokodil/desomorphine often involves mixing codeine with various chemicals such as gasoline, paint thinner, and heavy metals, thereby contaminating the end product, which can then potentially cause significant neurotoxicity and organ damage (Florez et al. 2017). Whereas desomorphine is illegal in the United States, kratom is still legal on a federal level and in most states. Kratom is readily available for purchase on the internet and is also sold in tobacco or smoke shops in some states. In addition to its recreational uses, kratom has been marketed as a remedy for chronic pain and to help manage opioid withdrawal, despite serious safety concerns and a lack of studies proving its efficacy (Pourmand et al. 2018). As with opioids, kratom or krokodil intoxication is managed supportively. Naloxone can be used to reverse CNS and respiratory depression associated with severe intoxication or overdose.

Phenibut (β-phenyl-γ-aminobutyric acid) is a $GABA_B$ agonist that was initially developed in Russia, where it is still prescribed for anxiolysis, among other indications. It is readily available for purchase via the internet and is also available in over-the-counter dietary supplements, which are often marketed as anxiolytics, sleep aids, and nootropic agents (Cohen et al. 2022; Owen et al. 2016). Because of the ready availability and unregulated status of phenibut, the potential for abuse and dependence is high. Phenibut intoxication can manifest with drowsiness, lethargy, tachycardia, confusion, agitation, delirium, coma, and death (Graves et al. 2020). Patients who are regular or heavy users of phenibut can experience withdrawal with abrupt discontinuation or dosage reduction. Phenibut withdrawal is similar to withdrawal from other GABAergic agents and can result in worsening anxiety, psychomotor agitation, tachycardia, hypertension, insomnia, perceptual disturbances, and frank delirium. Given the substance's structural and mechanistic similarity to baclofen, phenibut withdrawal has been successfully treated with baclofen, which can be considered especially if symptoms are unresponsive to benzodiazepine administration (Ahuja et al. 2018).

Concomitant with the spread of prescription drug abuse, over-the-counter medications that contain DXM (present in cough syrup and cold remedies) and pseudoephedrine (present in allergy and cold medications) have become quite popular, particularly among teenagers. This seems to be primarily due to their ease of access and has prompted stricter monitoring guidelines regarding their purchase in most states. DXM has a multimodal mechanism of action that involves serotonergic, noradrenergic, and glutamatergic (NMDA receptor antagonist) pathways (Pourmand et al. 2018). Intoxication results in hypertension, tachycardia, mydriasis, diaphoresis, and nystagmus, as well as neuropsychiatric symptoms ranging from mild agitation, euphoria, and hallucinations to severe agitation and frank dissociation at higher doses (Pourmand et al. 2018). DXM also carries a risk of serotonin syndrome, particularly when used in high doses or when used in combination with other serotonergic agents. Pseudoephedrine has stimulant properties and is converted into methamphetamine and methcathinone. Management of DXM and pseudoephedrine toxicity is analogous to management of hallucinogen (as well as MDMA) and stimulant toxicity, respectively. Primary interventions are supportive and include ensuring adequate hydration. Benzodiazepines are preferred as first-line agents in managing associated agitation.

It is also important to mention that the recreational use and abuse of gabapentin, pregabalin, and quetiapine have been on the rise, largely because of an increase in prescribing and use for off-label indications. Furthermore, these medications are commonly encountered in medically ill patients. Because of its more rapid absorption and higher bioavailability, pregabalin appears to have a higher abuse potential than gabapentin (Hägg et al. 2020). Additionally, quetiapine is the most abused or misused second-generation antipsychotic (Klein et al. 2017). Intoxication with these agents can cause significant CNS depression, especially if ingested with other depressant-like substances. This underscores the need to exercise caution when prescribing these medications, particularly for patients with a history of substance use disorders and/or for whom there is concern about synergistic polypharmacy.

Last, the recreational use or abuse of inhalants is common, particularly among adolescents and young adults. These agents include various hydrocarbon-containing solvents such as paint thinners, gasoline, and glues; nitrites that are sometimes sold in adult novelty stores (also known as poppers) and found in certain air fresheners; propellants containing hydrocarbons and fluorocarbons (used in compressed air duster cans); and inhaled anesthetic gases such as nitrous oxide (N_2O, also known as laughing gas), which is commonly used as an anesthetic during dental procedures. N_2O is also found in pressurized cans of whipped cream and is often distributed in canisters known as whippets that are subsequently cracked open and inhaled for recreational purposes. Inhalant intoxication can result in euphoria, headache, dizziness, nausea, lack of coordination, arrhythmias, and pulmonary inflammation, as well as profound alterations in mental status ranging from disorientation, dissociation, and frank confusion to coma (Filley 2013; van Amsterdam et al. 2015). Toluene, a solvent found in spray paint, paint thinner, glues, and gasoline, has been associated with toxic leukoencephalopathy (Filley 2013). Furthermore, heavy use of N_2O can result in irreversible inactivation of vitamin B_{12}, causing megaloblastic anemia and neuronal demyelination that can result in peripheral neuropathy, paralysis, and altered mental status (van Amsterdam et al. 2015). If N_2O is suspected as the offending agent, treatment typically involves vitamin B_{12} repletion (van Amsterdam et al. 2015). Otherwise, inhalant intoxication is managed supportively.

Neuropsychiatric Adverse Effects of Drugs Used for Substance-Related Disorders

Table 18–1 lists the more common neuropsychiatric adverse effects of drugs used to manage substance-related disorders.

Drug-Drug Interactions

Acamprosate and varenicline have no significant drug-drug interactions. Furthermore, baclofen, gabapentin, pregabalin, and topiramate are primarily renally excreted and therefore have minimal drug-drug interactions. Table 18–2 lists some of the more common drug-drug interactions between psychotropics and medications used for substance-related disorders.

Key Points

- Although only 3%–5% of patients admitted for alcohol withdrawal syndrome (AWS) progress to delirium tremens, mortality rates due to delirium tremens can be as high as 20% in hospitalized medically ill patients.

- Despite evidence suggesting a possible adjunctive role for anticonvulsants and α_2 agonists, benzodiazepines remain the gold standard in the management of moderate and severe AWS.

Table 18–1.   Neuropsychiatric adverse effects of medications that treat substance-related disorders

Medication	Neuropsychiatric adverse effects
Acamprosate	Common: anxiety, insomnia, anorexia Serious: suicidality, clinical depression
α_2 Agonists (e.g., clonidine, guanfacine, lofexidine, dexmedetomidine)	Common: drowsiness, sedation, nervousness, agitation, sexual dysfunction Serious: clinical depression
Anticonvulsants (e.g., carbamazepine, valproic acid, topiramate, gabapentin)	Common: sedation, confusion, fatigue, appetite or weight changes, psychomotor slowing, cognitive blunting Serious: paresthesias (with topiramate), clinical depression, seizure exacerbation, suicidality, psychosis, delirium
Baclofen	Common: sedation, psychomotor slowing, fatigue, cognitive blunting Serious: respiratory depression, withdrawal with discontinuation, seizures, delirium, agitation, mania, catatonia
Barbiturates (e.g., phenobarbital)	Common: somnolence, psychomotor slowing, amnesia Serious: dependence, withdrawal seizures, suicidality, clinical depression, respiratory depression, delirium
Benzodiazepines (e.g., lorazepam, diazepam)	Common: somnolence, lethargy, psychomotor slowing Serious: dependence, withdrawal seizures, clinical depression, delirium, amnesia
β-Blockers (e.g., propranolol)	Common: fatigue, sexual dysfunction, psychomotor slowing Serious: no serious neuropsychiatric adverse effects
Buprenorphine	Common: sedation, insomnia, depression Serious: withdrawal, seizures, respiratory depression, delirium
Bupropion	Common: anxiety, insomnia, appetite suppression Serious: seizures, suicidality, agitation, hallucinations, paranoia, delirium

Table 18–1. Neuropsychiatric adverse effects of medications that treat substance-related disorders *(continued)*

Medication	Neuropsychiatric adverse effects
Disulfiram	Common: alcohol-disulfiram reaction, drowsiness, anxiety or panic symptoms Serious: optic neuritis and other multiple sclerosis–like symptoms, psychosis, respiratory depression, seizures
Flumazenil	Common: agitation, anxiety, fatigue, confusion Serious: seizures, re-sedation (due to short half-life), iatrogenic precipitation of benzodiazepine withdrawal syndrome
Methadone	Common: somnolence or sedation, psychomotor slowing, cognitive blunting Serious: respiratory depression or arrest, withdrawal, seizures, delirium, coma
Nalmefene	Common: insomnia Serious: delirium, hallucinations, precipitation of opioid withdrawal
Naloxone	Common: muscle weakness and fatigue Serious: hallucinations, delirium, coma, precipitation of opioid withdrawal resulting in severe agitation
Naltrexone	Common: insomnia, anxiety, fatigue, somnolence Serious: suicidality, clinical depression, iatrogenic precipitation of opioid withdrawal syndrome
Nicotine replacement therapy (e.g., transdermal patch, lozenge, gum, spray)	Common: insomnia, vivid dreams or nightmares Serious: clinical depression
Propofol	Common: sedation, cognitive impairment Serious: respiratory depression or arrest, propofol infusion syndrome, opisthotonus, delirium, coma
Varenicline	Common: insomnia, abnormal dreams, appetite suppression, somnolence Serious: suicidality, severe clinical depression, agitation or hostility, behavioral disturbances, exacerbation of underlying psychiatric disorder, seizures, hallucinations

Source. Adapted from McEvoy 2008.

Table 18–2.   Interactions between psychotropic medications and medications for substance-related disorders

Medication	Interaction mechanism	Effects on psychotropic medications and management
Buprenorphine	Similar to methadone (see below)	Similar drug interaction profile to methadone, although generally attenuated effects; fewer drug-drug interactions; and less concomitant sedation, respiratory depression, and QT prolongation
	Opioid receptor occupation and partial agonism	May induce withdrawal in patients taking opioid analgesics and methadone
Clonidine, dexmedetomidine, guanfacine, and lofexidine	Additive hypotensive effect	Increased risk of hypotensive effects with antipsychotics, TCAs, and MAOIs; increased risk of dry mouth and eyes with TCAs and antipsychotics
	Inhibit norepinephrine release	May decrease the therapeutic effect of TCAs and NRIs, including atomoxetine. Similarly, TCAs and NRIs may decrease the effects of clonidine.
Disulfiram	Inhibits CYP2E1, CYP1A2, and possibly other CYP enzymes	Increased levels and toxicity of phenytoin (and possibly mephenytoin and fosphenytoin), olanzapine, and risperidone
	Inhibits acetaldehyde metabolism	Many oral medications in liquid form and some intravenous infusions contain small amounts of alcohol, which would provoke a disulfiram reaction.
	Inhibits dopamine β-hydroxylase	Increased seizure potential with illicit cocaine use

Table 18–2. Interactions between psychotropic medications and medications for substance-related disorders *(continued)*

Medication	Interaction mechanism	Effects on psychotropic medications and management
Flumazenil	GABA antagonism	Contraindicated in patients receiving a benzodiazepine for control of intracranial pressure or status epilepticus or in cases of TCA overdose
Methadone	Opioid receptor occupation or blockade	Decreased methadone effect and possibly withdrawal in combination with naloxone, naltrexone, pentazocine, nalbuphine, butorphanol, and buprenorphine
	Induces CYP3A4	Decreased serum levels of methadone and possible withdrawal in combination with phenytoin, St. John's wort, phenobarbital, carbamazepine, rifampin, and some antiretroviral medications (see Chapter 12, "Infectious Diseases")
	Inhibits CYP3A4	Increased serum levels of methadone and potential excessive sedation and respiratory suppression with CYP3A4 inhibitors such as fluvoxamine and nefazodone
	Potentiation of opioid sedation and respiratory depression	Coadministration with benzodiazepines or strong antihistamines (e.g., tertiary-amine TCAs, quetiapine, diphenhydramine) can potentiate opioid sedation and respiratory depression.

Table 18–2. Interactions between psychotropic medications and medications for substance-related disorders *(continued)*

Medication	Interaction mechanism	Effects on psychotropic medications and management
Methadone *(continued)*	QT prolongation	Additive risk for QT prolongation and electrolyte disturbances with psychotropics that increase QT interval, including TCAs, typical antipsychotics, pimozide, risperidone, paliperidone, iloperidone, quetiapine, ziprasidone, and lithium (also see Chapter 6, "Cardiovascular Disorders")
Naltrexone	Opioid antagonism	Blocks the effect of opioids administered for pain, cough, and diarrhea; use should be avoided in patients dependent on opioids for control of severe pain
	Unknown	Increases area under the plasma concentration–time curve of acamprosate by 25%[a]

Note. CYP = cytochrome P450; MAOIs = monoamine oxidase inhibitors; NRIs = norepinephrine reuptake inhibitors; TCAs = tricyclic antidepressants.
[a]Acamprosate product monograph (Mason et al. 2002).

- High-dose thiamine should be administered parenterally to high-risk patients with a history of heavy alcohol use who are presenting with altered mental status, patients with drastic weight loss and malnutrition, and patients with poor oral intake or prominent evidence of cachexia.

- Methadone can significantly prolong the QTc interval and should be used with extreme caution in cardiac patients.

- By virtue of its partial agonism, buprenorphine has less risk of respiratory depression with dosage escalation as compared with methadone.

- Buprenorphine is regarded as a safer and equally efficacious alternative to methadone for pregnant patients.

- It is no longer recommended to hold or avoid use of buprenorphine in the acute perioperative setting.

- Varenicline is shown to be the most effective pharmacotherapy for smoking cessation.

- Varenicline can be used safely in patients with comorbid psychiatric illness, although caution is still advised if their psychiatric illness is not well controlled.

- Cocaine and amphetamine-like agents carry significant risks for cardiovascular and neurological sequelae, even for younger patients without other risk factors.

- Synthetic cannabinoids represent a group of agents with more potent cannabinoid receptor agonism and more profound toxidromes.

- The use of e-cigarettes and vaping products containing Δ-9-tetrahydrocannabinol has been associated with lung injury that is thought to be secondary to the presence of vitamin E acetate in vaping cartridges.

- The increase in prescribing of and off-label uses for gabapentin, pregabalin, and quetiapine has resulted in these agents being readily available and more commonly misused, especially among patients with substance use disorders.

References

ACOG Committee on Health Care for Underserved Women; American Society of Addiction Medicine: ACOG Committee Opinion No. 524: opioid abuse, dependence, and addiction in pregnancy. Obstet Gynecol 119(5):1070–1076, 2012 22525931

Addolorato G, Leggio L, Abenavoli L, et al: Baclofen in the treatment of alcohol withdrawal syndrome: a comparative study vs diazepam. Am J Med 119(3):276.e13–276.e18, 2006 16490478

Addolorato G, Lesch OM, Maremmani I, et al: Post-marketing and clinical safety experience with sodium oxybate for the treatment of alcohol withdrawal syndrome and maintenance of abstinence in alcohol-dependent subjects. Expert Opin Drug Saf 19(2):159–166, 2020 31876433

Ahmed S, Bhivandkar S, Lonergan BB, et al: Microinduction of buprenorphine/naloxone: a review of literature. Am J Addict 30(4):305–315, 2021 33378137

Ahuja T, Mgbako O, Katzman C, Grossman A: Phenibut (β-phenyl-γ-aminobutyric acid) dependence and management of withdrawal: emerging nootropics of abuse. Case Rep Psychiatry 2018:9864285, 2018 29854531

Ait-Daoud N, Hamby AS, Sharma S, et al: A review of alprazolam use, misuse, and withdrawal. J Addict Med 12(1):4–10, 2018 28777203

American Psychiatric Association: Diagnostic and Statistical Manual of Mental Disorders, 5th Edition. Arlington, VA, American Psychiatric Publishing, 2013

Andorn AC, Haight BR, Shinde S, et al: Treating opioid use disorder with a monthly subcutaneous buprenorphine depot injection: 12-month safety, tolerability, and efficacy analysis. J Clin Psychopharmacol 40(3):231–239, 2020 32282418

Anthenelli RM, Benowitz NL, West R, et al: Neuropsychiatric safety and efficacy of varenicline, bupropion, and nicotine patch in smokers with and without psychiatric disorders (EAGLES): a double-blind, randomised, placebo-controlled clinical trial. Lancet 387(10037):2507–2520, 2016 27116918

Armenian P, Vo KT, Barr-Walker J, et al: Fentanyl, fentanyl analogs and novel synthetic opioids: a comprehensive review. Neuropharmacology 134(Pt A):121–132, 2018 29042317

Asconape JJ: Use of antiepileptic drugs in hepatic and renal disease, in Handbook of Clinical Neurology: Neurologic Aspects of Systemic Disease, Part I. Edited by Biller J, Ferro J. Amsterdam, The Netherlands, Elsevier, 2014, pp 417–432

Asghar MU, Cheema HA, Tanveer K, et al: Propofol infusion and acute pancreatitis: a review. Am J Ther 27(4):e371–e374, 2020 31283535

Avetian GK, Fiuty P, Mazzella S, et al: Use of naloxone nasal spray 4 mg in the community setting: a survey of use by community organizations. Curr Med Res Opin 34(4):573–576, 2018 28535115

Balakirouchenane D, Khoudour N, Chouchana L, et al: Pharmacokinetics of baclofen in a full-term newborn after intrauterine exposure: a case report. Neonatology 118(5):624–627, 2021 34569533

Bellantuono C, Tofani S, Di Sciascio G, et al: Benzodiazepine exposure in pregnancy and risk of major malformations: a critical overview. Gen Hosp Psychiatry 35(1):3–8, 2013 23044244

Benowitz NL, Pipe A, West R, et al: Cardiovascular safety of varenicline, bupropion, and nicotine patch in smokers: a randomized clinical trial. JAMA Intern Med 178(5):622–631, 2018 29630702

Blanc J, Tosello B, Ekblad MO, et al: Nicotine replacement therapy during pregnancy and child health outcomes: a systematic review. Int J Environ Res Public Health 18(8):4004, 2021 33920348

Blodgett JC, Del Re AC, Maisel NC, et al: A meta-analysis of topiramate's effects for individuals with alcohol use disorders. Alcohol Clin Exp Res 38(6):1481–1488, 2014 24796492

Bohn MJ, Babor TF, Kranzler HR: The Alcohol Use Disorders Identification Test (AUDIT): validation of a screening instrument for use in medical settings. J Stud Alcohol 56(4):423–432, 1995 7674678

Bolton M, Hodkinson A, Boda S, et al: Serious adverse events reported in placebo randomised controlled trials of oral naltrexone: a systematic review and meta-analysis. BMC Med 17(1):10, 2019 30642329

Buckley MS, Smithburger PL, Wong A, et al: Dexmedetomidine for facilitating mechanical ventilation extubation in difficult-to-wean ICU patients: systematic review and meta-analysis of clinical trials. J Intensive Care Med 36(8):925–936, 2021 32627672

Buoli M, Serati M, Botturi A, et al: The risk of thrombocytopenia during valproic acid therapy: a critical summary of available clinical data. Drugs R D 18(1):1–5, 2018 29260458

Buresh M, Ratner J, Zgierska A, et al: Treating perioperative and acute pain in patients on buprenorphine: narrative literature review and practice recommendations. J Gen Intern Med 35(12):3635–3643, 2020 32827109

Caine D, Halliday GM, Kril JJ, et al: Operational criteria for the classification of chronic alcoholics: identification of Wernicke's encephalopathy. J Neurol Neurosurg Psychiatry 62(1):51–60, 1997 9010400

Castaneto MS, Gorelick DA, Desrosiers NA, et al: Synthetic cannabinoids: epidemiology, pharmacodynamics, and clinical implications. Drug Alcohol Depend 144:12–41, 2014 25220897

Castells X, Cunill R, Pérez-Mañá C, et al: Psychostimulant drugs for cocaine dependence. Cochrane Database Syst Rev 9(9):CD007380, 2016 27670244

Centers for Disease Control and Prevention: WISQARS Injury Data. Atlanta, GA, Centers for Disease Control and Prevention, 2020. Available at: www.cdc.gov/injury/wisqars/index.html. Accessed March 25, 2023.

Chan B, Kondo K, Freeman M, et al: Pharmacotherapy for cocaine use disorder—a systematic review and meta-analysis. J Gen Intern Med 34(12):2858–2873, 2019 31183685

Cheng HY, McGuinness LA, Elbers RG, et al: Treatment interventions to maintain abstinence from alcohol in primary care: systematic review and network meta-analysis. BMJ 371:m3934, 2020 33239318

Cherian SV, Kumar A, Estrada-Y-Martin RM: E-cigarette or vaping product-associated lung injury: a review. Am J Med 133(6):657–663, 2020 32179055

Ciraulo DA, Hitzemann RJ, Somoza E, et al: Pharmacokinetics and pharmacodynamics of multiple sublingual buprenorphine tablets in dose-escalation trials. J Clin Pharmacol 46(2):179–192, 2006 16432270

Cohen PA, Ellison RR, Travis JC, et al: Quantity of phenibut in dietary supplements before and after FDA warnings. Clin Toxicol (Phila) 60(4):486–488, 2022 34550038

Cornelius ME, Wang TW, Jamal A, et al: Tobacco product use among adults—United States. MMWR Morb Mortal Wkly Rep 69(46):1736–1742, 2020 33211681

Cunningham FE, Baughman VL, Peters J, et al: Comparative pharmacokinetics of oral versus sublingual clonidine. J Clin Anesth 6(5):430–433, 1994 7986518

Curatolo C, Trinh M: Challenges in the perioperative management of the patient receiving extended-release naltrexone. A A Case Rep 3(11):142–144, 2014 25612099

DeCarolis DD, Rice KL, Ho L, et al: Symptom-driven lorazepam protocol for treatment of severe alcohol withdrawal delirium in the intensive care unit. Pharmacotherapy 27(4):510–518, 2007 17381377

DeVido J, Bogunovic O, Weiss RD: Alcohol use disorders in pregnancy. Harv Rev Psychiatry 23(2):112–121, 2015 25747924

de Wit M, Jones DG, Sessler CN, et al: Alcohol-use disorders in the critically ill patient. Chest 138(4):994–1003, 2010 20923804

Dhalwani NN, Szatkowski L, Coleman T, et al: Nicotine replacement therapy in pregnancy and major congenital anomalies in offspring. Pediatrics 135(5):859–867, 2015 25847803

Dietze P, Jauncey M, Salmon A, et al: Effect of intranasal vs intramuscular naloxone on opioid overdose: a randomized clinical trial [Erratum in: JAMA Netw Open 3(4):e206593, 2020]. JAMA Netw Open 2(11):e1914977, 2019 31722024

Dominici P, Kopec K, Manur R, et al: Phencyclidine intoxication case series study. J Med Toxicol 11(3):321–325, 2015 25502414

Edwards S, Kenna GA, Swift RM, et al: Current and promising pharmacotherapies, and novel research target areas in the treatment of alcohol dependence: a review. Curr Pharm Des 17(14):1323–1332, 2011 21524263

Evins AE, Benowitz NL, West R, et al: Neuropsychiatric safety and efficacy of varenicline, bupropion, and nicotine patch in smokers with psychotic, anxiety, and mood disorders in the EAGLES trial. J Clin Psychopharmacol 39(2):108–116, 2019 30811371

Fareed A, Patil D, Scheinberg K, et al: Comparison of QTc interval prolongation for patients in methadone versus buprenorphine maintenance treatment: a 5-year follow-up. J Addict Dis 32(3):244–251, 2013 24074190

Farkas A, Lynch MJ, Westover R, et al: Pulmonary complications of opioid overdose treated with naloxone. Ann Emerg Med 75(1):39–48, 2020 31182316

Filley CM: Toluene abuse and white matter: a model of toxic leukoencephalopathy. Psychiatr Clin North Am 36(2):293–302, 2013 23688693

Fishman M, Tirado C, Alam D, et al: Safety and efficacy of lofexidine for medically managed opioid withdrawal: a randomized controlled clinical trial. J Addict Med 13(3):169–176, 2019 30531234

Florez DHA, Dos Santos Moreira AM, da Silva PR, et al: Desomorphine (Krokodil): an overview of its chemistry, pharmacology, metabolism, toxicology and analysis. Drug Alcohol Depend 173:59–68, 2017 28199917

Frazee EN, Personett HA, Leung JG, et al: Influence of dexmedetomidine therapy on the management of severe alcohol withdrawal syndrome in critically ill patients. J Crit Care 29(2):298–302, 2014 24360597

Gandhi KD, Mansukhani MP, Karpyak VM, et al: The impact of varenicline on alcohol consumption in subjects with alcohol use disorders: systematic review and meta-analysis. J Clin Psychiatry 81(2):19r12924, 2020 32097546

Garbutt JC: Efficacy and tolerability of naltrexone in the management of alcohol dependence. Curr Pharm Des 16(19):2091–2097, 2010 20482515

Goel N, Pullman JM, Coco M: Cocaine and kidney injury: a kaleidoscope of pathology. Clin Kidney J 7(6):513–517, 2014 25859366

Gowing L, Farrell M, Ali R, et al: Alpha2-adrenergic agonists for the management of opioid withdrawal. Cochrane Database Syst Rev (5):CD002024, 2016 27140827

Gowing L, Ali R, White JM, et al: Buprenorphine for managing opioid withdrawal. Cochrane Database Syst Rev 2(2):CD002025, 2017 28220474

Graves JM, Dilley J, Kubsad S, et al: Notes from the field: phenibut exposures reported to poison centers—United States, 2009–2019. MMWR Morb Mortal Wkly Rep 69(35):1227–1228, 2020 32881852

Greenwald MK, Comer SD, Fiellin DA: Buprenorphine maintenance and mu-opioid receptor availability in the treatment of opioid use disorder: implications for clinical use and policy. Drug Alcohol Depend 144:1–11, 2014 25179217

Grigoriadis S, Graves L, Peer M, et al: Benzodiazepine use during pregnancy alone or in combination with an antidepressant and congenital malformations: systematic review and meta-analysis. J Clin Psychiatry 80(4):e1–e11, 2019 31294935

Grigoriadis S, Graves L, Peer M, et al: Pregnancy and delivery outcomes following benzodiazepine exposure: a systematic review and meta-analysis. Can J Psychiatry 65(12):821–834, 2020 32148076

Gulati P, Chavan BS, Sidana A: Comparative efficacy of baclofen and lorazepam in the treatment of alcohol withdrawal syndrome. Indian J Psychiatry 61(1):60–64, 2019 30745655

Hägg S, Jönsson AK, Ahlner J: Current evidence on abuse and misuse of gabapentinoids. Drug Saf 43(12):1235–1254, 2020 32857333

Haight BR, Learned SM, Laffont CM, et al: Efficacy and safety of a monthly buprenorphine depot injection for opioid use disorder: a multicentre, randomised, double-blind, placebo-controlled, phase 3 trial. Lancet 393(10173):778–790, 2019 30792007

Hamilton RJ, Olmedo RE, Shah S, et al: Complications of ultrarapid opioid detoxification with subcutaneous naltrexone pellets. Acad Emerg Med 9(1):63–68, 2002 11772672

Hammond CJ, Niciu MJ, Drew S, et al: Anticonvulsants for the treatment of alcohol withdrawal syndrome and alcohol use disorders. CNS Drugs 29(4):293–311, 2015 25895020

Hammond DA, Rowe JM, Wong A, et al: Patient outcomes associated with phenobarbital use with or without benzodiazepines for alcohol withdrawal syndrome: a systematic review. Hosp Pharm 52(9):606–616, 2017 29276297

Harper C, Fornes P, Duyckaerts C, et al: An international perspective on the prevalence of the Wernicke-Korsakoff syndrome. Metab Brain Dis 10(1):17–24, 1995 7596325

Hartmann-Boyce J, Chepkin SC, Ye W, et al: Nicotine replacement therapy versus control for smoking cessation. Cochrane Database Syst Rev 5(5):CD000146, 2018 29852054

Hartmann-Boyce J, McRobbie H, Butler AR, et al: Electronic cigarettes for smoking cessation. Cochrane Database Syst Rev (9):CD010216, 2021 33913154

Hasan A, von Keller R, Friemel CM, et al: Cannabis use and psychosis: a review of reviews. Eur Arch Psychiatry Clin Neurosci 270(4):403–412, 2020 31563981

Heavner JJ, Akgün KM, Heavner MS, et al: Implementation of an ICU-specific alcohol withdrawal syndrome management protocol reduces the need for mechanical ventilation. Pharmacotherapy 38(7):701–713, 2018 29800507

Hedegaard H, Minino AM, Warner M: Drug overdose deaths in the United States, 1999–2019. NCHS Data Brief, No 394. Hyattsville, MD, National Center for Health Statistics, 2020. Available at: www.cdc.gov/nchs/products/databriefs/db394.htm. Accessed March 25, 2023.

Hemphill S, McMenamin L, Bellamy MC, et al: Propofol infusion syndrome: a structured literature review and analysis of published case reports. Br J Anaesth 122(4):448–459, 2019 30857601

Hickey T, Abelleira A, Acampora G, et al: Perioperative buprenorphine management: a multidisciplinary approach. Med Clin North Am 106(1):169–185, 2022 34823729

Hoch E, Bonnet U, Thomasius R, et al: Risks associated with the non-medicinal use of cannabis. Dtsch Arztebl Int 112(16):271–278, 2015 25939318

Horinek EL, Kiser TH, Fish DN, et al: Propylene glycol accumulation in critically ill patients receiving continuous intravenous lorazepam infusions. Ann Pharmacother 43(12):1964–1971, 2009 19920159

Houthoff Khemlani K, Weibel S, Kranke P, et al: Hypnotic agents for induction of general anesthesia in cesarean section patients: a systematic review and meta-analysis of randomized controlled trials. J Clin Anesth 48:73–80, 2018 29778972

Howes S, Hartmann-Boyce J, Livingstone-Banks J, et al: Antidepressants for smoking cessation. Cochrane Database Syst Rev 4(4):CD000031, 2020 32319681

Hughes DW, Vanwert E, Lepori L, et al: Propofol for benzodiazepine-refractory alcohol withdrawal in a non-mechanically ventilated patient. Am J Emerg Med 32(1):112.e3–112.e4, 2014 24075805

Isenberg-Grzeda E, Chabon B, Nicolson SE: Prescribing thiamine to inpatients with alcohol use disorders: how well are we doing? J Addict Med 8(1):1–5, 2014 24343128

Jarvis BP, Holtyn AF, Subramaniam S, et al: Extended-release injectable naltrexone for opioid use disorder: a systematic review. Addiction 113(7):1188–1209, 2018 29396985

Jonas AM, Raj R: Vaping-related acute parenchymal lung injury: a systematic review. Chest 158(4):1555–1565, 2020 32442559

Jonas DE, Amick HR, Feltner C, et al: Pharmacotherapy for adults with alcohol use disorders in outpatient settings: a systematic review and meta-analysis. JAMA 311(18):1889–1900, 2014 24825644

Jones HE, Kaltenbach K, Heil SH, et al: Neonatal abstinence syndrome after methadone or buprenorphine exposure. N Engl J Med 363(24):2320–2331, 2010 21142534

Karila L, Gorelick D, Weinstein A, et al: New treatments for cocaine dependence: a focused review. Int J Neuropsychopharmacol 11(3):425–438, 2008 17927843

Katz G, Durst R, Shufman E, et al: Substance abuse in hospitalized psychiatric patients. Isr Med Assoc J 10(10):672–675, 2008 19009943

Keating GM: Sodium oxybate: a review of its use in alcohol withdrawal syndrome and in the maintenance of abstinence in alcohol dependence. Clin Drug Investig 34(1):63–80, 2014 24307430

Kelty E, Terplan M, Greenland M, et al: Pharmacotherapies for the treatment of alcohol use disorders during pregnancy: time to reconsider? Drugs 81(7):739–748, 2021 33830479

Kesner AJ, Lovinger DM: Cannabis use, abuse, and withdrawal: cannabinergic mechanisms, clinical, and preclinical findings. J Neurochem 157(5):1674–1696, 2021 33891706

Kim HK, Nelson LS: Reducing the harm of opioid overdose with the safe use of naloxone: a pharmacologic review. Expert Opin Drug Saf 14(7):1137–1146, 2015 25865597

Klaman SL, Isaacs K, Leopold A, et al: Treating women who are pregnant and parenting for opioid use disorder and the concurrent care of their infants and children: literature review to support national guidance. J Addict Med 11(3):178–190, 2017 28406856

Klein L, Bangh S, Cole JB: Intentional recreational abuse of quetiapine compared to other second-generation antipsychotics. West J Emerg Med 18(2):243–250, 2017 28210359

Kohan L, Potru S, Barreveld AM, et al: Buprenorphine management in the perioperative period: educational review and recommendations from a multisociety expert panel. Reg Anesth Pain Med 46(10):840–859, 2021 34385292

Kranzler HR, Feinn R, Morris P, et al: A meta-analysis of the efficacy of gabapentin for treating alcohol use disorder. Addiction 114(9):1547–1555, 2019 31077485

Lai J, Kalk N, Roberts E: The effectiveness and tolerability of anti-seizure medication in alcohol withdrawal syndrome: a systematic review, meta-analysis, and GRADE of the evidence. Addiction 117(1):5–18, 2022 33822427

Lappin JM, Sara GE: Psychostimulant use and the brain. Addiction 114(11):2065–2077, 2019 31321819

Lindner BK, Gilmore VT, Kruer RM, et al: Evaluation of the Brief Alcohol Withdrawal Scale protocol at an academic medical center. J Addict Med 13(5):379–384, 2019 30741834

Link HM, Jones H, Miller L, et al: Buprenorphine-naloxone use in pregnancy: a systematic review and metaanalysis. Am J Obstet Gynecol MFM 2(3):100179, 2020 33345863

Liu J, Wang LN: Baclofen for alcohol withdrawal. Cochrane Database Syst Rev 2019(11):CD008502, 2019 31689723

Longmire AW, Seger DL: Topics in clinical pharmacology: flumazenil, a benzodiazepine antagonist. Am J Med Sci 306(1):49–52, 1993 8101045

Lu X, Wang X: Hyponatremia induced by antiepileptic drugs in patients with epilepsy. Expert Opin Drug Saf 16(1):77–87, 2017 27737595

Lund IO, Fischer G, Welle-Strand GK, et al: A comparison of buprenorphine + naloxone to buprenorphine and methadone in the treatment of opioid dependence during pregnancy: maternal and neonatal outcomes. Subst Abuse 7:61–74, 2013 23531704

Maldonado JR: Novel algorithms for the prophylaxis and management of alcohol withdrawal syndromes—beyond benzodiazepines. Crit Care Clin 33(3):559–599, 2017 28601135

Maldonado JR, Nguyen LH, Schader EM, et al: Benzodiazepine loading versus symptom-triggered treatment of alcohol withdrawal: a prospective, randomized clinical trial. Gen Hosp Psychiatry 34(6):611–617, 2012 22898443

Maldonado JR, Sher Y, Ashouri JF, et al: The "Prediction of Alcohol Withdrawal Severity Scale" (PAWSS): systematic literature review and pilot study of a new scale for the prediction of complicated alcohol withdrawal syndrome. Alcohol 48(4):375–390, 2014 24657098

Maldonado JR, Sher Y, Das S, et al: Prospective validation study of the Prediction of Alcohol Withdrawal Severity Scale (PAWSS) in medically ill patients: a new scale for the prediction of complicated alcohol withdrawal syndrome. Alcohol Alcohol 50(5):509–518, 2015 25999438

Manasco AT, Stephens RJ, Yaeger LH, et al: Ketamine sedation in mechanically ventilated patients: a systematic review and meta-analysis. J Crit Care 56:80–88, 2020 31865256

Mann K, Torup L, Sørensen P, et al: Nalmefene for the management of alcohol dependence: review on its pharmacology, mechanism of action and meta-analysis on its clinical efficacy. Eur Neuropsychopharmacol 26(12):1941–1949, 2016 27842940

Marik PE: Propofol: therapeutic indications and side-effects. Curr Pharm Des 10(29):3639–3649, 2004 15579060

Mason BJ, Goodman AM, Dixon RM, et al: A pharmacokinetic and pharmacodynamic drug interaction study of acamprosate and naltrexone. Neuropsychopharmacology 27(4):596–606, 2002 12377396

Mattick RP, Breen C, Kimber J, et al: Buprenorphine maintenance versus placebo or methadone maintenance for opioid dependence. Cochrane Database Syst Rev (2):CD002207, 2014 24500948

McCowan C, Marik P: Refractory delirium tremens treated with propofol: a case series. Crit Care Med 28(6):1781–1784, 2000 10890619

McEvoy GK: American Hospital Formulary Service (AHFS) Drug Information 2008. Bethesda, MD, American Society of Health-System Pharmacists, 2008

Meemken L, Hanhoff N, Tseng A, et al: Drug-drug interactions with antiviral agents in people who inject drugs requiring substitution therapy. Ann Pharmacother 49(7):796–807, 2015 25902733

Meyer MC, Johnston AM, Crocker AM, et al: Methadone and buprenorphine for opioid dependence during pregnancy: a retrospective cohort study. J Addict Med 9(2):81–86, 2015 25622120

Minozzi S, Amato L, Vecchi S, et al: Anticonvulsants for alcohol withdrawal. Cochrane Database Syst Rev (3):CD005064, 2010 20238337

Minozzi S, Saulle R, Rösner S: Baclofen for alcohol use disorder. Cochrane Database Syst Rev 11(11):CD012557, 2018 30484285

Minozzi S, Amato L, Jahanfar S, et al: Maintenance agonist treatments for opiate-dependent pregnant women. Cochrane Database Syst Rev 11(11):CD006318, 2020 33165953

Mirijello A, D'Angelo C, Ferrulli A, et al: Identification and management of alcohol withdrawal syndrome. Drugs 75(4):353–365, 2015 25666543

Mosoni C, Dionisi T, Vassallo GA, et al: Baclofen for the treatment of alcohol use disorder in patients with liver cirrhosis: 10 years after the first evidence. Front Psychiatry 9:474, 2018 30327620

Moss M, Burnham EL: Alcohol abuse in the critically ill patient. Lancet 368(9554):2231–2242, 2006 17189035

Mueller SW, Preslaski CR, Kiser TH, et al: A randomized, double-blind, placebo-controlled dose range study of dexmedetomidine as adjunctive therapy for alcohol withdrawal. Crit Care Med 42(5):1131–1139, 2014 24351375

Mueller S, Luderer M, Zhang D, et al: Open-label study with nalmefene as needed use in alcohol-dependent patients with evidence of elevated liver stiffness and/or hepatic steatosis. Alcohol Alcohol 55(1):63–70, 2020 31713583

Mujtaba S, Romero J, Taub CC: Methadone, QTc prolongation and torsades de pointes: current concepts, management and a hidden twist in the tale? J Cardiovasc Dis Res 4(4):229–235, 2013 24653586

Murphy CE IV, Wang RC, Montoy JC, et al: Effect of extended-release naltrexone on alcohol consumption: a systematic review and meta-analysis. Addiction 117(2):271–281, 2022 34033183

Muzyk AJ, Fowler JA, Norwood DK, et al: Role of α2-agonists in the treatment of acute alcohol withdrawal. Ann Pharmacother 45(5):649–657, 2011 21521867

Nejad S, Nisavic M, Larentzakis A, et al: Phenobarbital for acute alcohol withdrawal management in surgical trauma patients: a retrospective comparison study. Psychosomatics 61(4):327–335, 2020 32199629

Nguyen TA, Lam SW: Phenobarbital and symptom-triggered lorazepam versus lorazepam alone for severe alcohol withdrawal in the intensive care unit. Alcohol 82:23–27, 2020 31326601

Nielsen S, Gowing L, Sabioni P, et al: Pharmacotherapies for cannabis dependence. Cochrane Database Syst Rev 1(1):CD008940, 2019 30687936

Nisavic M, Nejad SH, Isenberg BM, et al: Use of phenobarbital in alcohol withdrawal management: a retrospective comparison study of phenobarbital and benzodiazepines for acute alcohol withdrawal management in general medical patients. Psychosomatics 60(5):458–467, 2019 30876654

O'Brien JM Jr, Lu B, Ali NA, et al: Alcohol dependence is independently associated with sepsis, septic shock, and hospital mortality among adult intensive care unit patients. Crit Care Med 35(2):345–350, 2007 17205003

Owen DR, Wood DM, Archer JRH, et al: Phenibut (4-amino-3-phenyl-butyric acid): availability, prevalence of use, desired effects and acute toxicity. Drug Alcohol Rev 35(5):591–596, 2016 26693960

Pandharipande P, Shintani A, Peterson J, et al: Lorazepam is an independent risk factor for transitioning to delirium in intensive care unit patients. Anesthesiology 104(1):21–26, 2006 16394685

Pandharipande PP, Pun BT, Herr DL, et al: Effect of sedation with dexmedetomidine vs lorazepam on acute brain dysfunction in mechanically ventilated patients: the MENDS randomized controlled trial. JAMA 298(22):2644–2653, 2007 18073360

Pandharipande PP, Sanders RD, Girard TD, et al: Effect of dexmedetomidine versus lorazepam on outcome in patients with sepsis: an a priori-designed analysis of the MENDS randomized controlled trial. Crit Care 14(2):R38, 2010 20233428

Passie T, Halpern JH: Hallucinogens and related drugs, in Clinical Manual of Addiction Psychopharmacology, 2nd Edition. Edited by Kranzler HR, Ciraulo DA, Zindel LR. Washington, DC, American Psychiatric Publishing, 2014, pp 261–320

Pecoraro A, Ewen E, Horton T, et al: Using the AUDIT-PC to predict alcohol withdrawal in hospitalized patients. J Gen Intern Med 29(1):34–40, 2014 23959745

Penninga EI, Graudal N, Ladekarl MB, et al: Adverse events associated with flumazenil treatment for the management of suspected benzodiazepine intoxication—a systematic review with meta-analyses of randomised trials. Basic Clin Pharmacol Toxicol 118(1):37–44, 2016 26096314

Pérez-Mañá C, Castells X, Torrens M, et al: Efficacy of psychostimulant drugs for amphetamine abuse or dependence. Cochrane Database Syst Rev (9):CD009695, 2013 23996457

Phillips K, Luk A, Soor GS, et al: Cocaine cardiotoxicity: a review of the pathophysiology, pathology, and treatment options. Am J Cardiovasc Drugs 9(3):177–196, 2009 19463023

Pierce M, Sutterland A, Beraha EM, et al: Efficacy, tolerability, and safety of low-dose and high-dose baclofen in the treatment of alcohol dependence: a systematic review and meta-analysis. Eur Neuropsychopharmacol 28(7):795–806, 2018 29934090

Pizon AF, Lynch MJ, Benedict NJ, et al: Adjunct ketamine use in the management of severe ethanol withdrawal. Crit Care Med 46(8):e768–e771, 2018 29742583

Plosker GL: Acamprosate: a review of its use in alcohol dependence. Drugs 75(11):1255–1268, 2015 26084940

Pourmand A, Armstrong P, Mazer-Amirshahi M, et al: The evolving high: new designer drugs of abuse. Hum Exp Toxicol 33(10):993–999, 2014 24501103

Pourmand A, Mazer-Amirshahi M, Chistov S, et al: Designer drugs: review and implications for emergency management. Hum Exp Toxicol 37(1):94–101, 2018 28764574

Quigley MA, Boyce SH: Unintentional rapid opioid detoxification. Emerg Med J 18(6):494–495, 2001 11696513

Rastegar DA, Applewhite D, Alvanzo AAH, et al: Development and implementation of an alcohol withdrawal protocol using a 5-item scale, the Brief Alcohol Withdrawal Scale (BAWS). Subst Abus 38(4):394–400, 2017 28699845

Rastegar DA, Jarrell AS, Chen ES: Implementation of a protocol using the 5-item Brief Alcohol Withdrawal Scale for treatment of severe alcohol withdrawal in intensive care units. J Intensive Care Med 36(11):1361–1365, 2021 32851920

Rigotti NA, Munafo MR, Stead LF: Smoking cessation interventions for hospitalized smokers: a systematic review. Arch Intern Med 168(18):1950–1960, 2008 18852395

Rojo-Mira J, Pineda-Alvarez M, Zapata-Ospina JP: Efficacy and safety of anticonvulsants for the inpatient treatment of alcohol withdrawal syndrome: a systematic review and meta-analysis. Alcohol Alcohol 57(2):155–164, 2022 34396386

Romito JW, Turner ER, Rosener JA, et al: Baclofen therapeutics, toxicity, and withdrawal: a narrative review. SAGE Open Med 9:2050312121211022197, 2022 34158937

Rosenson J, Clements C, Simon B, et al: Phenobarbital for acute alcohol withdrawal: a prospective randomized double-blind placebo-controlled study. J Emerg Med 44(3):592.e2–598.e2, 2013 22999778

Ross S, Peselow E: Pharmacotherapy of addictive disorders. Clin Neuropharmacol 32(5):277–289, 2009 19834993

Saitz R, Mayo-Smith MF, Roberts MS, et al: Individualized treatment for alcohol withdrawal: a randomized double-blind controlled trial. JAMA 272(7):519–523, 1994 8046805

Sanchez-Ramos J: Neurologic complications of psychomotor stimulant abuse. Int Rev Neurobiol 120:131–160, 2015 26070756

Schellhorn SE, Barnhill JW, Raiteri V, et al: A comparison of psychiatric consultation between geriatric and non-geriatric medical inpatients. Int J Geriatr Psychiatry 24(10):1054–1061, 2009 19326400

Schnoll RA, Goelz PM, Veluz-Wilkins A, et al: Long-term nicotine replacement therapy: a randomized clinical trial. JAMA Intern Med 175(4):504–511, 2015 25705872

Schoenfeld A, Friedman S, Stein LB, et al: Severe hypertensive reaction after naloxone injection during labor. Arch Gynecol 240(1):45–47, 1987 3827314

Schuckit MA: Recognition and management of withdrawal delirium (delirium tremens). N Engl J Med 371(22):2109–2113, 2014 25427113

Seger DL: Flumazenil: treatment or toxin. J Toxicol Clin Toxicol 42(2):209–216, 2004 15214628

Shah P, McDowell M, Ebisu R, et al: Adjunctive use of ketamine for benzodiazepine resistant severe alcohol withdrawal: a retrospective evaluation. J Med Toxicol 14(3):229–236, 2018 29748926

Sills GJ, Rogawski MA: Mechanisms of action of currently used antiseizure drugs. Neuropharmacology 168:107966, 2020 32120063

Singh M, Keer D, Klimas J, et al: Topiramate for cocaine dependence: a systematic review and meta-analysis of randomized controlled trials. Addiction 111(8):1337–1346, 2016 26826006

Skinner MD, Lahmek P, Pham H, et al: Disulfiram efficacy in the treatment of alcohol dependence: a meta-analysis. PLoS One 9(2):e87366, 2014 24520330

Skolnik P: Treatment of overdose in the synthetic opioid era. Pharmacol Ther 233:108019, 2022 34637841

Soares J, Costa VM, Bastos ML, et al: An updated review on synthetic cathinones. Arch Toxicol 95(9):2895–2940, 2021 34100120

Sobieraj DM, White WB, Baker WL: Cardiovascular effects of pharmacologic therapies for smoking cessation. J Am Soc Hypertens 7(1):61–67, 2013 23266101

Soderstrom CA, Smith GS, Kufera JA, et al: The accuracy of the CAGE, the Brief Michigan Alcoholism Screening Test, and the Alcohol Use Disorders Identification Test in screening trauma center patients for alcoholism. J Trauma 43(6):962–969, 1997 9420113

Sorensen CJ, DeSanto K, Borgelt L, et al: Cannabinoid hyperemesis syndrome: diagnosis, pathophysiology, and treatment—a systematic review. J Med Toxicol 13(1):71–87, 2017 28000146

Sterling LH, Windle SB, Filion KB, et al: Varenicline and adverse cardiovascular events: a systematic review and meta-analysis of randomized controlled trials. J Am Heart Assoc 5(2):e002849, 2016 26903004

Substance Abuse and Mental Health Services Administration: 2020 NSDUH Annual National Report. Rockville, MD, Substance Abuse and Mental Health Services Administration, 2021. Available at: www.samhsa.gov/data/report/2020-nsduh-annual-national-report. Accessed November 17, 2021.

Sullivan JT, Sykora K, Schneiderman J, et al: Assessment of alcohol withdrawal: the revised Clinical Institute Withdrawal Assessment for Alcohol Scale (CIWA-Ar). Br J Addict 84(11):1353–1357, 1989 2597811

Tetrault JM, Fiellin DA: Current and potential pharmacological treatment options for maintenance therapy in opioid-dependent individuals. Drugs 72(2):217–228, 2012 22235870

Thomas KH, Dalili MN, Lopez-Lopez JA, et al: Comparative clinical effectiveness and safety of tobacco cessation pharmacotherapies and electronic cigarettes: a systematic review and network meta-analysis of randomized controlled trials. Addiction 117(4):861–876, 2022

Thomson AD: Mechanisms of vitamin deficiency in chronic alcohol misusers and the development of the Wernicke-Korsakoff syndrome. Alcohol Alcohol Suppl 35(1):2–7, 2000 11304071

Thomson AD, Cook CCH, Touquet R, et al: The Royal College of Physicians report on alcohol: guidelines for managing Wernicke's encephalopathy in the accident and emergency department. Alcohol Alcohol 37(6):513–521, 2002 12414541

Tomson T, Battino D, Bonizzoni E, et al: Comparative risk of major congenital malformations with eight different antiepileptic drugs: a prospective cohort study of the EURAP registry. Lancet Neurol 17(6):530–538, 2018 29680205

Tomson T, Battino D, Perucca E: Teratogenicity of antiepileptic drugs. Curr Opin Neurol 32(2):246–252, 2019 30664067

Turner E, Jones M, Vaz LR, et al: Systematic review and meta-analysis to assess the safety of bupropion and varenicline in pregnancy. Nicotine Tob Res 21(8):1001–1010, 2019 29579233

U.S. Department of Health and Human Services: The health consequences of smoking—50 years of progress: a report of the Surgeon General. Washington, DC, U.S. Department of Health and Human Services, 2014. Available at: https://www.ncbi.nlm.nih.gov/books/NBK179276/pdf/Bookshelf_NBK179276.pdf. Accessed January 11, 2022.

van Amsterdam J, Nabben T, van den Brink W: Recreational nitrous oxide use: prevalence and risks. Regul Toxicol Pharmacol 73(3):790–796, 2015 26496821

Veroniki AA, Cogo E, Rios P, et al: Comparative safety of anti-epileptic drugs during pregnancy: a systematic review and network meta-analysis of congenital malformations and prenatal outcomes. BMC Med 15(1):95, 2017 28472982

Volkow ND, Baler RD, Compton WM, et al: Adverse health effects of marijuana use. N Engl J Med 370(23):2219–2227, 2014 24897085

Walsh SL, Comer SD, Lofwall MR, et al: Effect of buprenorphine weekly depot (CAM2038) and hydromorphone blockade in individuals with opioid use disorder: a randomized clinical trial. JAMA Psychiatry 74(9):894–902, 2017 28655025

Weimer MB, Guerra M, Morrow G, et al: Hospital-based buprenorphine micro-dose initiation. J Addict Med 15(3):255–257, 2021 32960820

Weinberg JA, Magnotti LJ, Fischer PE, et al: Comparison of intravenous ethanol versus diazepam for alcohol withdrawal prophylaxis in the trauma ICU: results of a randomized trial. J Trauma 64(1):99–104, 2008 18188105

Weinbroum AA, Flaishon R, Sorkine P, et al: A risk-benefit assessment of flumazenil in the management of benzodiazepine overdose. Drug Saf 17(3):181–196, 1997 9306053

Welsh CJ, Suman M, Cohen A, et al: The use of intravenous buprenorphine for the treatment of opioid withdrawal in medically ill hospitalized patients. Am J Addict 11(2):135–140, 2002 12028743

Westover AN, McBride S, Haley RW: Stroke in young adults who abuse amphetamines or cocaine: a population-based study of hospitalized patients. Arch Gen Psychiatry 64(4):495–502, 2007 17404126

Whiting PF, Wolff RF, Deshpande S, et al: Cannabinoids for medical use: a systematic review and meta-analysis. JAMA 313(24):2456–2473, 2015 26103030

Wiegand SL, Stringer EM, Stuebe AM, et al: Buprenorphine and naloxone compared with methadone treatment in pregnancy. Obstet Gynecol 125(2):363–368, 2015 25569005

Woods AD, Giometti R, Weeks SM: The use of dexmedetomidine as an adjuvant to benzodiazepine-based therapy to decrease the severity of delirium in alcohol withdrawal in adult intensive care unit patients: a systematic review. JBI Database System Rev Implement Rep 13(1):224–252, 2015 26447017

Yavarovich ER, Bintvihok M, McCarty JC, et al: Association between dexmedetomidine use for the treatment of alcohol withdrawal syndrome and intensive care unit length of stay. J Intensive Care 7:49, 2019 31700642

Zelner I, Matlow J, Hutson JR, et al: Acute poisoning during pregnancy: observations from the Toxicology Investigators Consortium. J Med Toxicol 11(3):301–308, 2015 25783189

Index

*Page numbers printed in **boldface** type refer to figures and tables.*